Clinical Dermatology

Clinical Dermatology

Editor: Maximus Turner

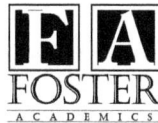

FA
FOSTER
ACADEMICS

www.fosteracademics.com

www.fosteracademics.com

FA
FOSTER
ACADEMICS

Cataloging-in-Publication Data

Clinical dermatology / edited by Maximus Turner.
    p. cm.
Includes bibliographical references and index.
ISBN 978-1-63242-619-2
1. Dermatology. 2. Skin--Diseases. I. Turner, Maximus.
RL72 .C55 2019
616.5--dc23

Foster Academics,
118-35 Queens Blvd., Suite 400,
Forest Hills, NY 11375, USA

ISBN 978-1-63242-619-2 (Hardback)

Contents

Preface

The purpose of the book is to provide a glimpse into the dynamics and to present opinions and studies of some of the scientists engaged in the development of new ideas in the field from very different standpoints. This book will prove useful to students and researchers owing to its high content quality.

Dermatology is a branch of medicine, which deals with the conditions of the nails, scalp, hair and skin. It is a vast subject, which has a number of significant sub-disciplines. Some of the specializations in dermatology include cosmetic dermatology, immunodermatology, dermatopathology, pediatric dermatology and dermatoepidemiology. Cosmetic surgeries like blepharoplasty, liposuction and face-lift are within the scope of this field. It can also include the use of botulinum toxins, fillers and laser surgery. The field of immunodermatology is concerned with the treatment of various immune-mediated skin disorders such as pemphigus vulgaris, lupus, bullous pemphigoid, etc. This book explores all the important aspects of clinical dermatology in the present day scenario. It attempts to understand the multiple branches that fall under this discipline. As this field is emerging at a rapid pace, the contents of this book will help the readers understand the modern concepts and principles of the subject.

At the end, I would like to appreciate all the efforts made by the authors in completing their chapters professionally. I express my deepest gratitude to all of them for contributing to this book by sharing their valuable works. A special thanks to my family and friends for their constant support in this journey.

Editor

Facial L*a*b* values and preferred base makeup products among native Korean women

In Jung, Aha Ryoung Jo, Yu Jeong Kwon, Seungbin Kwon and In-Sook An[*] 🔟

Abstract

Background: Bare face L*a*b* values are needed to serve as a standard reference point for the development of base makeup products for Korean women.

Methods: A total of 543 Korean women ranging in age from their 20s to 50s underwent spectrophotometer skin analysis under constant temperature (22 ± 2%) and humidity (50 ± 5%) conditions. Eight parts of each subject's face (center of the forehead, right cheekbone, right cheek, under the chin, left cheek, left cheekbone, philtrum, and under the lips) were measured, and average values were calculated. Subjects were then asked to complete questionnaires regarding their use and preferences for base makeup products.

Results: Skin tone was classified into three categories (dark, normal, bright) based on L* values. Compared with the contrast value, the dark group L* was 60.66 and the normal group L* was 63.87 (with a difference of 3.21), and the bright group L* was 66.66 (with a difference of 2.79 from the normal group). According to the survey responses regarding preferences and use of base makeup products, the most common answer for all respondents regardless of age was that their skin tone was average or slightly darker than that of their peers. Preferred base makeup products usually were found to be of slightly brighter color than actual skin tone. As in previous studies, the most frequently used base makeup product regardless of age was BB cream.

Conclusions: Given that the average L* standard deviation between groups was 3, a difference of one step in skin tone may be considered to be equivalent to this L* value difference. The survey results suggest that target colors for base makeup product development should be brighter than bare face tones.

Keywords: Skin color, Skin tone, Native Korean women, L*a*b* values, Base makeup products

Background

Skin tone provides not only a reflection of individual heritage, but over the course of human history, certain variations in tone have been accepted as standards of beauty (Wagatsuma 1967). In East Asian more than Western cultures, a particular reverence for white skin has unfortunately contributed to the widespread use of lead-containing cosmetics, resulting in lead poisoning becoming a social issue (Dunbabin et al. 1992; Witkowski and Parish 2001). Bleaching agents classified as medicinal ingredients are also illegally added to some cosmetics that target consumers seeking substantially whiter skin (Desmedt et al. 2014).

Skin color is influenced by complicated interactions among a considerable number of factors including skin pigmentation; thickness; water content; relative proportions of melanin, hemoglobin, and bilirubin; seasonal environment; genetic factors; ultraviolet ray exposure; and personal health status (Jablonski 2006; Muehlenbein 2010). Melanin is the black or brown pigment directly responsible for skin color that is present in the skin, hair, and tissues of plants and animals. Melanin undergoes oxidation according to the following process: tyrosine → 3,4-dihydroxyphenylalanine (DOPA) → DOPA quinone → melanin (Kang et al. 2007). Research on melanin inhibition for medicinal, cosmetic, and food applications is being actively pursued. Among

* Correspondence: anis@skinresearch.or.kr
Korea Institute of Dermatological Sciences, 6F, Tower A, 25, Beobwon-ro 11-gil, Songpa-gu, Seoul, Republic of Korea

these, whitening cosmetics and base makeup products are worth looking at more closely.

Attempts to achieve consistent skin tone have led to breakthroughs in base makeup products that can mask skin imperfections and correct skin tone (Couteau et al. 2016). In the cosmetic industry, Korean products are currently leading the global market, with popular items ranging from blemish balm (BB) cream to the cushion compact (Park and Chin 2010; Baek 2015). To permit further advances in skin tone matching and enhancement, it has therefore become necessary to establish L*a*b* value ranges to inform the coloring of base makeup products.

Previous studies measuring skin tone variations among Korean women were conducted mainly for personal color and color research in the fashion industry. The numbers of subjects in these studies were extremely limited, making it somewhat difficult to interpret and generalize these data. Until now, there has been limited utilization of these findings in the field of cosmetic science. In addition, as data from various age groups were not collected, average values could not be calculated. In this study, facial L*a*b* values were measured for 543 Korean women residing in one metropolitan (Seoul, the capital of Republic of Korea) area who ranged in age from their 20s to 50s, and their use of base makeup products was surveyed.

Methods

Measurement of facial tone L*a*b* values

Clinical testing of facial tone L*a*b* values was performed for 543 Korean women ranging in age from their 20s to 50s under constant conditions of temperature (22 ± 2%) and humidity (50 ± 5%) (Park et al. 2015). All clinical research was based on the revised Declaration of Helsinki (Shin 2009), and the study protocol was

Table 1 L*a*b* values by lightness group

		ΔL*	Δa*	Δb*
Mean ± SD	Dark	60.66 ± 2.16	12.63 ± 1.36	17.82 ± 0.65
	Normal	63.87 ± 2.27	11.10 ± 1.67	18.12 ± 0.54
	Bright	66.66 ± 2.34	9.84 ± 1.62	17.47 ± 0.64

approved by the institutional review board (IRB) of the Korea Institute of Dermatological Sciences (IRB no. KIDS2016W217). All subjects used the same facial cleanser to clean off their makeup and sunscreen to reveal a bare face. After cleansing, subjects rested for 30 min before testing (Binggeli et al. 2003). Then, using a spectrophotometer (CM-2600D, Konica Minolta, Japan), an experienced lab technician measured eight selected parts of the face for each subject: center of the forehead, right cheekbone, right cheek, under the chin, left cheek, left cheek bone, philtrum, and under the lips. Each measurement was taken three times consecutively, and an average was calculated (Weatherall and Coombs 1992; Piérard 1998; Ahn et al. 2002; Latreille et al. 2007).

The spectrophotometer is a device that measures chromaticity coordinates by measuring the intensity of wavelengths on a sample surface. Measurement modes include Specular Component Inclusion (SCI), which is a total reflection mode that measures both specular reflections (as from a glass-like surface) and diffuse reflections (as from a coarse surface), and Specular Component Exclusion (SCE), which is a mode measuring only diffuse reflections while excluding specular reflections. L*a*b* values indicate the error of color, and one can quickly see the direction of the conversion. This method is therefore widely accepted as a method based on the complementary relationships between yellow, blue, green, and red, whereby humans perceive color. L* (lightness) values are luminosity indices, expressed as

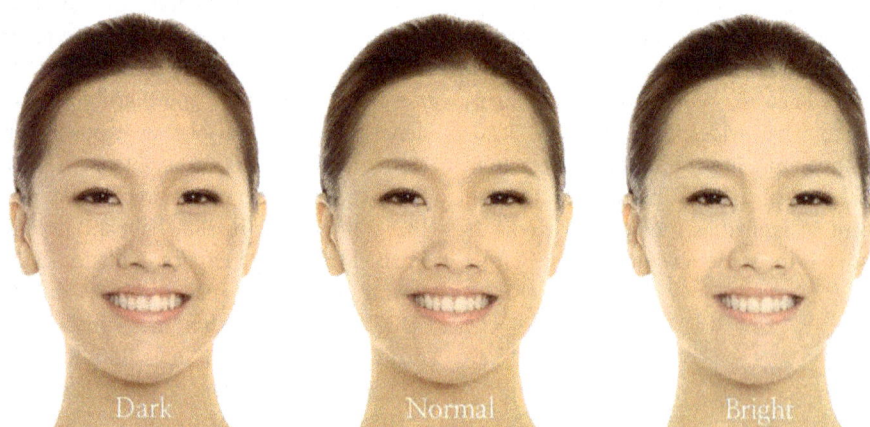

Fig. 1 Facial color simulation using an Asian model. Using Adobe Photoshop® CS5, average values were applied to the face of an Asian model. The image mode was set to Lab Color, and after loading a picture, a new transparency layer was created and overlaid using the Paint Bucket tool

Table 2 Differences in preferred products by age (N (%))

		BB cream	CC cream	Foundation	Cushion compact	Tinted moisturizer	Tinted sunscreen	Powder	χ^2 (p)
Age	20s–30s	101 (47.6)	17 (37.8)	63 (64.3)	59 (48.4)	3 (100.0)	15 (25.9)	1 (20.0)	28.51 (0.000)
	40s–50s	111 (52.4)	28 (62.2)	35 (35.7)	63 (51.6)	0 (0)	43 (74.1)	4 (80.0)	
Total		212 (39.0)	45 (8.3)	98 (18.0)	122 (22.5)	3 (0.6)	58 (10.7)	5 (0.9)	

numbers from 0 to 100, with more black colors closer to 0 and more white colors closer to 100. The a* (redness) values and b* (yellowness) values are indices representing saturation. Therefore, high values for a* indicate red, while low values indicate change to green. High values for b* indicate yellow, and low values indicate change to blue (Baulieu et al. 2000; Lee et al. 2002; Armas et al. 2007).

As described in a previous study, L* values sorted in ascending order were used to divide the study subjects into three groups, each including 181 participants (Jung et al. 2013). The group in which the L* values were darkest was designated dark; the middle group, normal; and the brightest group, bright. Face color was not divided by age because there were subjects who were much brighter or darker than their peers within the same age group, and base makeup products on the market are divided by facial color rather than by age.

Questionnaire responses

In order to investigate use and preferences for base makeup products, following completion of facial color measurements, subjects were asked to complete a questionnaire consisting of nine items. The questionnaire included three items requesting information on demographic characteristics, three on skin color, and three on base makeup product use and preferences. To compare questionnaire responses by age, subjects were divided into two age groups: subjects between 20 and 39 years old (20s–30s) and subjects between 40 and 59 years old (40s–50s) (Shin and Park 2015).

SPSS, version 18.0 (SPSS Inc., Chicago), was used after data coding for data processing, and statistical results were considered significant when $p < 0.05$. Frequency analysis was performed for the demographic analysis of the subjects, and the χ^2 goodness of fit and

independence tests were used to compare the actual use and preferences for base makeup products by age.

Results

Facial color L*a*b* values among native Korean women

Measured L* values, which is the parameter representing lightness, were 60.66 ± 2.16 for the dark group, 63.87 ± 2.27 for the normal group (with a difference of 3.21 compared with the dark group), and 66.66 ± 2.34 for the bright group (with a difference of 2.79 compared with the normal group). The a* values, which is the parameter representing redness, decreased as skin color became brighter: 12.63 ± 1.36 for the dark group, 11.10 ± 1.67 for the normal group, and 9.84 ± 1.62 for the bright group. The b* values, which is the parameter representing yellowness, were 17.82 ± 0.65 for the dark group, 18.12 ± 0.54 for the normal group, and 17.47 ± 0.64 for the bright group, with no significant differences found among groups (Table 1).

When looking at these results, significant differences in yellowness were not found among subjects of the same race, but differences in redness were observed. In comparison, values measured in a previous study including 110 Korean women were the following: L* was 63.4 ± 2.5 (similar to the normal group in this study), a* was 13.0 ± 1.8 (slightly more red than the dark group in this study), and b* was 15.3 ± 1.9 (more blue than all groups in this study). Only the L* values were similar between studies (Jung et al. 2013).

Facial color simulation using an Asian model

Using Adobe Photoshop® CS5, average values were applied to the face of an Asian model. The image mode was set to Lab Color, and after loading a picture, a new transparency layer was created and overlaid using the Paint Bucket tool. The overlay was created using the

Table 3 Notation of products used by age (N (%))

		Specific code notation by numbering	Notation by Korean	Notation by English	Unique notation depends on the company	No notation for all skin types	χ^2 (p)
Age	20s–30s	183 (44.9)	18 (39.1)	28 (65.1)	20 (90.9)	10 (41.7)	24.72 (0.000)
	40s–50s	225 (55.1)	28 (60.9)	15 (34.9)	2 (9.1)	14 (58.3)	
Total		408 (75.1)	46 (8.5)	43 (7.9)	22 (4.1)	24 (4.4)	

Table 4 Differences in skin color perception by age (N (%))

		Perception of much darker skin color than others	Perception of slightly darker skin color than others	Perception of average skin color	Perception of slightly lighter skin color than others	Perception of much lighter skin color than others	χ^2 (p)
Age	20s–30s	9 (45.0)	88 (48.9)	105 (46.4)	54 (49.5)	3 (37.5)	0.781 (0.941)
	40s–50s	11 (55.0)	92 (51.1)	121 (53.5)	55 (50.5)	5 (62.5)	
Total		20 (3.7)	180 (33.1)	226 (41.6)	109 (20.1)	8 (1.5)	

layer settings and was able to generate the picture sequence shown in Fig. 1, which presents dark, normal, and bright facial color examples.

Differences in base makeup product use for skin color correction by age

In order of use, the products applied for skin color correction in the 20s–30s group were BB cream, foundation, and cushion compact, whereas in the 40s–50s group, the order was BB cream, cushion compact, and tinted sunscreen (Table 2). BB cream was reported as the most frequently used product regardless of age. As in previous studies, all ages reported the highest preference for BB cream, which confirms a previous report that BB cream is preferred over other base makeup products.

Color notation of main base makeup products for skin color correction by age

A specific system for expressing skin color by numbering exists only in Korea. This system uses two digits to indicate differences in color. A first number of 1 refers to pink, 2 refers to beige, and 3 refers to brown. The second number is the lightness value, indicating brightness, with smaller numbers indicating brighter coloration and larger numbers indicating darker shades (Shin 2016). Although there were some differences in the color notation of the most frequently used base makeup products between the two groups, 75.1% of respondents reported using base makeup products no. 13, no. 21, and no. 23, respectively (Table 3). This suggests that additional research is needed in order to determine whether the subjects perceive their skin color brightness as a number.

Differences in perceived skin color brightness by age

Subjects in both the 20s–30s and 40s–50s groups reported most frequently that they perceive themselves to have average skin color compared to their peers, and the

next most common answer was that they perceive themselves to have slightly darker skin than others (Table 4). Among all subjects, 36.8% responded that they had slightly or much darker skin color than others, but 21.6% responded that they perceived themselves to have slightly lighter or much lighter skin color than others.

Comparing self-perceived skin color with the color of base makeup products currently in use

Both age groups were found to use a slightly brighter product color that would be entirely consistent with their actual skin color (Table 5). There were very few respondents using far darker or brighter colors, but it is meaningful to note that the coloring of the base makeup products was most often chosen to make the skin color lighter than natural skin color.

Comparing the most important considerations when selecting base makeup products for skin color correction by age

Makeup product measurement items from previous research papers were reviewed (Lee et al. 2014). In order of response frequency, the 20s–30s group answered that they are worried about product adhesion, long-lasting effect, and coverage (Table 6). The 40s–50s group answered that their most important considerations are coverage, product adhesion, and color matching with the skin. There was a limit to the degree of equivalence with the other five view items because the coverage effect surveyed in this item did not ask each subject whether they have their own reference point and prefer if it is weaker or, on the contrary, stronger.

Discussion

The face, which is always exposed, is continuously tanned by ultraviolet rays, and the lightness or redness of the skin may be further influenced by whitening cosmetics, dermatological procedures, or other variables.

Table 5 Comparison of color matching between skin color and product by age (N (%))

		Product color much darker than skin color	Product color slightly darker than skin color	Product color same as skin color	Product color slightly lighter than skin color	Product color much lighter than skin color	χ^2 (p)
Age	20s–30s	0 (0.0)	15 (30.6)	75 (42.9)	165 (52.9)	4 (66.7)	12.51 (0.014)
	40s–50s	1 (100.0)	34 (69.4)	100 (57.1)	147 (47.1)	2 (33.3)	
Total		1 (0.2)	49 (9.0)	175 (32.2)	312 (57.5)	6 (1.1)	

Table 6 The most important considerations when selecting products by age (N (%))

		Color matching with skin	Effect of coverage	Effect of long-lasting	Effect of adhesion	Skin trouble	Nothing here	χ^2 (p)
Age	20s–30s	34 (35.1)	51 (34.7)	52 (58.4)	104 (56.2)	17 (77.3)	1 (33.3)	33.63 (0.000)
	40s–50s	63 (64.9)	96 (65.3)	37 (41.6)	81 (43.8)	5 (22.7)	2 (66.7)	
Total		97 (17.9)	147 (27.1)	89 (16.4)	185 (34.1)	22 (4.1)	3 (0.6)	

Therefore, when measuring facial color, even for the same subject, the season, weather, recently used whitening cosmetics, and any dermatological treatments are among the factors which may affect facial skin L*a*b* values. Therefore, defining a measurement time interval and specifying subject selection criteria are considered among the minimum preparatory steps for starting an experiment. This study only completed a one-time measurement, but in order to generate a more objective skin color chart, further studies will be needed to follow up with subjects and to study deviations by re-measuring the same subjects' skin tones.

One limitation of this study was that only the L* values were used to divide subjects into the three skin color groups. In a previous study on color preference among Korean women, b* values affected certain color preferences among 180 subjects ranging in age from their 30s to 40s (Kang et al. 2014). Although skin color is somewhat difficult to define simply using L* values, there are hundreds of unique skin colors if a* and b* values are included. Therefore, setting a certain reference point appears to be meaningful.

In the questionnaire evaluation, the fact that responses might vary by occupation or living environment within the same age range was not taken into account. Furthermore, it is necessary to separate preferences among subjects in their 20s, 30s, 40s, and 50s to grasp a better understanding. Finally, most respondents used the color notation (for example, no. 21, no. 23) from a numbering system that is used for base makeup products only in Korea. Further research is needed to investigate whether subjects perceive their skin color by the notation created by cosmetic companies, instead of having subjective standards about their skin color, such as perceiving that one's skin color is dark or bright.

Conclusions

In this study, facial colors among Korean women were classified into three colors: dark, normal, and bright. The color L*a*b* values of the bare face could be used as a reference for coloring base makeup products. When looking at the contrast value that was set as a reference point, the dark group was 60.66 and the normal group was 63.87, with a difference of 3.21. The bright group was 66.66, with a difference of 2.79 compared with the normal group. Considering that the average standard deviation for the L* values among the groups was 3, it can be assumed that a one-step difference in skin tone is equivalent to the addition or subtraction of 3 to the L* value.

Similarities and differences among the age groups were compared using a questionnaire, and in their responses regarding product preference and usage of base makeup products, most subjects gave a common answer that their skin color is average or slightly darker than their peers, regardless of age. It was also found that subjects selected base makeup products that were slightly brighter than their skin color. Therefore, it would be meaningful to aim for a color that is brighter than the bare face when developing base makeup products. As found in previous studies, the most frequently used base makeup product in all age groups was BB cream.

Abbreviations
BB: Blemish balm; DOPA: 3,4-Dihydroxyphenylalanine; IRB: Institutional review board; SCE: Specular Component Exclusion; SCI: Specular Component Inclusion

Funding
This work was supported by a grant from the Ministry of Trade, Industry & Energy (MOTIE), Korea Institute for Advancement of Technology (KIAT) through the Encouragement Program for The Industries of Economic Cooperation Region (Grant R0003962) and a grant from the Marine Biotechnology Program (20150184) funded by the Ministry of Oceans and Fishers, Republic of Korea.

Authors' contributions
IJ, ARJ, and YJK performed the experiments. YJK and SK carried out the experimental design and advising. IJ and ISA analyzed the data and wrote the manuscript. All authors read and approved the final manuscript.

Competing interests
The authors declare that they have no competing interests.

References
Ahn BT, Moon EB, Song KS. Study of skin colors of Korean women. Proc SPIE. 2002. https://doi.org/10.1117/12.464600.
Armas LA, Dowell S, Akhter M, Duthuluru S, Huerter C, Hollis BW, et al. Ultraviolet-B radiation increases serum 25-hydroxyvitamin D levels: the effect of UVB dose and skin color. J Am Acad Dermatol. 2007;57:588–93.
Baek YR. Going to New York where K-beauty is trendy. Economy Chosun. 2015. http://economychosun.com/special/special_view_past.php?boardName=C11&t_num=8664&img_ho=130. Accessed 27 July 2015.
Baulieu EE, Thomas G, Legrain S, Lahlou N, Roger M, Debuire B, et al. Dehydroepiandrosterone (DHEA), DHEA sulfate, and aging: contribution of the DHEAge study to a sociobiomedical issue. Proc Natl Acad Sci U S A. 2000;97:4279–84.
Binggeli C, Spieker LE, Corti R, Sudano I, Stojanovic V, Hayoz D, et al. Statins enhance postischemic hyperemia in the skin circulation of hypercholesterolemic patients: a monitoring test of endothelial dysfunction for clinical practice? J Am Coll Cardiol. 2003;42:71–7.

Couteau C, Paparis E, Coiffard LJ. BB creams and their photoprotective effect. Pharm Dev Technol. 2016;21:39–42.

Desmedt B, Van Hoeck E, Rogiers V, Courselle P, De Beer JO, De Paepe K, et al. Characterization of suspected illegal skin whitening cosmetics. J Pharm Biomed Anal. 2014;90:85–91.

Dunbabin DW, Tallis GA, Popplewell PY, Lee RA. Lead poisoning from Indian herbal medicine (Ayurveda). Med J Aust. 1992;157:835–6.

Jablonski NG. Skin: a natural history. 1st ed. Berkeley: University of California Press; 2006.

Jung YC, Lee MR, Kim EH, Cho JC, Lee HK. Comparison between face color change and its recognition difference on Asian: Korean, Indonesian and Vietnamian. J Soc Cosmet Sci Korea. 2013;39:323–7.

Kang NG, Kwak TJ, Kim JA, Kim TH, Moon TK, Park SG, et al. A preferred skin color by Korean female in the age between 30s~40s. J Soc Cosmet Sci Korea. 2014;40:373–82.

Kang WK, Hwang SD, Kim HS, Jeung JS, Lee BU. The development of whitening cosmetic ingredient having activity of melanin degradation. KSBB Journal. 2007;22:7–15.

Latreille J, Gardinier S, Ambroisine L, Mauger E, Tenenhaus M, Guéhenneux S, et al. Influence of skin colour on the detection of cutaneous erythema and tanning phenomena using reflectance spectrophotometry. Skin Res Technol. 2007;13:236–41.

Lee SY, Baek JH, Shin MK, Koh JS. The quantitative analysis of spreadability, coverage, and adhesion effect after application of the base make-up product. Skin Res Technol. 2014;20:341–6.

Lee YK, Yoon TH, Lim BS, Kim CW, Powers JM. Effects of colour measuring mode and light source on the colour of shade guides. J Oral Rehabil. 2002;29:1099–107.

Muehlenbein M. Human evolutionary biology. New York: Cambridge University Press; 2010. p. 192–213.

Park HK, Kim NS, Moon TK, Kim B, Jung HY. A comparison study between image analysis and conventional methods in the evaluation of Asian skin color. J Soc Cosmet Sci Korea. 2015;41:97–103.

Park YE, Chin CH. Analysis of B.B cream used condition. AJBC. 2010;8:63–74.

Piérard GE. EEMCO guidance for the assessment of skin colour. J Eur Acad Dermatol Venereol. 1998;10:1–11.

Shin HM. Why do we use cosmetics only No.21? MBC NEWS. 2016. http://imnews.imbc.com. Accessed 13 Oct 2016.

Shin HS, Park YS. A comparative analysis on complexion and skin color in 20s-30s and 40s-50s by frequency of L*a*b values. JKSCS. 2015;29:103–13.

Shin HY. The revised Declaration of Helsinki and clinical research. Transl Clin Pharmacol. 2009;17:152–63.

Wagatsuma H. The social perception of skin color in Japan. Daedalus. 1967;96:407–43.

Weatherall IL, Coombs BD. Skin color measurements in terms of CIELAB color space values. J Invest Dermatol. 1992;99:468–73.

Witkowski JA, Parish LC. You've come a long way baby: a history of cosmetic lead toxicity. Clin Dermatol. 2001;19:367–70.

2

Photodamage attenuation effect by angelic acid in UVA irradiation-induced damages in normal human dermal fibroblast

Jung-Eun Ku

Abstract

Background: Among various extra stimuli of humans, ultraviolet (UV) has been the most studied factor because it arouses not only internal but also external irritation in the body. UVA, one type of UV rays, has a wavelength between 320 and 400 nm and capacity to penetrate the skin dermal layer. Therefore, studies on how to reduce UVA-induced maleficence have been investigated vibrantly. Angelic acid has been demonstrated to aid in wound healing and exhibited sedative and psychotropic properties. But there have not been sufficient reports whether angelic acid has potential properties in the cosmeceutical aspect.

Methods: To investigate protective effects of angelic acid on UVA-induced oxidative stress and disruption of extracellular matrix, researchers analyzed cell proliferation rate, intracellular reactive oxygen species (ROS) scavenging capacity, cellular senescence, transcriptional activity of activating protein-1 (AP-1) transcription factor, and gene expression of antioxidant enzymes and connective tissue-related proteins.

Results: Pretreatment of angelic acid in normal human dermal fibroblasts (NHDFs) showed protective effect on UVA-induced proliferative inhibition. Via estimating ROS scavenging activity, angelic acid represented a scavenging effect of excessive increased intracellular ROS which is induced by UVA irradiation. Through quantitative real-time polymerase reaction, antioxidant enzyme and extracellular matrix (ECM)-related protein coded gene expressions were analyzed. Analysis of senescent cell and AP-1 promoter activity by beta-galactosidase assay and luciferase reporter gene assay, respectively, indicated how angelic acid regulates cellular mechanisms associated with connective tissue density.

Conclusions: Through the present study, researchers verify that angelic acid has dermal protective effect against UVA and suggest angelic acid as an efficacious cosmetic material preventing dermal cellular damages.

Keywords: Angelic acid, Human dermal fibroblast, Reactive oxygen species, Ultraviolet A, Senescence, Connective tissue

Background

In human skin, exposure of solar ultraviolet (UV) rays leads to physiological damages, DNA disorder, formation of intracellular reactive oxygen species (ROS), and collapse of connective tissue density via degradation of extracellular matrix (ECM) components (Yel et al., 2014; Bae et al., 2017; Kohl et al., 2011). Three types of UV rays, UVA (315–400 nm), UVB (280–315 nm), and UVC (200–280 nm), compose solar radiation and only UVA and UVB inflict damage to ground surface because UVC is screened out by the ozone layer (Ko, 2015). The deepest penetration is from UVA; even relative intensity is not more energetic than UVB, which can reach deeper skin layers (Binic et al., 2013; Kim et al., 2016; Song et al., 2016). Increased substantial ROS by UV irradiation in the cells augment proteins that deplete ECM components (Binic et al., 2013; Song et al., 2016; Rittié & Fisher, 2002; Tsuji et al., 2001).

Cells that are building connective tissue synthesize ECM components which are composed of structural and biochemical proteins to influence cellular function

Correspondence: jungeunku@hanmail.net
Department of Cosmetology, Kyung-In Women's University, 63, Gyeyangsan-ro, Gyeyang-gu, Incheon, Republic of Korea

reciprocally against diverse cell biology (Hynes, 2009; Lu et al., 2011). Collagen is one of the main extracellular structural components which is responsible for structural integrity and stability with various biological functions like cell growth, differentiation, migration, and even skin aging (Ricard-Blum, 2011; Kim et al., 2017; Jabłońska-Trypuć et al., 2016; Quan et al., 2006). For the importance of structural proteins, especially diverse types of collagen, studies focused on understanding its regulating mechanisms have been pursued.

Angelic acid is a substance found in the essential oil of *Anthemis nobilis*, a plant from the *Asteraceae* family, or *Angelica* from the *Apiaceae* family, and it exists in an ester form (Ernest, 2006; Craker & Simon, 1986). It is also isolated from carrots, *Euphorbia* species and *Alkanna tinctoria* (Sonobe et al., 1981; Sosath et al., 1988; Papageorgiou, 1978). It has been reported to aid in wound healing in clinical study (Papageorgiou, 1978) and used as sedative and antispasmodic (Ernest, 2006) and psychotropic (Rhind, 2012), but not in skin aspects such as for therapeutic and cosmeceutical use. Thus, the present study is designed to determine the role of angelic acid on UVA-induced oxidative stress and dermal senescence in normal human dermal fibroblasts (NHDFs) by assessing its excessive ROS scavenging capacity and ECM deterioration.

Methods
Chemicals and reagents
Angelic acid was purchased from Santa Cruz Biotechnology (Dallas, TX, USA) and was dissolved in dimethyl sulfoxide (DMSO; Sigma Aldrich, St. Louis, MO, USA) to obtain a 1 mM stock solution that was stored at 4 °C until used. Dulbecco's modified Eagle's medium (DMEM), 1% penicillin/streptomycin, and TRIzol reagent were purchased from Gibco/Life Technologies (Carlsbad, CA, USA). The 10% fetal bovine serum (FBS), 3-(4,5-dimethylthiazol-2-yl)-2,5-diphenyl-tertazolium bromide (MTT), 2,7-dichlorofluorescin diacetate (DCFH-DA), glutathione (GSH) assay kit, and L-ascorbic acid were purchased from Sigma-Aldrich. The activating protein-1 (AP-1) reporter kit was purchased from BPS Bioscience (San Diego, CA, USA). The miScript II RT kit was purchased from Qiagen (Hilden, Germany) and the Evagreen dye was from Solis BioDyne (Tartu, Estonia). The senescence-associated β-galactosidase (SA-β-gal) staining kit was obtained from Biovision (Milpitas, CA, USA), and the manufactured primers for the quantitative real-time polymerase chain reaction (RT-qPCR) analysis were purchased from Macrogen (Seoul, Korea).

Cell culture
The NHDF derived from human skin cells were obtained from the Lonza Group (Basel, Switzerland) and were maintained in DMEM supplemented with 10% heat-inactivated FBS, 100 units/ml penicillin, and 100 μg/ml streptomycin in a humidified atmosphere of 5% CO_2 at 37 °C. For subculture, the medium was eliminated and cells were rinsed with phosphate-buffered saline (PBS) twice. Then, the cells were detached using trypsin-EDTA and were cultured with fresh complete growth medium in a ratio of 1:5 every 72 h. The reagents such as angelic acid and L-ascorbic acid were diluted with the culture medium before treatment, and final concentrations were adjusted using DMSO.

UVA irradiation
The cells were plated until they had attained 80–90% confluence, rinsed with phosphate-buffered saline (PBS), and then were exposed to UVA light in fresh PBS-filled wells without the lid. UVA irradiation was carried out in a closed chamber using UVA lamps (UVP, Upland, CA, USA), and the intensity was detected using a fiberoptic spectrometer system USB2000 (Ocean Optics, Dunedin, FL, USA). After irradiation, the PBS was aspirated from each well and a pre-warmed complete growth medium was immediately added to the wells. The control cells were operated under the same culture conditions except for the UVA exposure.

Cell cytotoxicity
The cytotoxicity was determined using an MTT assay kit following the manufacturer's protocol. Briefly, the cells were seeded in the culture plate, incubated for 24 h, and then were pretreated for 6 h with diverse concentrations of angelic acid (5, 10, 15, and 30 μM) before UVA irradiation. Then, 24 h after UVA irradiation, the content of each well was changed to a serum-free medium containing 5 mg/ml MTT and incubated for 4 h, and then the formazan blue crystals that were formed in the cells after the medium was removed were dissolved with DMSO. The absorbance of the reaction solution was subsequently measured at 540 nm using an iMark microplate reader (Bio-Rad, Hercules, CA, USA).

DCFH-DA scavenging assay
The intracellular ROS generation was measured using the fluorescence dye DCFH-DA, which produces a detectable fluorescence when the non-fluorescent DCFH reacts with ROS in cells. The treated cells were incubated with 25 μM DCFH-DA at 37 °C for 1 h, and then the fluorescence intensity was measured using a BD fluorescence-activated cell sorting calibur (FACSCalibur, flow cytometer, BD Biosciences, San Jose, CA, USA), at excitation and emission wavelengths of 485 and 535 nm, respectively.

Intercellular GSH content

GSH content of the cells was measured using the Thiol-Tracker Violet GSH detection reagent (Invitrogen/Molecular probes, Eugene, OR) according to the manufacturer's protocol. Cells were seeded in six-well plates, incubated overnight, and treated the following day. Subsequent to treatment of angelic acid and UVA exposure for the indicated dose, the cells were washed with PBS once and incubated in PBS containing 10 μM (final concentration) ThiolTracker Violet for 30 min at 37 °C. Then, cells were semiquantified using a FACSCalibur (BD Biosciences).

RNA isolation and qRT-PCR

The total RNA of each sample was isolated using the TRIzol reagent following the manufacturer's protocol. After the purified RNA had been validated using a spectrophotometer (MaestroNano, Maestrogen, NV, USA), 1 μg of the total RNA was used for cDNA synthesis using a miScript II RT kit. The mRNA expression was quantitatively assessed using Evagreen dye with the Line-Gene K software (BioER, Hangzhou, China), according to the manufacturer's protocol. The primer list for the qRT-PCR is provided in Table 1, and this experiment was performed in triplicate.

SA-β-gal activity

The SA-β-gal staining was carried out according to the manufacturer's instructions, and senescence cell staining was detected 24 h after UVA irradiation. Briefly, the cells were rinsed twice with PBS, fixed with 0.5 ml fixative solution (4% formaldehyde and 0.5% glutaraldehyde in PBS, pH 7.2) for 20 min, rinsed again with PBS, and then were incubated with the staining solution for 24 h at 37 °C. Then, the staining solution was removed, and 70% glycerol was added to each well before the stained cells were examined for senescence using a microscope (Olympus Microscope System IX51, Olympus, Japan).

AP-1 promoter luciferase assay

For the AP-1 reporter luciferase assays, AP-1 luciferase reporter vectors were transiently transfected with the pSV-β-galactosidase (pSV-β-gal) plasmid into the cells. Then, luciferase activity and β-galactosidase activity were assayed as described previously (Choi et al., 2012). Briefly, after transfection, cells were treated with angelic acid for 6 h and irradiated with UVA before 24 h incubation. Then, the cells were re-suspended in Passive Lysis Buffer (Promega Corp., Madison, WI, USA), and the luciferase activity was measured with a Veritas Luminometer (Turnur Designs, Sunnyvale, CA, USA). β-galactosidase activity was measured using Luminescent β-galactosidase Detection Kit II (Clontech Laboratories, Inc., Mountain View, CA, USA) according to the manufacturer's protocol. The relative luciferase activity was normalized to β-galactosidase activity. The results are the averages of three independent experiments.

Statistics

All the results are presented as the mean percentage ± standard deviation (M ± SD) of three independent experiments. p values <0.05, 0.01, and 0.001 were considered statistically significant and were determined using Student's t test.

Results

Pretreatment with angelic acid inhibits UVA-induced cytotoxicity in HDFs

Prior to estimating protective effect on UVA-induced cytotoxicity, researchers examine whether angelic acid has cytotoxicity as the concentration range is tested. Fibroblast cells were treated with angelic acid (0–30 μM) for 24 h, and viability was determined using the MTT assay (Fig. 1a). Then, cells were exposed to 10 J/cm^2 UVA after 3 h pretreatment with angelic acid to investigate UVA-induced cytoprotective effect. Cyto-protective effect of angelic acid was also measured using the MTT assay (Fig. 1b). As shown in Fig. 1, angelic acid has no significant cytotoxicity with indicated concentrations. Though there was no significant

Table 1 Overview of qRT-PCR primer sequences

Gene name (symbol)	Forward primer	Reverse primer
β-actin	GGATTCCTATGTGGGCGACGA	CGCTCGGTGAGGATCTTCATG
GPx1	TTCCCGTGCAACCAGTTTG	GGACGTACTTGAGGGAATTCAGA
SOD1	GGGAGATGGCCCAACTACTG	CCAGTTGACATGCAACCGTT
SOD2	GCCCTGGAACCTCACATCAA	GGTACTTCTCCTCGGTGACGTT
CAT	ATGGTCCATGCTCTCAAACC	CAGGTCATCCAATAGGAAGG
NRF2	TACTCCCAGGTTGCCCACA	CATCTACAAACGGGAATGTCTGC
HO-1	GCCTGCTAGCCTGGTTCAAG	AGCGGTGTCTGGGATGAACTA
uPA	CCACCAAAATGCTGTGTGCT	GCTTGTCCTTCAGGGCACAT
COL1A1	AGGGCCAAGACGAAGACATC	AGATCACGTCATCGCACAACA
MMP1	TCTGACGTTGATCCCAGAGAGCAG	CAGGGTGACACCAGTGACTGCAC

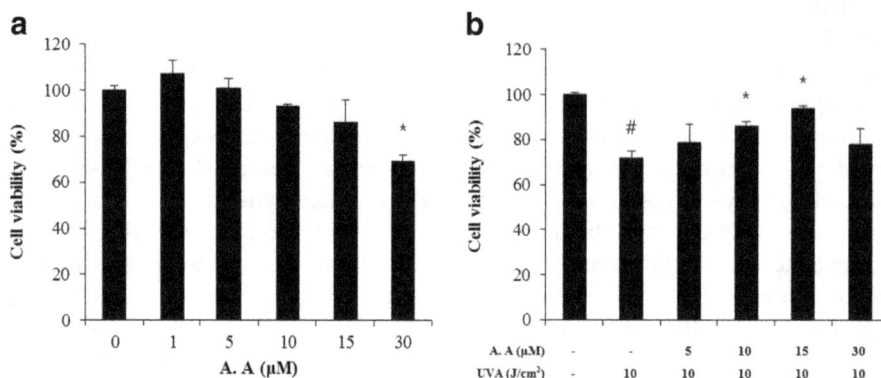

Fig. 1 Determination of NHDF cell viability via MTT assay. **a** Effect of angelic acid on NHDF cell viability at the indicated concentrations, up to 30 μM. **b** Protective effect of angelic acid on UVA-induced cellular cytotoxicity in NHDF cells. Cell viability was expressed as a percentage of control and values are M ± SD; *$p \leq 0.05$ compared with irradiated cells without angelic acid treatment and #$p \leq 0.05$ compared with negative control cells that were not treated with angelic acid and UVA irradiation

cytotoxicity within 30 μM angelic acid, UVA irradiation which reduced cell viability and cells treated with 30 μM of angelic acid represented no UVA-induced cytotoxic protective effect. In accordance with these results, researchers investigated diverse effects of angelic acid against UVA irradiation at concentrations up to 15 μM, in sequence.

Pretreatment with angelic acid reduces UVA-induced intracellular ROS generation in HDFs

On account of inducing ROS, UVA is regarded as one of major extrinsic factors leading the aging phenomena. Pursuantly, we investigated protective effects of angelic acid on UVA-induced oxidative stress through ROS scavenging efficacy on HDFs, and regulation capacity of GSH and glutathione peroxidase 1 (GPx1) transcriptional expression. As shown in Fig. 2a, cells were pre-treated angelic acid before UVA irradiation described reduced DCF fluorescence levels in a dose-dependent manner while UVA-irradiated cells showed increased levels. Furthermore, relative contents of GSH also appeared to have conspicuous antioxidant efficiency, in a dose-dependent manner by angelic acid (Fig. 2b). In the current study, irradiation of UVA reduced the mRNA expression of *GPx1* by 0.68, compared with their respective control values ($p < 0.05$, Fig. 2c). Prior to UVA irradiation, cells were treated with angelic acid at the dose of 5, 10, and 15 μM for 6 h then irradiated with UVA with indicated dosage. Following this treatment, researchers identified the mRNA expression level of *GPx1* via qRT-PCR and observed photo-protective effect of angelic acid by increasing *GPx1* mRNA expression level as significantly within 15 μM ($p < 0.05$, except not significant at 5 μM, Fig. 2c).

Angelic acid activates antioxidant gene expression against UVA irradiation in HDFs

As indicated by the ROS scavenging assay, UVA increased the intracellular ROS levels in HDF cells compared with the non-irradiated cells. Following this treatment, researchers investigated an intrinsic enzyme defense system against UVA-induced oxidative stress, additionally. To evaluate antioxidant gene expression under UVA irradiation, the mRNA expression status of HDF cells were measured using reverse transcriptase PCR and qRT-PCR assay. As presented in Fig. 3, expression levels of superoxide dismutase 1 (*SOD1*) and 2 (*SOD2*), catalase (*CAT*), nuclear factor erythroid 2-related factor 2 (*NRF2*), and Heme oxygenase 1 (*HO-1*) mRNA were assessed in UVA-irradiated and co-treated with UVA and angelic acid HDFs. Cells were co-treated with angelic acid before UVA radiation, in accordance with the above experiments. Relative mRNA expression of *SOD1* and *SOD2* revealed that pretreatment with angelic acid stimulated transcriptional levels of SOD1 and SOD2 against UVA-induced ROS generation (Fig. 3a). In detail, the rate of *SOD1* mRNA expression was decreased by UVA irradiation while cells which were co-treated with angelic acid and UVA showed increased mRNA levels in a dose-dependent manner by angelic acid ($p < 0.05$, not significant in 5 μM angelic acid). *SOD2* mRNA expression increased as concentration of angelic acid increased to 0.80, 0.89, and 0.97, respectively. Following UVA irradiation, relative *CAT* mRNA expression was decreased to 0.53 but angelic acid improved *CAT* mRNA expression levels against UVA irradiation. In this experiment, *CAT* mRNA expression was revealed at 0.61, 0.78, and 0.97 compared with the level of the control HDFs (Fig. 3b). *NRF2* mRNA expression levels showed as similar in *SOD1*, *SOD2*, and *CAT*. UVA-irradiated cells showed a significantly attenuated

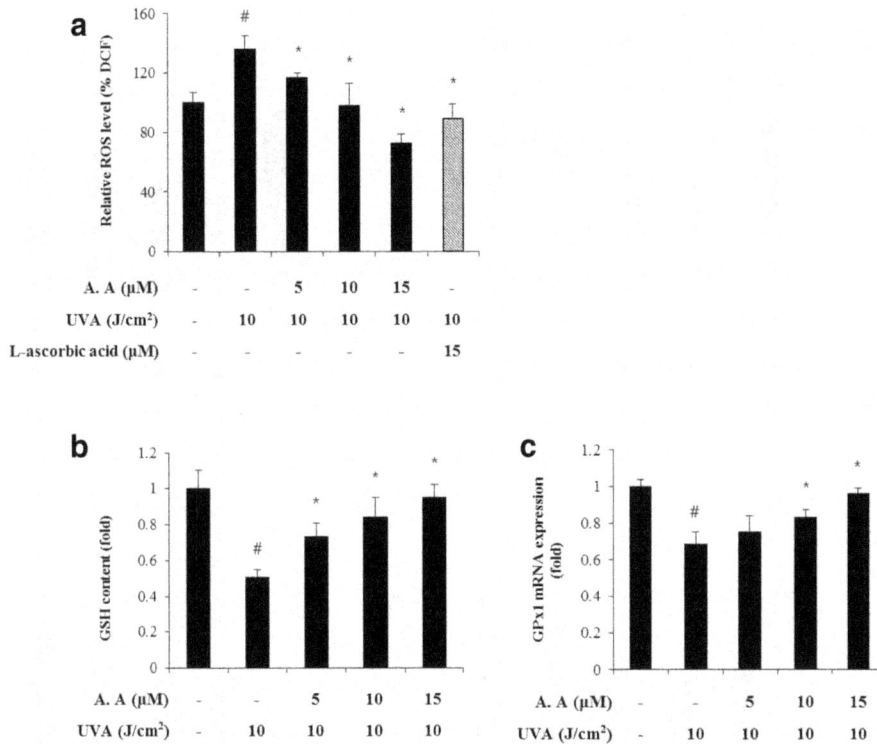

Fig. 2 ROS scavenging capacities of angelic acid and intracellular GSH content estimation. **a** Effect of angelic acid on DCF fluorescence intensity in NHDF cells. Ascorbic acid was used as positive control, and UVA irradiation (10 J/cm²) was performed as inducing intracellular ROS in NHDFs. **b** Effect of angelic acid on intracellular glutathione contents under UVA irradiation. **c** Effect of angelic acid on *GPx1* mRNA expression levels against UVA irradiation. Data were expressed as a percentage of control and values are M ± SD; *$p \leq 0.05$ compared with irradiated cells without angelic acid treatment and #$p \leq 0.05$ compared with negative control cells that were not treated with angelic acid and UVA irradiation

expression of *NRF2* mRNA compared with the control HDFs. Interestingly, the pretreatment of HDFs with angelic acid significantly showed protective effect against UVA-induced ROS via upregulating *NRF2* expression levels (Fig. 3c). Furthermore, *HO-1*, one of representative NRF2 downstream targets which regulate inflammatory cytokine production and catalyzes the degradation of free heme molecules, also showed increased mRNA expression via angelic acid pretreatment (Fig. 3d).

Pretreatment with angelic acid retards UVA-induced cellular senescence and acid protects UVA-induced extracellular matrix decomposition in HDFs

The above results indicated the protective effects of angelic acid against UVA-induced ROS via scavenging overgenerated intracellular ROS and promoting transcriptional levels of antioxidant enzymes. These consequences led us to examine whether angelic acid regulates cellular senescence which was derived by UVA irradiation in HDF cells. To test this, researchers used a senescence-associated-β-galactosidase staining kit (BioVision) and HDFs were also operated according to the above procedure. As indicated in Fig. 4a, cells treated with 15 μM of angelic acid had no significant difference

in cellular senescence. However, 10 J/cm² UVA led cellular senescence 11-fold more than control HDFs significantly. The interesting point was that pretreatment of angelic acid reduced UVA-induced cellular senescence by indicated angelic acid concentration gradient. Though 5 μM angelic acid-treated cells presented no significantly reduced data, 10 and 15 μM angelic acid-treated cells showed remarkable decreased senescent cell population of 34.67 and 21.67%, individually. Following evaluation on cellular senescence, researchers conducted quantitative real-time polymerase chain reaction and luciferase reporter gene activity to investigate alterative mRNA expression of urokinase plasminogen activator (*uPA*), collagen type I, alpha 1 chain (*COL1A1*) and matrix metalloproteinase-1 (*MMP1*), and transcriptional level transition of activator protein 1 (AP-1). To demonstrate whether angelic acid protects ECM from UVA-induced collapse via modulating ECM-associated gene transcriptional level, cells were pretreated angelic acid before UVA irradiation, like the above experiments. After cell harvest and extraction mRNA, synthesis of cDNA also operated through reverse transcription polymerase chain reaction. Then, quantitative polymerase chain reaction was performed to estimate how angelic acid regulates

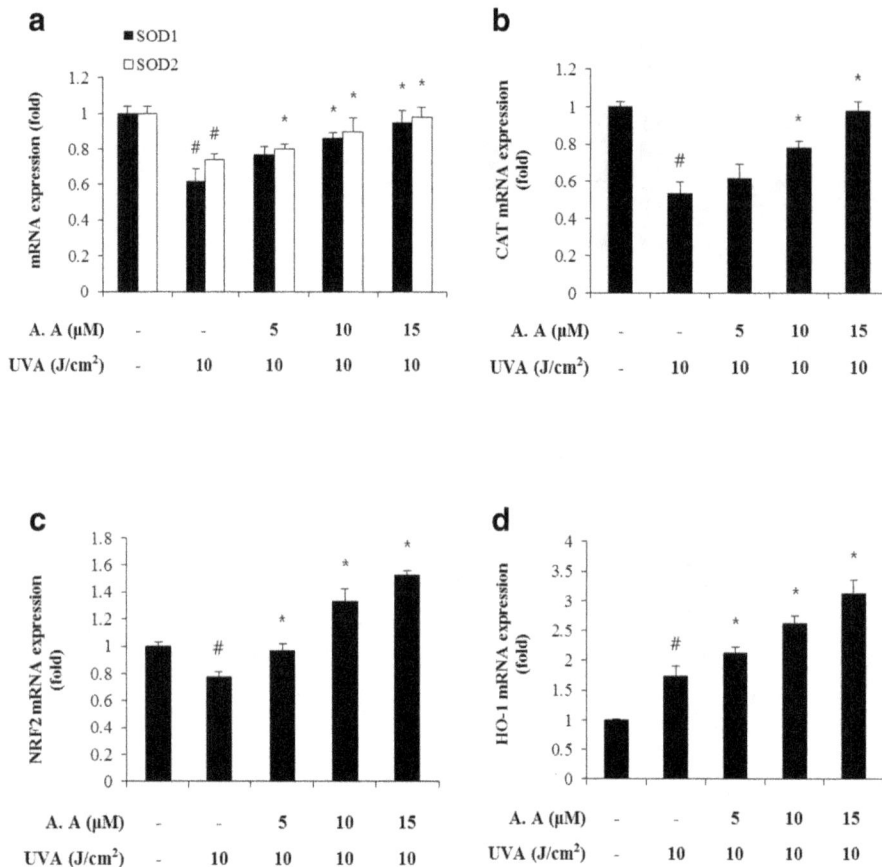

Fig. 3 Analysis of antioxidant gene expression modulating efficacy of angelic acid in NHDF cells. Effect of angelic acid on controlling mRNA expression levels of **a** *SOD1* and *SOD2*, **b** *CAT*, **c** *NRF2*, and **d** *HO-1* in NHDFs, in opposition to UVA. Data were expressed as a percentage of control and values are M ± SD; *$p \leq 0.05$ compared with irradiated cells without angelic acid treatment and #$p \leq 0.05$ compared with negative control cells that were not treated with angelic acid and UVA irradiation

gene expression against UVA irradiation in NHDF cells. As shown in Fig. 4b–d, *uPA*, *COL1A1*, and *MMP1* gene expression levels in NHDFs adduced that pretreatment of angelic acid was efficacious on UVA irradiation which induces breakdown of ECM. Further interesting point is AP-1 promoter luciferase activity. In this experiment, the AP-1 promoter contains luciferase reporter vector which transfected into the NHDF cells. Similar patterns were obtained with ECM regulating gene expression and luciferase activity estimated cells (Fig. 4e). In conclusion, the effect of angelic acid dominates in controlling the transcriptional activity of genes which reconstructs ECM.

Discussion

ROS generation occurs in respiratory chain from molecular oxygen and mitochondrial metabolism of mammals. But this natural production as a byproduct of homeostasis is important on pathological elimination (Zorov et al., 2014; Murphy, 2009). Exposure to UVA radiation also induces ROS production while it causes oxidative stress and initiates senescence response

(Bickers & Athar, 2006; Berneburg et al., 2004a; Yin & Jiang, 2013; Yang et al., 2015), because this stimulus is excessive ROS production. Against stimuli like these, there are enzymatic or non-enzymatic mechanisms that defend against oxidative stress-induced damages by scavenging intracellular ROS levels. In this study, researchers investigate angelic acid to approach as a novel material in therapeutic cosmetic ingredients.

We estimated the cytotoxicity of angelic acid in indicated concentration at first and then demonstrated the protective effect by UVA-induced photo-damages. At 5, 10, and 15 μM, angelic acid-pretreated cells showed attenuated cytotoxic damages which influence cell proliferation by 10 mJ/cm^2 of UVA irradiation in HDFs. But in 30 μM, angelic acid has no significant protective effect, compared with cells only UVA-irradiated.

Subsequently, we demonstrated the intracellular ROS scavenging effect of angelic acid on UVA-induced generation, via analysis of DCF-DA fluorescent intensity, reduced GSH contents, and *GPx1* mRNA expression. Pretreatment of angelic acid modulates UVA-induced

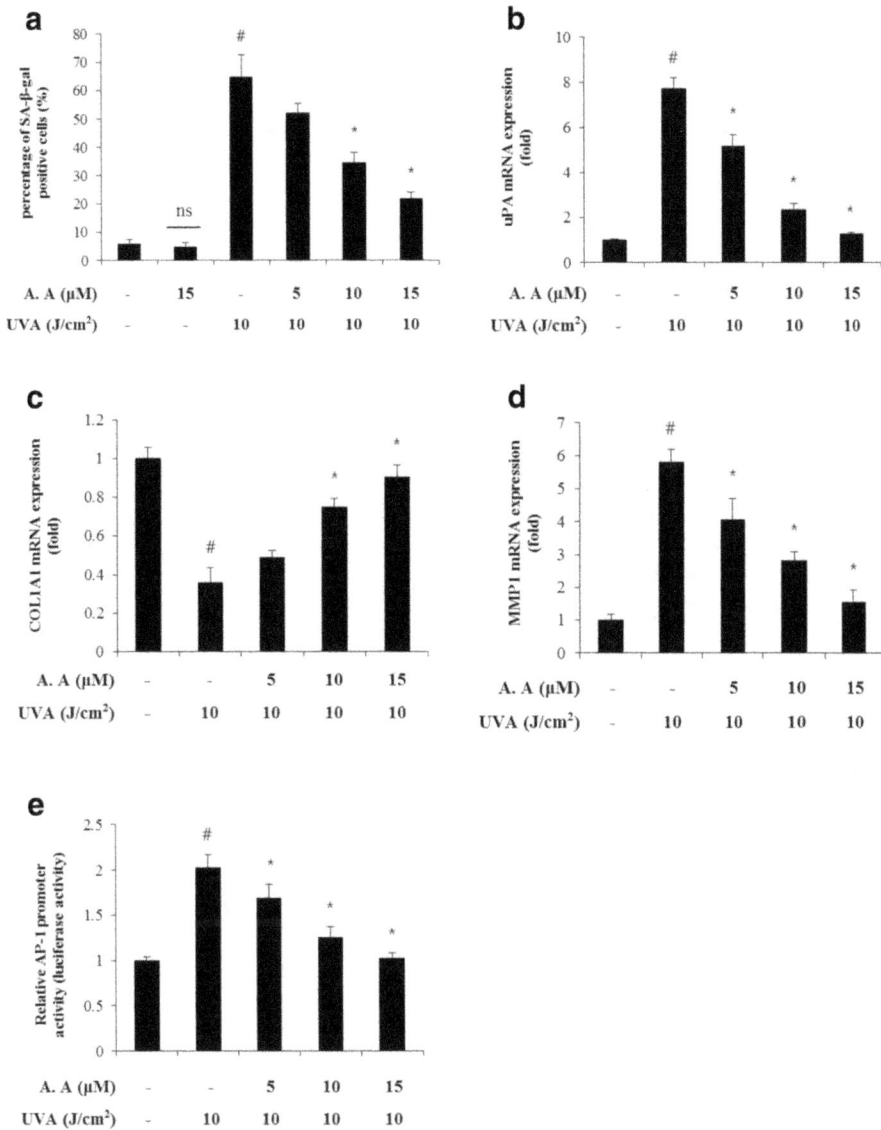

Fig. 4 Protective effect of angelic acid on UVA-induced cellular senescence and ECM controlling gene expression in NHDF cells. **a** Effect of angelic acid on cellular senescence using SA-β-gal assay. Effects of angelic acid on gene expression of **b** *uPA*, **c** *COL1A1*, and **d** *MMP1*. **e** Relative AP-1 promoter luciferase reporter activity using fluorescent intensity. Gene expression of *uPA*, *COL1A1*, and *MMP1* was evaluated using RT-qPCR with the $2^{-\Delta\Delta Ct}$ method and data presented were normalized to β-actin; *$p \leq 0.05$ compared with irradiated cells without angelic acid treatment and #$p \leq 0.05$ compared with negative control cells that were not treated with angelic acid and UVA irradiation

ROS levels through activating an internal cellular excessive ROS scavenging mechanism. To research how angelic acid controls other enzymatic defense mechanisms, researchers conducted mRNA expression analysis of *SOD1* and *SOD2*, *CAT*, *NRF2*, and *HO-1* using qRT-PCR. At the test concentration of angelic acid, especially 10 and 15 μM, above antioxidant enzyme coded gene expressions were significantly increased in dose-dependent manners.

The fibroblasts, one of the major components of the skin, are intimately related with the ECM by synthesizing and secreting matrix macromolecules, such as collagen, elastin, laminin, and fibronectin (Alberts et al., 2002; Khavkin & Ellis, 2011; Saito et al., 2015). Previous reports have revealed and studied characteristics of the fibroblasts and the relation with various stimuli including intrinsic and extrinsic. Following the precedent study, it has been suggested that UVA and oxidative stress induced by the ray irradiation lead to collapse of ECM via decomposing collagen fibers (Rittié & Fisher, 2002; Polte & Tyrrell, 2004; Berneburg et al., 2004b). MMPs, typical enzymes which degrade ECM proteins including collagen and gelatin, are considered responsible as a key regulator in ECM decomposition (Jabłońska-

Trypuć et al., 2016). Having views on those reports, we aimed at demonstrating whether angelic acid protects UVA-induced ECM decomposition as modulating gene expression which coded ECM proteins, uPA, COL1A1, and MMP1 especially. Further experiments investigated influence on cellular senescence via SA-β-gal assay and promoter activity of AP-1 which is upstream of the senescence mechanism. As a result, cells treated with angelic acid prior to UVA irradiation showed retardation of UVA-induced cellular senescence and regulated gene expression of ECM proteins, which were intimately related to construction or disruption of connective tissue.

Conclusions

In conclusion, we verified that angelic acid has photoprotective effect on the HDFs against UVA-induced cytotoxicity, oxidative stress, and cellular senescence. This study elucidates how angelic acid, a new material which has suggestive cosmeceutical applications, militates against UVA-induced damages via revealing unknown cellular mechanisms presented above. Further investigations such as protein level evaluation including in vivo experiments are needed to substantiate biological roles of angelic acid; this study suggests that angelic acid has potential value in the implementation of new therapeutic and cosmetic strategies for skin aging.

Abbreviations

A.A: Angelic acid; AP-1: Activating protein-1; *CAT*: Catalase; *COL1A1*: Collagen type I, alpha 1 chain; DCFH-DA: 2,7-Dichlorofluorescin diacetate; DMSO: Dissolved in dimethyl sulfoxide; ECM: Extracellular matrix; FBS: Fetal bovine serum; *GPx1*: Glutathione peroxidase 1; GSH: Glutathione; *HO-1*: Heme oxygenase 1; M ± SD: Mean percentage ± standard deviation; *MMP1*: Matrix metalloproteinase-1; MTT: 3-(4,5-Dimethylthiazol-2-yl)-2,5-diphenyl-tertazolium bromide; NHDFs: Normal human dermal fibroblasts; *NRF2*: Nuclear factor erythroid 2-related factor 2; PBS: Phosphate-buffered saline; pSV-β-gal: pSV-β-galactosidase; ROS: Intracellular reactive oxygen species; RT-qPCR: Quantitative real-time polymerase chain reaction; SA-β-gal: Senescence-associated β-galactosidase; *SOD1*: Superoxide dismutase 1; *uPA*: Urokinase plasminogen activator; UV: Ultraviolet

Acknowledgements

The author thanks all the study subjects and research staff who participated in this work.

Funding

Not applicable.

Authors' contributions

JK performed the experiments, data analysis, and drafted the manuscript. The author read and approved the final manuscript.

Competing interests

The author declares no competing interests.

References

Alberts B, Johnson A, Lewis J, Raff M, Roberts K, Walter P. Molecular biology of the cell. 4th ed. New York: Garland Science; 2002.

Bae JS, Han M, Shin HS, Kim MK, Shin CY, Lee DH, et al. Perilla frutescens leaves extract ameliorates ultraviolet radiation-induced extracellular matrix damage in human dermal fibroblasts and hairless mice skin. J Ethnopharmacol. 2017; 195:334–42.

Berneburg M, Plettenberg H, Medve-König K, Pfahlberg A, Gers-Barlag H, Gefeller O, et al. Induction of the photoaging-associated mitochondrial common deletion in vivo in normal human skin. J Invest Dermatol. 2004;122:1277–83.

Bickers DR, Athar M. Oxidative stress in the pathogenesis of skin disease. J Invest Dermatol. 2006;126:2565–75.

Binic I, Lazarevic V, Ljubenovic M, Mojsa J, Sokolovic D. Skin ageing: natural weapons and strategies. Evid Based Complement Alternat Med. 2013;2013:827248.

Choi YM, An S, Lee EM, Kim K, Choi SJ, Kim JS, et al. CYP1A1 is a target of miR-892a-mediated post-transcriptional repression. Int J Oncol. 2012;41:331–6.

Craker LE, Simon JE. Herbs, spices, and medicinal plants: recent advances in botany, horticulture, and pharmacology. Binghamton: Haworth Press Inc; 1986.

Ernest S. Culinary herbs. 2nd ed. National Research Council: Canada; 2006.

Hynes RO. The extracellular matrix: not just pretty fibrils. Science. 2009;326:1216–9.

Jabłońska-Trypuć A, Matejczyk M, Rosochacki S. Matrix metalloproteinases (MMPs), the main extracellular matrix (ECM) enzymes in collagen degradation, as a target for anticancer drugs. J Enzyme Inhib Med Chem. 2016;31(Suppl 1):177–83.

Khavkin J, Ellis DA. Aging skin: histology, physiology, and pathology. Facial Plast Surg Clin North Am. 2011;19:229–34.

Kim KS, Han SH, An IS, Ahn KJ. Protective effects of ellagic acid against UVA-induced oxidative stress in human dermal papilla. Asian J Beauty Cosmetol. 2016;14:191–200.

Kim MK, Kim EJ, Cheng Y, Shin MH, JH O, Lee DH, et al. Inhibition of DNA methylation in the COL1A2 promoter by anacardic acid prevents UV-induced decrease of type I procollagen expression. J Invest Dermatol. 2017;137:1343–52.

Ko JM. Protective effects of α-mangostin on UVB-induced oxidative stress and cellular senescence. Asian J Beauty Cosmetol. 2015;13:813–8.

Kohl E, Steinbauer J, Landthaler M, Szeimies RM. Skin ageing. J Eur Acad Dermatol Venereol. 2011;25:873–84.

Lu P, Takai K, Weaver VM, Werb Z. Extracellular matrix degradation and remodeling in development and disease. Cold Spring Harb Perspect Biol. 2011; https://doi.org/10.1101/cshperspect.a005058.

Murphy MP. How mitochondria produce reactive oxygen species. Biochem J. 2009;417:1–13.

Papageorgiou VP. Wound healing properties of naphthaquinone pigments from Alkanna Tinctoria. Experientia. 1978;34:1499–501.

Polte T, Tyrrell RM. Involvement of lipid peroxidation and organic peroxides in UVA-induced matrix metalloproteinase-1 expression. Free Radic Biol Med. 2004;36:1566–74.

Quan T, He T, Shao Y, Lin L, Kang S, Voorhees JJ, et al. Elevated cysteine-rich 61 mediates aberrant collagen homeostasis in chronologically aged and photoaged human skin. Am J Pathol. 2006;169:482–90.

Rhind JP. Essential oils: a handbook for aromatherapy practice. 2nd ed. London: Singing Dragon; 2012.

Ricard-Blum S. The collagen family. Cold Spring Harb Perspect Biol. 2011; https://doi.org/10.1101/cshperspect.a004978.

Rittié L, Fisher GJ. UV-light-induced signal cascades and skin aging. Ageing Res Rev. 2002;1:705–20.

Saito Y, Tsuruma K, Ichihara K, Shimazawa M, Hara H. Brazilian green propolis water extract up-regulates the early expression level of HO-1 and accelerates Nrf2 after UVA irradiation. BMC Complement Altern Med. 2015;15:421.

Song E, Chung H, Shim E, Jeong JK, Han BK, Choi HJ, et al. Gastrodia elata Blume extract modulates antioxidant activity and ultraviolet A-irradiated skin aging in human dermal fibroblast cells. J Med Food. 2016;19:1057–64.

Sonobe H, Kamps LR, Mazzola EP, Roach JA. Isolation and identification of a new conjugated carbofuran metabolite in carrots: angelic acid ester of 3-hydroxycarbofuran. J Agric Food Chem. 1981;29:1125–9.

Sosath S, Ott HH, Hecker E. Irritant principles of the spurge family (Euphorbiaceae). XIII. Oligocyclic and macrocyclic diterpene esters from latices of some euphorbia species utilized as source plants of honey. J Nat Prod. 1988;51:1062–74.

Tsuji N, Moriwaki S, Suzuki Y, Takema Y, Imokawa G. The role of elastases secreted by fibroblasts in wrinkle formation: implication through selective inhibition of elastase activity. Photochem Photobiol. 2001;74:283–90.

Yang SR, Park JR, Kang KS. Reactive oxygen species in mesenchymal stem cell aging: implication to lung diseases. Oxidative Med Cell Longev. 2015;2015:486263.

Yel M, Güven T, Türker H. Effects of ultraviolet radiation on the stratum corneum of skin in mole rats. J Radiat Res. 2014;7:506–11.

3

Perspectives of aging study on stem cell

Sang-Hun Bae[1†], Chun-Hyung Kim[2†], Pierre Leblanc[3], Jisook Moon[1*] and Kwang-Soo Kim[3*]

Abstract

Aging is the result of a complex polygenetic trait characterized by decreased regeneration capacity and increased vulnerability to external and internal perturbations. Consequently, the inevitable process critically influences longevity, health, and disease susceptibility, ultimately leading to age-related pathologies and death. Gaining insights into inherent properties of aging and identifying definitive biomarkers and/or signatures are prerequisites for a better understanding and for the design of therapeutics for a wide range of age-related diseases that would improve the quality of life of the elderlies. However, a comprehensive understanding of the molecular mechanisms underlying aging has been hampered by its complex nature. Although the process has been subjected to substantial data-driven analyses including genomics, transcriptomics, and proteomics in a systemic manner, aging's complexity hampers proper analysis as well as interpretation of the resulting outputs. Therefore, we review recent consequences focused on stem cell aging and age-related diseases.

Keywords: Aging, Stem cell, OMICS technology, Target therapy

Background

Multicellular organisms experience a gradual loss of repair potential and tissue homeostasis with age, consequently resulting in age-related decline in organ function and intractable age-related diseases. The progressive deterioration in regenerative potential with age is closely linked to a time-dependent decrease in functionality of tissue-specific stem cells including endogenous stem cell exhaustion, aberrant changes in the supporting niches, and functional attrition. Thus, aging can be defined as a process involving the progressive inability of tissue-resident stem cells to replace damaged cells with age, which stresses the need for more complete analyses of stem cell aging in an age-dependent context. The analysis of aged stem cells leverages rapid advancements in the field including the identification of various cell types clearly defined in terms of lineage progression facilitating their characterization in the context of aging. Based on the conceptual framework of stem cell aging, the analysis of aged stem cells has been recently postulated to be one of the more promising approaches to

decipher the fundamental aspects of aging. However, the significant challenge remaining is a better translation of our knowledge of aged stem cells to the general process of aging (Jones and Rando 2011). Here, we discuss recent findings on stem cell aging and ask whether clinical manipulation of stem cells in particular or multiple tissues reverses or counteracts age-related pathological changes. These novel approaches may lead to new biological themes of the stem cell aging, which can be generalized to studies of the general aging process and potential identification of the underlying molecular pathways and therapeutic targets.

Investigation of stem cell aging provides new insights into understanding aging

Complex biological systems are designed to be robust against internal and external challenges to maintain the homeostasis of their functions (Kitano 2004). Aging process seriously compromises this fundamental feature and leaves aged organisms highly susceptible to lesser/minimal changes and damages, as manifested by a reduced capacity of resident stem cells to replenish cells lost to age-related pathological changes (Oh et al. 2014). Stem cell exhaustion with age is consistently observed in diverse tissue-specific stem cells including muscle (Cerletti et al. 2008), hematopoietic (Kollman et al. 2001), and neural stem cells (Enwere et al. 2004), necessitating

* Correspondence: jmoon@cha.ac.kr; kskim@mclean.harvard.edu
[†]Equal contributors
[1]Department of biotechnology, College of Life Science, CHA University, Pangyo-Ro 335, Bundang-gu, Seongnam-si, Seoul, South Korea
[3]Molecular Neurobiology Laboratory, McLean Hospital, Harvard Medical School, 115 Mill St., Belmont, MA 02478, USA
Full list of author information is available at the end of the article

studies for a comprehensive understanding of aged stem cells associated with the progressive regenerative deterioration. A parabiosis study showed that when exposed to the niche of young mice's muscles, aged mice are able to ameliorate the age-related cognitive impairments, suggesting therapeutic potential for enhancing or replacing aged stem cells and significance of stem cell aging study (Villeda et al. 2014). Many molecular processes implicated in stem cell aging are evolutionarily conserved such as the accumulation of damaged macromolecules, DNA damage, reactive oxygen species (ROS) production, TOR, and WNT signaling (Jones and Rando 2011; Oh et al. 2014). To facilitate the clinical translation of knowledge acquired from the study of aged stem cells to the process of aging, an exploration of the overlapping or conserved processes between aging and stem cells would yield interesting leads. Therefore, a comprehensive understanding of the molecular mechanisms regulating stem cell aging and their surrounding niches will provide a valuable clue for developing therapeutic strategies to delay or reverse age-related diseases. Hereafter, we will focus on the important molecular processes regulating stem cell aging before discussing the integration of OMICS technology with stem cell aging research.

Biological process underlying stem cell aging

As organisms age, somatic stem cells progressively lose their competence to deal with a battery of cell-intrinsic and cell-extrinsic challenges, which is mainly attributed to a decline in stem cell functionality. Tissue-resident stem cells frequently encounter accumulated toxic molecules generated by normal metabolism and environmental interventions, but to ensure the maintenance of cellular function, the cells must adopt appropriate strategies to respond to the damage accumulation. Among many risk drivers for the accumulation, ROS have been implicated as disrupting stem cell function and fate decision, implying that redox status in the cells may determine in part their regenerative potential (Pervaiz et al. 2009). In support of this notion, a study on the conditional ablation of Foxo family, playing a crucial role in dealing with oxidative environments, displayed that deregulation of ROS levels in hematopoietic stem cells leads to aberrant proliferation and impaired self-renewal ability (Tothova et al. 2007). Moreover, in antioxidant enzyme deficient mice, hematopoietic systems are particularly vulnerable to oxidative stress (Melov et al. 1999). Several studies suggest that regulation of toxic molecules by antioxidant agents hold great therapeutic promise for age-related pathologies (Drowley et al. 2010; Ito et al. 2006). However, studies of ROS in terms of stem cell aging require cautious interpretation, given that ROS has pleiotropic activity and exhibits the effects in a context-dependent manner (Finkel 2011). For example, an experiment on unexpected roles of ROS using neural stem cells (NSC) suggests that high levels of ROS enhance self-renewal and neurogenesis of neural stem cells in a proliferative state through PI3K pathway signaling (Le Belle et al. 2011). In the case of hematopoietic stem cells, a choice between quiescence and proliferation is likely to be determined by the extent of ROS levels (Owusu-Ansah and Banerjee 2009). With so much conflicting evidence, there is a clear consensus that when reaching a certain threshold, ROS significantly impair cellular architectures enough to induce cellular dysfunction (Hekimi et al. 2011).

The ROS theory can relate mitochondrial dysfunction to stem cell aging, although many other risk factors contribute to the functional decline in the organelle. Respiratory chain system in mitochondria becomes less efficient at generating ATP with age, resulting in elevated levels of ROS which in turn deteriorate mitochondrial genomic integrity in a vicious cycle manner (Harman 1965). Mitochondrial DNA mutations in somatic stem cells lead to impaired neural and hematopoietic progenitor, contributing to progeroid symptoms which can be reversible by altering redox states (Ahlqvist et al. 2012). Taken together, maintaining a balanced regulation of redox state in cellular compartments can have potential therapeutic values for age-induced phenotypes.

Due to a relatively frequent transition from quiescence to proliferation or vice versa, mainly in a quiescent state, tissue-resident stem cells persisting throughout life are continuously exposed to genotoxic challenges, jeopardizing genetic stability (Oh et al. 2014). As a result, it has been suggested that accumulation of genetic damage with age is a principal mechanism underlying aging stem cells by which the aged cells reduce the capacity to maintain homeostasis and fail to return to a more youthful state. Several experimental interventions which disrupt the pathways involved in DNA damage response have suggested that reduced regenerative potential with age is largely attributed to genomic instability induced by accumulation of DNA damage in stem cells (Rübe et al. 2011; Ito et al. 2004; Rossi et al. 2007). Similar to ROS, DNA damage can be transient as part of normal processes (Larsen et al. 2010) and reversed (Beerman et al. 2014) such that context-dependent interpretation must be needed in associating the damage with stem cell aging. During aging, toxic molecules ranging from damaged DNA to metabolites inevitably accumulate in multiple tissues, ultimately leading to death, suggesting that developing ways to minimize or attenuate the unavoidable phenomenon can be an efficient therapeutic avenue for age-related diseases.

Calorie restriction (CR) is considered one of the dietary interventions that can delay or reduce age-dependent pathologies (Mair and Dillin 2008). A mouse model of young vs. aged mice revealed that short-term CR improved functionality of muscle stem cells, through enhanced mitochondrial function and metabolic benefits (Cerletti et al. 2012). In *Drosophila*, CR counteracts an age-dependent decrease in germline stem cells and extends lifespan, implying that dietary intervention can reverse the decline of adult stem cells (Mair et al. 2010). Moreover, CR enhances brain plasticity in adult rats by increasing neurogenesis and influencing production of neurotrophic factors (Lee et al. 2000). These effects have been reported to act through mTOR signaling, a converging pathway sensing and integrating intracellular and extracellular cues, deregulation of which leads to a number of pathological conditions including neurodegenerative disease, cancer, and metabolic disease (Laplante and Sabatini 2012). Accordingly, it is reasonable to propose that reducing activity of mTOR signaling could attenuate as age-dependent decline in stem cell functionality, although little is known about beneficial effects of the intervention on aged stem cells. The hypothesis is supported by the observation that age-related impairments in hematopoietic system are reversed by suppressing mTOR activity with increased life span, implicating manipulation of mTOR signaling as therapeutic potential for disrupted hematopoiesis of the elderly (Chen et al. 2009). Further studies are needed to point toward a direct link between reduced mTOR signaling and aging stem cells rescue.

Tissue homeostasis requires maintenance of a stem cell pool by fine-tuning cellular states balance between self-renewal and differentiation. The fate control rate determines the population size of a stem cell pool. A series of studies have underscored the roles of metabolic pathways in stem cell transition and homeostasis, highlighting the importance of bioenergetics in stem cells biology (Ito et al. 2004; Gan et al. 2010). Stem cells in multiple tissues are mainly in a quiescent state for prolonged periods preferring glycolysis to mitochondrial oxidative phosphorylation to generate ATP (Ito and Suda 2014). An untargeted metabolomics study of human-induced pluripotent stem cells (iPSCs) showed that somatic cells are reprogrammed into iPSCs by a transition toward a glycolytic state (Panopoulos et al. 2012). Interestingly, many metabolic properties of cancer cells are shared with those of stem cells such as TCA cycle and Gln metabolism, suggesting that a fundamental similarity exists even at the metabolic level between the two cell types (Ito and Suda 2014). Recent research into aging has extensively characterized individual variations in human blood metabolites, some of which are clearly relevant to elderly subjects, implying that metabolites can serve as an important source of information with which to explore the aging process (Chaleckis et al. 2016). Even though comprehensive metabolic profiling of stem cell aging is still lacking, rapid advances in metabolomics will provide new mechanical insights into metabolic characteristics in age-related dysfunction in regenerative potential.

OMICS technology and future study of stem cell aging

The process of aging broadly and progressively influences biological components ranging from micromolecules to cellular structures to organ systems. The time-dependent impact and complexity of the process require a novel study approach. Conventional aging research strategies accounting only for a few features of aging have been replaced by OMICS technologies, which are designed to collectively characterize and quantify pools of molecules at different levels including genomics, proteomics, and metabolomics (Sondheimer et al. 2011; Hannum et al. 2013). The massive amount of data-driven analysis could allow for exploration of age-related molecular changes in a multifactorial manner. Increased number of manually curated databases of aging in the public domain may accelerate biological data-centered studies (Craig et al. 2015; Tacutu et al. 2013). However, most OMICS studies have focused on one technology, limiting biological meaningful interpretations of the complex property, although the different OMICS data are strongly inter-correlated (Zierer et al. 2015). Moreover, many aging OMICS studies are restricted to blood analysis due to its easier accessibility, although the aging process exerts its detrimental effects across multiple tissues (Valdes et al. 2013). Despite rapid advances in OMICS technologies, a conspicuous lack of integrative methods for different OMICS data and the complexity of the aging process hinder a more system-level understanding of aging. Nonetheless, systems biology has provided a rich collection of integrative methods to overcome the obstacles, and one of the efficient methods is the integration of OMICS profiling with network approaches where molecular components such as genes or gene products are represented as nodes and mutual dependencies between them as edges (Fig. 1) (Zierer et al. 2015). Research on neurodegenerative diseases successfully adopted the integrative strategy while leveraging the availability of high-throughput neurobiology data to gain a better understanding of the complex nature of these diseases (Parikshak et al. 2015). Intriguingly, a series of studies revealed that a hierarchical structure is embedded in many biological networks including multiple molecular levels, indicating that molecular components of aging also can be modeled as networks to identify main drivers of aging. As discussed above, one of the greatest challenges lies in inferring causal links between aging and dynamic molecular changes mainly due to the inherent nature of the aging process and the lack of current biological knowledge about the progressive decline process. Accordingly, studies on stem cell aging must be carried out with

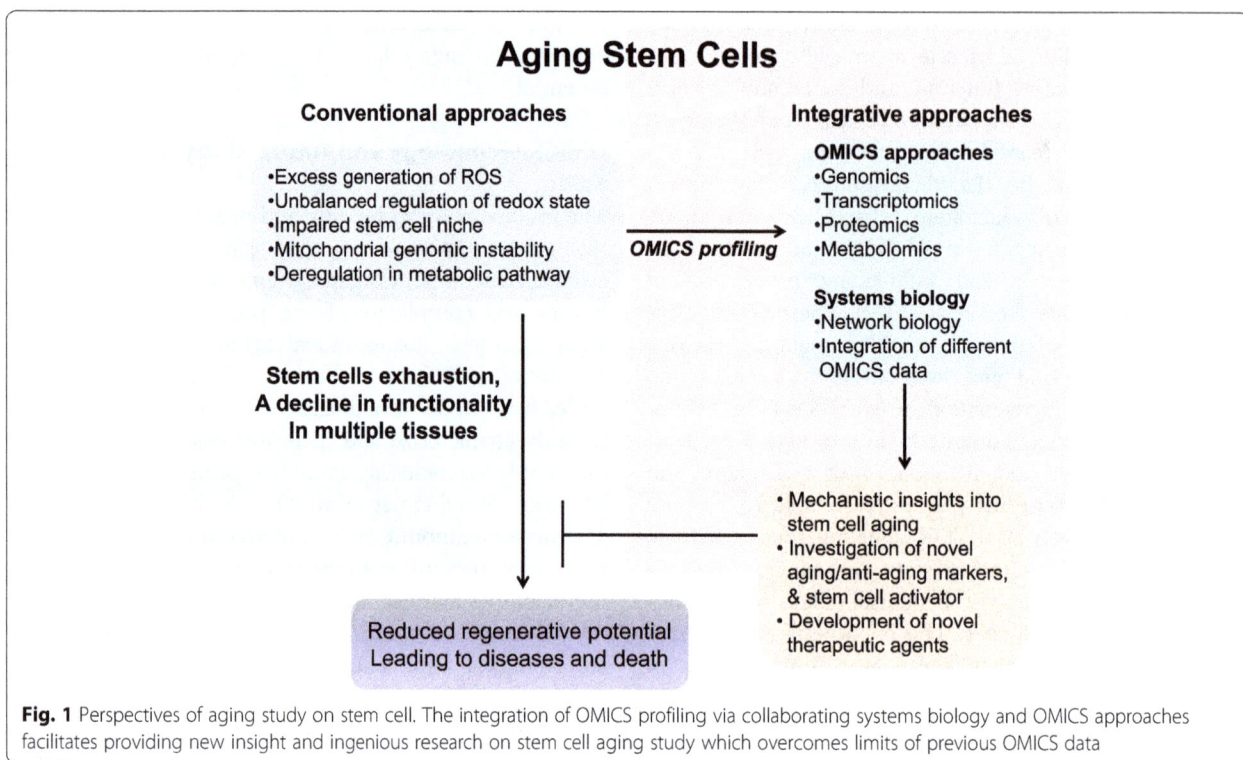

Fig. 1 Perspectives of aging study on stem cell. The integration of OMICS profiling via collaborating systems biology and OMICS approaches facilitates providing new insight and ingenious research on stem cell aging study which overcomes limits of previous OMICS data

rigorous data-driven analysis and integrative approaches to be a step beyond understanding one feature of the process at a time (Moon and Bae 2015). We strongly suggest that clarifying the fundamental aspects of stem cell aging with OMICS technologies and combining them with integrated analyses will deepen our understanding of aging. Elucidating the mechanistic insights will facilitate the development of therapeutic agents that delay or attenuate age-related functional deterioration that occurs in multiple organs including the skin, heart, and brain, improving quality of life in the elderly and lessening the economic burden of age-related diseases.

Conclusions

Many molecular variants with age influence tissue-specific stem cell populations, residing in adult tissues such as the skin, liver, muscle and brain, in a way that leads to a progressive decline in regenerative capacity. Understanding the mechanisms underlying stem cell aging with the integrative approaches will enable us to make significant progress toward providing precision, preventive, and personalized medicine for aging.

Abbreviations
CR: Calorie restriction; Gln: Glutamine; iPSCs: Induced pluripotent stem cells; NSC: Neural stem cells; ROS: Reactive oxygen species; TCA: Tricarboxylic acid cycle; TOR: Target of rapamycin

Acknowledgements
We greatly appreciate the support received through the collaborative work undertaken between CHA University and McLean Hospital.

Funding
This work was supported by the National Research Foundation of Korea (NRF-2016R1A2B4007640) and (NRF-2017M3A9B4025699 and NRF-2017M3A9B4025709).

Authors' contributions
SHB and CHK designed the study and wrote the manuscript. PL revised the article. JM and KSK reviewed the study and edited the manuscript. All authors read and approved the final manuscript.

Competing interests
The authors declare that they have no competing interests.

Author details
[1]Department of biotechnology, College of Life Science, CHA University, Pangyo-Ro 335, Bundang-gu, Seongnam-si, Seoul, South Korea. [2]Paean Biotechnology, Daejeon, South Korea. [3]Molecular Neurobiology Laboratory, McLean Hospital, Harvard Medical School, 115 Mill St., Belmont, MA 02478, USA.

References
Ahlqvist KJ, Hämäläinen RH, Yatsuga S, Uutela M, Terzioglu M, Götz A, Forsström S, Salven P, Angers-Loustau A, Kopra OH, Tyynismaa H, Larsson NG, Wartiovaara K, Prolla T, Trifunovic A, Suomalainen A. Somatic progenitor cell vulnerability to mitochondrial DNA mutagenesis underlies progeroid phenotypes in Polg mutator mice. Cell Metab. 2012;15:100–9.
Beerman I, Seita J, Inlay MA, Weissman IL, Rossi DJ. Quiescent hematopoietic stem cells accumulate DNA damage during aging that is repaired upon entry into cell cycle. Cell Stem Cell. 2014;15:37–50.
Cerletti M, Jang YC, Finley LW, Haigis MC, Wagers AJ. Short-term calorie restriction enhances skeletal muscle stem cell function. Cell Stem Cell. 2012;10:515–9.

Cerletti M, Shadrach JL, Jurga S, Sherwood R, Wagers AJ. Regulation and function of skeletal muscle stem cells. Cold Spring Harb Symp Quant Biol. 2008;73:317–22.

Chaleckis R, Murakami I, Takada J, Kondoh H, Yanagida M. Individual variability in human blood metabolites identifies age-related differences. Proc Natl Acad Sci U S A. 2016;113:4252–9.

Chen C, Liu Y, Zheng P. mTOR regulation and therapeutic rejuvenation of aging hematopoietic stem cells. Sci Signal. 2009;2:ra75.

Craig T, Smelick C, Tacutu R, Wuttke D, Wood SH, Stanley H, Janssens G, Savitskaya E, Moskalev A, Arking R, de Magalhães JP. The Digital Ageing Atlas: integrating the diversity of age-related changes into a unified resource. Nucleic Acids Res. 2015;43:D873–8.

Drowley L, Okada M, Beckman S, Vella J, Keller B, Tobita K, Huard J. Cellular antioxidant levels influence muscle stem cell therapy. Mol Ther. 2010;18:1865–73.

Enwere E, Shingo T, Gregg C, Fujikawa H, Ohta S, Weiss S. Aging results in reduced epidermal growth factor receptor signaling, diminished olfactory neurogenesis, and deficits in fine olfactory discrimination. J Neurosci. 2004;24:8354–65.

Finkel T. Signal transduction by reactive oxygen species. J Cell Biol. 2011;194:7–15.

Gan B, Hu J, Jiang S, Liu Y, Sahin E, Zhuang L, Fletcher-Sananikone E, Colla S, Wang YA, Chin L, Depinho RA. Lkb1 regulates quiescence and metabolic homeostasis of haematopoietic stem cells. Nature. 2010;468:701–4.

Hannum G, Guinney J, Zhao L, Zhang L, Hughes G, Sadda S, Klotzle B, Bibikova M, Fan JB, Gao Y, Deconde R, Chen M, Rajapakse I, Friend S, Ideker T, Zhang K. Genome-wide methylation profiles reveal quantitative views of human aging rates. Mol Cell. 2013;49:359–67.

Harman D. The free radical theory of aging: effect of age on serum copper levels. J Gerontol. 1965;20:151–3.

Hekimi S, Lapointe J, Wen Y. Taking a "good" look at free radicals in the aging process. Trends Cell Biol. 2011;21:569–76.

Ito K, Hirao A, Arai F, Matsuoka S, Takubo K, Hamaguchi I, Nomiyama K, Hosokawa K, Sakurada K, Nakagata N, Ikeda Y, Mak TW, Suda T. Regulation of oxidative stress by ATM is required for self-renewal of haematopoietic stem cells. Nature. 2004;431:997–1002.

Ito K, Hirao A, Arai F, Takubo K, Matsuoka S, Miyamoto K, Ohmura M, Naka K, Hosokawa K, Ikeda Y, Suda T. Reactive oxygen species act through p38 MAPK to limit the lifespan of hematopoietic stem cells. Nat Med. 2006;12:446–51.

Ito K, Suda T. Metabolic requirements for the maintenance of self-renewing stem cells. Nat Rev Mol Cell Biol. 2014;15:243–56.

Jones DL, Rando TA. Emerging models and paradigms for stem cell ageing. Nat Cell Biol. 2011;13:506–12.

Kitano H. Biological robustness. Nat Rev Genet. 2004;5:826–37.

Kollman C, Howe CW, Anasetti C, Antin JH, Davies SM, Filipovich AH, Hegland J, Kamani N, Kernan NA, King R, Ratanatharathorn V, Weisdorf D, Confer DL. Donor characteristics as risk factors in recipients after transplantation of bone marrow from unrelated donors: the effect of donor age. Blood. 2001;98:2043–51.

Laplante M, Sabatini DM. mTOR signaling in growth control and disease. Cell. 2012;149:274–93.

Larsen BD, Rampalli S, Burns LE, Brunette S, Dilworth FJ, Megeney LA. Caspase 3/caspase-activated DNase promote cell differentiation by inducing DNA strand breaks. Proc Natl Acad Sci U S A. 2010;107:4230–5.

Le Belle JE, Orozco NM, Paucar AA, Saxe JP, Mottahedeh J, Pyle AD, Wu H, Kornblum HI. Proliferative neural stem cells have high endogenous ROS levels that regulate self-renewal and neurogenesis in a PI3K/Akt-dependant manner. Cell Stem Cell. 2011;8:59–71.

Lee J, Duan W, Long JM, Ingram DK, Mattson MP. Dietary restriction increases the number of newly generated neural cells, and induces BDNF expression, in the dentate gyrus of rats. J Mol Neurosci. 2000;15:99–108.

Mair W, Dillin A. Aging and survival: the genetics of life span extension by dietary restriction. Annu Rev Biochem. 2008;77:727–54.

Mair W, McLeod CJ, Wang L, Jones DL. Dietary restriction enhances germline stem cell maintenance. Aging Cell. 2010;9:916–8.

Melov S, Coskun P, Patel M, Tuinstra R, Cottrell B, Jun AS, Zastawny TH, Dizdaroglu M, Goodman SI, Huang TT, Miziorko H, Epstein CJ, Wallace DC. Mitochondrial disease in superoxide dismutase 2 mutant mice. Proc Natl Acad Sci U S A. 1999;96:846–51.

Moon J, Bae SH. Antiaging—effect of stem cells on aging and stem cell aging. InTech; 2015. doi:10.5772/60637.

Oh J, Lee YD, Wagers AJ. Stem cell aging: mechanisms, regulators and therapeutic opportunities. Nat Med. 2014;20:870–80.

Owusu-Ansah E, Banerjee U. Reactive oxygen species prime Drosophila haematopoietic progenitors for differentiation. Nature. 2009;461:537–41.

Panopoulos AD, Yanes O, Ruiz S, Kida YS, Diep D, Tautenhahn R, Herrerías A, Batchelder EM, Plongthongkum N, Lutz M, Berggren WT, Zhang K, Evans RM, Siuzdak G, Izpisua Belmonte JC. The metabolome of induced pluripotent stem cells reveals metabolic changes occurring in somatic cell reprogramming. Cell Res. 2012;22:168–77.

Parikshak NN, Gandal MJ, Geschwind DH. Systems biology and gene networks in neurodevelopmental and neurodegenerative disorders. Nat Rev Genet. 2015;16:441–58.

Pervaiz S, Taneja R, Ghaffari S. Oxidative stress regulation of stem and progenitor cells. Antioxid Redox Signal. 2009;11:2777–89.

Rossi DJ, Bryder D, Seita J, Nussenzweig A, Hoeijmakers J, Weissman IL. Deficiencies in DNA damage repair limit the function of haematopoietic stem cells with age. Nature. 2007;447:725–9.

Rübe CE, Fricke A, Widmann TA, Fürst T, Madry H, Pfreundschuh M, Rübe C. Accumulation of DNA damage in hematopoietic stem and progenitor cells during human aging. PLoS One. 2011;6:e17487.

Sondheimer N, Glatz CE, Tirone JE, Deardorff MA, Krieger AM, Hakonarson H. Neutral mitochondrial heteroplasmy and the influence of aging. Hum Mol Genet. 2011;20:1653–9.

Tacutu R, Craig T, Budovsky A, Wuttke D, Lehmann G, Taranukha D, Costa J, Fraifeld VE, de Magalhães JP. Human Ageing Genomic Resources: integrated databases and tools for the biology and genetics of ageing. Nucleic Acids Res. 2013;41:D1027–33.

Tothova Z, Kollipara R, Huntly BJ, Lee BH, Castrillon DH, Cullen DE, McDowell EP, Lazo-Kallanian S, Williams IR, Sears C, Armstrong SA, Passegué E, DePinho RA, Gilliland DG. FoxOs are critical mediators of hematopoietic stem cell resistance to physiologic oxidative stress. Cell. 2007;128:325–39.

Valdes AM, Glass D, Spector TD. OMICS technologies and the study of human ageing. Nat Rev Genet. 2013;14:601–7.

Villeda SA, Plambeck KE, Middeldorp J, Castellano JM, Mosher KI, Luo J, Smith LK, Bieri G, Lin K, Berdnik D, Wabl R, Udeochu J, Wheatley EG, Zou B, Simmons DA, Xie XS, Longo FM, Wyss-Coray T. Young blood reverses age-related impairments in cognitive function and synaptic plasticity in mice. Nat Med. 2014;20:659–63.

Zierer J, Menni C, Kastenmüller G, Spector TD. Integration of 'omics' data in aging research: from biomarkers to systems biology. Aging Cell. 2015;14:933–44.

4

Annona muricata L. extracts decrease melanogenesis in B16F10 mouse melanoma cells

Dahye Joo[1], Seonghee Jeong[1], Hyun Kyung Lee[1], Shang Hun Shin[1], Seong Jin Choi[1], Karam Kim[1], In-Sook An[1], Kyung-Yun Kim[2], Jung-Eun Ku[3], Sun-Hee Jeong[4] and Hwa Jun Cha[5,6]*

Abstract

Background: *Annona muricata* (*A. muricata*) L. (also known as graviola) contains various antioxidants that have beneficial effects on headaches, hypertension, coughs and asthma. *A. muricata* L. also has various other physiological effects, such as antispasmodic effects for the treatment of heart conditions, and sedative and nervine effects. In the present study, the effect of *A. muricata* L. extracts on melanogenesis was investigated and the ensuing inhibitory mechanisms were determined.

Methods: The inhibitory effects of *A. muricata* L. extracts on melanogenesis were initially investigated by measuring melanin contents. Subsequently, the ensuing mechanisms were characterized by determining changes in the activity of tyrosinase, which is the rate-limiting step of melanogenesis. Finally, mRNA and protein expression levels of tyrosinase and the melanogenesis-associated transcription factor (MITF) were determined.

Results: Decreased melanin contents after treatments with *A. muricata* L. extracts suggested skin-whitening effects, and these changes were reflected by decreased tyrosinase activities. In addition, tyrosinase mRNA and protein expression levels were regulated by *A. muricata* L. extracts. MITF is a known key transcription factor of tyrosinase and was transcriptionally regulated by *A. muricata* L. extracts. Specifically, MITF mRNA expression levels were decreased in the presence of *A. muricata* L. extracts. Taken together, the melanogenesis-moderating effects of *A. muricata* L. extracts follow suppression of MITF mRNA expression and subsequent transactivation of tyrosinase.

Conclusions: The results of the present study confirm the skin-whitening effects of *A. muricata* L. and characterize the related molecular mechanisms. These data indicate that *A. muricata* L. has high potential as an ingredient of skin-whitening cosmetics.

Keywords: *Annona muricata*, Melanogenesis, B16F10, MITF, Tyrosinase

Background

Annona muricata (*A. muricata*) L. is an evergreen tree of about 5–6 m in height that is best known as graviola and is prevalent in tropical regions of South America and North America, especially in the Amazon. The sweet oval fruit is prickly and has white flesh inside a dark green or yellow green rind. Bark, leaves, roots and seeds of graviola have been used as traditional medicines, and parts of the plant have differing effects and methods of utilization (Asare et al. 2015). Graviola has excellent antioxidant effects due to the abundance of polyphenols and is effective against headaches, hypertension, coughs and asthma. In recent applications, graviola has been used as an antispasmodic agent for the treatment of heart conditions, as well as a sedative and nervine agent (Lans 2006; Baskar et al. 2007). In addition, active components of the leaves and seeds are known to have cytotoxic effects against cancer cells (Baskar et al. 2007).

Over the past century, environmental pollution from rapid industrialization led to depletion of the ozone layer, and the increased ultraviolet irradiation (Yu et al. 2005)

* Correspondence: hjcha@osan.ac.kr
[5]Department of Skin Care and Beauty, Osan University, Osan-si, Gyeonggi-do 18119, Republic of Korea
[6]Department of Skin Care and Cosmetics, Osan University, 45 Cheonghak-ro, Osan-si, Gyeonggi-do 18119, Republic of Korea
Full list of author information is available at the end of the article

has known effects on the colour of human skin. The natural skin pigment melanin is the fundamental internal factor that determines human skin colour (Jeong et al. 2005). Excessive melanin synthesis due to sun exposure is known to cause melasma, freckles and spots and promotes skin aging and may be involved in dermal carcinogenesis (Chen et al. 1991; Urabe et al. 1994). The rate-limiting step in the biosynthesis of melanin (Hearing and Tsukamoto 1991) involves the initial hydroxylation of tyrosine by tyrosinase, which produces 3,4-dihydroxy-phenylalanine (DOPA) (Jimenez-Cervantes et al. 1994). Recently, studies of melanogenesis have been conducted following inhibition of tyrosinase, microphthalmia-associated transcription factor (MITF) and the tyrosinase-related proteins 1 (TRP-1) and 2 (TRP-2) (Parvez et al. 2006). Melanin synthesis is sensitive to various intracellular signal pathways, including (1) the cyclic adenosine monophosphate/protein kinase A (cAMP/PKA) pathway; (2) the cyclic guanosine monophosphate pathway, which is based on nitric oxide; (3) the protein kinase C pathway; and (4) the p38 MAP kinase pathway. Among these, the cAMP/PKA pathway is central to melanogenesis and follows induction of MITF expression by the cAMP response element binding protein (CREB) after exposure to UV (Busca and Ballotti 2000; Sassone 1998). As a central melanogenesis transcription factor, MITF induces tyrosinase, TRP-1 and TRP-2 transcription (Busca and Ballotti 2000; Saha et al. 2006). Arbutin, which is the most frequently used skin-whitening agent, is an inhibitor that competes with l-tyrosine. Moreover, arbutin and ascorbic acid chelate copper atoms from the active site of tyrosinase and inhibit the conversion of tyrosine to DOPA and DOPA to DOPA quinone (Maeda and Fukuda 1996; Battaini et al. 2000). However, limited quantities of arbutin are currently used in medicines and cosmetics, because of issues involving skin safety and formulation stability (Chun et al. 2002; Curto et al. 1999). Therefore, further studies of natural skin-whitening agents are warranted. Herein, we verified the skin-whitening effects of A. muricata L. and characterized the ensuing intracellular signalling mechanisms.

Methods

Cells and cell culture

B16F10 cells were cultured in Dulbecco's modified Eagle's medium (DMEM; HyClone, USA) containing foetal bovine serum (FBS; HyClone), which was purchased from Gibco (USA), and the antibiotics penicillin and streptomycin, which were purchased from Invitrogen™ (USA). HaCaT cells were cultured at 37 °C in an incubator containing 5% CO_2 at 100% relative humidity.

Preparation of A. muricata L. extracts

Dried A. muricata L. tissues were pulverized and extracted in 10 volumes of 70% ethanol for 1 h in a sonicator. The mixture was then filtered with Whatman No. 2 filter paper, and the resulting filtrate was freeze-dried using a freeze-dryer (PVTFD-10R; IlShinBioBase, Dongducheon, Korea) and was stored at − 20 °C until analysis.

Cytotoxicity assays

Cytotoxic activities of A. muricata L. extracts were determined using 3-[4,5-dimethylthiazol-2-yl]-2,5-diphenyl-tetrazolium bromide (MTT) assays as described previously (Mosmann 1983). Briefly, B16F10 cells were seeded into 96-well plates at 5×10^3 cells/well and then cultured for 24 h. Culture solutions were then replaced with serum-free DMEM, and samples were treated with A. muricata L. extracts at various concentrations for 48 h. The cells were then washed with phosphate-buffered saline (PBS; Thermo Fisher Scientific, USA), and MTT (Sigma-Aldrich, USA) solution was added to each well and incubated for 1–2 h at 37 °C. After removing the MTT solution, 200 μL of DMSO (Sigma-Aldrich, USA) was added to dissolve the formed formazan crystals and absorbance was determined using an ELISA reader at 540 nm.

Measurements of melanin contents

Melanin contents of cells were determined using the method described by Hosoi et al. (1985) with slight modifications. Briefly, cells were washed with PBS three times and then centrifuged to obtain cell pellets. The pellets were then placed in 200-μL aliquots of 1-N NaOH containing 10% DMSO and were incubated at 80 °C for 1 h. Subsequently, absorbance was measured at 405 nm using the ELISA reader, and total melanin contents were expressed as percentages of the control group.

In vitro tyrosinase activity assays

Tyrosinase is the rate-limiting enzyme in melanogenesis and catalyses the oxidation of tyrosine to 3,4-dihydroxyphenylalanine (DOPA) and then to DOPA quinone. In previous studies of skin-whitening activities, melanin absorbance was measured before and after oxidation reactions to investigate the capacity of samples to inhibit tyrosinase activity (Kwon et al. 2014). Herein, 1.7-mM l-tyrosine was completely dissolved in 10-mM sodium phosphate buffer (pH 6.8). Subsequently, 5-μL aliquots of A. muricata L. extracts at various concentrations of up to 0.3 mg/mL were added to 450-μL aliquots of l-tyrosine. Mushroom tyrosinase (250 U/mL; 50 μL) was then added, mixed and incubated at 37 °C for 60 min, and absorbance was measured at 475 nm.

Tyrosinase activity assays

Tyrosinase activities were measured using the methods described by Choi et al. (1998). Briefly, treated cells were lysed in 100-μL aliquots of cell lysis solution and then centrifuged. Subsequently, 50-μL aliquots of the resulting supernatants were added to 450-μL solutions of 1.7-mM

-tyrosine and 0.1-M PBS and incubated at 37 °C for 15 min prior to measurements of absorbance at 490 nm using an ELISA reader. Enzyme activities were expressed as percentages of those in the control group. Tyrosinase inhibitory activities of extracts were expressed as percentage absorbance decreases relative to the untreated control group.

qRT-PCR analysis
B16F10 cells were pretreated with extracts for 3 h and then incubated with 200-nM α-MSH for 48 h. After removing the culture solution, RNA extraction was performed using TRIzol (Invitrogen™, USA). RNA contents were then measured by a NanoDrop spectrophotometer (Thermo Scientific, USA), and equal amounts of RNA were used to synthesize cDNA with PrimeScript Reverse Transcriptase (Takara, Japan). Subsequently, gene expression was determined using qRT-PCR with the HOT FIREPol EvaGreen PCR Mix Plus (Solis BioDyne) and the primers presented in a StepOnePlus Real-Time PCR System (Applied Biosystems, Thermo Fisher Scientific, USA). PCR was performed with denaturation at initial denaturation at 94 °C for 3 min, followed by 40 cycles of denaturation (94 °C, 30 s), annealing (58 °C, 30 s) and polymerization (72 °C, 30 s). Data were analysed using the exclusive software program (ver. 2.0.6) provided by Applied Biosystems (USA).

Promoter activity assays
B16F10 cells were seeded into 60-mm culture dishes and cultured for 24 h and then transfected with a vector for the expression of the pGL-MITF reporter. Transfected

B16F10 cells were then treated with the extracts for 24 h, and luciferase activities were measured according to the protocol provided by the manufacturer of the luciferase assay system. Inhibitory activities were expressed relative to controls that were treated with α-MSH.

Western blotting analysis
After cell treatments, culture media were removed and the cells were washed twice in ice-cold PBS (pH 7.4) and then incubated on ice for 20 min in a radioimmunoprecipitation assay buffer (Sigma-Aldrich, USA) containing protease inhibitors (Roche, Germany). Lysates were then centrifuged at 10,000g for 15 min at 4 °C, and protein concentrations of supernatants were measured using the Bradford method. After adjusting protein concentrations of all samples, equal quantities of protein were mixed with 5× sodium dodecyl sulphate (SDS) sample buffer (Sigma-Aldrich) and boiled at 100 °C for 5 min. SDS–protein samples were then electrophoresed on 8–10% SDS polyacrylamide gels using a Mini-PROTEAN system (Bio-Rad, USA). Protein bands were then transferred to cellulose membranes (GE Healthcare Life Sciences, UK) and blocked in Tris-buffered saline (TBST, pH 8.0) containing 0.1% Tween-20 and 5% skim milk at room temperature for 1 h. Membranes were probed with anti-MMP-1 and anti-type-1 procollagen, anti-MMP-3 (Santa Cruz Biotechnology, USA) or anti-β-actin (Sigma-Aldrich) primary antibodies in blocking solution at 4 °C for 18 h. Membranes were then washed in TBST and exposed to the following secondary antibodies for 2 h at room temperature: Horseradish peroxidase-conjugated anti-rabbit IgG and anti-goat IgG (Santa Cruz Biotechnology), anti-mouse IgG

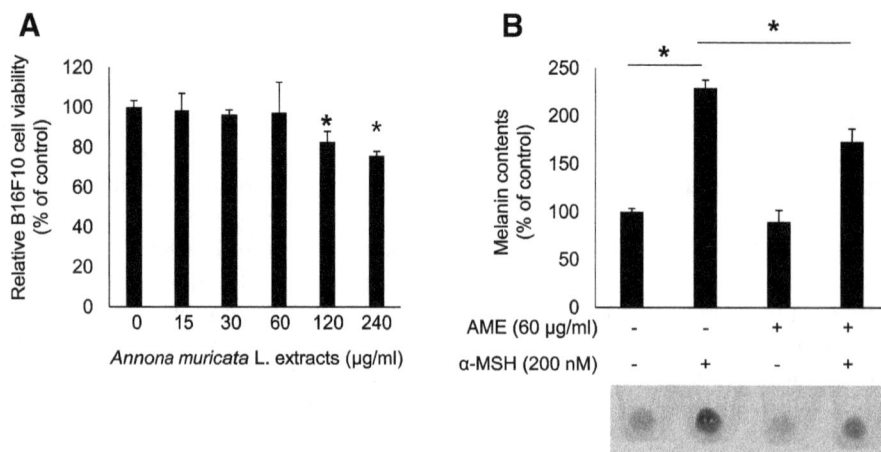

Fig. 1 Effects of *A. muricata* L. extracts on melanin production and cell viability in B16F10 melanoma cells. **a** Effects of *A. muricata* extracts on cytotoxicity in B16F10 melanoma cells. MTT assays were used to determine cytotoxic activities and appropriate concentration ranges in B16F10 cells. In these experiments, survival rates were 90% or higher after treatments with *A. muricata* L. extracts at 60 μg/mL or less. **b** Effects of *A. muricata* extracts on melanin contents in B16F10 melanoma cells; *p < 0.05. Melanin contents of mouse melanoma cells were determined after treatment with *A. muricata* L. extracts at 60 μg/mL. In these experiments, α-MSH-induced melanogenesis was reduced to 24.42% in cells treated with *A. muricata* L. extracts compared to those treated with α-MSH only

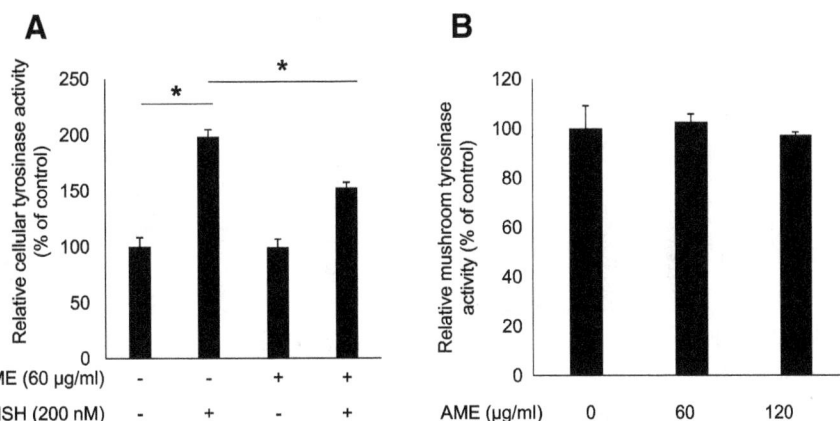

Fig. 2 Effects of *A. muricata* L. extracts on tyrosinase activities. **a** Effects of *A. muricata* L. extracts on cellular tyrosinase activity in B16F10 melanoma cells. *A. muricata* L. extracts decreased tyrosinase activities to 23.24% at 60 μg/mL. **b** Effects of *A. muricata* L. extracts on mushroom tyrosinase activity; *$p < 0.05$

(Sigma-Aldrich) After washing, ECL solution (Pierce, USA) was sprayed onto the membranes, and bands were identified and quantified using an LAS-3000 Luminescent Image Analyser (Fujifilm, Japan).

Statistical analysis

Data are presented as means ± standard deviations, and differences were identified using Student's *t* test. Differences were considered significant when $p < 0.05$.

Results

Cytotoxicity assays of *A. muricata* L. extracts

MTT assays were used to determine cytotoxic activities and appropriate concentration ranges in B16F10 cells. In these experiments, survival rates were 90% or higher after treatments with *A. muricata* L. extracts at 60 μg/mL or less (Fig. 1a). Therefore, subsequent experiments were performed with extracts at ≤ 60 μg/mL.

Measurement of skin-whitening effects of *A. muricata* L. extracts

To assess the skin-whitening effects of *A. muricata* L. extracts, melanin contents of mouse melanoma cells were determined after treatment with *A. muricata* L. extracts at 60 μg/mL. In these experiments, α-MSH-induced melanogenesis was reduced to 24.42% in cells treated with *A. muricata* L. extracts compared to those treated with α-MSH only (Fig. 1b).

Changed tyrosinase activities and expression levels in the presence of *A. muricata* L. extracts

A. muricata L. extracts decreased tyrosinase activities to 23.24% at 60 μg/mL (Fig. 2a). To determine whether *A. muricata* L. extracts inhibit tyrosinase directly (Fig. 2b), we measured changes in the expression of tyrosinase mRNA and protein (Fig. 3) and showed 23.24 and 48.13% decrease, respectively, following treatment with *A. muricata* L. extracts. These data suggest that

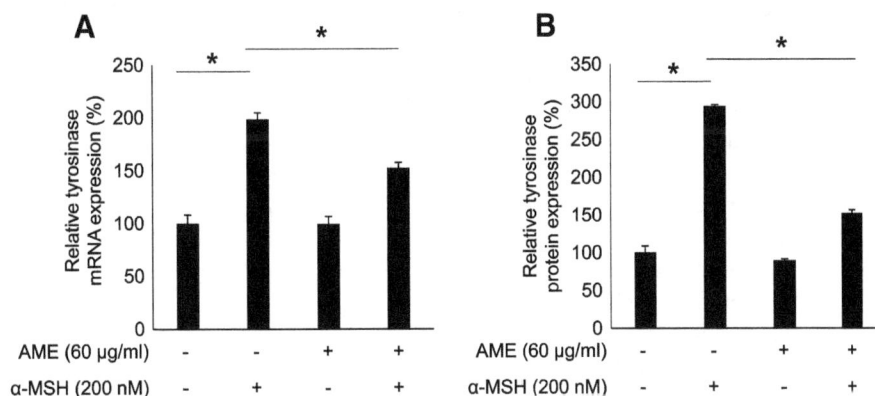

Fig. 3 Effects of *A. muricata* L. extracts on tyrosinase expression levels in B16F10 melanoma cells. **a** Effects of *A. muricata* L. extracts on tyrosinase mRNA and **b** protein expression in B16F10 melanoma cells. *$p < 0.05$. The expression of tyrosinase mRNA and protein were decreased by 23.24 and 48.13%, respectively, following treatment with *A. muricata* L. extracts

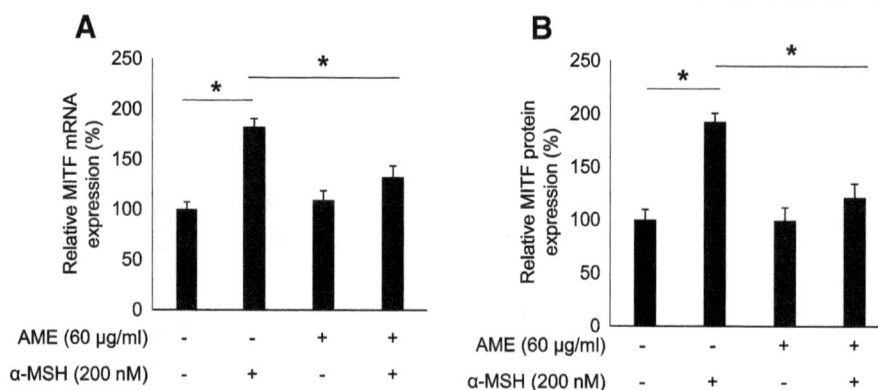

Fig. 4 Effects of *A. muricata* L. extracts on MITF expression in B16F10 melanoma cell. **a** Effects of *A. muricata* L. extracts on MITF mRNA and **b** protein expression in B16F10 melanoma cells. *$p < 0.05$. To confirm the mechanisms by which *A. muricata* L. extracts inhibit melanogenesis, we determined MITF mRNA and protein expression levels using qRT-PCR and Western blotting analyses, respectively. These experiments demonstrated that treatments with *A. muricata* L. lead to decreased expression of MITF

the effects of the present extracts on tyrosinase activities are transcriptional.

Changes in MITF transcription and protein expression in the presence of *A. muricata* L. extracts

To confirm the mechanisms by which *A. muricata* L. extracts inhibit melanogenesis, we determined MITF mRNA and protein expression levels using qRT-PCR and Western blotting analyses, respectively. These experiments demonstrated that treatments with *A. muricata* L. lead to decreased expression of MITF, likely leading to decreased transcriptional activation of tyrosinase (Fig. 4).

Discussion

During in vivo melanogenesis, tyrosinase performs the rate-limiting step in the production of melanin by hydroxylating tyrosine to L-DOPA and then L-DOPA quinone (Saha et al. 2006). Melanin is subsequently synthesized by polymerization of amino acids and proteins (Maeda and Fukuda 1996). In the present MTT assays, *A. muricata* L. extracts had weak cytotoxicity in B16F10 cells when added at 120 μg/mL and no detectable cytotoxicity at 60 μg/mL (Fig. 1a). As shown in Fig. 1b, melanin contents in B16F10 cells were decreased in an extract concentration-dependent manner to 24.46% of that in the α-MSH-treated control group.

In subsequent investigations of the mechanisms behind the effects of *A. muricata* L. extracts on melanogenesis, we showed that decreased tyrosinase activities reflected decreased tyrosinase mRNA and protein expression (Fig. 2), and these effects were concentration dependent. In agreement, we showed that the expression of the major tyrosinase, TRP-1 and TRP-2 transcription factor MITF (Battaini et al. 2000; Chun et al. 2002; Curto et al. 1999), was decreased in the presence of *A. muricata* L. extracts. Collectively, the present data indicate the potential of *A.*

muricata L. extracts as a skin-whitening ingredient for functional cosmetics.

Conclusions

Herein, we investigated the effects of *A. muricata* L. extracts on melanogenesis and elucidated the ensuing mechanisms. Our experiments showed that treatment with *A. muricata* L. extracts decreases melanogenesis in a concentration-dependent manner by inhibiting the expression of intracellular tyrosinase and MITF. In detail, it has been demonstrated that 60 μg/mL of *A. muricata* L. extracts reduced α-MSH-inducing melanin contents, via diminishing mRNA and protein levels of tyrosinase and MITF in B16F10 melanoma cells, in vitro. Additional in vitro and in vivo studies will be necessary to identify the signalling pathways involved in *A. muricata* L. extract-mediated molecular mechanisms, but these preliminary results suggest that *A. muricata* L. extracts regulate MITF expression and can be used as a functional skin-whitening material that inhibits melanogenesis via direct transcriptional effects.

Abbreviations
A. muricata: *Annona muricata*; cAMP: Cyclic adenosine monophosphate; CREB: cAMP response element binding protein; DMEM: Dulbecco's modified Eagle's medium; DOPA: 3,4-dihydroxyphenylalanine; MITF: Microphthalmia-associated transcription factor; MTT: 3-[4,5-dimethylthiazol-2-yl]-2,5-diphenyltetrazolium bromide; PBS: Phosphate-buffered saline; PKA: Protein kinase A; SDS: Sodium dodecyl sulphate; TBST: Tris-buffered saline; TRP-1: Tyrosinase-related protein 1

Funding
This work was supported by a grant from the Ministry of Trade, Industry and Energy (MOTIE), Korea Institute for Advancement of Technology (KIAT) through the Encouragement Program for The Industries of Economic Cooperation Region (Grant R0003962) and a grant from the Marine Biotechnology Program (20150184) funded by the Ministry of Oceans and Fishers, Republic of Korea and a grant from the Korean Health Technology R&D Project (Grant No. HN13C0075), Ministry of Health & Welfare, Republic of Korea.

Authors' contributions

DJ, SJ, HKL, SHS, SJC and KK performed the experiments. KYK, JEK, SHJ and HJC were involved in the experimental design and advising. DJ, ISA and HJC analysed the data and wrote the manuscript. All authors have read and approved the final manuscript.

Competing interests

The authors declare that there are no competing interests.

Author details

[1]Korea Institute of Dermatological Sciences, Cheongju-si, Chungcheongbuk-do 28160, Republic of Korea. [2]URG Inc., URG Building, Seochogu, Seoul 06753, Republic of Korea. [3]Department of Cosmetology, Kyung-In Women's University, Incheon 21014, Republic of Korea. [4]Department of Beauty Art, Faculty of Art, Suwon Women's University, Suwon-si, Gyeonggi-do 16632, Republic of Korea. [5]Department of Skin Care and Beauty, Osan University, Osan-si, Gyeonggi-do 18119, Republic of Korea. [6]Department of Skin Care and Cosmetics, Osan University, 45 Cheonghak-ro, Osan-si, Gyeonggi-do 18119, Republic of Korea.

References

Asare GA, Afriyie D, Ngala RA, Abutiate H, Doku D, Mahmood SA, et al. Antiproliferative activity of aqueous leaf extract of Annona muricata L. on the prostate, BPH-1 cells, and some target genes. Integr Cancer Ther. 2015;14:65–74.

Baskar R, Rajeswari V, Kumar TS. In vitro antioxidant studies in leaves of Annona species. Indian J Exp Biol. 2007;45:480–5.

Battaini GE, Monzani L, Casella L, Santagostini R, Pagliarin R. Inhibition of the catecholase activity of biomimetic dinuclear copper complexes by kojic acid. J Biol Inorg Chem. 2000;5:262–8.

Busca R, Ballotti R. Cyclic AMP a key messenger in the regulation of skin pigmentation. Pigment Cell Res. 2000;13:60–9.

Chen JS, Wei C, Marxhall MR. Inhibition mechanism of koji acid on polyphenol oxidase. J Agr Food Chem. 1991;58:79–110.

Choi BW, Lee BH, Kang KJ, Lee ES, Lee NH. Screening of the tyrosinase inhibitors from marine algae and medicinal plants. Kor J Pharmacogn. 1998;29:237–43.

Chun HJ, Chli WH, Baek SH, Woo WH. Effect of quercetin on melanogenesis in melan-a melanocyte cells. Korean J Pharmacogn. 2002;33:245–51.

Curto EV, Kwong C, Hermersdorfer H, Glatt C, Santis V, Virador VJ, et al. Inhibitions of mammalian melanocytes tyrosinase: in vitro comparisons of alkyl esters of gentiic acid with other putative inhibitors. Biochem Pharmacol. 1999;57:663–72.

Hearing VJ, Tsukamoto K. Enzymatic control of pigmentation in mammals. FASEB J. 1991;5:2902–9.

Hosoi J, Abe T, Suda T, Kuroki T. Regulation of melanin synthesis of B16 mouse melanoma cells by 1 alpha, 25-dihydroxyvitamin D3 and retinoic acid. Cancer Res. 1985;45:1474–8.

Jeong MH, Kim SS, Kim JS, Lee HJ, Chio GP, Lee HY. Skin whitening and skin immune activities of different parts of Acer mono and Acer okamotoanum. Korean For Soc. 2005;99:470478.

Jimenez-Cervantes C, Solano F, Kobayashi T, Urabe K, Hearing VJ, Lezano JA, et al. A new enzymatic function in the melanogenic pathway. J Biol Chem. 1994; 269:17993–8000.

Kwon KJ, Bae S, Kim K, An IS, Ahn KJ, An S, et al. Asiaticoside, a component of Centella asiatica, inhibits melanogenesis in B16F10 mouse melanoma. Mol Med Rep. 2014;10:503–7.

Lans CA. Ethnomedicines used in trinidad and tobago for urinary problems and diabetes mellitus. J Ethnobiol Ethnomedicine. 2006;2:45–55.

Maeda K, Fukuda M. Arbutin: mechanism of its depigmenting action in human melanocyte culture. J Phamacol Exp Ther. 1996;276:765–9.

Mosmann T. Rapid colorimetric assay for cellular growth and survival: application to proliferation and cytotoxicity assays. J Immunol Meth. 1983;65:55–63.

Parvez S, Malik K, Ah KS, Kim HY. Probiotics and their fermented food products are beneficial for health. J Appl Microbiol. 2006;100:1171–85.

Saha B, Singh SK, Sarkar C, Bera R, Ratha J, Tobin DJ, et al. Activation of the Mitf promoter by lipid-stimulated activation of p38-stress signalling to CREB. Pigment Cell Res. 2006;29:595–605.

Sassone CP. Coupling gene expression to cAMP signalling: role of CREB and CREM. Int J Biochem Cell B. 1998;30:27–38.

Urabe K, Aroca P, Tsukamoto K, Mascagna D, Paulumbo A, Prota G, et al. The inherent cytotoxicty of melanin precursors. Biochim Biophys Acta. 1994;1221: 272–8.

Yu YG, Jeong MS, Choe JY, Kim JY. A study on whitening effect of Ephedra sinica extracts. Korean J Design Cult Soc. 2005;31:153–9.

5

Importance of the immune response to *Mycobacterium leprae* in the skin

Song-Hyo Jin[1], Kyu Joong Ahn[2] and Sungkwan An[3*] (iD)

Abstract

The causative agent of leprosy is *Mycobacterium leprae* (*M. leprae*), which establishes infectious lesions in the skin. Leprosy is classified based on the clinical manifestation, the host's immune response and skin symptoms. *M. leprae* is an intracellular pathogen that invades keratinocytes, macrophages, dendritic cells and Schwann cells and replicates within these cells. *M. leprae*-infected keratinocytes secrete various cytokines and chemokines and induce highly effective immune responses. Understanding the mechanisms by which *M. leprae* establishes an infection within the skin and the associated immune response may be of great help in the early detection and treatment of the disease.

Keywords: *Mycobacterium leprae*, Leprosy, Immune response, Keratinocytes

Background

Leprosy is a chronic granulomatous infection caused by an intracellular organism, *Mycobacterium leprae* (*M. leprae*), which primarily affects the skin and peripheral nerves (Walker and Lockwood 2006). *M. leprae* is a unique type of bacteria as it has a long generation time and does not grow on an artificial medium. In addition, *M. leprae* is 0.3–7.0 μm in size and is an exclusively intracellular parasite that grows extremely slowly with a generation time of 12–14 days (Sasaki et al. 2001). The most striking feature of the *M. leprae* genome is the extensive deletion and inactivation of genes, referred to as gene degradation (Cole et al. 2001). These characteristics of the *M. leprae* genome can explain its slow growth and failure to proliferate in synthetic media. The human genomes PARK2 and PACRG are associated with increased susceptibility to leprosy or more severe forms of leprosy.

The host's immune system affects the clinical manifestation of leprosy. Strong cell-mediated immunity and low humoral immunity characterise the response to tuberculoid (TT) leprosy, whereas in lepromatous (LL) leprosy, the opposite is observed. Leprosy can be classified more precisely in an immunological context based on skin findings, motor and sensory changes and biopsy findings as indeterminate (I), TT, borderline tuberculoid (BT), mid-borderline (BB), borderline lepromatous (BL) and LL (Jacobson and Krahenbuhl 1999). In addition, *M. leprae* invades and survives within macrophages, dendritic cells and Schwann cells. Interleukin 2 (IL-2) and interferon gamma (IFN-γ) are markedly dominant in TT lesions, whereas IL-4, IL-5 and IL-10 are characteristic of LL lesions (Salgame et al. 1991; Yamamura et al. 1991).

Leprosy is a disease that manifests as skin lesions, and keratinocytes and the epidermis play an important role in the innate immune response to *M. leprae* (Lyrio et al. 2015). Moreover, while some evidence indicates a role for dendritic cells (DCs) in the immune response to *M. leprae* (Santos et al. 2001), another cell type important for epidermal defence, the keratinocyte, is also a source of cytokines and chemokines, which are critical for recruiting DCs, T cells and neutrophils to the site of infection (Lyrio et al. 2015). In addition, human keratinocytes have been shown to phagocytose *M. leprae* in vitro and subsequently exhibit changes in the expression of surface molecules and cathelicidin as well as secrete tumour necrosis factor (TNF)-α and IL-1β *(Lyrio et al. 2015)*. In addition, the invasion of keratinocytes and the secretion of cytokines and chemokines by immune cells were reported. This suggests that keratinocytes play an important role in the immune response to an infection with *M. leprae*.

* Correspondence: ansungkwan@konkuk.ac.kr
[3]Department of Cosmetics Engineering, Konkuk University, 120 Neungdong-ro, Gwangjin-gu, Seoul 05029, Republic of Korea
Full list of author information is available at the end of the article

Pathophysiology of leprosy

M. leprae is an intracellular parasitic pathogen, and attempts to cultivate in artificial medium have failed since 1874 when it was first identified by Armauer Hansen (Walker and Lockwood 2006). In addition, it multiplies extensively in the footpads of nude mice (Shepard 1960), nine-banded armadillos (Kirchheimer and Storrs 1971) and, to a limited extent, in the footpads of normal mice (Sasaki et al. 2001). *M. leprae* bacilli are 0.3–0.4 × 4.0–7.0 μm in size and multiplies very slowly, with a generation time of 12–14 days. Optimal growth occurs at approximately 30 °C; hence, *M. leprae* prefers the cooler areas of the human body. The cell wall is gram-positive and highly complex and contains proteins, phenolic glycolipids, arabinoglycan, peptidoglycan and mycolic acid (Sasaki et al. 2001).

The host's immune system affects the clinical manifestation of leprosy. Strong cell-mediated immunity and low humoral immunity characterises the response to TT leprosy, whereas the opposite is observed in cases of LL leprosy (Jacobson and Krahenbuhl 1999).

The most striking feature of the *M. leprae* genome is the extensive deletion and inactivation of genes, referred to as gene degradation; only 49.5% of the genome contains protein-coding genes and 27% contains recognisable pseudogenes (inactive reading frames with functional counterparts in the tuberculosis bacillus). Moreover, an analysis of the genomic sequence revealed that the genes encoding various enzymes have been replaced by pseudogenes, which suggests limited metabolic activity of *M. leprae* (Cole et al. 2001). This genomic feature might correspond to its unique bacteriological characteristics, including its exceptionally slow growth rate and failure to multiply in synthetic media (Sasaki et al. 2001).

There are various genes and regions of the human genome that have been associated with susceptibility to leprosy or more severe forms of the disease (Walker and Lockwood 2006). For example, Mira et al. (Mira et al. 2004) identified certain alleles in the PARK2 and PACRG region of chromosome 6 to be associated with susceptibility to leprosy in Vietnamese and Brazilian cohorts. Moreover, PARK2 is expressed by both Schwann cells and macrophages. It is an ubiquitination E3 ligase involved in the delivery of polyubiquitinated proteins to the proteasome complex for protein degradation (Ciechanover 2006). An Indian cohort demonstrated that homozygotes expressing different alleles of the vitamin D receptor (VDR) gene were associated with either TT or LL leprosy (Roy et al. 1999). In addition, the upregulation of the VDR gene on macrophages is associated with enhanced intracellular killing of *M. tuberculosis* (Liu et al. 2006).

Classification of leprosy

Leprosy is classified according to the WHO guidelines (World Health Organization 2012). Patients with only one skin lesion are categorised as a single lesion paucibacillary; however, paucibacillary leprosy is defined as five or fewer skin lesions without bacilli in the skin smears. Multibacillary denotes more than six lesions and may be skin smear positive. TT leprosy is characterised by a minor loss of nerve, the presence of few bacilli and strong cell-mediated immunity (i.e. IFN-γ and IL-2) and weak humoral immunity. In contrast, LL leprosy induces strong bacterial immunity (i.e. IFN-beta, IL-4 and IL-10) and cell-mediated immunity exhibited by a wide range of lesions, multiple bacteria as well as lesions with extensive skin and nerve involvement.

TT

In TT, patients have one or two larger macular hypopigmented or erythematous anaesthetic lesions that have a well-defined and often raised margin or appear as scaly plaques (Jacobson and Krahenbuhl 1999). The first type of lesion is a macule that has erythema or hypochloremesis and has a dry, hairless surface and a well-defined outer edge and sensory damage. Foci of well-developed epithelioid cells, with or without Langhans giant cells, are encompassed by a zone of dense lymphocyte infiltration. The granuloma, which extends up to the epidermis, is without an intervening clear zone (Ridley and Jopling 1966).

BT

In BT, the macules or plaques resemble TT leprosy in appearance and sensory loss but can be differentiated by the fact that they have a smaller average size, are more numerous, the surface is less dry, the outer edges are less defined, hair growth is less affected and nerves are thickened. The cytology and composition of the granuloma are typically indistinguishable from those of TT. The most distinguishing characteristic is the presence of a clear subepidermal zone; however, it is very narrow. Moreover, the granulomas can be distinguished from BB based on epithelial cell focalization near the peripheral lymphocyte region or occasionally by the presence of Langhans giant cells. The nerve bundles within the granuloma are generally grossly swollen and infiltrated, and innervation is greatly diminished (Ridley and Jopling 1966).

BB

In cases of BB, the lesion size and number is between that of TT and LL, moderate anaesthesia and exhibits a typical 'punched-out' or 'hole-in-cheese' appearance. The essential defining characteristic is the presence of epithelial cells diffused throughout the granuloma and not by the lymphocyte zone. The epithelial cells are well-developed but generally not as large as those in TT leprosy. BB lesions contain no Langhans giant cells, and if lymphocytes are present, they are highly diffuse. In addition, the nerve bundles exhibit moderate Schwann cell proliferation but they are usually recognisable without much difficulty (Ridley and Jopling 1966).

BL

BL lesions tend to be numerous and particularly macular and consist of lacerations, papules and nodules. There are two types of BL leprosy: (1) granulomas that consist of histiocytic cells that cannot be classified as epithelial cells but tend to evolve into epithelial cells and (2) the *M. leprae* host cells that consist of histiocytes that tend to exhibit foamy changes; however, they do not produce large globes. The granulomas can be distinguished from LL granulomas by the presence of dense lymphocytic infiltration (Ridley and Jopling 1966).

LL

LL lesions typically consist of erythematous macules, papules and/or nodules, which are widespread and can occasionally become diffuse without defined lesions. In addition, the lesions may appear similar to TT but with more BT and BL characteristics. Sensory and/or motor loss usually occurs in the nerves near TT lesions but may be more prevalent in BL and LL leprosy. In addition, nerve damage is a common form of sensory loss and occurs at the final stages of LL leprosy. The ulnar and median (clawed hands), the common peroneal (foot drop), the posterior tibial (claw toes and plantar insensitivity) and the facial, radial cutaneous and great auricular nerves are involved. Occasionally, progressive multibacillary LL leprosy can result in the loss of the eyebrows and eyelashes, nasal septal perforation with a collapsed nose and hoarseness (Jacobson and Krahenbuhl 1999). Moreover, the granuloma is composed of histiocytes that exhibit a varying degree of fatty changes, characterised by the production of foam cells and globi. Numerous globi or heavy foamy changes are only found in LL leprosy. Lymphocytes are usually deficient and diffuse if they are present. Nerves can show structural damage but do not exhibit cell penetration or cuffing (Ridley and Jopling 1966).

Immunology of leprosy

Leprosy exhibits a wide variety of clinical features that are dependent on the host's immune response and has an apparent polarity in the form of TT and LL leprosy. The major defence against *M. leprae* is achieved by cell-mediated immunity, and the outcome of the infection depends on how the host responds to the infection (Modlin 1994).

M. leprae invades and survives within macrophages, DCs and Schwann cells. Entry into the host cell is the first step in the intracellular lifecycle of *M. leprae*, which

is achieved via several different methods. In particular, the phenolic glycolipid 1 (PGL 1) expressed on the cell wall of *M. leprae* is recognised by complement, and the complement receptor (CR) 1, CR 3 and CR 4 assist in phagocytosis of the bacilli (Schlesinger and Horwitz 1991). Host cells recognise many pathogens through general molecular pattern recognition; however, the complement and toll-like receptors (TLRs) expressed on macrophages and DCs are important for the recognition of microbial, including mycobacterial, pathogens (Nath et al. 2015).

IL-2 and IFN-γ are markedly dominant in TT lesions, whereas IL-4, IL-5 and IL-l0 are characteristic of LL lesions (Salgame et al. 1991; Yamamura et al. 1991). Moreover, the T helper type 1 (Th1) subset, characterised by the predominant secretion of IL-2 and IFN-γ, preferentially elicits cell-mediated immunity, whereas Th2 cells, which produce IL-4, IL-5 and IL-10, augment the humoral immune response. Both the classic reciprocal relationship between antibody production and cell-mediated immunity and the resistance or susceptibility to *M. leprae* can be explained by T cell subsets differing in the pattern of cytokine production (Sasaki et al. 2001). The mechanism of T cell activation in response to mycobacteria is highlighted by the CD1-mediated lipid antigen presentation pathway (Moody et al. 1996) as it represents an aspect of host defence independent of classical peptide antigen presentation via major histocompatibility complex (MHC) molecules (Sasaki et al. 2001).

M. leprae activates TLR2 and TLR1 in Schwann cells, which specifically leads to TT leprosy. Although this cell-mediated immune response is most active in TT leprosy, it can also activate apoptosis genes and consequently cause nerve damage in cases of TT leprosy. In addition, the alpha-2 laminin receptors found in the basal lamina of Schwann cells are also an entry target for *M. leprae* in these cells, while the activation of the ErbB2 receptor tyrosine kinase signalling pathway has been identified as a mediator of demyelination in leprosy (Tapinos et al. 2006). The activation of macrophages and DCs, which are antigen-presenting cells, is associated with the initiation of the host immune response to *M leprae*. Moreover, IL-1β produced by antigen-presenting cells has been shown to impair the maturation and function of DCs (Makino et al. 2006). Another mechanism is the ubiquitin-proteasome pathway, which causes immune cell death and tumour necrosis factor (TNF)-α/IL-10 secretion (Fulco TO et al. 2007). Vitamin D can contribute to the intrinsic response through the production of antimicrobial peptides and is differentially expressed in TT leprosy compared to that in LL leprosy. On the other hand, IL-10 can induce phagocytosis. In addition, it has been shown that IL-15 induced the vitamin D antimicrobial pathway and decreased phagocytosis (Nath et al. 2015). While TT leprosy is the result of a high cell-mediated immunity with a Th1-type immune response, LL leprosy is characterised by a low level of cellular immunity due to an increased humoral Th2 response (Modlin 1994). Because *M. leprae* is present in the skin, nerve tissue and endothelium of the nasal mucosa, it is thought that endothelial cells contribute to the pathogenesis of leprosy.

Keratinocytes and leprosy

Keratinocytes express mannose-binding receptors (KCMR), TLRs and Class II MHC antigens and have also been identified as a source of cytokines, chemokines and antimicrobial peptides. In addition, keratinocytes may play an important role in leprosy by participating in the epidermal immune response to *M. leprae* (Mutis et al. 1993). Thus, this cell type possesses a highly sophisticated innate pattern recognition system in which the simultaneous recognition of a pathogen by different classes of pattern recognition receptors can provide a specific immune response or, in the case of commensals, a lack of a response to microorganisms (Lyrio et al. 2015). Furthermore, keratinocytes can distinguish between pathogenic and commensal microorganisms (Pivarcsi et al. 2005). In skin biopsy sections obtained from an LL leprosy patient, *M. leprae* were found in macrophages as well as in smooth muscle cells and keratinocytes, suggesting that the skin is a potential route of leprosy transmission (Satapathy et al. 2005). Keratinocytes also spontaneously express CD80 (B7–1) on their surface. A reduction of CD80 surface expression also occurs on monocytes after LPS exposure during hypoxia (Lahat et al. 2003). Moreover, Nickoloff et al. reported that keratinocytes can regulate T cells through both cytokine expression and CD80 and CD28 interactions (Nickoloff et al. 1995).

It has been established that epidermal keratinocytes express human beta-defensin (HBD) 2 and that this expression is upregulated by TNF-α stimulation (Yang et al. 1999). TNF-α induces MIP-3α in human keratinocytes and recruits Langerhans cells to the epidermis (Tohyama et al. 2001). Additionally, TNF-α has a synergistic effect on Th1 pattern maintenance as IFN-γ in synergy with TNF-α activates infected macrophages. As a result, it induces a major effect on cell-mediated immunity (Tohyama et al. 2001). Most recently, Cogen et al. have demonstrated that *M. leprae* induced HBD 2 and 3 in keratinocytes but not in macrophages (Cogen et al. 2012).

Okada et al. suggested that *M. leprae* can be phagocytosed by keratinocytes (Okada et al. 1978). Epidermal changes, Ia (HLA-DR) expression on keratinocytes, Langerhans cell (LC) hyperplasia and lymphocyte infiltration were identified in the skin lesions of leprosy patients (Rea et al. 1986). Seo et al. reported that the bacilli are located within typical epidermal cells, which exhibit tonofilaments and melanosomes in their cytoplasm as well as desmosomes at the junction of each of the cells (Seo et al. 1995). Human keratinocytes have been shown to phagocytose *M. leprae* in vitro, which induces changes in the expression of various surface molecules and cathelicidin as well as the secretion of TNF-α and IL-1β by these cells (Lyrio et al. 2015). Cytokines and chemokines derived from keratinocytes are important for the mobilisation of LCs, DCs, T cells and neutrophils to the site of infection, where they can mediate microbial killing and initiate a more efficient immune response against *M. leprae*.

Conclusions

Leprosy exhibits a wide variety of clinical features depending on the host's immune response and has an apparent polarity in the form of TT and LL leprosy. A majority of individuals do not develop leprosy or become infected following regular exposure. Those who have a latent *M. leprae* infection for years may have only single lesions, which is often self-healing. If the lesion does not self-heal and the single lesion is not treated, the disease can progress to the paucibacillary or multibacillary stage (Jacobson and Krahenbuhl 1999).

Research to uncover new targets for the early detection and treatment of an *M. leprae* infection should continue to gain insight into the pathophysiology of leprosy. The most recent studies have included interferon (Teles et al. 2013), vitamin D-dependent antimicrobial pathways (Liu et al. 2012), NOD2-mediated signalling (Netea et al. 2010) and the role of T regulatory cells, Th-17/IL-17a/IL-17F cytokines, CD163 and galectin-3 (Polycarpou et al. 2013). A deeper understanding of the *M. leprae* genome will provide insight into the mechanism by which this organism avoids immune surveillance.

M. leprae invades the skin and peripheral nerves, causing leprosy. Thus, the skin epithelial cells and keratinocytes are important in the innate immune response towards this bacterium. Because keratinocytes express mannose-binding receptors (KCMR), TLRs and Class II MHC antigens as well as produce cytokines, chemokines and antimicrobial peptides, they may play an important role and participate in the epidermal immune response to *M. leprae* (Mutis et al. 1993). It has been demonstrated in vitro that human keratinocytes can phagocytose *M. leprae* and subsequently exhibit the expression of the surface molecules CD80, CD209 and cathelicidin as well as secrete TNF-α and IL-1β (Lyrio et al. 2015). *M. leprae* induces the production of cytokines and chemokines in keratinocytes, which mediates mycobacterial killing and results in a more efficient immune response that is important for the recruitment of LCs, DCs, T cells and neutrophils. Because keratinocytes play an important role in the immune response against mycobacteria, we will present basic data for the early detection and treatment of leprosy by studying the interaction between keratinocytes and *M. leprae*.

Abbreviations

IFN-γ: Interferon gamma; BB: Mid-borderline; BL: Borderline lepromatous; BT: Borderline tuberculoid; CR: Complement receptor; DCs: Dendritic cells; HBD: Human beta-defensin; KCMR: Keratinocytes express mannose-binding receptors; LC: Langerhans cells; LL: Lepromatous; IL-2: Interleukin 2; *M. leprae*: *Mycobacterium leprae*; MHC: Major histocompatibility complex; PGL 1: Phenolic glycolipid 1; Th1: T helper type 1; TLRs: Toll-like receptors; TNF: Tumour necrosis factor; TT: Tuberculoid; VDR: Vitamin D receptor

Acknowledgements

Not applicable.

Funding

Not applicable.

Authors' contributions

SHJ, KJA and SA analysed the data, reviewed the literatures and wrote the manuscript. All authors read and approved the final manuscript.

Competing interests

The authors declare that they have no competing interests.

Author details

[1]Department of Pathology College of Medicine, Institute of Hansen's Disease, The Catholic University of Korea, Seoul 06591, Republic of Korea. [2]Department of Dermatology, Konkuk University School of Medicine, Seoul 05029, Republic of Korea. [3]Department of Cosmetics Engineering, Konkuk University, 120 Neungdong-ro, Gwangjin-gu, Seoul 05029, Republic of Korea.

References

Ciechanover A. The ubiquitin proteolytic system: from a vague idea, through basic mechanisms, and onto human diseases and drug targeting. Neurology. 2006;66(Suppl 1):7–19.

Cogen AL, Walker SL, Roberts CH, Hagge DA, Neupane KD, Khadge S, et al. Human beta-defensin 3 is up-regulated in cutaneous leprosy type 1 reactions. PLoS Negl Trop Dis. 2012;6:e1869.

Cole ST, Eiglmeier K, Parkhill J, James KD, Thomson NR, Wheeler PR, et al. Massive gene decay in the leprosy bacillus. Nature. 2001;409:1007–11.

Fulco TO, Lopes UG, Sarno EN, Sampaio EP, Saliba AM. The proteasome function is required for mycobacterium leprae-induced apoptosis and cytokine secretion. Immunol Lett. 2007;110:82–5.

Jacobson RR, Krahenbuhl JL. Leprosy. Lancet. 1999;353:655–60.

Kirchheimer WF, Storrs EE. Attempts to establish the armadillo (Dasypus novemcinctus Linn.) as a model for the study of leprosy. I. Report of lepromatoid leprosy in an experimentally infected armadillo. Int J Lepr Other Mycobact Dis. 1971;39:693–702.

Lahat N, Rahat MA, Ballan M, Weiss-Cerem L, Engelmayer M, Bitterman H. Hypoxia reduces CD80 expression on monocytes but enhances their LPS-stimulated TNF-alpha secretion. J Leukoc Biol. 2003;74:197–205.

Liu PT, Stenger S, Li H, Wenzel L, Tan BH, Krutzik SR, et al. Toll-like receptor triggering of a vitamin D-mediated human antimicrobial response. Science. 2006;311:1770–3.

Liu PT, Wheelwright M, Teles R, Komisopoulou E, Edfeldt K, Ferguson B, et al. MicroRNA-21 targets the vitamin D-dependent antimicrobial pathway in leprosy. Nat Med. 2012;18:267–73.

Lyrio EC, Campos-Souza IC, Corrêa LC, Lechuga GC, Verícimo M, Castro HC, et al. Interaction of Mycobacterium leprae with the HaCaT human keratinocyte cell line: new frontiers in the cellular immunology of leprosy. Exp Dermatol. 2015; 24:536–42.

Makino M, Maeda Y, Mukai T, Kaufmann SH. Impaired maturation and function of dendritic cells by mycobacteria through IL-1beta. Eur J Immunol. 2006;36:1443–52.

Mira MT, Alcaïs A, Nguyen VT, Moraes MO, Di Flumeri C, HT V, et al. Susceptibility to leprosy is associated with PARK2 and PACRG. Nature. 2004;427:636–40.

Modlin RL. Th1-Th2 paradigm: insights from leprosy. J Invest Dermatol. 1994;102: 828–32.

Moody DB, Sugita M, Peters PJ, Brenner MB, Porcelli SA. The CD1-restricted T-cell response to mycobacteria. Res Immunol. 1996;147:550–9.

Mutis T, De Bueger M, Bakker A, Ottenhoff THHLA. Class II+ human keratinocytes present Mycobacterium leprae antigens to CD4+ Th1-like cells. Scand J Immunol. 1993;37:43–51.

Nath I, Saini C, Valluri VL. Immunology of leprosy and diagnostic challenges. Clin Dermatol. 2015;33:90–8.

Netea MG, Kullberg BJ, van der Meer JW. Genomewide association study of leprosy. N Engl J Med. 2010;362:1447–8.

Nickoloff BJ, Turka LA, Mitra RS, Nestle FO. Direct and indirect control of T-cell activation by keratinocytes. J Invest Dermatol. 1995;105(Suppl1):25–9.

Okada S, Komura J, Nishiura M. Mycobacterium leprae found in epidermal cells by electron microscopy. Int J Lepr Other Mycobact Dis. 1978;46:30–4.

Pivarcsi A, Nagy I, Kemeny L. Innate immunity in the skin: how keratinocytes fight against pathogens. Curr Immunol Rev. 2005;1:29–42.

Polycarpou A, Walker SL, Lockwood DN. New findings in the pathogenesis of leprosy and implications for the management of leprosy. Curr Opin Infect Dis. 2013;26:413–9.

Rea TH, Shen JY, Modlin RL. Epidermal keratinocyte Ia expression, Langerhans cell hyperplasia and lymphocytic infiltration in skin lesions of leprosy. Clin Exp Immunol. 1986;65:253–9.

Ridley DS, Jopling WH. Classification of leprosy according to immunity. A five-group system. Int J Lepr Other Mycobact Dis. 1966;34:255–73.

Roy S, Frodsham A, Saha B, Hazra SK, Mascie-Taylor CG, Hill AV. Association of vitamin D receptor genotype with leprosy type. J Infect Dis. 1999;179:187–91.

Salgame P, Abrams JS, Clayberger C, Goldstein H, Convit J, Modlin RL, et al. Differing lymphokine profiles of functional subsets of human CD4 and CD8 T cell clones. Science. 1991;254:279–82.

Santos DO, Santos SL, Esquenazi D, Nery JA, Defruyt M, Lorré K, et al. Evaluation of B7-1 (CD80) and B7-2 (CD86) costimulatory molecules and dendritic cells on the immune response in leprosy. Nihon Hansenbyo Gakkai Zasshi. 2001;70:15–24.

Sasaki S, Takeshita F, Okuda K, Ishii N. Mycobacterium leprae and leprosy: a compendium. Microbiol Immunol. 2001;45:729–36.

Satapathy J, Kar BR, Job CK. Presence of mycobacterium leprae in epidermal cells of lepromatous skin and its significance. Indian J Dermatol Venereol Leprol. 2005;71:267–9.

Schlesinger LS, Horwitz MA. Phenolic glycolipid-1 of Mycobacterium leprae binds complement component C3 in serum and mediates phagocytosis by human monocytes. J Exp Med. 1991;174:1031–8.

Seo VH, Cho W, Choi HY, Hah YM, Cho SN. Mycobacterium leprae in the epidermis: ultrastructural study I. Int J Lepr Other Mycobact Dis. 1995;63:101–4.

Shepard CC. The experimental disease that follows the injection of human leprosy bacilli into foot-pads of mice. J Exp Med. 1960;112:445–54.

Tapinos N, Ohnishi M, Rambukkana A. ErbB2 receptor tyrosine kinase signaling mediates early demyelination induced by leprosy bacilli. Nat Med. 2006;12:961–6.

Teles RM, Graeber TG, Krutzik SR, Montoya D, Schenk M, Lee DJ, et al. Type I interferon suppresses type II interferon-triggered human anti-mycobacterial responses. Science. 2013;339:1448–53.

Tohyama M, Shirakara Y, Yamasaki K, Sayama K, Hashimoto K. Differentiated keratinocytes are responsible for TNF-alpha regulated production of macrophage inflammatory protein 3alpha/CCL20, a potent chemokine for Langerhans cells. J Dermatol Sci. 2001;27:130–9.

Walker SL, Lockwood DN. The clinical and immunological features of leprosy. Br Med Bull. 2006;77–78:103–21.

World Health Organization. WHO expert committee on leprosy. World Health Organ Tech Rep Ser. 2012;968:1–61.

Yamamura M, Uyemura K, Deans RJ, Weinberg K, Rea TH, Bloom BR, et al. Defining protective responses to pathogens: cytokine profiles in leprosy lesions. Science. 1991;254:277–9.

Yang D, Chertov O, Bykovskaia SN, Chen Q, Buffo MJ, Shogan J, et al. Beta-defensins: linking innate and adaptive immunity through dendritic and T cell CCR6. Science. 1999;286:525–8.

6

Direct conversion from skin fibroblasts to functional dopaminergic neurons for biomedical application

Yongwoo Jang and Jin Hyuk Jung[*]

Abstract

Recent progress in tissue engineering research led to the generation of different types of cells from a handful of skin tissue. Lineage reprogramming is a nascent field, which holds great potential to expand its use in regenerative medicine and disease modeling. The concept of somatic cell epigenetic stability has been fundamentally reshaped through the report of direct conversion of somatic identity to another lineage by introducing transcription factors. Here, we review recent advances in lineage reprogramming research, especially direct conversion into dopamine neurons from fibroblasts.

Keywords: Direct conversion, Dopamine neurons, Fibroblasts and iPSC

Background

Parkinson's disease (PD) is a movement disorder that is caused by chronic and progressive degeneration of midbrain dopamine (mDA) neurons in substantia nigra of brain (de Lau and Breteler 2006; Betarbet et al. 2000). Because there is no cure for PD patients, researchers have developed alternative ways to cure PD using cell-based transplantation therapy (Barker et al. 2015; Olanow et al. 1996). Fetal cell transplantation demonstrated that cell-based transplantation therapy is a viable therapeutic approach, showing improvement of PD-related symptoms in some patients (Mendez et al. 2005; Li et al. 2008; Kordower et al. 1996; Kordower et al. 1998; Kordower et al. 2008; Hagell et al. 1999). However, there are significant shortcomings including ethical, technical, and practical issues, as well as variable ranges in effectiveness (Olanow et al. 2003; Freed et al. 2001). After introduction of induced pluripotent stem cell (iPSC) technology by Shinya Yamanaka and his colleagues a decade ago, patient-derived iPSCs have been extensively investigated to generate functional autologous mDA neurons for clinical and research use (Takahashi and Yamanaka 2006; Tapia and Scholer 2016; Takahashi and Yamanaka 2016; Li and Izpisua Belmonte 2016; Karagiannis and Eto

2016; Mertens et al. 2016; Hotta and Yamanaka 2015). Consequently, concept of iPSC generation that somatic tissues can be reprogrammed to early embryonic-like cells by transcription factors raised the question of whether transcription factors could reprogram somatic cell differentiation. This concept was originally demonstrated by the conversion of fibroblasts into myoblasts by introducing expressing plasmid containing *MyoD* (Davis et al. 1987). Subsequently, introduction of transcription factors induces direct conversion of different cell types: (1) glial cells into neuronal cells, (2) liver into pancreas, and (3) B cells into macrophages (Heins et al. 2002; Kulessa et al. 1995; Shen et al. 2000; Xie et al. 2004). Moreover, induction of neuronal cells from fibroblasts using defined transcription factors showed that the direct conversion could be manipulated across different germ layers (Vierbuchen et al. 2010). Transcription factors known to serve crucial roles in dopamine neuron specification and maturation are required for direct conversion of dopamine neurons from fibroblasts (Caiazzo et al. 2011; Pfisterer et al. 2011; Kim et al. 2014; Kim et al. 2011). Subsequently, combination of microRNA (miRNA) and small molecules are being investigated along with the key transcription factors to generate efficient and non-viral integrating neurons (Yoo et al. 2011; Jiang et al. 2015; Lau et al. 2014) (Fig. 1). In this review, we discuss the recent research progress of the direct conversion from fibroblasts to mDA neurons.

* Correspondence: jjung@mclean.harvard.edu
Molecular Neurobiology Laboratory, McLean Hospital and Program in Neuroscience, Harvard Medical School, 115 Mill St. Mail stop 149, Belmont, MA 02478-1064, USA

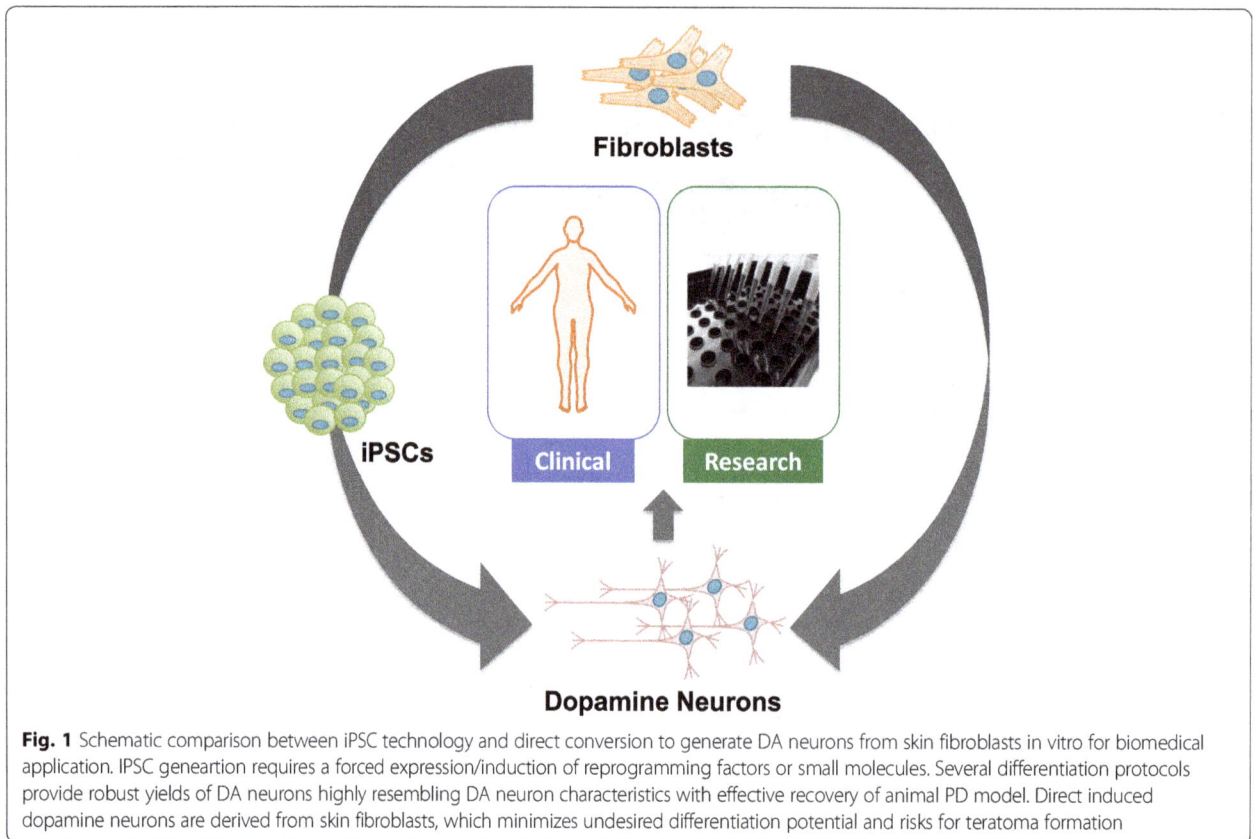

Fig. 1 Schematic comparison between iPSC technology and direct conversion to generate DA neurons from skin fibroblasts in vitro for biomedical application. IPSC geneartion requires a forced expression/induction of reprogramming factors or small molecules. Several differentiation protocols provide robust yields of DA neurons highly resembling DA neuron characteristics with effective recovery of animal PD model. Direct induced dopamine neurons are derived from skin fibroblasts, which minimizes undesired differentiation potential and risks for teratoma formation

Key transcription factors during dopamine neuron development

Mash1 (also known as achaete-scute homolog 1, Ascl1)

Mash1 (mammalian achaete scute homolog-1) is a pro-neural transcription factor, which serves multiple roles in neuronal commitment. In brain development, neurogenesis is an essential process that drives neural progenitors into functional differentiated neurons. This neurogenesis is coordinated by pro-neural transcription factors including Mash1, Ngn1, and Ngn2. Especially, Mash1 is responsible for the neuronal cell specification, by binding with other neural pro-neural genes such as Ngn1 and Ngn2 (Parras et al. 2002; Cau et al. 2002). In sympathetic ganglia, Mash1 facilitates noradrenergic neuron differentiation by inducing expression of the homeobox gene Phox2a and the noradrenaline-synthesizing enzyme dopamine β-hydroxylase 1 (DBH1) (Lo et al. 1998; Hirsch et al. 1998). In the neuroepithelium of the hindbrain, Mash1 is indispensible for the differentiation of central serotonergic neurons (Pattyn et al. 2004). Genome-wide analysis of Mash1-mediated target genes in neural tube during murine embryogenesis revealed that Mash1 directly regulates numerous genes involved in proliferation, differentiation, and maturation of neurons by binding to the specific sequence, E-Box motif (CAGCTG) (Borromeo et al. 2014). Indeed, Mash1-deficient mice exhibit a severe loss of

neural progenitors in the subventricular zone and abnormal ventral forebrain differentiation (Casarosa et al. 1999; Horton et al. 1999). Therefore, Mash1 is an important transcription factor, which promotes the neural lineage differentiation and context-dependent proliferation (Vasconcelos and Castro 2014).

Lmx1a and Foxa2

During early brain development, mDA neurons are derived from the ventral midline of the mesencephalon by the combined action of morphogen molecules and transcriptional factors. The initial event of mDA neuron development is regulated by sonic hedgehog (SHH) and wingless-related MMTV integration site 1 (Wnt1) (Arenas et al. 2015). The morphogen, SHH, directly induces the expression of *Foxa2* in the ventral mesencephalon (VM) at embryonic day 8 (E8). Foxa2 regulates the extent of neurogenesis of mDA progenitors by inducing *Ngn2* (Neurog 2) and sequentially differentiates immature mDA neurons by inducing *Nurr1* (Sasaki et al. 1997; Ferri et al. 2007) (Fig. 2). Meanwhile, the glycoprotein Wnt1 secreted from midbrain-hindbrain border (MHB) directly induces the expression *Lmx1* through the β-catenin complex. Lmx1 sequentially induces the expression of *Nurr1* and *Pitx3* for mDA neurons differentiation (Chung et al. 2009; Wurst and Prakash 2014) (Fig. 2). Therefore, transcriptional activity of Lmx1 and

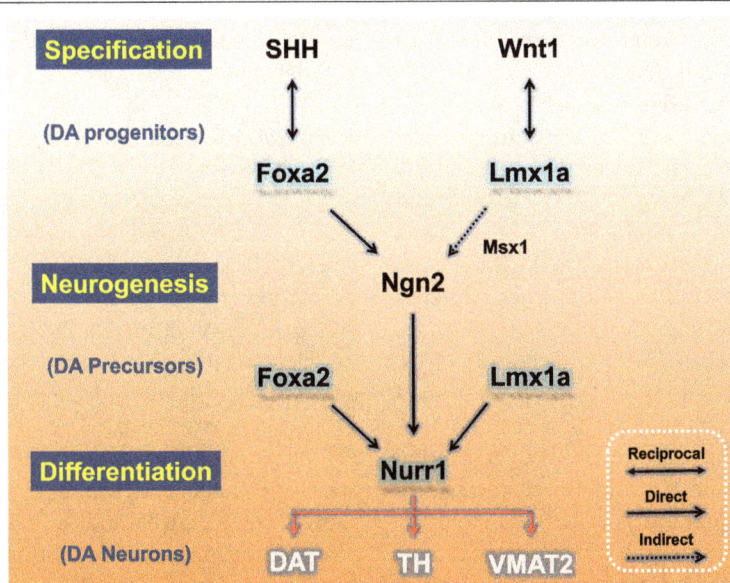

Fig. 2 Schematic interactions between transcription factors and morphogen molecules in the process of the specification, neurogenesis, and differentiation of mDA neurons. Two secreted morphogen molecules (SHH, Wnt1) control the patterning of dopaminergic progenitors through a reciprocal induction of Foxa2 and Lmx1a transcription factors. Subsequently, essential proneural gene, Ngn2, is induced by directly Foxa2 and indirectly Lmx1a (through Msx1) to promote the neurogenesis of dopaminergic precursor cells. Meanwhile, the sustained expression of Foxa2 and Lmx1a begins to induce the dopaminergic differentiation by increasing Nurr1 transcription. The evoked Nurr1 directly leads to the expression of various essential enzymes and transporters in dopaminergic differentiation. The abbreviated designations are the following: sonic hedgehog (SHH), wingless-related MMTV integration site 1 (Wnt1), Msh homeobox homolog (Msx1), neurogenin 2 (Ngn2), nuclear receptor-related factor 1 (Nurr1), dopamine transporter (DAT), tyrosine hydrolase (TH), and vesicular monoamine transporter 2 (VMAT2)

Foxa2 is required in floor-plate formation as well as mDA progenitor induction. Lmx1a is a protein that is involved in the proliferation, specification, and early differentiation of the mesodiencephalic DA progenitors into mDA neurons. In the murine brain development, *Lmx1a* is expressed by E.8.5 in the dorsal midline (roof plate) of the neural tube and in the optic vesicles (Failli et al. 2002). Thereafter, *Lmx1a* is highly expressed in the DA progenitors arising from the VM floor plate. During early neurogenesis of DA progenitors, Lmx1a induces *Msx1* (Msh homeobox homolog 1) expression, which drives the expression of *neurogenin 2* (Ngn2), a key transcription factor involved in neurogenesis and neural specification (Parras et al. 2002; Andersson et al. 2006; Roybon et al. 2008) (Fig. 2). Indeed, a severe reduction in the midbrain is observed in Lmx1a-deficient mice and dreher mutant mice, which are Lmx1a functional mutants (Mishima et al. 2009; Millonig et al. 2000). Therefore, Lmx1a is necessary for mDA neuron characterization. Foxa2 is a transcriptional factor that serves crucial role in mDA neuron specification during E7.5–E9.5. During mDA neuronal development, Foxa1 and Foxa2 are key regulatory factors, which regulate neurogenesis in the mDA progenitors by inducing the expression of *Lmx1a* and *Ngn2* (Ferri et al. 2007; Lin et al. 2009). Lmx1a and Ngn2 cooperatively facilitate mDA neuronal differentiation. Moreover, Foxa1 and Foxa2-induced *Nurr1* and engrailed 1 (*en-1*) increase the expression of aromatic l-amino acid decarboxylase

(*AADC*) and tyrosine hydrolase (*TH*) in immature dopaminergic neurons (Ferri et al. 2007). The genetic ablation of Foxa1 and Foxa2 causes a severe loss of TH-positive mDA neurons (Stott et al. 2013). Moreover, a conditional deletion of Foxa1 and Foxa2 in adulthood also leads to the reduction of TH-positive adult dopaminergic neurons in ventral midbrain (Domanskyi et al. 2014). Therefore, the transcriptional activity of Foxa1 and Foxa2 is required in the mDA neuronal development.

Nurr1 (also known as NR4A2)

Nurr1 is an orphan nuclear receptor that serves essential roles for the differentiation, maturation, and maintenance of mDA neurons. In the murine brain development, *Nurr1* is expressed around E10.5 in the ventral midbrain prior to expression of *TH*, which is a key enzyme to generate dopamine at E11.5. Nurr1 expression is retained in DA neurons of the substantia nigra and ventral tegmental area (SN-VTA) throughout adulthood. Therefore, Nurr1 may be involved in the early stage of mDA neuronal differentiation as well as in the postnatal stage of mDA neuron maintenance. Moreover, SHH-Foxa2 and Wnt1-Lmx1 axis orchestrate the expression of *Nurr1*, suggesting that *Nurr1* expression is a molecular cue for the development of mDA neurons.

Three conserved DNA-binding domains of Nurr1 are important for its transcriptional activity. NGFI-B response element (NBRE, AAAGGTCA) is crucial for Nurr1 function as a monomer, Nurr response element (NurRE, AAAT(G/A)(C/T)CA) is important for homodimers or heterodimers with NR4A family (Nur77 or Nor1), and direct repeat of AGGTCA with a five-base-pair spacer (DR5) is required for heterodimer with RXR (Campos-Melo et al. 2013). Importantly, Nurr1 induces the expression of *TH* as well as dopamine transporter (*DAT*) to maintain dopamine levels in synaptic cleft (Sakurada et al. 1999; Schimmel et al. 1999; Sacchetti et al. 2001). Subsequent studies have revealed that Nurr1 induces essential genes for the mDA neuronal function such as vesicular monoamine transporter 2 (*VMAT2*), aromatic amino acid carboxylase (*AADC*), and Ret (*GDNF* receptor) (Hermanson et al. 2003; Smits et al. 2003; Li et al. 2009).

Indeed, Nurr1-deficient mice are incapable of generating mDA neurons in the SN and VTA. However, these mice eventually died within the first 2 days of birth due to milk-suckling difficulty (Zetterstrom et al. 1997). A study using conditional *Nurr1*-gene targeted mice, in which *Nurr1* is selectively ablated in mature DA neurons, showed progressive reduction in both developing and adult striatal DA neurons (Kadkhodaei et al. 2013). Moreover, selective *Nurr1* deletion in mature DA neurons at adulthood (~ 5 weeks) results in typical pathological phenotypes seen in PD patients: (1) degeneration of DA neurons, (2) reduced dopamine and dopamine-related metabolites, and (3) impaired motor behaviors. Collectively, Nurr1 plays an indispensable role for generating and maintaining DA neurons by regulating numerous genes including dopamine-related enzymes, transporters, and transcription factors.

Generation of DA neurons from fibroblasts

Research on the generation of DA neurons from fibroblasts was inspired from the finding of direct conversion that generation of neurons using three transcription factors Ascl1, Brn2 and Myt1l (Vierbuchen et al. 2010). To determine which transcription factor is required for induced mDA neuron generation, Pfisterer and colleagues examined 10 genes involved in patterning and specification of DA neurons (*En1, Foxa2, Gli1, Lmx1a, Lmx1b, Msx1, Nurr1, Otx1, Pax2*, and *Pax5*). They found that Foxa2 and Lmx1a in combination with the three known genes (*Ascl1, Brn2,* and *Myt1l*) are required for induced DA neuron generation (Pfisterer et al. 2011). Consequently, Caiazzo and colleagues reported the minimal transcription factor combination (*Ascl1, Nurr1,* and *Lmx1a*) for generating induced DA neurons from mouse and human fibroblasts (Caiazzo et al. 2011). Induced DA neurons from murine fibroblasts alleviate symptoms in a mouse model of PD (Kim et al. 2011). Transcription factors including Axcl1, Nurr1, and Lmx1b induce direct conversion into DA neurons from astrocytes (Addis et al. 2011). Collectively, the ectopic expression of genes that are known to serve crucial function in the DA neuron specification and development is required for the generation of induced DA neurons.

MicroRNA-mediated conversion into dopamine neurons from fibroblasts

miRNA is an endogenous small non-coding molecule found in many organisms including plants, animals, and viruses (Dethoff et al. 2012). miRNA regulates gene expression by binding to complementary sequences (Vidigal and Ventura 2015). Numerous studies showed the close relationship between microRNA and neuronal development (Behm and Ohman 2016). Especially, miR-133b is expressed in the DA neurons and is deficient in PD patients. MiR-133b regulates function and maturation of DA neurons (Kim et al. 2007). Subsequent study showed that miR-9 and miR-124 repress BAF53a in post-mitotic neurons, regulating essential transition of neurogenesis (Yoo et al. 2011; Yoo et al. 2009). Interestingly, ectopic expression of miR-9 and miR-124 induces neuron-like morphological change in fibroblasts (Yoo et al. 2009). Combination of miR-124 and two transcriptional factors, Ascl1 and Myt1l, promote into human-induced neuron (ihN) generation from human primary dermal fibroblasts (Yoo et al. 2011). Collectively, these studies suggest that miRNAs involved in neuronal development could play an important role for generating neurons directly from fibroblasts. A more rigorous approach will be required to elucidate molecular mechanism of miRNA-mediated neuronal differentiation, specifically DA neuron differentiation.

Recent studies of induced DA neurons

The lentiviral vector system has been widely used to generate induced neurons from fibroblasts (Caiazzo et al. 2011; Pfisterer et al. 2011; Kim et al. 2014; Kim et al. 2011). Although this system is efficient to generate induced neurons, it is not safe for clinical use due to the possibility of transformation by lentiviral elements. Thus, alternative methods including non-integrating vector and chemical (small molecules) combinations have been investigated (Yoo et al. 2011; Jiang et al. 2015; Lau et al. 2014). The advantage of small molecules is the rapid, reversible, and dose-dependent effect, which allows control of the outcome by applying different concentration and combinations. Small molecules target key factors including transcription factors that regulate cell differentiation and reprogramming. Thus, small molecules have been widely used for generating iPSC and iPSC-derived DA neurons (Hou et al. 2013; Zhu et al. 2010; Li et al. 2011; Chen et al. 2011; Huangfu et al. 2008; Mali et al. 2010; Kriks et al. 2011; Studer 2012; Sundberg et al. 2013; Doi et al. 2014; Kirkeby et al. 2012; Ma et al. 2011). For example, epigenetic-related small molecules including

HDAC inhibitors promote mouse embryonic fibroblasts reprogramming into iPSC (Huangfu et al. 2008; Mali et al. 2010). GSK3 inhibitors support embryonic stem cell (ESC) self-renewal and also facilitate rapid and efficient generation of iPSC (Li et al. 2009). Furthermore, there are small molecules that induce neural differentiation. SMAD inhibitors efficiently drive hESC to neural precursors through floor plate. SHH and FGF8 accelerates efficient generation of DA neuron precursors (Chambers et al. 2009). For ALK2, 3 and 6 inhibitors, LDN193189 facilitates neural conversion of human fibroblasts (Dai et al. 2015). Multiple studies have demonstrated direct conversion of DA neurons from fibroblasts using combination of small molecules and known transcription factors (summarized in Table 1).

iPSC-derived DA neuron vs. induced DA neuron

James Thompson and his colleagues established human embryonic stem cells (hESC) in 1998 (Thomson et al. 1998). hESC offers unlimited cell source not only for the inaccessible tissue but also for the development of diverse protocols including efficient generation of DA neurons. These efficient protocols are being used to generate iPSC-derived DA neurons, but there is a variation in differentiation potential of iPSCs (Hu et al. 2010). A subsequent study showed that treatment by a combination of small molecules efficiently induces

hESC, iPSC, and PiPSC-derived DA neurons that (1) express dopamine neuronal markers in vitro, (2) exhibit robust TH positive neuritis innervation of the host striatum, and (3) show recovery in 6-OHDA PD rat model (Sundberg et al. 2013). This result indicated that iPSC-derived DA neurons could be a potent alternative cell source for PD. However, eliminating undifferentiated and undesired cell populations during iPSC-derived DA neuron generation is one of the major hurdles for clinical use of iPSC-derived DA neuron (Trounson and DeWitt 2016; Gutierrez-Aranda et al. 2010; Katsukawa et al. 2016; Lu and Zhao 2013). Especially, undifferentiated autologous iPSC can form teratoma, which does not fulfill clinical criteria. Induced neurons directly generated from fibroblasts that undergo senescence after several passages do not require cell proliferation, which is a necessary condition for iPSC reprogramming, eliminating the risk of teratoma. Although generation of DA neurons by direct conversion is faster compared to iPSC-derived DA neuron generation, there is a practical limitation to generate sufficient numbers of induced neurons by direct conversion for therapeutic use (Yang et al. 2011). Based on postmortem analysis from fetal VM transplantation in PD patients, large numbers of TH-positive cells (200,000~400,000) are required (Mendez et al. 2005; Li et al. 2008; Kordower et al. 1996; Hagell et al. 1999; Mendez et al. 2008). Therefore, it

Table 1 Summary of studies on induced mDA neuron differentiation from fibroblasts

Reference	Dopamine neuron differentiation				
	Transcription factor	miRNA	Chemical	Characteristics	Functional test
Pfisterer et al. 2011	Ascl1, Brn2, Myt1l, Foxa2, and Lmx1a	N/A	N/A	-16.43 ± 4.3% conversion efficiency to neuron -Less than 10% of TH+ cells among neurons	-Electrophysiology -Spontaneous action potentials and rebound action potentials are comparable with mDA neuron
Caiazzo et al. 2011	Ascl1, Nurr1, and Lmx1a	N/A	N/A	-ICC TH+ (~ 5%), VMAT2, DAT, ALDH1A1, and calbindin -Gene expression pattern	-Electrophysiology -Spontaneous action potentials and rebound action potentials are comparable with mDA neuron -HPLC:DA release
Kim et al. 2011	Ascl1 and Pitx3	N/A	Shh + FGF in N3 media (N2 + bFGF)	-ICC TH+ (~ 5%), Tuj, DAT, and AADC -Gene expression pattern	-Electrophysiology -HPLC:DA release -About 50% recovery in amphetamine-induced rotation -About 2000 TH+ cells in grafted with elevated dopamine level
Addis et al. 2011	Ascl1, Lmx1b, and Nurr1	N/A	N/A	-ICC 35.15% of Tuj1+ 50.9 ± 3.3% of TH+ among Tuj1+ cells (18.2 ± 1.5% conversion rate) -Gene expression pattern	-Electrophysiology -HPLC:DA release
Jiang et al. 2015	Ascl1, Lmx1a, Nurr1, and p53 shRNA	miR-124	Y27632/CHIR/VC/DM/SB/BDNF/PMN/NGF/GDNF/TGF-β	-ICC 93.3 ± 1.6% of Tuj1+, 59.2 ± 3.7% TH+	-Electrophysiology -HPLC:DA release

would be desirable to generate DA neuron precursors from fibroblasts that are expendable (Kim et al. 2014; Tian et al. 2015; Lim et al. 2015).

Conclusions

Despite the short amount of time since the report of direct conversion into neuronal cells from fibroblasts, it already represents a significant shift that cell fate plasticity can be manipulated by transcription factors (Vierbuchen et al. 2010; Pfisterer et al. 2011; Kim et al. 2011). Although the molecular mechanism is still poorly understood, this new methodology may be a strong and attractive tool to expand our knowledge on the relationship between transcription factors and various repressive/active chromatin states to regulate cell fate decision. Moreover, direct conversion of DA neurons provides an alternative for the cell-based therapy using iPSC technology. Recently, disease modeling using iPSC-derived neurons has provided new insights into the cellular aspect of diseases by recapitulating patient derived cells (Nishizawa et al. 2016; Mucci et al. 2016; Li et al. 2016; Heman-Ackah et al. 2016; Jang and Ye 2016; Choi et al. 2016; Mekhoubad et al. 2012; Marchetto et al. 2011; Soldner and Jaenisch 2012). Consequently, progerin-mediated late-onset disease modeling provides the possibility of using iPSC-derived DA neurons in late-onset age-related diseases (e.g., Parkinson's diseases) (Miller et al. 2013). Along with the advance of iPSC-based disease modeling, induced mDA neurons from patient-derived fibroblasts will be beneficial for recapitulating diseases in vitro. Although small molecule-mediated generation of functional DA neuron from iPSC has been established, direct conversion of fibroblasts into DA neurons using only small molecules has not been established. This may be due to the different epigenetic control and chromatin statuses that are involved in cell fate plasticity, compared to those in iPSCs. Thus, more rigorous approaches are required to screen effective small molecules that regulate epigenetic changes in fibroblasts. Recent studies showed the close relationship between metabolites and epigenetic control in stem cell self-renewal and differentiation (Donohoe and Bultman 2012; Inagaki et al. 2016; Ryall et al. 2015; Berger and Sassone-Corsi 2015; Menendez 2015; Ryall et al. 2015; Ost and Pospisilik 2015; Meier 2013; Agathocleous and Harris 2013; Kaelin and McKnight 2013; Lu and Thompson 2012; Hanover et al. 2012). Acetyl-CoA, methionine, and α-ketoglutarate are the key metabolites that are either a source or cofactor of acetylation, methylation, and dimethylation. Moreover, metabolites like glucosamine-induced stem cell proliferation and differentiation by regulating both epigenetic control and anabolic metabolism (Hwang et al. 2016; TeSlaa et al. 2016; Carey et al. 2015; Jung et al. 2016; Jang et al. 2012). Thus, metabolic reprogramming is one of the candidates

to further examine for regulation of cell fate plasticity. Future investigation will need to overcome the low efficiency of induced DA neurons from adult human fibroblasts.

Abbreviations

6-OHDA: 6-Hydroxydopamine; AADC: Aromatic l-amino acid decarboxylase; ALK2: Activin A receptor type 2; BAF53a: BAF complex 53 KDa subunit; BDNF: Brain-derived neurotrophic factor; Brn2 also POU3F2: POU class 3 homeobox 2; CHIR: CHIR99021; DA neurons: Dopamine neurons; DAT: Dopamine transporter; DBH1: Noradrenaline-synthesizing enzyme dopamine β-hydroxylase 1; DM: Dorsomorphin; DR5: Five-base-pair spacer; en-1: Engrailed 1; FGF8: Fibroblast growth factor 8; Foxa2: Forkhead Box A2; GDNF: Glial cell line-derived neurotrophic factor; Gli1: Gli family zinc finger1; GSK3: Glycogen synthase kinase 3; HDAC: Histone deacetylase; ihN: Human-induced neuron; iPSC: Induced pluripotent stem cell; Lmx1a: LIM homeobox transcription factor 1 α; Mash1 also known as Ascl1: Mammalian achaete scute homolog-1; mDA neuron: Midbrain dopamine neuron; MHB: Midbrain-hindbrain border; miRNA: MicroRNA; Msx1: Msh homeobox homolog 1; MyoD: Myogenic differentiation 1; Myt1l: Myelin transcription factor 1 like; NGF: Nerve growth factor; Ngn1: Neurogenin 1; Ngn2: Neurogenin 2; Nurr1: Nuclear receptor-related 1 protein; Otx1: Orthodenticle homeobox1; Pax2: Paired box 2; Pax5: Paired box 5; PD: Parkinson's disease; Phox2a: Paired like homeodomain 2a; PiPSC: Primate iPSC; PMN: Purmorphamine; RXR: Retinoic X receptor; SB: SB431542; SHH: Sonic hedgehog; SN: Substantia nigra; TH: Tyrosine hydrolase; VC: Vitamin C; VM: Ventral mesencephalon; VTA: Ventral tegmental area; Wnt1: Wingless-related MMTV integration site 1; Y27632: Rock inhibitor

Acknowledgements

We thank Dr. Jeha Jeon for editing the figures. We are grateful to Dabin Hwang for the proofreading of the manuscript.

Funding

Not applicable.

Authors, contributions

YJ and JHJ wrote the manuscript and figures. JHJ decided on the content, had editorial input on all sections, and designed the layout of figures. All authors read and approved the final manuscript.

Competing interests

The authors declare that they have no competing interests.

References

Addis RC, Hsu FC, Wright RL, Dichter MA, Coulter DA, Gearhart JD. Efficient conversion of astrocytes to functional midbrain dopaminergic neurons using a single polycistronic vector. PLoS One. 2011;6(12):e28719.

Agathocleous M, Harris WA. Metabolism in physiological cell proliferation and differentiation. Trends Cell Biol. 2013;23(10):484–92.

Andersson E, Tryggvason U, Deng Q, Friling S, Alekseenko Z, Robert B, Perlmann T, Ericson J. Identification of intrinsic determinants of midbrain dopamine neurons. Cell. 2006;124(2):393–405.

Arenas E, Denham M, Villaescusa JC. How to make a midbrain dopaminergic neuron. Development. 2015;142(11):1918–36.

Barker RA, Drouin-Ouellet J, Parmar M. Cell-based therapies for Parkinson disease-past insights and future potential. Nat Rev Neurol. 2015;11(9):492–503.

Behm M, Ohman M. RNA editing: a contributor to neuronal dynamics in the mammalian brain. Trends Genet. 2016;32(3):165–75.

Berger SL, Sassone-Corsi P. Metabolic signaling to chromatin. Cold Spring Harb Perspect Biol. 2015;

Betarbet R, Sherer TB, MacKenzie G, Garcia-Osuna M, Panov AV, Greenamyre JT. Chronic systemic pesticide exposure reproduces features of Parkinson's disease. Nat Neurosci. 2000;3(12):1301–6.

Borromeo MD, Meredith DM, Castro DS, Chang JC, Tung KC, Guillemot F, Johnson JE. A transcription factor network specifying inhibitory versus excitatory neurons in the dorsal spinal cord. Development. 2014;141(14):2803–12.

Caiazzo M, Dell'Anno MT, Dvoretskova E, Lazarevic D, Taverna S, Leo D, Sotnikova TD, Menegon A, Roncaglia P, Colciago G, et al. Direct generation of functional dopaminergic neurons from mouse and human fibroblasts. Nature. 2011;476(7359):224–7.

Campos-Melo D, Galleguillos D, Sanchez N, Gysling K, Andres ME. Nur transcription factors in stress and addiction. Front Mol Neurosci. 2013;6:44.

Carey BW, Finley LW, Cross JR, Allis CD, Thompson CB. Intracellular alpha-ketoglutarate maintains the pluripotency of embryonic stem cells. Nature. 2015;518(7539):413–6.

Casarosa S, Fode C, Guillemot F. Mash1 regulates neurogenesis in the ventral telencephalon. Development. 1999;126(3):525–34.

Cau E, Casarosa S, Guillemot F. Mash1 and Ngn1 control distinct steps of determination and differentiation in the olfactory sensory neuron lineage. Development. 2002;129(8):1871–80.

Chambers SM, Fasano CA, Papapetrou EP, Tomishima M, Sadelain M, Studer L. Highly efficient neural conversion of human ES and iPS cells by dual inhibition of SMAD signaling. Nat Biotechnol. 2009;27(3):275–80.

Chen G, Gulbranson DR, Hou Z, Bolin JM, Ruotti V, Probasco MD, Smuga-Otto K, Howden SE, Diol NR, Propson NE, et al. Chemically defined conditions for human iPSC derivation and culture. Nat Methods. 2011;8(5):424–9.

Choi IY, Lim H, Estrellas K, Mula J, Cohen TV, Zhang Y, Donnelly CJ, Richard JP, Kim YJ, Kim H, et al. Concordant but varied phenotypes among Duchenne muscular dystrophy patient-specific myoblasts derived using a human iPSC-based model. Cell Rep. 2016;15(10):2301–12.

Chung S, Leung A, Han BS, Chang MY, Moon JI, Kim CH, Hong S, Pruszak J, Isacson O, Kim KS. Wnt1-lmx1a forms a novel autoregulatory loop and controls midbrain dopaminergic differentiation synergistically with the SHH-FoxA2 pathway. Cell Stem Cell. 2009;5(6):646–58.

Dai P, Harada Y, Takamatsu T. Highly efficient direct conversion of human fibroblasts to neuronal cells by chemical compounds. J Clin Biochem Nutr. 2015;56(3):166–70.

Davis RL, Weintraub H, Lassar AB. Expression of a single transfected cDNA converts fibroblasts to myoblasts. Cell. 1987;51(6):987–1000.

de Lau LM, Breteler MM. Epidemiology of Parkinson's disease. Lancet Neurol. 2006;5(6):525–35.

Dethoff EA, Chugh J, Mustoe AM, Al-Hashimi HM. Functional complexity and regulation through RNA dynamics. Nature. 2012;482(7385):322–30.

Doi D, Samata B, Katsukawa M, Kikuchi T, Morizane A, Ono Y, Sekiguchi K, Nakagawa M, Parmar M, Takahashi J. Isolation of human induced pluripotent stem cell-derived dopaminergic progenitors by cell sorting for successful transplantation. Stem Cell Reports. 2014;2(3):337–50.

Domanskyi A, Alter H, Vogt MA, Gass P, Vinnikov IA. Transcription factors Foxa1 and Foxa2 are required for adult dopamine neurons maintenance. Front Cell Neurosci. 2014;8:275.

Donohoe DR, Bultman SJ. Metaboloepigenetics: interrelationships between energy metabolism and epigenetic control of gene expression. J Cell Physiol. 2012;227(9):3169–77.

Failli V, Bachy I, Retaux S. Expression of the LIM-homeodomain gene Lmx1a (dreher) during development of the mouse nervous system. Mech Dev. 2002;118(1-2):225–8.

Ferri AL, Lin W, Mavromatakis YE, Wang JC, Sasaki H, Whitsett JA, Ang SL. Foxa1 and Foxa2 regulate multiple phases of midbrain dopaminergic neuron development in a dosage-dependent manner. Development. 2007;134(15):2761–9.

Freed CR, Greene PE, Breeze RE, Tsai WY, DuMouchel W, Kao R, Dillon S, Winfield H, Culver S, Trojanowski JQ, et al. Transplantation of embryonic dopamine neurons for severe Parkinson's disease. N Engl J Med. 2001;344(10):710–9.

Gutierrez-Aranda I, Ramos-Mejia V, Bueno C, Munoz-Lopez M, Real PJ, Macia A, Sanchez L, Ligero G, Garcia-Parez JL, Menendez P. Human induced pluripotent stem cells develop teratoma more efficiently and faster than human embryonic stem cells regardless the site of injection. Stem Cells. 2010;28(9):1568–70.

Hagell P, Schrag A, Piccini P, Jahanshahi M, Brown R, Rehncrona S, Widner H, Brundin P, Rothwell JC, Odin P, et al. Sequential bilateral transplantation in Parkinson's disease: effects of the second graft. Brain. 1999;122(Pt 6):1121–32.

Hanover JA, Krause MW, Love DC. Bittersweet memories: linking metabolism to epigenetics through O-GlcNAcylation. Nat Rev Mol Cell Biol. 2012;13(5):312–21.

Heins N, Malatesta P, Cecconi F, Nakafuku M, Tucker KL, Hack MA, Chapouton P, Barde YA, Gotz M. Glial cells generate neurons: the role of the transcription factor Pax6. Nat Neurosci. 2002;5(4):308–15.

Heman-Ackah SM, Bassett AR, Wood MJ. Precision modulation of neurodegenerative disease-related gene expression in human iPSC-derived neurons. Sci Rep. 2016;6:28420.

Hermanson E, Joseph B, Castro D, Lindqvist E, Aarnisalo P, Wallen A, Benoit G, Hengerer B, Olson L, Perlmann T. Nurr1 regulates dopamine synthesis and storage in MN9D dopamine cells. Exp Cell Res. 2003;288(2):324–34.

Hirsch MR, Tiveron MC, Guillemot F, Brunet JF, Goridis C. Control of noradrenergic differentiation and Phox2a expression by MASH1 in the central and peripheral nervous system. Development. 1998;125(4):599–608.

Horton S, Meredith A, Richardson JA, Johnson JE. Correct coordination of neuronal differentiation events in ventral forebrain requires the bHLH factor MASH1. Mol Cell Neurosci. 1999;14(4-5):355–69.

Hotta A, Yamanaka S. From genomics to gene therapy: induced pluripotent stem cells meet genome editing. Annu Rev Genet. 2015;49:47–70.

Hou P, Li Y, Zhang X, Liu C, Guan J, Li H, Zhao T, Ye J, Yang W, Liu K, et al. Pluripotent stem cells induced from mouse somatic cells by small-molecule compounds. Science. 2013;341(6146):651–4.

Hu BY, Weick JP, Yu J, Ma LX, Zhang XQ, Thomson JA, Zhang SC. Neural differentiation of human induced pluripotent stem cells follows developmental principles but with variable potency. Proc Natl Acad Sci U S A. 2010;107(9):4335–40.

Huangfu D, Maehr R, Guo W, Eijkelenboom A, Snitow M, Chen AE, Melton DA. Induction of pluripotent stem cells by defined factors is greatly improved by small-molecule compounds. Nat Biotechnol. 2008;26(7):795–7.

Hwang IY, Kwak S, Lee S, Kim H, Lee SE, Kim JH, Kim YA, Jeon YK, Chung DH, Jin X, et al. Psat1-dependent fluctuations in alpha-ketoglutarate affect the timing of ESC differentiation. Cell Metab. 2016;

Inagaki T, Sakai J, Kajimura S. Transcriptional and epigenetic control of brown and beige adipose cell fate and function. Nat Rev Mol Cell Biol. 2016;17(8):480–95.

Jang H, Kim TW, Yoon S, Choi SY, Kang TW, Kim SY, Kwon YW, Cho EJ, Youn HD. O-GlcNAc regulates pluripotency and reprogramming by directly acting on core components of the pluripotency network. Cell Stem Cell. 2012;11(1):62–74.

Jang YY, Ye Z. Gene correction in patient-specific iPSCs for therapy development and disease modeling. Hum Genet. 2016;135(9):1041–58.

Jiang H, Xu Z, Zhong P, Ren Y, Liang G, Schilling HA, Hu Z, Zhang Y, Wang X, Chen S, et al. Cell cycle and p53 gate the direct conversion of human fibroblasts to dopaminergic neurons. Nat Commun. 2015;6:10100.

Jung JH, Iwabuchi K, Yang Z, Loeken MR. Embryonic stem cell proliferation stimulated by altered anabolic metabolism from glucose transporter 2-transported glucosamine. Sci Rep. 2016;6:28452.

Kadkhodaei B, Alvarsson A, Schintu N, Ramskold D, Volakakis N, Joodmardi E, Yoshitake T, Kehr J, Decressac M, Bjorklund A, et al. Transcription factor Nurr1 maintains fiber integrity and nuclear-encoded mitochondrial gene expression in dopamine neurons. Proc Natl Acad Sci U S A. 2013;110(6):2360–5.

Kaelin WG Jr, McKnight SL. Influence of metabolism on epigenetics and disease. Cell. 2013;153(1):56–69.

Karagiannis P, Eto K. Ten years of induced pluripotency: from basic mechanisms to therapeutic applications. Development. 2016;143(12):2039–43.

Katsukawa M, Nakajima Y, Fukumoto A, Doi D, Takahashi J. Fail-safe therapy by gamma-ray irradiation against tumor formation by human-induced pluripotent stem cell-derived neural progenitors. Stem Cells Dev. 2016;25(11):815–25.

Kim HS, Kim J, Jo Y, Jeon D, Cho YS. Direct lineage reprogramming of mouse fibroblasts to functional midbrain dopaminergic neuronal progenitors. Stem Cell Res. 2014;12(1):60–8.

Kim J, Inoue K, Ishii J, Vanti WB, Voronov SV, Murchison E, Hannon G, Abeliovich A. A microRNA feedback circuit in midbrain dopamine neurons. Science. 2007;317(5842):1220–4.

Kim J, Su SC, Wang H, Cheng AW, Cassady JP, Lodato MA, Lengner CJ, Chung CY, Dawlaty MM, Tsai LH, et al. Functional integration of dopaminergic neurons directly converted from mouse fibroblasts. Cell Stem Cell. 2011;9(5):413–9.

Kirkeby A, Grealish S, Wolf DA, Nelander J, Wood J, Lundblad M, Lindvall O, Parmar M. Generation of regionally specified neural progenitors and functional neurons from human embryonic stem cells under defined conditions. Cell Rep. 2012;1(6):703–14.

Kordower JH, Chu Y, Hauser RA, Freeman TB, Olanow CW. Lewy body-like pathology in long-term embryonic nigral transplants in Parkinson's disease. Nat Med. 2008;14(5):504–6.

Kordower JH, Freeman TB, Chen EY, Mufson EJ, Sanberg PR, Hauser RA, Snow B, Olanow CW. Fetal nigral grafts survive and mediate clinical benefit in a patient with Parkinson's disease. Mov Disord. 1998;13(3):383–93.

Kordower JH, Rosenstein JM, Collier TJ, Burke MA, Chen EY, Li JM, Martel L, Levey AE, Mufson EJ, Freeman TB, et al. Functional fetal nigral grafts in a patient with Parkinson's disease: chemoanatomic, ultrastructural, and metabolic studies. J Comp Neurol. 1996;370(2):203–30.

Kriks S, Shim JW, Piao J, Ganat YM, Wakeman DR, Xie Z, Carrillo-Reid L, Auyeung G, Antonacci C, Buch A, et al. Dopamine neurons derived from human ES cells efficiently engraft in animal models of Parkinson's disease. Nature. 2011; 480(7378):547–51.

Kulessa H, Frampton J, Graf T. GATA-1 reprograms avian myelomonocytic cell lines into eosinophils, thromboblasts, and erythroblasts. Genes Dev. 1995; 9(10):1250–62.

Lau S, Rylander Ottosson D, Jakobsson J, Parmar M. Direct neural conversion from human fibroblasts using self-regulating and nonintegrating viral vectors. Cell Rep. 2014;9(5):1673–80.

Li JY, Englund E, Holton JL, Soulet D, Hagell P, Lees AJ, Lashley T, Quinn NP, Rehncrona S, Bjorklund A, et al. Lewy bodies in grafted neurons in subjects with Parkinson's disease suggest host-to-graft disease propagation. Nat Med. 2008;14(5):501–3.

Li L, Su Y, Zhao C, Xu Q. Role of Nurr1 and Ret in inducing rat embryonic neural precursors to dopaminergic neurons. Neurol Res. 2009;31(5):534–40.

Li M, Izpisua Belmonte JC. Looking to the future following 10 years of induced pluripotent stem cell technologies. Nat Protoc. 2016;11(9):1579–85.

Li M, Zhao H, Ananiev GE, Musser MT, Ness KH, Maglaque DL, Saha K, Bhattacharyya A, Zhao X. Establishment of reporter lines for detecting fragile X mental retardation (FMR1) gene reactivation in human neural cells. Stem Cells. 2016;

Li W, Wei W, Zhu S, Zhu J, Shi Y, Lin T, Hao E, Hayek A, Deng H, Ding S. Generation of rat and human induced pluripotent stem cells by combining genetic reprogramming and chemical inhibitors. Cell Stem Cell. 2009;4(1):16–9.

Li Y, Zhang Q, Yin X, Yang W, Du Y, Hou P, Ge J, Liu C, Zhang W, Zhang X, et al. Generation of iPSCs from mouse fibroblasts with a single gene, Oct4, and small molecules. Cell Res. 2011;21(1):196–204.

Lim MS, Chang MY, Kim SM, Yi SH, Suh-Kim H, Jung SJ, Kim MJ, Kim JH, Lee YS, Lee SY, et al. Generation of dopamine neurons from rodent fibroblasts through the expandable neural precursor cell stage. J Biol Chem. 2015; 290(28):17401–14.

Lin W, Metzakopian E, Mavromatakis YE, Gao N, Balaskas N, Sasaki H, Briscoe J, Whitsett JA, Goulding M, Kaestner KH, et al. Foxa1 and Foxa2 function both upstream of and cooperatively with Lmx1a and Lmx1b in a feedforward loop promoting mesodiencephalic dopaminergic neuron development. Dev Biol. 2009;333(2):386–96.

Lo L, Tiveron MC, Anderson DJ. MASH1 activates expression of the paired homeodomain transcription factor Phox2a, and couples pan-neuronal and subtype-specific components of autonomic neuronal identity. Development. 1998;125(4):609–20.

Lu C, Thompson CB. Metabolic regulation of epigenetics. Cell Metab. 2012; 16(1):9–17.

Lu X, Zhao T. Clinical therapy using iPSCs: hopes and challenges. Genomics Proteomics Bioinformatics. 2013;11(5):294–8.

Ma L, Liu Y, Zhang SC. Directed differentiation of dopamine neurons from human pluripotent stem cells. Methods Mol Biol. 2011;767:411–8.

Mali P, Chou BK, Yen J, Ye Z, Zou J, Dowey S, Brodsky RA, Ohm JE, Yu W, Baylin SB, et al. Butyrate greatly enhances derivation of human induced pluripotent stem cells by promoting epigenetic remodeling and the expression of pluripotency-associated genes. Stem Cells. 2010;28(4):713–20.

Marchetto MC, Brennand KJ, Boyer LF, Gage FH. Induced pluripotent stem cells (iPSCs) and neurological disease modeling: progress and promises. Hum Mol Genet. 2011;20(R2):R109–15.

Meier JL. Metabolic mechanisms of epigenetic regulation. ACS Chem Biol. 2013; 8(12):2607–21.

Mekhoubad S, Bock C, de Boer AS, Kiskinis E, Meissner A, Eggan K. Erosion of dosage compensation impacts human iPSC disease modeling. Cell Stem Cell. 2012;10(5):595–609.

Mendez I, Sanchez-Pernaute R, Cooper O, Vinuela A, Ferrari D, Bjorklund L, Dagher A, Isacson O. Cell type analysis of functional fetal dopamine cell suspension transplants in the striatum and substantia nigra of patients with Parkinson's disease. Brain. 2005;128(Pt 7):1498–510.

Mendez I, Vinuela A, Astradsson A, Mukhida K, Hallett P, Robertson H, Tierney T, Holness R, Dagher A, Trojanowski JQ, et al. Dopamine neurons implanted into people with Parkinson's disease survive without pathology for 14 years. Nat Med. 2008;14(5):507–9.

Menendez JA. Metabolic control of cancer cell stemness: lessons from iPS cells. Cell Cycle. 2015;14(24):3801–11.

Mertens J, Marchetto MC, Bardy C, Gage FH. Evaluating cell reprogramming, differentiation and conversion technologies in neuroscience. Nat Rev Neurosci. 2016;17(7):424–37.

Miller JD, Ganat YM, Kishinevsky S, Bowman RL, Liu B, Tu EY, Mandal PK, Vera E, Shim JW, Kriks S, et al. Human iPSC-based modeling of late-onset disease via progerin-induced aging. Cell Stem Cell. 2013;13(6):691–705.

Millonig JH, Millen KJ, Hatten ME. The mouse dreher gene Lmx1a controls formation of the roof plate in the vertebrate CNS. Nature. 2000;403(6771):764–9.

Mishima Y, Lindgren AG, Chizhikov VV, Johnson RL, Millen KJ. Overlapping function of Lmx1a and Lmx1b in anterior hindbrain roof plate formation and cerebellar growth. J Neurosci. 2009;29(36):11377–84.

Mucci A, Kunkiel J, Suzuki T, Brennig S, Glage S, Kuhnel MP, Ackermann M, Happle C, Kuhn A, Schambach A, et al. Murine iPSC-derived macrophages as a tool for disease modeling of hereditary pulmonary alveolar proteinosis due to Csf2rb deficiency. Stem Cell Reports. 2016;7(2):292–305.

Nishizawa M, Chonabayashi K, Nomura M, Tanaka A, Nakamura M, Inagaki A, Nishikawa M, Takei I, Oishi A, Tanabe K, et al. Epigenetic variation between human induced pluripotent stem cell lines is an indicator of differentiation capacity. Cell Stem Cell. 2016;

Olanow CW, Goetz CG, Kordower JH, Stoessl AJ, Sossi V, Brin MF, Shannon KM, Nauert GM, Perl DP, Godbold J, et al. A double-blind controlled trial of bilateral fetal nigral transplantation in Parkinson's disease. Ann Neurol. 2003; 54(3):403–14.

Olanow CW, Kordower JH, Freeman TB. Fetal nigral transplantation as a therapy for Parkinson's disease. Trends Neurosci. 1996;19(3):102–9.

Ost A, Pospisilik JA. Epigenetic modulation of metabolic decisions. Curr Opin Cell Biol. 2015;33:88–94.

Parras CM, Schuurmans C, Scardigli R, Kim J, Anderson DJ, Guillemot F. Divergent functions of the proneural genes Mash1 and Ngn2 in the specification of neuronal subtype identity. Genes Dev. 2002;16(3):324–38.

Pattyn A, Simplicio N, van Doorninck JH, Goridis C, Guillemot F, Brunet JF. Ascl1/ Mash1 is required for the development of central serotonergic neurons. Nat Neurosci. 2004;7(6):589–95.

Pfisterer U, Kirkeby A, Torper O, Wood J, Nelander J, Dufour A, Bjorklund A, Lindvall O, Jakobsson J, Parmar M. Direct conversion of human fibroblasts to dopaminergic neurons. Proc Natl Acad Sci U S A. 2011;108(25):10343–8.

Roybon L, Hjalt T, Christophersen NS, Li JY, Brundin P. Effects on differentiation of embryonic ventral midbrain progenitors by Lmx1a, Msx1, Ngn2, and Pitx3. J Neurosci. 2008;28(14):3644–56.

Ryall JG, Cliff T, Dalton S, Sartorelli V. Metabolic reprogramming of stem cell epigenetics. Cell Stem Cell. 2015;17(6):651–62.

Ryall JG, Dell'Orso S, Derfoul A, Juan A, Zare H, Feng X, Clermont D, Koulnis M, Gutierrez-Cruz G, Fulco M, et al. The NAD(+)-dependent SIRT1 deacetylase translates a metabolic switch into regulatory epigenetics in skeletal muscle stem cells. Cell Stem Cell. 2015;16(2):171–83.

Sacchetti P, Mitchell TR, Granneman JG, Bannon MJ. Nurr1 enhances transcription of the human dopamine transporter gene through a novel mechanism. J Neurochem. 2001;76(5):1565–72.

Sakurada K, Ohshima-Sakurada M, Palmer TD, Gage FH. Nurr1, an orphan nuclear receptor, is a transcriptional activator of endogenous tyrosine hydroxylase in neural progenitor cells derived from the adult brain. Development. 1999; 126(18):4017–26.

Sasaki H, Hui C, Nakafuku M, Kondoh H. A binding site for Gli proteins is essential for HNF-3beta floor plate enhancer activity in transgenics and can respond to Shh in vitro. Development. 1997;124(7):1313–22.

Schimmel JJ, Crews L, Roffler-Tarlov S, Chikaraishi DM. 4.5 kb of the rat tyrosine hydroxylase 5′ flanking sequence directs tissue specific expression during development and contains consensus sites for multiple transcription factors. Brain Res Mol Brain Res. 1999;74(1-2):1–14.

Shen CN, Slack JM, Tosh D. Molecular basis of transdifferentiation of pancreas to liver. Nat Cell Biol. 2000;2(12):879–87.

Smits SM, Ponnio T, Conneely OM, Burbach JP, Smidt MP. Involvement of Nurr1 in specifying the neurotransmitter identity of ventral midbrain dopaminergic neurons. Eur J Neurosci. 2003;18(7):1731–8.

Soldner F, Jaenisch R. Medicine. iPSC disease modeling. Science. 2012;338(6111):1155–6.

Stott SR, Metzakopian E, Lin W, Kaestner KH, Hen R, Ang SL. Foxa1 and foxa2 are required for the maintenance of dopaminergic properties in ventral midbrain neurons at late embryonic stages. J Neurosci. 2013;33(18):8022–34.

Studer L. Derivation of dopaminergic neurons from pluripotent stem cells. Prog Brain Res. 2012;200:243–63.

Sundberg M, Bogetofte H, Lawson T, Jansson J, Smith G, Astradsson A, Moore M, Osborn T, Cooper O, Spealman R, et al. Improved cell therapy protocols for Parkinson's disease based on differentiation efficiency and safety of hESC-, hiPSC-, and non-human primate iPSC-derived dopaminergic neurons. Stem Cells. 2013;31(8):1548–62.

Takahashi K, Yamanaka S. Induction of pluripotent stem cells from mouse embryonic and adult fibroblast cultures by defined factors. Cell. 2006;126(4):663–76.

Takahashi K, Yamanaka S. A decade of transcription factor-mediated reprogramming to pluripotency. Nat Rev Mol Cell Biol. 2016;17(3):183–93.

Tapia N, Scholer HR. Molecular obstacles to clinical translation of iPSCs. Cell Stem Cell. 2016;

TeSlaa T, Chaikovsky AC, Lipchina I, Escobar SL, Hochedlinger K, Huang J, Graeber TG, Braas D, Teitell MA. Alpha-ketoglutarate accelerates the initial differentiation of primed human pluripotent stem cells. Cell Metab. 2016;

Thomson JA, Itskovitz-Eldor J, Shapiro SS, Waknitz MA, Swiergiel JJ, Marshall VS, Jones JM. Embryonic stem cell lines derived from human blastocysts. Science. 1998;282(5391):1145–7.

Tian C, Li Y, Huang Y, Wang Y, Chen D, Liu J, Deng X, Sun L, Anderson K, Qi X, et al. Selective generation of dopaminergic precursors from mouse fibroblasts by direct lineage conversion. Sci Rep. 2015;5:12622.

Trounson A, DeWitt ND. Pluripotent stem cells progressing to the clinic. Nat Rev Mol Cell Biol. 2016;17(3):194–200.

Vasconcelos FF, Castro DS. Transcriptional control of vertebrate neurogenesis by the proneural factor Ascl1. Front Cell Neurosci. 2014;8:412.

Vidigal JA, Ventura A. The biological functions of miRNAs: lessons from in vivo studies. Trends Cell Biol. 2015;25(3):137–47.

Vierbuchen T, Ostermeier A, Pang ZP, Kokubu Y, Sudhof TC, Wernig M. Direct conversion of fibroblasts to functional neurons by defined factors. Nature. 2010;463(7284):1035–41.

Wurst W, Prakash N. Wnt1-regulated genetic networks in midbrain dopaminergic neuron development. J Mol Cell Biol. 2014;6(1):34–41.

Xie H, Ye M, Feng R, Graf T. Stepwise reprogramming of B cells into macrophages. Cell. 2004;117(5):663–76.

Yang N, Ng YH, Pang ZP, Sudhof TC, Wernig M. Induced neuronal cells: how to make and define a neuron. Cell Stem Cell. 2011;9(6):517–25.

Yoo AS, Staahl BT, Chen L, Crabtree GR. MicroRNA-mediated switching of chromatin-remodelling complexes in neural development. Nature. 2009;460(7255):642–6.

Yoo AS, Sun AX, Li L, Shcheglovitov A, Portmann T, Li Y, Lee-Messer C, Dolmetsch RE, Tsien RW, Crabtree GR. MicroRNA-mediated conversion of human fibroblasts to neurons. Nature. 2011;476(7359):228–31.

Zetterstrom RH, Solomin L, Jansson L, Hoffer BJ, Olson L, Perlmann T. Dopamine neuron agenesis in Nurr1-deficient mice. Science. 1997;276(5310):248–50.

Zhu S, Li W, Zhou H, Wei W, Ambasudhan R, Lin T, Kim J, Zhang K, Ding S. Reprogramming of human primary somatic cells by OCT4 and chemical compounds. Cell Stem Cell. 2010;7(6):651–5.

7

Anti-inflammatory and ECM gene expression modulations of β-eudesmol via NF-κB signaling pathway in normal human dermal fibroblasts

Kyung Yun Kim

Abstract

Background: β-eudesmol is a kind of aromatic compound belonging to sesquiterpenoid which exists within not only the bark of *magnolia* but also *Nardostachys jatamansi*, *Atractylodes lancea*, *Pterocarpus santalinus*, *Ginkgo bilobal*, *Cryptomeria japonica*, etc., and there has been progress in medical and pharmaceutic researches on antitumor, anticancer, and anti-inflammatory effects; nervous system stabilization; and vasodilator effects, etc., but not in researches on skin cares and cosmetics at all. Therefore, this study pretreated β-eudesmol with human dermal fibroblasts (HDFs) and then gave oxidative stresses with H_2O_2 to examine antioxidation, anti-inflammatory, and cell preservation effects. Through this process, it proves the possibility of β-eudesmol as cosmetic materials.

Methods: This study verified the effectiveness of β-eudesmol through cell viability analysis, reactive oxygen estimation, associated β-galactosidase assay, nuclear factor-kappa B (NF-κB) luciferase assay, and quantitative real-time polymerase chain reaction (qRT-PCR).

Results: The cell viability which decreased due to H_2O_2 increased as per dose-dependent manners of β-eudesmol. Also, at the 2,2-diphenyl-1-picrylhydrazyl (DPPH) radical scavenging activity assay, intracellular reactive oxygen species (ROS) quantitative analysis and glutathione (GSH) estimation, the relative levels which were changed by H_2O_2 treatment, showed attenuated or protective transition forms, depending on the concentration of β-eudesmol. Additionally, reduced superoxide dismutase 1 (*SOD1*) and catalase (*CAT*) gene expression by H_2O_2 were increased by β-eudesmol. As the result of the promoter activity analysis of NF-κB which has a key role in inflammation and skin aging, NF-κB activity decreases as β-eudesmol concentration increases, and also this study proves that gene expression of interleukin 1 beta (*IL-1β*) which is a downstream gene of NF-κB related to inflammatory response decreases as well as tumor necrosis factor-alpha (*TNF-α*) gene expression depending on the concentration of β-eudesmol.

Conclusions: Through these results, this study suggests there are anti-inflammatory effects by shutting out the NF-κB pathway. Following the results of the extracellular matrix (ECM) regulating gene expression analysis, this study proves that oxidative stress-induced increased *MMP1* levels were decreased depending on the concentration of β-eudesmol and verifies that it hinders the collapse of collagen through inhibition of transcriptional activity of NF-κB. From the result of β-eudesmol regulating tissue inhibitors of metalloproteinase (*TIMP*)-1 gene expression which hinders matrix metalloproteinase (MMP), activation and alteration of gene expression of collagen type I alpha 1 (*COL1A1*) underpins the above consequences. Through this research, it is considered that β-eudesmol as one of natural cosmetic materials with such effects as antioxidation, anti-inflammation, and cell preservation is worthy of notice.

Keywords: β-eudesmol, Antioxidant, Anti-inflammation, Cellular senescence, Fibroblast, Extra cellular matrix

Correspondence: skykkr00@nate.com
URG Inc (2F, URG B/D), 28, Yangjaecheon-ro 19-gil, Seocho-gu, Seoul, Republic of Korea

Background

The bark of *magnolia* and *magnolia obovata* which is the dried rhizodermis have been used as a traditional medicine for medical treatment of bronchitis, asthma, stomach disease, emotional instability disorder, and allergy in Korea, Japan, and China (Hoang et al. 2010). On the basis of this folk remedy, the research on central sedation of central nervous system through *magnolia* bark extract was reported in 1973 (Watanabe et al. 1973). Various biologically active substances extracted from the bark and rhizodermis of *magnolia* are essential oils such as β-eudesmol, α-pinenes, β-pinenes, and bornyl acetate and diphenyl compounds such as magnolol, honokiol, and alkaloids; magnocurarine; and magnoflorine. It is reported that some of these ingredients has pharmacologic effects on the nervous system (Watanabe et al. 1983; Chiou et al. 1997).

In this experiment, β-eudesmol is used among those biologically active substances of *magnolia*, and β-eudesmol is a kind of aromatic compound belonging to sesquiterpenoid which exists not only in the bark of *magnolia* but also in medical herbs such as *Nardostachys jatamansi*, *Atractylodes lancea*, *Pterocarpus santalinus*, *Ginkgo biloba*, and *Cryptomeria japonica* etc. (Li et al. 2013), and its chemical formula is $C_{15}H_{26}O$ and its molecular mass is 222. β-eudesmol has antimutagenic effects (Miyazawa et al. 1996) and nervous system sedation effects too. It has been proved that β-eudesmol has effects to shut off nicotinic acetylcholine receptor in the neuromuscular junction (Kimura et al. 1991), to control neuromuscular disorder caused by neostigmine (Chiou and Chang 1992), and to control activities of Na^+, K^+-ATPase, and H^+ (Satoh et al. 1992). Also, it has been reported that β-eudesmol controls fatal toxicity caused by organophosphorus compound (Chiou et al. 1995), induces outgrowing of neurite in pheochromocytoma (PC12) cells through activation of mitogen-activated protein kinases (MAPK) (Obara et al. 2002), and has vasodilator effects through shutting off adrenaline α-1 receptor (Lim and Kee 2005). It has been reported that β-eudesmol controls interleukin (IL)-6 and receptor interacting protein-2 in mast cell, activates p38 MAPK, and has anti-inflammation effects through process to control caspase-1 (Seo et al. 2011). Recently, researches on effectiveness of β-eudesmol to blood vessels on the nervous system and also antitumor and anticancer effects have been largely in progress. Apoptotic effect through neovascular control effect of β-eudesmol has been reported (Ikeda and Nagase 2002; Ma et al. 2008). And it has been proved that β-eudesmol has apoptotic effect through caspase-3 via caspase-9 caused by cytochrome in HL-60 cells (Hoang et al. 2010), c-Jun N-terminal kinase (JNK)-dependent apoptotic effect through mitochondria passage in HL-60 cells (Li et al. 2013), and anticancer effects in the experiment of nude mouse to whom it implanted through the method of heterotransplantation of human cholangiocarcinoma (Plengsuriyakarn et al. 2015).

Looking at existing studies on β-eudesmol, there have been reports about medical and pharmacologic researches on its anti-inflammation, antimutagenicity, nervous system stabilization, vasodilator, antitumor, and anticancer effects (Li et al. 2013; Miyazawa et al. 1996; Kimura et al. 1991; Chiou and Chang 1992; Satoh et al. 1992; Chiou et al. 1995; Obara et al. 2002; Lim and Kee 2005; Seo et al. 2011; Ikeda and Nagase 2002; Ma et al. 2008; Plengsuriyakarn et al. 2015). However, research on the mechanism of β-eudesmol in human dermal fibroblast has not been reported yet, and also, there have been no researches on β-eudesmol as skin care and cosmetic compounds. Therefore, this research intends to verify antioxidation, anti-inflammation, and cell preservation effects of β-eudesmol in human dermal fibroblast through studying the intracellular mechanism. Therefore, this study aims to suggest possibility of β-eudesmol as natural cosmetic materials.

Methods

Cell culture

For this research, we purchased and used human dermal fibroblasts (HDFs) from Lonza Inc. (Basel, Switzerland) and cultured it using Dulbecco's modified Eagle's medium (DMEM; Hyclone, Logan, UT, USA) as culture medium which contains 10% fetal bovine serum (FBS; Hyclone) and 1% penicillin/streptomycin (penicillin 100 IU/mL, streptomycin 100 μg/mL; Invitrogen/Life Technologies, Carlsbad, CA, USA). Cultured cells within an incubator where we kept in a temperature of 37 °C and 5% CO_2.

Sample treatment

We purchased β-eudesmol in the form of powder which is refined (> 90%) from Sigma-Aldrich Inc. (St. Louis, MO, USA). When we used it in the experiment, we dissolved it in dimethyl sulfoxide (DMSO; Sigma-Aldrich) in optimal concentration. After, we cultured HDFs (1×10^6 cells/well) in a 60-mm cell culture dish for 24 h; we added β-eudesmol as per indicated concentration to the culture medium and pretreated for 24 h, treated H_2O_2 in an appropriate concentration, and then used them for analysis after 3 h. For the experiment of gene level, after culturing HDFs (2×10^5 cells/well) in a cell culture medium, we treated β-eudesmol as per indicated concentration for 24 h when the plate's density is more than 85–90%. We treated H_2O_2 and collected cells after 3 h, and from these cells, we extracted RNA; then on the basis of this RNA, we identified gene expression through quantitative real-time polymerase chain reaction (qRT-PCR).

Cell viability estimation

We used the principle of water-soluble tetrazolium salt (WST-1) assay for evaluating cell viability. After we inoculated each HDF of 100 μL in density of 3×10^3 cells/well in 96-well plates and cultured for 24 h, we treated H_2O_2 and every kind of sample, in cell culture plates. After we added 10 μL of EZ-Cytox cell viability assay kit reagent (ItsBio, Seoul, Korea) in the cultured cell and cultured for 1 h, we used a microplate reader (Bio-Rad, Hercules, CA, USA) to estimate absorbance in the scale of 490 nm and repeated three times and deduced the average value and standard deviation of cell viability.

cDNA manufacturing
After using Trizol reagent (Invitrogen/Life Technologies) to dissolve cells which we obtained through cell culture, we added 0.2 mL of chloroform (Biopure, Tulln, Austria) and then centrifuged for 20 min at 12,000 rpm at 4 °C to divide into pellets which include protein and supernatant which include mRNA. For the supernatant, we added 0.5 mL of isopropanol (Biopure) and left at room temperature for 10 min, and then centrifuged it at 12,000 rpm at 4 °C to precipitate RNA. Next, we used 75% ethanol to wash, and then we removed ethanol and dried at room temperature. We dissolved dried RNA in diethylpyrocarbonate (DEPC; Biopure) water, and among the extracted RNA, we only used pure RNA whose purity is more than a ratio 1.8 of 260/280 nm using Nanodrop (Maestrogen, Las Vegas, NV, USA).

For cDNA synthesis, we manufactured total 10 μL of 1 μg RNA, 0.5 ng oligo dT18, and DEPC water in a PCR tube, and then we treated them for 10 min at the degree of 70 °C to induce RNA denaturation. Next, we used M-MLV reverse transcriptase (Enzynomics, Dajeon, Korea) to react for 1 h at 37 °C to synthesize cDNA.

Quantitative real-time PCR
To analyze gene expression pattern quantitatively within HDFs caused by β-eudesmol, we used qRT-PCR method. The qRT-PCR is to synthesize 0.2 μM primers, 50 mM KCl, 20 mM Tris/HCl pH 8.4, 0.8 mM dNTP, 0.5 U Taq DNA polymerase, 3 mM $MgCl_2$, and 1× SYBR green (Invitrogen/Life Technologies) in a PCR tube to manufacture the reaction solution, and is to use Linegene K (BioER,

Hangzhou, China). To denature DNA, the mixture is heated for 3 min at 94 °C, and then 40 cycles of denaturation (94 °C, 30 s), annealing (58 °C, 30 s), and polymerization (72 °C, 30 s) were performed. We used SYBR green to identify changing of each gene expression and verified effectiveness of PCR through the melting curve. We standardized expression of β-actin for comparative analysis on each gene expression. The primer used in the experiment is shown in Table 1.

DPPH radical scavenging activity assay
DPPH assay is a method to inject a sample diluent of 100 μL of each concentration respectively on a 96-well plate and add 50 μL of DPPH of 0.2 mM, and then shut off the light at room temperature and neglect it for 30 min. We used a microplate reader (Bio-Rad) to estimate absorbance caused by DPPH reduction in the scale of 514 nm and repeated to perform estimation three times and deduced average value and standard deviation of absorbance.

Intracellular reactive oxygen species (ROS) quantitative analysis
To estimate the changing of concentration of ROS within cells, we inoculated HDFs of 2×10^5 cells/well in a 60-mm culture medium and cultured for 24 h and afterwards we treated cells properly and then cultured for 24 h. Then we added 10 μM of dichlorofluorescein diacetate (DCF-DA; Sigma-Aldrich) which is needed to estimate ROS within cells and cultured for 30 min. Subsequently, we added phosphate buffered saline (PBS) to obtained cells and set them free; finally, we estimated amount of changing of ROS by using a flow cytometer (BD Biosciences, San Jose, CA, USA). To verify ROS scavenging effects of β-eudesmol, we also treated L-ascorbic acid which acts as an ROS scavenger, and then we estimated through the same process.

Glutathione (GSH) estimation
As an indicator for toxicity reaction inducing apoptotic and oxidative stress, GSH level change has been estimated (Esposito et al. 2000; Zhang et al. 2010; Kil et al.

Table 1 Lists of primers used in this study

Gene	Forward primer	Reverse primer
β-actin	GGATTCCTATGTGGGCGACGA	CGCTCGGTGAGGATCTTCATG
SOD1	GGGAGATGGCCCAACTACTG	CCAGTTGACATCGAACCGTT
CAT	ATGGTCCATGCTCTCAAACC	CAGGTCATCCAATAGGAAGG
TNF-α	CCCAGGGACCTCTCTCTAATC	GGTTTGCTACAACATGGGCTACA
IL-1β	GATCCATTCTCCAGCTGCA	CAACCAAGTATTCTCCATG
COL1A1	AGGGCCAAGACGAAGACATC	AGATCACGCATCGCACAACA
MMP1	GGGCTTAGATCATTCCTCAGTGCC	CAGGGTGACACCAGTGACTGCAC
TIMP1	AACCCACCCACAGACA	ACCCATGAATTTAGCCCTTA

2012). We used ThiolTracker™ Violet Glutathione Detection Reagent (Invitrogen) to estimate the amount of reduced GSH. Before pretreatment of β-eudesmol for 24 h, HDF cells were seeded as 2×10^5 cells/well in a 60-mm culture dish and cultured for 24 h. Next cells were treated 500 μM H_2O_2 and cultured for 3 h more. After we obtained cultured cells, we centrifuged them at 5000 rpm at 4 °C for 5 min to precipitate cells, and we removed supernatant and set cell pellet free through PBS of 300 μL. Then we added ThiolTracker™ Violet dye of 300 μL to cells. After blending softly, we cultured in the darkroom at room temperature for 30 min. And then, we washed cells through PBS, and in the condition of 5000 rpm at 4 °C, cells were centrifuged for 5 min and supernatant removed. Using excitation and emission at 405 and 525 nm each, a flow cytometer (BD Biosciences) was used to estimate fluorescent value.

Cellular senescence estimation

We estimated senescence by using senescence-associated beta-galactosidase (SA-β-gal) assay which is a method using a senescence detection kit (Biovision, Milpitas, CA, USA). After we inoculated HDFs of 2×10^5 cells/well in a 60-mm culture dish and cultured for 24 h, we treated cells properly and cultured for 24 h more. Then we eliminated a culture medium from the plates and washed with 1 mL PBS, and added 0.5 mL fixing solution for 15 min. Next, we added 0.5 mL mixed staining solution (staining solution 470 μL, staining supplement 5 μL, 20 mg/mL X-gal in dimethylformamide (DMF) 25 μL) to each fixed HDFs and cultured for 24 h at 37 °C. After washing dyed cells with PBS, we estimated numbers of dyed cells through an optical microscope (Olympus, Tokyo, Japan) to analyze senescent cell portion. We calculated the numbers of total cells and dyed cells and figured out the ratio of senescent cells to identify.

NF-κB luciferase assay

To identify influence of β-eudesmol on NF-κB activity, we used NF-κB promoter luciferase assay in this experiment. We used NF-κB reporter NIH-3T3 stable cell line (Panomics, Fermont, CA, USA) including reporter gene (luciferase gene) which contains NF-κB promoter consensus sequence at the promoter region. As for the promoter activity of NF-κB, the transcription factor is proportional to the amount of luciferase gene expression; therefore, through this, we identified activity of such a transcription factor as NF-κB has an influence on skin inflammatory and skin aging.

After we seeded NF-κB reporter NIH-3T3 stable cell of 2×10^5 cells/well in a 60-mm culture dish and cultured for 24 h, we treated cells in the proper condition like the above experiments, and cultured for 24 h more. Then we obtained cultured cells, added passive lysis buffer (Promega, Madison, WI, USA), on ice for 10 min to dissolve; next, we centrifuged for 30 min in the condition of 12,000 rpm at 4 °C and collected supernatant. After aliquoting 80 μL of the supernatant which contains the same amount of protein in each black 96-well plate, we added and mixed luciferin (Promega) subsequently. Because luciferin is sensitive to the light, we used a Veritas luminometer (Turner Designs, Sunnyvale, CA, USA) to estimate luminance of luciferin right after adding it to the sample.

Statistical process

All experiments of this research were performed more than three times separately under the same condition to get experimental results, and we used Student's t test for every experiment and analyzed that it is statistically significant when p value of every experimental result is less than 0.05.

Results

Cell viability

After we treated each HDF through β-eudesmol in various concentrations of 5, 10, 20, 40, and 80 μM and cultured for 24 h, we used WST-1 assay to estimate cell viability. As the result that we identified cell viability, it showed viability of 101, 107, 98, 91, and 83%, respectively. For concentration of 20 μM, it hardly had an influence on viability, and it showed that cell viability decreased at the case of treatment through β-eudesmol in their concentrations of 40 and 80 μM (Fig. 1a). After

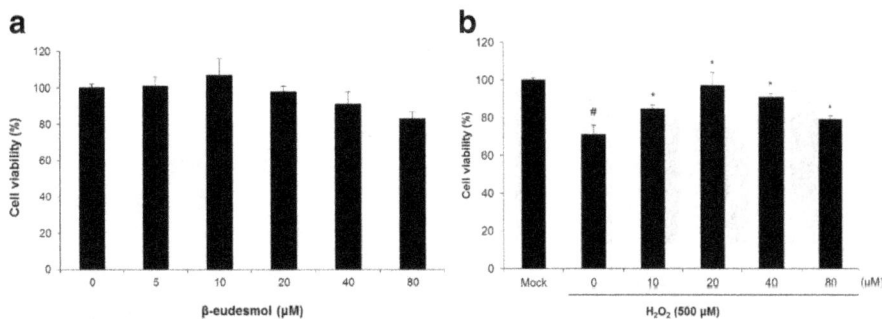

Fig. 1 Cell viability on β-eudesmol in HDFs. **a** Cytotoxicity on β-eudesmol in HDFs. **b** Cell viability on H_2O_2 in the HDFs pretreated with β-eudesmol. (*$p < 0.05$)

pretreating HDFs through β-eudesmol in concentrations of 5, 10, and 20 μM respectively for 24 h and treating with 500 μM H_2O_2 for 3 h, we made observations of cell viability. Assuming cell viability is 100%, in that case, we did not treat HDFs through both β-eudesmol and H_2O_2, cell viability decreased to 71% when we did not treat HDFs through β-eudesmol but H_2O_2 of 500 μM. However, cell viability was 85% at the case of pretreatment through β-eudesmol at 5 μM, 85% at the case of pretreatment through β-eudesmol of 10 μM, and 97% at the case of pretreatment through β-eudesmol of 20 μM; therefore, through this result, we identified that cell viability of HDFs recovered depending on concentrations. On the contrary, cell viability at the case of pretreatment through β-eudesmol of 40 and 80 μM was shown as 91 and 79% respectively; therefore, we identified that cell viability decreased in concentration more than 40 μM. So we used concentration of β-eudesmol to 20 μM at the most for HDFs in further experiments (Fig. 1b).

Antioxidative effects of β-eudesmol

Using DPPH radical scavenging activity assay, we identified radical scavenging effects of β-eudesmol. As positive control group, we performed comparative analysis on N-acetyl-L-cysteine (NAC) which is known as an ROS scavenger. At the case of treatment through β-eudesmol in concentrations of 5, 10, and 20 μM, radical scavenging effects increased to 5, 31, and 49% respectively depending on concentration. At the case of treatment through NAC as positive control group in concentrations of 5, 10, and 20 μM, we identified that radical scavenging effects are shown as 8, 25, and 46% respectively. Identified that β-eudesmol has similar radical scavenging effects with NAC, it can be admitted that β-eudesmol has positive radical scavenging effects (Fig. 2a). To identify effects of β-eudesmol on decrease of total amount of intracellular ROS which occurs in the course of cell metabolism and H_2O_2 addition, we used DCF-DA as a fluorescent probe to perform flow cytometry, and after pretreating HDFs through

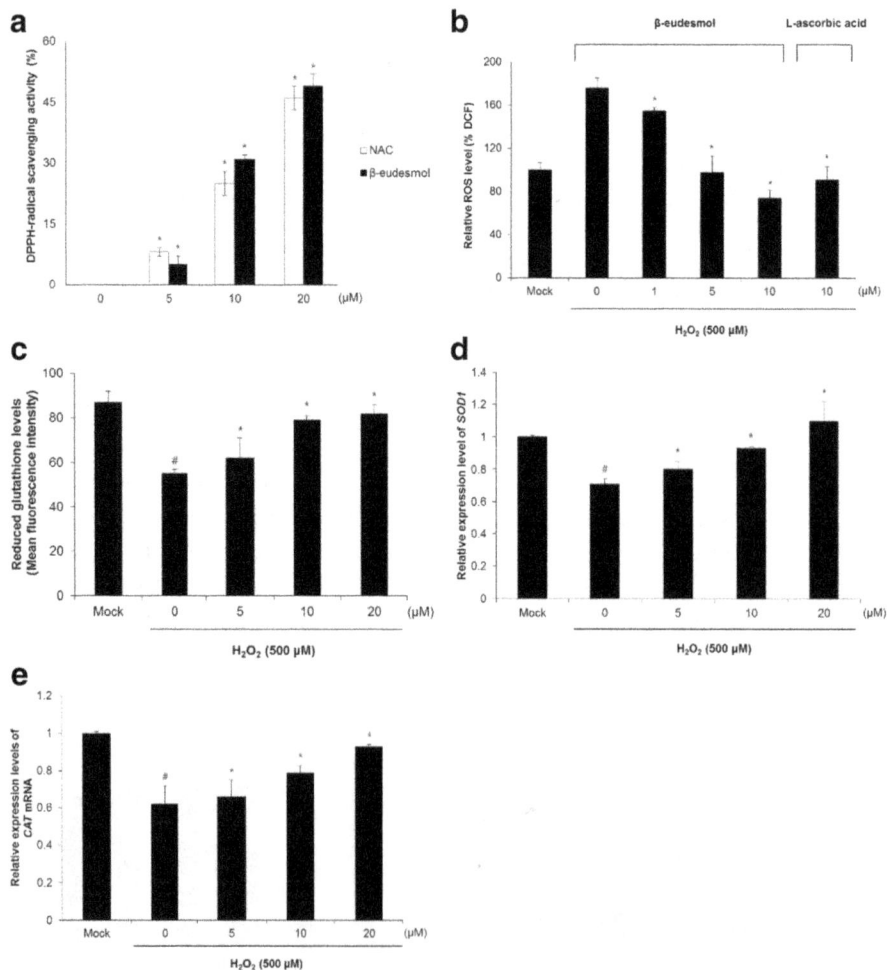

Fig. 2 Antioxidative effect of β-eudesmol against H_2O_2. **a** The DPPH radical scavenging activity of β-eudesmol. **b** H_2O_2-induced intracellular ROS scavenging activity of β-eudesmol in HDFs. **c** Reduced GSH level in HDFs with pretreated β-eudesmol before H_2O_2 treatment. **d** SOD1 and **e** CAT mRNA gene expression analysis in HDFs with β-eudesmol over H_2O_2 treatment. (*$p < 0.05$)

β-eudesmol for 24 h, we treated HDFs through H_2O_2 of 500 μM. Its results which we analyzed after 3 h are as follows: Assuming it is 100%, in that case, we did not treat HDFs through both β-eudesmol and H_2O_2, total amount of ROS increased to 176% at the case of treatment through H_2O_2. However, at the case of treatment through β-eudesmol in each concentration of 1, 5, and 10 μM, it was identified that the total amount of ROS decreases to 155, 98, and 74% respectively. At the case of L-ascorbic acid as the positive control group, total amount of ROS was shown as 91% when we treated in concentration of 10 μM. This result is similar to the case of treatment through β-eudesmol in concentration of 5 μM; therefore, we identified that β-eudesmol has an effect on decrease of total amount of intracellular ROS (Fig. 2b). Using the principle that ROS lowers intracellular GSH level through oxidative reaction or reaction to thiol group, we used Violet dye which reacts to thiol group to identify the glutathione level reduced form. As for the result that we pretreated HDFs through β-eudesmol for 24 h and then treated through H_2O_2 of 500 μM and analyzed 3 h later, when we treated nothing, GSH level was shown as 87, but at the case of treatment through H_2O_2, it decreases to 55. However, at the case of pretreatment through β-eudesmol in each concentration of 5, 10, and 20 μM, GSH level increased to 62, 79, and 82 respectively; therefore, we identified that both results were similar to each other and GSH levels recovered at the same level (Fig. 2c). To identify antioxidation effects of β-eudesmol at a gene level, we identified changing of antioxidation enzyme *SOD1* gene expression through qRT-PCR. Assuming *SOD1* gene expression level is 1 at the case of no treatment for both β-eudesmol and H_2O_2, *SOD1* gene expression decreased to 0.71 at the case of treatment through H_2O_2. However, when we pretreated through β-eudesmol in each concentration of 5, 10, and 20 μM for 24 h, treated through H_2O_2, and then analyzed 3 h later, *SOD1* gene expression increased to 0.8, 0.93, and 1.1 respectively. Through this result, we were able to identify that β-eudesmol increased *SOD1* gene expression to have an influence on antioxidation effects in this experiment (Fig. 2d). Catalase (CAT) as the antioxidation enzyme has a role as catalyst to react to intracellular H_2O_2 and extinct radical to change into H_2O. To identify antioxidation effects of β-eudesmol, we checked changing of catalase gene, *CAT* expression. Assuming *CAT* gene expression level is 1 at the case of no treatment through both β-eudesmol and H_2O_2, *CAT* gene expression decreased to 0.62 at the case of treatment through H_2O_2. However, when we pretreated through β-eudesmol in each concentration of 5, 10, and 20 μM and then treated through H_2O_2, *CAT* gene expression increased to 0.66, 0.79, and 0.93 respectively as per a dose-dependent manner of β-eudesmol. Through this result, we identified that β-eudesmol increased *CAT* gene expression to have intracellular antioxidation effects (Fig. 2e).

Anti-inflammatory effects of β-eudesmol

Through NF-κB luciferase assay, we identified promoter activity of NF-κB, the transcription factor. We used NIH-3T3 stable cell line including luciferase gene which contains NF-κB promoter consensus sequence in the field of promoter, added luciferin which reacts to luciferase to form fluorescer, and estimated the amount of luciferase gene expression through luciferin luminance estimation. When we treated through H_2O_2, luminance of luciferin increased to 7.9 times compared with control group which were non-treated with HDFs, but when we treated through H_2O_2 after pretreating β-eudesmol in a concentration of 5 μM, it decreased to 5.7 times. At the case of pretreatment through β-eudesmol in a concentration of 10 μM and treatment through H_2O_2, it decreased to 3.1 times; at the case of pretreatment through β-eudesmol in a concentration of 20 μM and treatment through H_2O_2, it decreased to 2.8 times; therefore, we identified that luciferin luminance decreased depending on the concentration of β-eudesmol. Therefore, we identified that β-eudesmol hindered transcriptional activity of NF-κB (Fig. 3a). We checked changing of *IL-1β* gene expression which is related to early inflammation reaction. *IL-1β* gene expression increased to 9.2 times when we treated through H_2O_2 than when we did not treat through both β-eudesmol and H_2O_2. However, when we pretreated through β-eudesmol in a concentration of 5 μM and then treated through H_2O_2, the amount of *IL-1β* gene expression depending on concentrations of β-eudesmol decreased to 7.3 times. At the case of pretreatment through β-eudesmol in a concentration of 10 μM and treatment through H_2O_2, it decreased to 3.1 times; at the case of pretreatment through β-eudesmol in a concentration of 20 μM and treatment through H_2O_2, it decreased to 2.4 times (Fig. 3b). Subsequently, after we pretreated HDFs through β-eudesmol in each concentration for 24 h and treated through H_2O_2 for 3 h, we analyzed changing of *TNF-α* gene expression. When we treated HDFs through H_2O_2, it increased to 6.6 times comparing with the control group which we did not treat through both β-eudesmol and H_2O_2. However, when we pretreated through β-eudesmol in a concentration of 5 μM for 24 h and then treated through H_2O_2, the amount of *TNF-α* gene expression depending on concentration of β-eudesmol decreased to 4.9 times; at the case of pretreatment through β-eudesmol in concentration of 10 μM for 24 h and treatment through H_2O_2, it decreased to 3.1 times; and at the case of pretreatment through β-eudesmol in concentration of 20 μM for 24 h and treatment through H_2O_2, it decreased to 2.3 times (Fig. 3c).

Cellular senescence and extracellular matrix (ECM) modulation gene expression analysis of β-eudesmol

SA β-gal assay is particularly observed in senescent cells and is largely used as an indicator of senescence (Dimri et al. 1995). When we did not treat HDFs through both

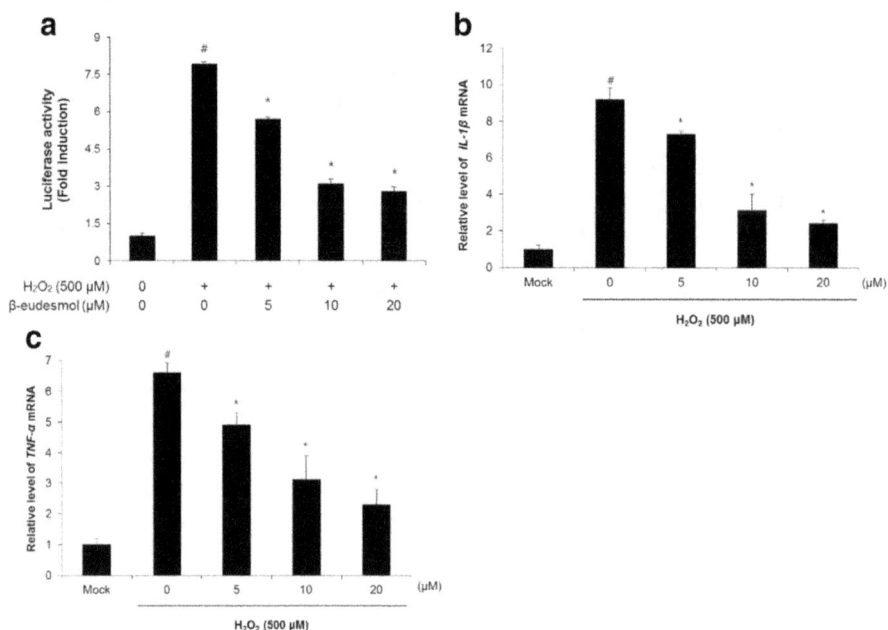

Fig. 3 Anti-inflammatory effect of β-eudesmol against H_2O_2 in HDFs. **a** Analysis of NF-κB promoter luciferase activity on H_2O_2-treated HDFs, pretreated with β-eudesmol. **b** *IL-1β* and **c** *TNF-α* mRNA gene expression levels on H_2O_2 HDFs, pretreated with β-eudesmol. Gene expression was evaluated using qRT-PCR with the $2^{-\Delta\Delta Ct}$ method and data presented were normalized to β-actin. (*$p < 0.05$)

β-eudesmol and H_2O_2, β-galactosidase activity was shown as 6, and at the case of treatment through H_2O_2, it increased to 69-folds. However, when we pretreated through β-eudesmol in a concentration of 5 μM for 24 h and then treated through H_2O_2, β-galactosidase activity depending on concentration of β-eudesmol decreased and was shown as 51; at the case of pretreatment through β-eudesmol in a concentration of 10 μM for 24 h and treatment through H_2O_2, it was shown as 27; and at the case of pretreatment through β-eudesmol in a concentration of 20 μM for 24 h and treatment through H_2O_2, it was shown as 18 (Fig. 4a). We used qRT-PCR method to identify changing of *COL1A1* gene expression which forms type I collagen constituting 80 to 85% of collagen. The relative *COL1A1* gene expression decreased to 0.39 at the case of treatment of H_2O_2 compared with non-treated cells. However, we identified that *COL1A1* gene expression increases depending on concentration of β-eudesmol, as the result that at the case of pretreatment through β-eudesmol in a concentration of 5 μM and treatment through H_2O_2, it was shown as 0.54; at the case of pretreatment through β-eudesmol in a concentration of 10 μM and treatment through H_2O_2, it was shown as 0.72; and at the case of pretreatment through β-eudesmol in a concentration of 20 μM and treatment through H_2O_2, it was shown as 0.88 (Fig. 4c). To identify changing of *MMP1* gene expression which decomposes type I collagen constituting most of dermis, we used qRT-PCR method to identify influence of β-

eudesmol on dermal tissue. When we did not treat HDFs through both β-eudesmol and H_2O_2, *MMP1* gene expression was 0.51, and *MMP1* gene expression was doubled to be shown as 1 at the case of treatment through H_2O_2. However, we identified that *MMP1* gene expression decreases depending on concentration, as the result that at the case of pretreatment through β-eudesmol in a concentration of 5 μM and treatment through H_2O_2, it was 0.84; at the case of pretreatment through β-eudesmol in a concentration of 10 μM and treatment through H_2O_2, it was 0.69; and at the case of pretreatment through β-eudesmol in a concentration of 20 μM and treatment through H_2O_2, it was 0.58. Particularly, *MMP1* gene expression at the case of treatment through β-eudesmol in a concentration of 20 μM was similar to the result at the case of no treatment (Fig. 4c). We identified changing of *TIMP1* (Fisher Jr and Zheng 1996; Enjoji et al. 2000) gene expression which is a hindrance factor to MMP1 and MMP9 to identify its influence on collagen metabolism. Assuming *TIMP1* gene expression is 1 when we did not treat HDFs through both β-eudesmol and H_2O_2, *TIMP1* gene expression decreased to 0.3 sharply at the case of treatment through H_2O_2. However, when we pretreated through β-eudesmol in a concentration of 5 μM and then treated though H_2O_2, *TIMP1* gene expression depending on concentration increased to be shown as 0.35; at the case of pretreatment through β-eudesmol in a concentration of 10 μM and treatment through H_2O_2, it

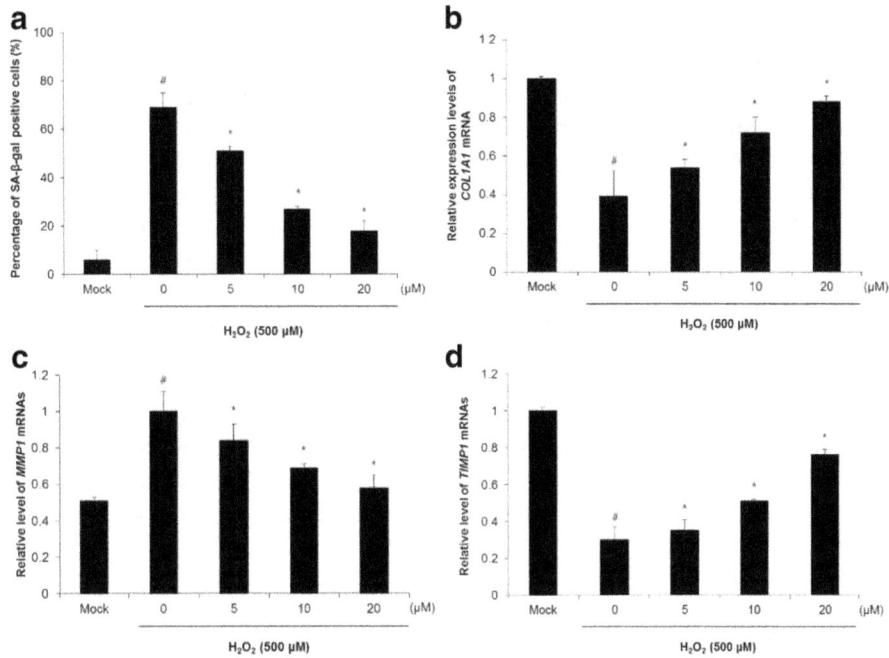

Fig. 4 Senescence attenuation effect of β-eudesmol against H_2O_2 in HDFs. **a** Protective effect of β-eudesmol on H_2O_2-induced cellular senescence in HDFs using SA-β-gal assay. **b** *COL1A1*, **c** *MMP1*, and **d** *TIMP1* mRNA gene expression levels on H_2O_2-treated HDFs, pretreated with β-eudesmol. Gene expression was evaluated using qRT-PCR with the $2^{-\Delta\Delta Ct}$ method and data presented were normalized to β-actin. (*$p < 0.05$)

was 0.51; and at the case of pretreatment through β-eudesmol in a concentration of 20 μM and treatment through H_2O_2, it was 0.76 (Fig. 4d).

Discussion

Antioxidation effects of β-eudesmol

When human skin is under oxidative stress caused by ROS, DNA, lipid, and protein damage can occur (Devasagayam and Kamat 2002). When intracellular ROS increases, through various intracellular signal transmission processes, it hinders collagen synthesis and promotes MMP expression which is an enzyme to decompose collagen to accelerate causing wrinkles and skin aging (Lavker and Kaidbey 1997). Also oxidative stress is deeply related to not only skin aging but also inflammation reaction so that it has an influence on controlling activity of various kinds of cells. If inflammation reaction is not controlled well, sometimes it will lead to a reaction to accelerate senescence (De Martinis et al. 2005).

To minimize damage caused by ROS, our body uses antioxidation enzymes such as SOD, CAT, and glutathione peroxidase (GPX) which are our defense mechanisms or methods to supply antioxidation substances such as vitamin (Vit) C, Vit E, and ubiquinone into our body, and research on development of antioxidation substances has been in progress continuously (Choi et al. 2007). In this research, we used β-eudesmol to apply to HDFs and identified its possibility as an antioxidant suitable for skin.

Through experimental methods such as DPPH radical activity assay, ROS quantitative analysis using DCF-DA, GSH estimation, *SOD1* gene expression, and *CAT* gene expression, we verified antioxidation effects of β-eudesmol. As the result of experiment through DPPH radical activity assay, we identified that radical extinction effects increase depending on concentration of β-eudesmol and that similar radical extinction effects appear comparing the case of N-acetyl-L-cysteine, the positive control group; therefore, we identified there were radical extinction effects. Although we identified antioxidation effects of β-eudesmol sample through DPPH radical activity assay, we also identified intracellular antioxidation effects through ROS quantitative analysis using DCF-DA and GHS estimation. The total amount of intracellular ROS in HDFs decreased depending on concentration of β-eudesmol, and particularly at the case of treatment through β-eudesmol in a concentration of 5 μM, it showed a similar result to a positive control group which we treated through L-ascorbic acid used as antioxidation effect marker in a concentration of 10 μM; therefore, it was considered that β-eudesmol had an effect to remove ROS. To identify effects of β-eudesmol to extinct intracellular H_2O_2 and hinder OH^- radical formation, we used a GSH measurement analysis method. As an indicator of toxicity reaction which induces apoptotic effect and oxidative stress, changing of GSH level has been estimated (Esposito et al. 2000; Zhang et al.

2010; Kil et al. 2012). It was identified that GSH level increased in accordance with an increase in concentration of β-eudesmol.

When human skin is under oxidative stress, signal transmission system is activated, in which cells react, increase radical formation, and decrease antioxidation enzyme expression (Masaki et al. 1995; Barber et al. 1998; Yasui and Sakurai 2000; Yamamoto and Gaynor 2001). To verify antioxidation effects of β-eudesmol at the gene level, we identified changing of antioxidation enzyme *SOD1* and *CAT* gene expression. It was identified that *SOD1* and *CAT* gene expression increased depending on concentration of β-eudesmol. Based on the above results, it was identified that β-eudesmol had not only antioxidation effects mediated with biological enzymes but also radical extinction effects with various methods. β-eudesmol sample itself had antioxidation effects and terminated intracellular ROS effectively. Also it was identified that it decreased antioxidation enzyme expression which is a ROS defense mechanism and controls ROS from the gene level to extinct ROS. Therefore, it was considered that β-eudesmol had hindrance effects to various damages and stimulations caused by oxidative stress on human skin (Fig. 5).

Anti-inflammation effects of β-eudesmol by controlling NF-κB promoter activity

NF-κB is the named transcription factor whose role is identified to be concerned with controlling immunoglobulin kappa chain gene expression in B cells (Sen and Baltimore 1986). Through classical pathway and alternative pathway, NF-κB has a decisive role of inflammation reaction, immune reaction, cell proliferation, and apoptotic effects in various processes, and it has been identified as a survival factor in various cells against lipopolysaccharide (LPS), cytokine, ROS, and stimulation by ultraviolet (UV) rays (Baeuerle and Henkel 1994; Siebenlist et al. 1994; Kopp and Ghosh 1995; Ghosh et al. 1998; Karin and Delhase 2000). NF-κB is composed of homo or hetero-dimer and formed with five subunits

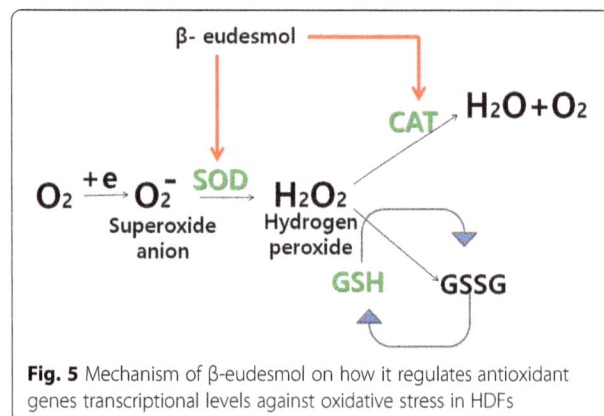

Fig. 5 Mechanism of β-eudesmol on how it regulates antioxidant genes transcriptional levels against oxidative stress in HDFs

such as p65 (RelA), RelB, c-Rel, p50 (NF-κB 1), and p52 (NF-κB 2) (Gilmore 2006). NF-κB is combined with inhibitor of NF-κB (IκB) to exist in the cytoplasm with its state of deactivation, but IκB kinase (IKK) is activated through stimulation of UV rays or ROS on cells and phosphorylates IκB to be separated. Phosphorylated IκB is decomposed by ubiquitination and separated from proteasome, and NF-κB flows into the nucleus and works as a transcription factor (Ghosh and Karin 2002; He and Karin 2011). TNF-α, IL, and chemokine, which are a product of inflammatory precursor, have a role to mediate an important course of cell activities such as cell proliferation, angiogenesis, and metastasis. Transcription of gene expression within which these molecules are coded is controlled by NF-κB (Gloire et al. 2006). Through intracellular signal transmission, NF-κB controls various cell metabolism, but in that case, it works as transcription factor of inflammation-mediated substances and it promotes transcription of COX2, E-selectin, inducible nitric oxide synthase (iNOS), intercellular adhesion molecule-1 (ICAM-1), IL-6, IL-12, IL-1β, MMP, TNF-α, and vascular cell adhesion molecular 1 (VCAM-1) to accelerate inflammation reaction and cause tissue damage (Limuro et al. 1997; Bukman et al. 1998; Chen et al. 1999; Suschek et al. 2004; Yamamoto and Gaynor 2001; Farooqui et al. 2007).

To identify that influence of β-eudesmol on control of NF-κB activity which has a significant role in inflammation reaction, we used NF-κB luciferase assay method to identify NF-κB activity, and it was found that NF-κB activity decreased depending on concentration of β-eudesmol. In this experiment, we examined effects to hinder NF-κB, and also, we checked changing of downstream gene expression which increases through NF-κB activation. Through a qRT-PCR method, we checked changing of gene expression of cytokine IL-1β, TNF-α (Fisher Jr and Zheng 1996; Dinarello 1991) which is a representative medium of early inflammation reaction. It was identified that *IL-1β*, *TNF-α* inflammation induction gene expression decreased as concentration of β-eudesmol increases. Through this experiment, we identified that β-eudesmol shut off the NF-κB pathway to hinder *IL-1β*, *TNF-α* gene expression and inflammation reaction.

Regulation mechanism of ECM gene expression of β-eudesmol

Increase in ROS within dermal tissue has an influence on intracellular transforming growth factor-beta (TGF-β) cytokine, activator protein 1 (AP-1) transcription factor, NF-κB transcription factor, and signal transmission pathway of Smad3/4; controls collagen formation gene expression; and increases gene expression of MMPs which is an enzyme-decomposing collagen so that it causes changing of ECM tissue and skin aging (Lee et al.

2012; Varani et al. 2002; Saito et al. 2004). AP-1, NF-κB, and Smad from increase in ROS are activated by MAPK which works as an intracellular signal transmission factor. MAP-kinase p38, JNK, and extracellular signal-regulated kinase (ERK) exist in MAPK, and MAPK is concerned with various intracellular mechanisms such as cell growth, division, apoptosis, and gene expression (Kohl et al. 2011). When MAPK is activated by ROS, it activates NF-κB to increase *MMP* gene expression and induce collagen decomposition (Lee et al. 2012; Bae et al. 2008). Moreover, it induces AP-1 activation, enters into cell nucleus, works as transcription factor to promote *MMP1*, *MMP3*, and *MMP9* gene expression, and hinders *COL1A1* gene expression (Quan et al. 2005; Lee et al. 2006). Increase in ROS causes hindering TGF-β which is a bifidus factor to control transcription activity of Smad (Leivonen and Kähäri 2007). Collagen gene expression which is one of their downstream genes is regulated and it induces collapse of ECM tissue within dermis to cause wrinkle, loss of elasticity, and skin aging (Quan et al. 2005). Within the dermis, TIMP which is an enzyme-hindering MMP activity, exists and with MMPs forms one to one complex to hinder MMP enzyme, and there are TIMP1, TIMP2, TIMP3, and TIMP4 as kinds of TIMP (Gomis-Rüth et al. 1997). MMP1 and MMP9 are enzymes which decompose type I collagen constituting 85% of collagen in the dermis, and it is TIMP1 enzyme which hinders MMP1 and MMP9 (Enjoji et al. 2000; Fisher et al. 1999). With its complicated mechanism, TIMPs control MMP activity, and when the balance between them is lost, it sometimes leads to tumor, and it has been reported that its gene expression increases through epidermal growth factor (EGF), TNF-α, IL-1, and TGF-β (Birkedal-Hansen 1993; Lee et al. 2016; Jang and Lee 2016).

Through changing of signal transmission process and gene expression of β-eudesmol in ECM, we identified its effects on human dermal fibroblast preservation and cell activation. Through experimental results, we identified that it controlled NF-κB activity, and we checked changing of *COL1A1*, *MMP1* gene expression which are downstream genes of NF-κB. *COL1A1* gene expression increased as concentration of β-eudesmol increased, and *MMP1* gene expression decreased depending on the concentration of β-eudesmol. We identified that *TIMP1* gene expression which hindered MMP1 increases depending on the concentration of β-eudesmol. Taking these experimental results together, it is identified that β-eudesmol shuts off the NF-κB pathway to regulate *MMP1* gene expression and that *COL1A1* gene expression increases as the concentration of β-eudesmol increases. According to existing researches related to *COL1A1* gene expression, when AP-1 is activated by ROS, it promotes *MMP1*, *MMP3*, and *MMP9* gene

expression and hinders *COL1A1* gene expression (Quan et al. 2005; Lee et al. 2006). Also, it has been reported that ROS hinders a bifidus factor such as TGF-β to regulate transcription activity of Smad (Leivonen and Kähäri 2007) and control collagen gene expression which is a downstream gene (Quan et al. 2005). Therefore, it is considered that by β-eudesmol, AP-1 activity is hindered to regulate *MMP1*, *MMP3*, and *MMP9* gene expression, that β-eudesmol increases *COL1A1* gene expression and activates TGF-β, and that *COL1A1* gene expression increases through transcription activity of Smad. Through this experimental result, it is considered that β-eudesmol preserves tissue within the dermis and has effects to promote ECM formation to protect dermal cells. It has been identified that β-eudesmol has effects on cell preservation within the dermis at the gene level, but to find out whether this result proves effects to regulate cell senescence actually, through SA-β-gal assay experimental method, we identified human dermal fibroblast cell senescence. As for the experimental result of SA-β-gal assay, β-galactosidase activity decreased depending on concentration of β-eudesmol. Namely, it is found that β-eudesmol has effects to regulate cell senescence. Therefore, it is considered that β-eudesmol is highly useful as a cosmetic compound because it has antioxidation and anti-inflammation effects, delays dermal cell senescence, and has cell preservation effects (Fig. 6).

Conclusions

In conclusion, the present study showed that β-eudesmol has several effects on anti-inflammatory and ECM constructed gene expression in human dermal fibroblasts. Our results represented the antioxidant effect of β-eudesmol through improving intracellular antioxidant molecule and gene expressions, scavenging excessive generated ROS, and

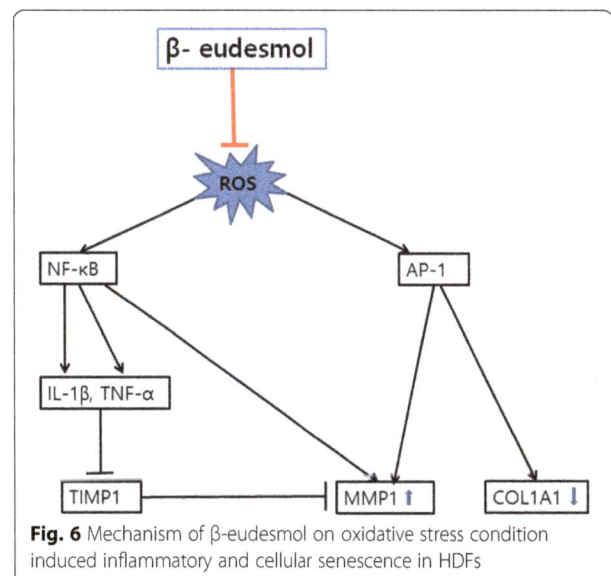

Fig. 6 Mechanism of β-eudesmol on oxidative stress condition induced inflammatory and cellular senescence in HDFs

radical scavenging capacity. Based on the above antioxidant results, we identified protective effect of β-eudesmol on NF-κB-mediated inflammatory signaling activities. These preliminary results provided an interesting point in HDF: β-eudesmol may have impediment action to aging. Thus, SA-β-gal assay and ECM-related gene expression analysis were conducted, which suggested effective senescence-hindering capacity of β-eudesmol in dermal fibroblast cells. Additional further studies, in vitro and in vivo, will be necessary to verify molecular pathways and mechanisms of β-eudesmol in detail, but this study suggests β-eudesmol as a "cosmeceutical" compound.

Abbreviations

AP-1: Activator protein 1; CAT: Catalase; COL1A1: Collagen, type I, alpha 1; DCF-DA: 2',7'-Dichlorofluorescin diacetate; DEPC: Diethylpyrocarbonate; DMEM: Dulbecco's modified Eagle's medium; DMF: Dimethylformamide; DMSO: Dimethyl sulfoxide; DPPH: 2,2-Diphenyl-1-picrylhydrazyl; ECM: Extracellular matrix; EGF: Epidermal growth factor; ERK: Extracellular signal-regulated kinase; FBS: Fetal bovine serum; GPX: Glutathione peroxidase; GSH: Glutathione; HDF: Human dermal fibroblast; ICAM-1: Intercellular adhesion molecule-1; IKK: IκB kinase; IL-12: Interleukin 12; IL-1β: Interleukin 1 beta; IL-6: Interleukin 6; iNOS: Inducible nitric oxide synthase; JNK: c-Jun N-terminal kinases; LPS: Lipopolysaccharide; MAPK: Mitogen-activated protein kinase; MMP: Matrix metalloproteinase; NAC: N-Acetyl-L-cysteine; NF-κB: Nuclear factor-kappa B; PC12: Pheochromocytoma; PBS: Phosphate buffered saline; qRT-PCR: Quantitative real-time polymerase chain reaction; ROS: Reactive oxygen species; SA-β-gal: Senescence-associated beta-galactosidase; SOD1: Superoxide dismutase 1; TIMP1: Tissue inhibitors of metalloproteinases-1; TNF-α: Tumor necrosis factor-alpha; TGF-β: Growth factor-beta; WST-1: Water-soluble tetrazolium salt; VCAM-1: Vascular cell adhesion molecular 1; Vit C: Vitamin C

Acknowledgements

The author thanks all the study subjects and research staff who participated in this work.

Funding

Not applicable

Author's contributions

KYK did all of research background such as experiments, data collecting, and statistical analysis as well as drafting the manuscript.

Competing interests

The author declares no competing interests.

References

Bae JY, Choi JS, Choi y, Shin SY, Kang SW, Han SJ, Kang YH. (−)Epigallocatechin gallate hampers collagen destruction and collagenase activation in ultraviolet-B-irradiated human dermal fibroblasts: involvement of mitogen-activated protein kinase. Food Chem Toxicol. 2008;46:1298–307.

Baeuerle PA, Henkel T. Function and activation of NF-kappa B in the immune system. Annu Rev Immunol. 1994;12:141–79.

Barber LA, Spandau DF, Rathman SC, Murphy RC, Johnson CA, Kelley SW, et al. Expression of the platelet-activating receptor results in enhanced ultraviolet B radiation-induced apoptosis in a human epidermal cell line. J Biol Chem. 1998;273:18891–7.

Birkedal-Hansen H. Role of matrix metalloproteinases in human periodontal disease. J Periodontol. 1993;64(Suppl 5):474–84.

Bukman SY, Gresham A, Hale P, Hruze G, Anast J, Masferrer J, et al. COX-2 expression is induced by UVB exposure in human skin: implications for the development of skin cancer. Carcinogenesis. 1998;19:723–9.

Chen F, Castranova V, Shi X, Demers LM. New insights into the role of nuclear factor-kappa B, a ubiquitous transcription factor in the initiation of diseases. Clin Chem. 1999;45:7–17.

Chiou LC, Chang CC. Antagonism by β-eudesmol of neostigmine-induced neuromuscular failure in mouse diaphragms. Eur J Pharmacol. 1992;216:199–206.

Chiou LC, Ling JY, Chang CC. β-Eudesmol as an antidote for intoxication from organophosphorus anticholinesterase agents. Eur J Pharmacol. 1995;292:151–6.

Chiou LC, Ling JY, Chang CC. Chinese herbs constituent β-eudesmol alleviated the electroshock seizures in mice and electrographic seizures in rat hippocampal slices. Neurosci Lett. 1997;231:171–4.

Choi CW, Jung HA, Kang SS, Choi JS. Antioxidant constituents and a new triterpenoid glycoside from Flos Lonicerae. Arch Parm Res. 2007;30:1–7.

De Martinis M, Franceschi C, Monti D, Ginaldi L. Inflamma-ageing and lifelong antigenic load as major determinants of ageing rate and longevity. FEBS Lett. 2005;579:2035–9.

Devasagayam TP, Kamat JP. Biological significance of singlet oxygen. Indian J Exp Biol. 2002;40:680–92.

Dimri GP, Lee X, Basile G, Acosta M, Scott G, Roskelley C, et al. A biomarker that identifies senescent human cells in culture and in aging skin in vivo. Proc Natl Acad Sci U S A. 1995;92:9363–7.

Dinarello CA. The proinflammatory cytokines interleukin-1 and tumor necrosis factor and treatment of the septic shock syndrome. J Infect Dis. 1991;163:1177–84.

Enjoji M, Kotoh K, Iwamoto H, Nakamuta M, Nawata H. Self-regulation of type I collagen degradation by collagen-induced production of matrix metalloproteinase-1 on cholangiocarcinoma and hepatocellular carcinoma cells. In Vitro Cell Dev Biol Anim. 2000;36:71–3.

Esposito LA, Kokoszka JE, Waymire KG, Cottrell B, MacGregor GR, Wallace DC. Mitochondrial oxidative stress in mice lacking the glutathione peroxidase-1 gene. Free Radic Biol Med. 2000;28:754–66.

Farooqui AA, Horrocks LA, Farooqui T. Modulation of inflammation in the brain; a matter of fat. J Neurochem. 2007;101:577–99.

Fisher GJ, Talwar HS, Voorhees JJ. Molecular mechanism of photoaging in human skin in vivo and their prevention by all trans retinoic acid. Photochem Photobiol. 1999;69:154–7.

Fisher CJ Jr, Zheng Y. Potential strategies for inflammatory mediator manipulation: retrospect and prospect. World J Surg. 1996;20:447–53.

Ghosh S, Karin M. Missing pieces in the NF-κB puzzle. Cell. 2002;109(Suppl 1):S81–96.

Ghosh S, May MJ, Kopp EB. NF-κB and Rel proteins: evolutionarily conserved mediators of immune responses. Annu Rev Immunol. 1998;16:255–60.

Gilmore TD. Introduction to NFkappaB: players, pathways, perspectives. Oncogene. 2006;25:6680–4.

Gloire G, Legrand-Poels S, Piette J. NF-κB activation by reactive oxygen species: fifteen years later. Biochem Pharmacol. 2006;72:1493–505.

Gomis-Rüth FX, Maskos K, Betz M, Bergner A, Huber R, Suzuki K, et al. Mechanism of inhibition of the human matrix metalloproteinase stromelysin-1 by TIMP-1. Nature. 1997;389:77–81.

He G, Karin M. NF-κB and STAT3 - key players in liver inflammation and cancer. Cell Res. 2011;21:159–68.

Hoang DM, Trung TN, He L, Ha DT, Lee MS, Kim BY. Eudesmols induce apoptosis through release of cytochrome c in HL-60 cells. Nat Prod Sci. 2010;16:88–92.

Ikeda K, Nagase H. Magnolol has the ability to induce apoptosis in tumor cells. Biol Pharm Bull. 2002;25:1546–9.

Jang HH, Lee SN. Epidermal skin barrier. Asian J Beauty Cosmetol. 2016;14:339–47.

Karin M, Delhase M. The IκB kinase (IKK) and NF-κB: key elements of proinflammatory signalling. Semin Immunol. 2000;12:85–98.

Kil IS, Lee SK, Ryu KW, Woo HA, Hu MC, Bae SH, et al. Feedback control of adrenal steroidogenesis via H_2O_2-dependent, reversible inactivation of peroxiredoxin III in mitochondria. Mol Cell. 2012;46:584–94.

Kimura M, Kimura I, Kondoh T, Tsuneki H. Noncontractile acetylcholine receptor-operated ca++ mobilization: suppression of activation by open channel blockers and acceleration of desensitization by closed channel blockers in mouse diaphragm muscle. J Pharmacol Exp Ther. 1991;256:18–23.

Kohl E, Steinbauer J, Landthaler M, Szeimies RM. Skin ageing. J Eur Acade Dermatol Venereol. 2011;25:873–84.

Kopp EB, Ghosh S. NF-κB and rel proteins in innate immunity. Adv Immunol. 1995;58:1–27.

Lavker R, Kaidbey K. The spectral dependence for UVA-induced cumulative damage in human skin. J Invest Dermatol. 1997;108:17–21.

Lee J, Jung E, Lee J, Huh S, Hwang CH, Lee HY, et al. Emodin inhibits TNF alpha-induced MMP-1 expression through suppression of activator protein-1 (AP-1). Life Sci. 2006;79:2480–5.

Lee S, Han HS, An IS, Ahn KJ. Effects of amentoflavone on anti-inflammation and cytoprotection. Asian J Beauty Cosmetol. 2016;14:201–11.

Lee YR, Noh EM, Han JH, Kim JM, Hwang BM, Cung EY, et al. Brazilin inhibits UVB-induced MMP-1/3 expressions and secretions by suppressing the NF-κB pathway in human dermal fibroblast. Eur J Pharmacol. 2012;674:80–6.

Leivonen SK, Kähäri VM. Transforming growth factor-β signaling in cancer invasion and metastasis. Int J Cancer. 2007;121:2119–24.

Li Y, Li T, Miao C, Li J, Xiao W, Ma E. β-Eudesmol induces JNK-dependent apoptosis through the mitochondrial pathway in HL60 cells. Phytother Res. 2013;27:338–43.

Lim DY, Kee YW. Infuence of β-eudesmol on blood pressure. Nat Prod Sci. 2005; 11:33–40.

Limuro Y, Gallucci RM, Luster MI, Kono H, Thurman RG. Antibodies to tumor necrosis factor alfa attenuate hepatic necrosis and inflammation caused by chronic exposure to ethanol in the rat. Hepatology. 1997;26:1530–7.

Ma EL, Li YC, Tsuneki H, Xiao JF, Xia MY, Wang MW, et al. β-Eudesmol suppresses tumour growth through inhibition of tumour neovascularisation and tumour cell proliferation. J Asian Nat Prod Res. 2008;10:159–68.

Masaki H, Atsumi T, Sakurai H. Detection of hydrogen peroxide and hydroxyl radicals in murine skin fibroblasts under UVB irradiation. Biochem Biophys Res Commun. 1995;206:474–9.

Miyazawa M, Shimamura H, Nakamura SI, Kameoka H. Antimutagenic activity of (+)-β-eudesmol and paeonol from *Dioscorea japonica*. J Agric Food Chem. 1996;44:1647–50.

Obara Y, Aoki T, Kusano M, Ohizumi Y. β-Eudesmol induces neurite outgrowth in rat pheochromocytoma cells accompanied by an activation of mitogen activated protein kinase. J Pharmacol Exp Ther. 2002;301:803–11.

Plengsuriyakarn T, Karbwang J, Na-Bangchang K. Anticancer activity using positron emission tomography-computed tomography and pharmacokinetics of β-eudesmol in human cholangiocarcinoma xenografted nude mouse model. Clin Exp Pharmacol Physiol. 2015;42:293–304.

Quan T, He T, Voorhees JJ, Fisher GJ. Ultraviolet irradiation induces Smad7 via induction of transcription factor AP-1 in human skin fibroblasts. J Biol Chem. 2005;280:8079–85.

Saito Y, Shiga A, Yoshida Y, Furuhashi T, Fujita Y, Niki E. Effects of a novel gaseous antioxidative system containing a rosemary extract on the oxidation induced by nitrogen dioxide and ultraviolet radiation. Biosci Biotechnol Biochem. 2004;68:781–6.

Satoh K, Nagai F, Ushiyama K, Yasuda I, Akiyama K, Kano I. Inhibition of Na+, K(+)-ATPase activity by β-eudesmol, a major component of atractylodis lanceae rhizoma, due to the interaction with enzyme in the Na.E1 state. Biochem Pharmacol. 1992;44:373–8.

Sen R, Baltimore D. Multiple nuclear factors interact with the immunoglobulin enhancer sequences. Cell. 1986;46:705–16.

Seo MJ, Kim SJ, Kang TH, Rim HK, Jeong HJ, Um JY. The regulatory mechanism of β-eudesmol is through the suppression of caspase-1 activation in mast cell-mediated inflammatory response. Immunopharm Immunot. 2011;33:178–85.

Siebenlist U, Franzoso G, Brown K. Structure, regulation and function of NF-κB. Annu Rev Cell Biol. 1994;10:405–55.

Suschek CV, Mahotka C, Schnorr o, Kolb-Bachofen V. UVB radiation-mediated expression of inducible nitric oxide synthase activity and the augmenting role of co-induced TNF-alpha in human skin endothelial cells. J Invest Dermatol. 2004;123:950–7.

Varani J, Perone P, Fligiel SE, Fisher GJ, Voorhees JJ. Inhibition of type I procollagen production in photodamage: corrclation between presence of high molecular weight collagen fragments and reduced procollagen synthesis. J Invest Dermatol. 2002;119:122–9.

Watanabe K, Goto Y, Yoshitomi K. Central depressant effects of the extracts of magnolia cortex. Chem Pham Bull. 1973;21:1700–8.

Watanabe K, Watanabe H, Goto Y, Yamaguchi N, Yamamoto N, Hagino K. Pharrmacologocal properties of magnolol and honokiol extracted from Magnolia officinalis: central depressant effects. Planta Med. 1983;49:103–8.

Yamamoto Y, Gaynor RB. Therapeutic potential of inhibition of the NF- κB pathway in the treatment of inflammation and cancer. J Clin Invest. 2001; 107:135–42.

Yasui H, Sakurai H. Chemiluminescent detection and imaging of reactive oxygen species in live mouse skin exposed to UVA. Biochem Biophys Res Commun. 2000;269:131–6.

Zhang Y, Zhang HM, Shi Y, Lustgarten M, Li Y, Qi W, et al. Loss of manganese superoxide dismutase leads to abnormal growth and signal transduction in mouse embryonic fibroblasts. Free Radic Biol Med. 2010;49:1255–62.

8

Sophora japonica extracts accelerates keratinocyte differentiation through miR-181a

Karam Kim[1†], Hwa Jun Cha[2†], Dahye Joo[1], Seong Jin Choi[1], In Sook An[1] and Sungkwan An[3*] (iD)

Abstract

Background: The *Sophora japonica* extracts contain flavonol triglycoside, isoflavonol, coumarone chromone, saponin, triterpene glucoside, phospholipids, alkaloids, amino acids, polysaccharides, and fatty acids. These components have physiological effects such as anti-infertility and anti-cancer activities. This study investigated the regulation of keratinocyte differentiation upon treatment with the *S. japonica* extracts in keratinocyte and the molecular cell biological mechanism involved.

Methods: To determine whether the *S. japonica* extracts or troxerutin, which is its main component, regulates keratinocyte differentiation, quantitative real-time polymerase chain reaction (qRT-PCR) was performed on keratinocyte differentiation markers such as keratin 1 (K1), keratin 10 (K10), involucrin, and filaggrin after treatment with the *S. japonica* extracts. miR-181a knockdown confirmed that keratinocyte differentiation was regulated by increased miR-181a expression upon treatment with the *S. japonica* extracts or troxerutin.

Results: The expression of keratinocyte differentiation markers such as K1, K10, involucrin, and filaggrin increased upon treatment with the *S. japonica* extracts and troxerutin. Furthermore, miR-181a expression, which is known to increase during keratinocyte differentiation, increased upon treatment with the *S. japonica* extracts and troxerutin. When miR-181a was knocked down, the increased expression of keratinocyte differentiation markers upon treatment with the *S. japonica* extracts and troxerutin decreased again. Finally, it was confirmed that miR-181a directly regulated and reduced the expression of Notch2, which reduces keratinocyte differentiation, and that the decrease in Notch2 expression by miR-181a regulated keratinocyte differentiation.

Conclusions: These results suggest that the *S. japonica* extracts or troxerutin accelerates keratinocyte differentiation through miR-181a. This accelerated keratinocyte differentiation was confirmed to have resulted from the regulation of Notch2 expression by miR-181a. The results of this study provide an opportunity to confirm the molecular cell biological mechanism of *S. japonica* extracts or troxerutin on skin keratinization, and we expected that this study contribute to develop a moisturizing cosmetic material that can strengthen the skin barrier through regulating keratinocyte differentiation.

Keywords: miR-181a, microRNA, Keratinocyte differentiation, *Sophora japonica*, Troxerutin

* Correspondence: ansungkwan@konkuk.ac.kr
†Equal contributors
3Department of Cosmetics Engineering, Konkuk University, 120 Neungdong-ro, Gwangjin-gu, Seoul 05029, Republic of Korea
Full list of author information is available at the end of the article

Background

The skin plays a role in protecting the body from external stimuli such as microbes and ultraviolet radiation (Chuong et al., 2002). These skin defense functions are mainly functions of the epidermis composed of keratinocytes and melanocytes. Among these cells, keratinocytes construct complicated structure by keratinocyte differentiation (Kalinin et al., 2002; Rice & Green, 1977). Basal layer keratinocyte was differentiated to corneocytes that exist in the outer layer of the epidermis, resulting in gene expression regulating differentiation, cell cycle, and cell morphology. Among these genes, transglutaminases 1 and 3, involucrin, cornifin, loricrin, filaggrin, and small proline-rich protein (SPR) are specifically regulated by keratinocyte differentiation (Fuchs, 1993; Steinert & Marekov, 1995). Factors affecting keratinocyte differentiation are known as calcium, retinoic acid, vitamin D, and 12-o-tetradecanoylphorbol-13-acetate (TPA). Among these, calcium is well known for promoting keratinocyte differentiation, which is known to increase the density of the upper epidermis (Menon et al., 1985; Hennings et al., 1980; Yuspa et al., 1989).

When keratinocyte differentiation proceeds, transglutaminase binds structural proteins, such as involucrin, cornifin, loricrin, and SPR, inside the cell membrane to form a cornified cell envelope, which is a solid structure that does not dissolve in water (Candi et al., 2005; Ishida-Yamamoto & Iizuka, 1998). When abnormal keratinocyte differentiation occurs, the skin barrier becomes defective, which causes dry skin, resulting in chronic skin diseases such as atopy. Therefore, many attempts have been made to control keratinocyte differentiation using chemical compounds or the extracts (Tsuchisaka et al., 2014).

Sophora japonica flowers and blooms are well-known traditional Chinese medicinal herbs (Ma & Lou, 2006; Lo et al., 2009) and have anti-infertility and anti-cancer effects (Ma & Lou, 2006; Wang et al., 2001). *S. japonica* components include flavonol triglycoside, isoflavonol, coumarone chromone, saponin, triterpene glucoside, phospholipids, alkaloids, amino acids, polysaccharides, and fatty acids (Grupp et al., 2001). The *S. japonica* extracts are commonly used to treat bleeding-related disorders such as hematochezia, hemorrhoidal bleeding, and uterine bleeding as well as diarrhea (Zhao, 2004). However, the effects of the *S. japonica* extracts on keratinocytes have yet to be extensively studied; therefore, this study was conducted to confirm that the *S. japonica* extracts regulate keratinocyte differentiation and to investigate the molecular cell biological mechanism involved.

Methods

Cell line

HaCaT cells were cultured in Dulbecco' s modified Eagle's medium (DMEM; Gibco, Thermo Fisher Scientific, USA) added with 1% penicillin/streptomycin (P/S; Gibco) and 10% fetal bovine serum (FBS; Gibco, USA) at 37 °C, 5% CO_2 incubator.

Cytotoxicity

Cytotoxicity was determined by EZ-cytox enhanced cell viability kit (Daeil Lab, Korea) based on water-soluble tetrazolium salt (WST). 5×10^4 cells/well and 1×10^5 cells/well HaCaT were plated in each 96-well plate and 24-well plate. And then the cells were incubated for 24 h. After 24 h, the cells were then treated at indicated concentrations of *Sophora japonica* extracts. At 24 h, EZ-cytox enhanced cell viability was added in each well. The cells were incubated for 1 h, and then absorbance was measured at 450 nm using a spectrophotometer (Bio-Rad, USA).

RNA isolation and qRT-PCR (quantitative real-time polymerase chain reaction)

RNA was isolated from HaCaT using the Trizol reagent (Invitrogen, USA) according to the manufacturer's protocol. RNA quality was assessed with nanodrop spectrophotometry (Maestrogen, Taiwan). cDNA was prepared using the M-MLV reverse transcriptase (Enzynomics, Korea) according to the manufacturer's instructions. All qPCR analyses were performed on a Linegene K (BioER, China) with HOT FIREPol EvaGreen PCR Mix Plus (Solis BioDyne). Sequences of forward and reverse primers used in real-time PCR reactions are listed in Table 1.

miRNA transfection

For miR-181a and Anti-miR-340 (Bioneer, Korea) transfection, HaCaT cells were plated into 60-mm culture plates and allowed to grow overnight. Then the cells were transiently transfected with negative scramble miRNA or miR-181a or Anti-miR-340 for 48 h using RNAi max (Invitrogen, USA) according to the manufacturer's instructions.

Table 1 The primers used in qRT-PCR

Gene	Primer sequence
K1	F: 5′-CAGCATCATTGCTGAGGTCAAGG-3′ R: 5′-CATGTCTGCCAGCAGTGATCTG-3′
K10	F: 5′-TGGTTCAATGAAAAGAGCAAGGA-3′ R: 5′-GGGATTGTTTCAAGGCCAGTT-3′
Involucrin	F: 5′-CAAAGAACCTGGAGCAGGAG-3′ R: 5′-CAGGGCTGGTTGAATGTCTT-3′
Filaggrin	F: 5′-GCAAGGTCAAGTCCAGGAGAA-3′ R: 5′-CCCTCGGTTTCCACTGTCTC-3′
β: 5′-C	F: 5′-GGATTCCTATGTGGGCGACGA-3′ R: 5′-CGCTCGGTGAGGATCTTCATG-3′

Statistical analyses

Statistical comparisons were performed with Microsoft Excel (Microsoft, USA), using Student's t test for two data sets.

Results

S. japonica extracts regulated keratinocyte differentiation in HaCaT cells

The WST assay was performed to determine the cytotoxicity of the *S. japonica* extracts and troxerutin, which is its main component, to keratinocytes and to determine the effective concentration range for experiments. According to the measurement of cytotoxicity on HaCaT cells, the viability of these cells was found to be 90% or more at an *S. japonica* extract concentration of 200 μg/mL or less and over 90% at a troxerutin concentration of 100 μM (data not shown). To evaluate whether the *S. japonica* extracts regulate keratinocyte differentiation, mRNA levels of keratinocyte differentiation markers, such as keratin 1 (K1), keratin 10 (K10), involucrin, and filaggrin, were measured using keratinocytes. According to the mRNA levels of K1, K10, involucrin, and filaggrin measured from collected cells treated with 200 μg/mL of the *S. japonica* extract, the increased expression of keratinocyte differentiation markers due to calcium was further increased upon treatment with the *S. japonica* extracts (Fig. 1). In addition, troxerutin, a representative

component of the *S. japonica* extract, further increased the expression of keratinocyte differentiation markers increased by calcium (Fig. 2).

S. japonica extracts regulated miR-181a expression in HaCaT cells

To determine whether keratinocyte differentiation upon treatment with the *S. japonica* extracts is regulated through miR-181a, the change in the expression of miR-181a associated with treatment with these extracts was measured. The results showed that the expression of miR-181a increased upon treatment with the *S. japonica* extracts (Fig. 3a). Additionally, the expression of miR-181a increased upon treatment with troxerutin (Fig. 3b).

Troxerutin, a major ingredient of *S. japonica* extracts, regulated keratinocyte differentiation and miR-181a expression in HaCaT cells

Because the expression of miR-181a, which is known to be closely related to keratinocyte differentiation due to its increased expression in a keratinocyte differentiation model, is regulated upon treatment with the *S. japonica* extracts and troxerutin (Hildebrand et al., 2011), this study specifically investigated whether keratinocyte differentiation regulated by treatment with the *S. japonica* extracts and troxerutin occurs through miR-181a. To achieve this, anti-miR-181a was used with the aim of

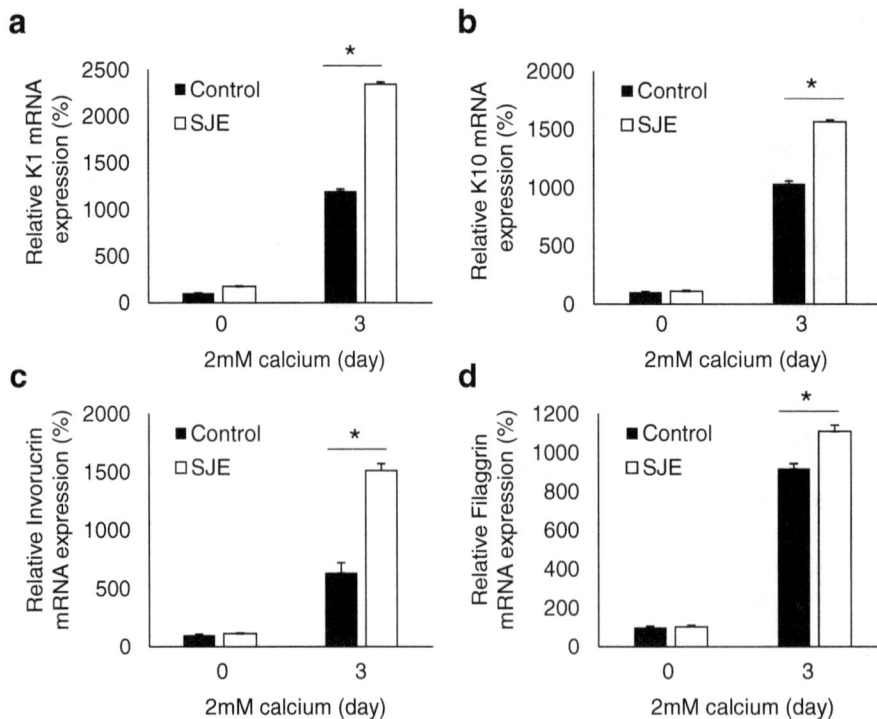

Fig. 1 *S. japonica* extracts regulated marker of keratinocyte differentiation in HaCaT cells. **a** *K1* mRNA expression. **b** *K10* mRNA expression. **c** *Involucrin* mRNA expression. **d** *Filaggrin* mRNA expression. SJE is *S. japonica* extracts. *<0.05

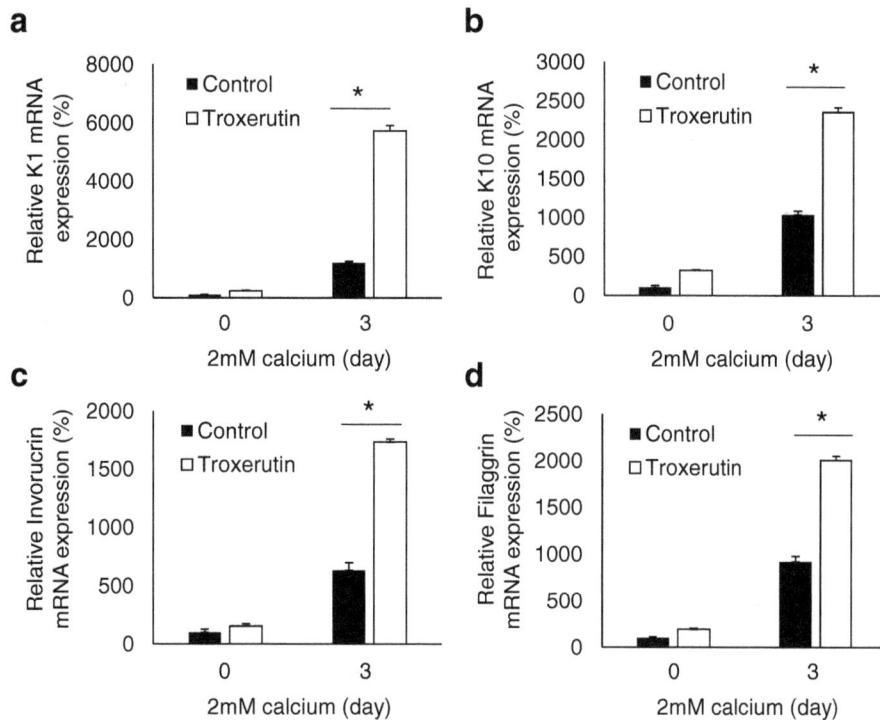

Fig. 2 Troxerutin regulated marker of keratinocyte differentiation in HaCaT cells. **a** *K1* mRNA expression. **b** *K10* mRNA expression. **c** *Involucrin* mRNA expression. **d** *Filaggrin* mRNA expression. *<0.05

inhibiting the acceleration of keratinocyte differentiation by the *S. japonica* extracts and troxerutin. The experimental results showed that keratinocyte differentiation was regulated upon treatment with the *S. japonica* extracts and troxerutin through miR-181a (Fig. 4).

Discussion

The stratum corneum is formed by keratinocytes in the epidermis and maintains the moisture of the epidermis and blocks external pollutants. The differentiation of keratinocytes can be easily confirmed using keratinocyte differentiation markers such as K1, K10, involucrin, and filaggrin.

The skin is the primary barrier to the external environment and plays a major role in protecting individuals. Keratinocytes are the main cells that constitute the epidermis of the skin and play a role in forming the skin barrier through division and differentiation. In case of skin diseases such as atopic dermatitis, a normal skin barrier is not produced and abnormal keratinocyte differentiation occurs; therefore, in such diseases, keratinocyte differentiation can be promoted to aid in the normal formation of the skin barrier (Leung et al., 2007).

The *S. japonica* extracts contain flavonol triglycoside, isoflavonol, coumarone chromone, saponin, triterpene glucoside, phospholipids, alkaloids, amino acids, polysaccharides, and fatty acids. These components have

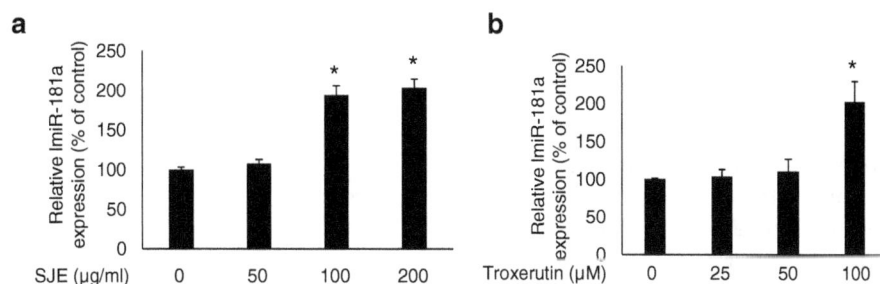

Fig. 3 *S. japonica* extracts and troxerutin regulated miR-181a expression in HaCaT cells. **a** *S. japonica* extract-mediated miRNA-181a expression change. SJE is *S. japonica* extracts. **b** Troxerutin-mediated miRNA-181a expression change. *< 0.05

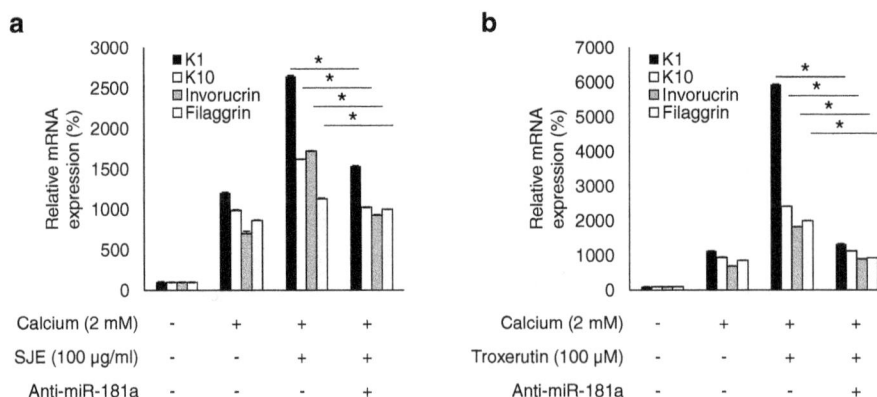

Fig. 4 *S. japonica* extracts and troxerutin regulated the marker of keratinocyte differentiation through miR-181a in HaCaT cells. **a** Anti-miRNA-181a effect to expression of keratinocyte differentiation markers in *S. japonica* extract-treated HaCaT cells. SJE is *S. japonica* extracts. **b** Anti-miRNA-181a effect to expression of keratinocyte differentiation markers in troxerutin-treated HaCaT cells. *< 0.05 compared with each calcium and *S. japonica* extracts or troxerutin-treated condition

physiological effects such as anti-infertility and anti-cancer activities. This study investigated the regulation of keratinocyte differentiation upon treatment with the *S. japonica* extracts and the molecular cell biological mechanism involved.

The expression of early differentiation markers such as K1, K10, and involucrin significantly increased upon treatment of cultured keratinocytes with the *S. japonica* extracts and troxerutin. In addition, the expression of late differentiation markers such filaggrin and loricrin significantly increased (Figs. 1 and 2). These results suggest that the *S. japonica* extracts and troxerutin activate the early and late signal transduction systems of keratinocyte differentiation. It is well known that keratinocyte differentiation plays an important role in activating the intracellular signal transduction system by delivering external stimuli. For example, keratinocyte differentiation-promoting factors, such as calcium, are known to activate protein kinase C and affect downstream signaling systems (Matsui et al., 1992; Dlugosz & Yuspa, 1993; Bollag et al., 1993; O'Driscoll et al., 1994). The activation of mitogen-activated protein kinases, such as ERK1/2 and p38, has also been shown to play a pivotal role in keratinocyte differentiation (Efimova et al., 2003; Eckert et al., 2002). These intracellular signal transduction activities increase the gene expression of keratinocyte differentiation markers by activating transcriptional regulatory factors such as AP-1, SP-1, and Ets (Nakamura et al., 2007; Jang & Steinert, 2002; Lee et al., 1996).

In the present study, the expression levels of early and late differentiation markers increased upon treatment with the *S. japonica* extracts and troxerutin; therefore, this study suggested that the effect of promoting keratinocyte differentiation was more related to the intracellular signal transduction system than to the increase in expression of a specific differentiation marker gene. In the future, it will be necessary to study the effect of

colostrum on the intracellular signal transduction system of keratinocytes.

Conclusions

In this study, keratinocyte differentiation markers were identified to investigate the possibility of the *S. japonica* extracts and troxerutin to be regulators of keratinocyte differentiation. The expression of keratinocyte differentiation markers K1, K10, involucrin, and filaggrin increased upon treatment with the *S. japonica* extracts and troxerutin. Therefore, the *S. japonica* extracts and troxerutin showed keratinocyte differentiation-regulating effects. In addition, the *S. japonica* extracts and troxerutin regulated miR-181a, which targets the keratinocyte differentiation regulator Notch2, thereby regulating keratinocyte differentiation. Through such regulation of keratinocyte differentiation, it is possible to control the skin barrier formed by keratinocyte differentiation in the epidermal layer, enhancing the moisturizing ability of the skin. Therefore, this study confirmed that the *S. japonica* extracts and troxerutin strengthen the skin barrier of the epidermis and enhance the moisturizing ability of the skin.

Abbreviations
DMEM: Dulbecco' s modified Eagle's medium; K1: Keratin 1; K10: Keratin 10; qRT-PCR: Quantitative real-time polymerase chain reaction; S. japonica: Sophora japonica; SPR: Proline-rich protein; TPA: 12-o-Tetradecanoylphorbol-13-acetate; WST: Water-soluble tetrazolium salt

Acknowledgements
Not applicable

Funding
This study was supported by a grant (no. HN13C0075) from the Korean Health Technology R&D Project, Ministry of Health & Welfare, Republic of Korea.

Authors' contributions

KK, HJC, DJ, and SJC performed the experiments. ISA and SA were involved in experimental design and advising. KK and HJC analyzed data and wrote the manuscript. All authors have read and approved the final manuscript.

Competing interests

The authors declare that they have no competing interests.

Author details

[1]Korea Institute of Dermatological Sciences, 6F Tower A, 25 Beobwon-ro 11-gil, Songpa-gu, Seoul 05836, Republic of Korea. [2]Department of Beauty Care, Osan University, 45 Cheonghak-ro, Osan-si, Gyeonggi-do 18119, Republic of Korea. [3]Department of Cosmetics Engineering, Konkuk University, 120 Neungdong-ro, Gwangjin-gu, Seoul 05029, Republic of Korea.

References

Bollag WB, Ducote J, Harmon CS. Effects of the selective protein kinase C inhibitor, Ro 31-7549, on the proliferation of cultured mouse epidermal keratinocytes. J Invest Dermatol. 1993;100:240–6.

Candi E, Schmidt R, Melino G. The cornified envelope: a model of cell death in the skin. Nat Rev Mol Cell Biol. 2005;6(4):328–40.

Chuong CM, Nickoloff BJ, Elias PM, Goldsmith LA, Macher E, Maderson PA, Sundberg JP, Tagami H, Plonka PM, Thestrup-Pederson K, Bernard BA, Schroder JM, Dotto P, Chang CM, Williams ML, Feingold KR, King LE, Kligman AM, Rees JL, Christophers E. What is the 'true' function of skin? Exp Dermatol. 2002;11:159–87.

Dlugosz AA, Yuspa SH. Coordinate changes in gene expression which mark the spinous to granular cell transition in epidermis are regulated by protein kinase C. J Cell Biol. 1993;120:217–25.

Eckert RL, Efimova T, Dashti SR, Balasubramanian S, Deucher A, Crish JF, Sturniolo M, Bone F. Keratinocyte survival, differentiation, and death: many roads lead to mitogen-activated protein kinase. J Investig Dermatol Symp Proc. 2002;7:36–40.

Efimova T, Broome AM, Eckert RL. A regulatory role for p38 delta MAPK in keratinocyte differentiation. Evidence for p38 delta-ERK1/2 complex formation. J Biol Chem. 2003;278:34277–85.

Fuchs E. Epidermal differentiation and keratin gene expression. J Cell Sci. 1993;17: 197–208.

Grupp C, John H, Hemprich U, Singer A, Munzel U, Muller GA. Identification of nucleated cells in urine using lectin staining. Am J Kidney Dis. 2001;37:84–93.

Hennings H, Michael D, Cheng C, Steinert P, Holbrook K, Yuspa SH. Calcium regulation of growth and differentiation of mouse epidermal cells in culture. Cell. 1980;19:245–54.

Hildebrand J, Rütze M, Walz N, Gallinat S, Wenck H, Deppert W, Grundhoff A, Knott A. A comprehensive analysis of microRNA expression during human keratinocyte differentiation in vitro and in vivo. J Invest Dermatol. 2011; 131(1):20–9.

Ishida-Yamamoto A, Iizuka H. Structural organization of cornified cell envelopes and alterations in inherited skin disorders. Exp Dermatol. 1998;7(1):1–10.

Jang SI, Steinert PM. Loricrin expression in cultured human keratinocytes is controlled by a complex interplay between transcription factors of the Sp1, CREB, AP1, and AP2 families. J Biol Chem. 2002;277:42268–79.

Kalinin AE, Kajava AV, Steinert PM. Epithelial barrier function: assembly and structural features of the cornified cell envelope. BioEssays. 2002;24:789–800.

Lee JH, Jang SI, Yang JM, Markova NG, Steinert PM. The proximal promoter of the human transglutaminase 3 gene. Stratified squamous epithelial-specific expression in cultured cells is mediated by binding of Sp1 and ets transcription factors to a proximal promoter element. J Biol Chem. 1996;271:4561–8.

Leung AK, Hon KL, Robson WL. Atopic dermatitis. Adv Pediatr Infect Dis. 2007;54: 241–73.

Lo YH, Lin RD, Lin YP, Liu YL, Lee MH. Active constituents from Sophora japonica exhibiting cellular tyrosinase inhibition in human epidermal melanocytes. J Ethnopharmacol. 2009;124(3):625–9.

Ma L, Lou FC. The anticancer activity in vitro of constituents from fruits of Sophora japonica. Chinese J of Nat Med. 2006;4:151–3.

Matsui MS, Chew SL, DeLeo VA. Protein kinase C in normal human epidermal keratinocytes during proliferation and calcium-induced differentiation. J Invest Dermatol. 1992;99:565–71.

Menon GK, Grayson S, Elias P. Ionic calcium reservoirs in mammalian epidermis: ultrastructural localization by ion-capture cytochemistry. J Invest Dermatol. 1985;84:508–12.

Nakamura Y, Kawachi Y, Xu X, Sakurai H, Ishii Y, Takahashi T, Otsuka F. The combination of ubiquitous transcription factors AP-1 and Sp1 directs keratinocytespecific and differentiation-specific gene expression in vitro. Exp Dermatol. 2007;16:143–50.

O'Driscoll KR, Madden PV, Christiansen KM, Viage A, Slaga TJ, Fabbro D, Powell CT, Weinstein IB. Overexpression of protein kinase C beta I in a murine keratinocyte cell line produces effects on cellular growth, morphology and differentiation. Cancer Lett. 1994;83:249–59.

Rice RH, Green H. The cornified envelope of terminally differentiated human epidermal keratinocytes consists of crosslinked protein. Cell. 1977;11:417–22.

Steinert PM, Marekov LN. The proteins elafin, filaggrin, keratin intermediate filaments, loricrin, and small prolinerich proteins 1 and 2 are isodipeptide cross-linked components of the human epidermal cornified cell envelope. J Biol Chem. 1995;270:17702–11.

Tsuchisaka A, Furumura M, Hashimoto T. Cytokine regulation during epidermal differentiation and barrier formation. J Invest Dermatol. 2014;134(5):1194–6.

Wang JH, Wang YL, Lou FC. Acacia trees the chemical constituents of the seeds. J China Pharma Univ. 2001;32:471.

Yuspa SH, Kilkenny AE, Steinert PM, Roop DR. Expression of murine epidermal differentiation markers is tightly regulated by restricted extracellular calcium concentrations in vitro. J Cell Biol. 1989;109:1207–17.

Zhao ZZ. An Illustrated Chinese Materia Medica in Hong Kong. School of Chinese Medicine. Hong Kong: Hong Kong Baptist University 2004.

9

Preservation effects of geniposidic acid on human keratinocytes (HaCaT) against UVB

Na Kyeong Lee

Abstract

Background: Geniposidic acid is a natural compound affiliated with iridoid glycoside which is contained in various plants such as *Gardenia* seeds, *Eucommia* bark, and *Psyllium*, and it is known that it has such effects as anti-inflammation, anti-virus, anti-cancer, anti-oxidation, suppression of stress, improvement of immune system, and relief of liver injury. However, there is a lack of research on action of geniposidic acid in dermal cells, so this research verifies effects of geniposidic acid on preservation of human keratinocytes, anti-oxidation, and DNA repair and finds out its mechanism.

Methods: This study demonstrated feasibility of geniposidic acid on cosmeceutical application via ultraviolet (UV) B-induced damage protective effects such as oxidative stress reduction, DNA repair, and decrease of apoptotic cell death. To investigate cytotoxicity of angelic acid and proliferation influence, researchers used formazan detection by water-soluble tetrazolium salts (WST). To examine cell cycle distribution and sub-G1 portion, fluorescence-activated cell sorting (FACS) analysis was used to the experiment. For further investigation, cleaved caspase-3 levels were determined in apoptotic cell death analysis. And we conducted comet assay, in vitro anti-oxidant effects using radical scavenging assay, lipid peroxidation analysis, and mRNA expression analysis.

Results: Geniposidic acid protects UVB-induced cytotoxic damage and reduces apoptotic cell death caused by UVB in human keratinocytes (HaCaT). Also, this research finds out that geniposidic acid decreases formation of cleaved caspase-3 increase and reduces both tailed DNA and cyclobutane pyrimidine dimer (CPD) which is increased by UVB. Through radical scavenging assay, we demonstrate in vitro anti-oxidant effect of geniposidic acid and, via quantitative real-time polymerase chain reaction (qRT-PCR), find out that gene expression of superoxide dismutase 1 and 2 (*SOD1* and *SOD2*) which are known as anti-oxidant gene increases dependently on concentration of geniposidic acid. Furthermore, geniposidic acid reduces lipid peroxidation to lead anti-oxidation effect. This research finds out that gene expression of *XPC* (XPC complex subunit, DNA damage recognition, and repair factor) and *PCNA* (proliferating cell nuclear antigen) which are DNA repair gene increases dependently on concentration of geniposidic acid.

Conclusions: Through this research, we verify that geniposidic acid has effects on anti-oxidation and DNA repair in human HaCaT damaged by UVB and suggest that geniposidic acid as a cosmetic material is fully worthy to use to delay dermal cellular senescence by UVB effectively.

Keywords: Geniposidic acid, HaCaT keratinocyte, Anti-oxidation, DNA repair, Ultraviolet B

Background

Dermal senescence is a complex phenomenon which is classified into intrinsic aging caused by the heredity and extrinsic aging through environmental exposure by UV (Jenkins 2002), and intrinsic aging is occurred by reactive oxygen species (ROS) which is formed in the course of cellular metabolism (Lee et al. 2012), and extrinsic aging occurs due to reactive oxygen which is formed by dermal permeation of UVB although there are several causes for extrinsic senescence (Kulms et al. 2002). Intracellular ROS causes damages on DNA and mitochondria and results in such intracellular damages as heterology in the course of energy metabolism as well as protein oxidation. The intracellular damages caused by oxidative stress occur cell cycle arrest, cellular senescence, and apoptosis which are shown on dermal keratinocyte to lead to dermal senescence (Cerella et al. 2009). DNA damage caused by

Correspondence: nklee2349@daum.net
JEI University, 808 Main Building, 178, Jaeneung-ro, Dong-gu, Incheon 22573, Republic of Korea

UV activates ATM (ataxia-telangiectasia mutated) and ATR (ATM- and Rad3-related) proteins, which activate p53. When DNA gets damaged, activation of p53 which is a transcription factor induces expression of p21 to stop cell cycle and hinder cell growth (Smits and Medema 2001). So in this experiment, to examine preservation effect on HaCaT against UVB, as object, I selected geniposidic acid which is anti-cancer, anti-oxidation, and anti-inflammatory properties.

Geniposidic acid as corresponding to (1S,4aS,7aS)-1-(β-D-glucopyranosyloxy)-7-(hydroxymethyl)-1,4a,5,7a-tet rahydrocyclopenta[c]pyran-4-carboxylic acid is a natural compound affiliated with iridoid glycoside which is contained in various plants such as *Gardenia* seeds, *Eucommia* bark, and *Psyllium*, and research on senescence-related insulin resistance improvement of genipin (Guan et al. 2013) and also research on airway inflammation and induction suppression of geniposide have been reported (Deng et al. 2013) with regard to biological action of *Gardenia* seeds. Also, the research on anti-oxidation and anti-inflammation action of manufactured *Gardenia* seeds and crocetin is known (Hong and Yang 2013). In the research on cancer cell proliferation suppression effect of *Eucommia* extract (Choi et al. 2003), geniposide and geniposidic acid were separated and refined respectively, and at the case of oral administration of these compounds, it significantly reduced tumor size of mouse in which cancer cell was transplanted (Hsu et al. 1997), and at in vitro experiment targeting C6 glioma cell, it induced apoptosis effectively (Chang et al. 2002). Also, in the experimental study depending on manufacturing of *eucommia*, as indicator substances, I selected geniposidic acid and geniposide which are mental stability factors in iridoid glycoside and examined its content depending on manufacturing, and through pharmacological experiment on catecholamine content within brain and plasma under the condition of pain, lipid metabolism, and restraint stress, it found out that it is significantly effective (Park and Kim 1992). Since the recent research trends on geniposidic acid, there has been a process of research on anti-cancer, anti-inflammation, and anti-oxidation, but nothing about research on application of geniposidic acid as cosmetic materials, and also, there have been no researches on mechanism in dermal cells. Also, researches on skin preservation against UV and about natural substances which delay cellular senescence have been increasing continuously in these days. So it is necessary to investigate various effects of geniposidic acid on usual action of keratinocyte in the course of dermal senescence. Therefore, this research intends to study effects of geniposidic acid such as cell preservation, anti-oxidation, and DNA repair and examine its effects to find out possibility for application of geniposidic acid as natural cosmetic materials which can help delaying dermal cellular senescence.

Methods

Cell culture

HaCaT cell line and HaCaT keratinocytes (ATCC, Manassas, VA, USA) were cultured using Dulbecco's modified Eagle's medium (DMEM; Hyclone, Logan, UT, USA) which contains 10% of fetal bovine serum (FBS; Hyclone) and 1% of penicillin/streptomycin (penicillin 100 IU/mL, streptomycin 100 μg/mL; Invitrogen/Life Technologies, Carlsbad, CA, USA) for HaCaT culture and cultured it within cell incubator kept under the condition of 5% of CO_2 with the temperature at 37 °C.

Sample treatment

I purchased geniposidic acid which is refined in the form of powder from Santa Cruz Biotech (Santa Cruz, CA, USA) and dissolved it in dimethyl sulfoxide (DMSO; Sigma-Aldrich, St. Louis, MO, USA) in a proper density to use it in the experiment. After I cultured HaCaT cell (1×10^6 cells/well) in the cell medium for 24 h, I added geniposidic acid in a proper density to culture medium and pretreated for 3 h, and for ultraviolet B test on cells, I used UV-B lamp (UVP, Upland, CA, USA) to examine. I used fiber optic Spectrometer System USB2000 (Ocean Optics, Dunedin, FL, USA) to estimate UVB wavelength, and at the UVB test on HaCaT, I washed it twice with phosphate-buffered saline (PBS; (Thermo Fisher Scientific, USA) in a pH of 7.4 to remove culture medium of cell culture dish. To prevent drying of cell, I opened cell culture dish lid for UVB test after adding 1 mL of PBS to cell culture dish, removed PBS after UVB testing, added culture medium again to culture in the culture incubator for 24 h, and then used in the experiment.

Cell viability estimation

I used the principle of WST assay to estimate cell viability. I used EZ-Cytox cell viability assay kit (Itsbio, Seoul, Korea), and after inoculating HaCaT (3×10^3 cells/well) in 96-well plate and cultured for 24 h, I treated HaCaT with geniposidic acid of each density of 5, 10, 20, 30, and 40 μM respectively, tested 40 mJ/cm^2 of UVB, and then cultured for 24 h. After I added 10 μL of EZ-Cytox cell viability assay kit reagent (ItsBio) into cultured well and cultured for 1 h, I used microplate reader (Bio-Rad, Hercules, CA, USA). I estimated the absorbance in the scale of 490 nm, repeated each experiments three times separately, and derived average value and standard deviation of cell viability.

Cell cycle analysis

I used an equipment of BD FACS Calibur Flow Cytometer (BD Biosciences, San Jose, CA, USA). I estimated the number of cells in sub-G1, G1, S, and G2/M cell cycle to analyze cell cycle. After I inoculated 2×10^5 cells/well of HaCaT in 60 mm of culture dish, I cultured it for 24 h, and then, I pretreated it with geniposidic acid for 3 h. After testing UVB, I cultured it for 24 h more and obtained cultured cells, and then, I centrifuged it at 5000 rpm with temperature at 4 °C for 5 min and precipitated cells. After I removed the supernatant and dissolved the cell pellet with 300 μL of PBS, I slowly added 700 μL of absolute ethanol (Biopure, Canada) while vortexing, and I refrigerated it with temperature at 4 °C for 3 h to fix cells. I added 1 mL of PBS, centrifuged at 5000 rpm with temperature at 4 °C for 5 min to remove supernatant, dissolved the pellet with 200 μL of propidium iodide (PI) staining buffer (PI 50 μg/mL, RNase 0.1 μg/mL, 0.05% Triton X-100; Sigma Aldrich), and then settled with temperature at 37 °C for 1 h. Afterward, I centrifuged HaCaT cells at 5000 rpm with temperature at 4 °C for 5 min to remove supernatant and washed with PBS, and then, I dissolved the pellet with 1 mL of PBS and through Flow Cytometer estimated the number of cells in each cell cycle.

qRT-PCR analysis

To analyze and find out gene expression occurred within HaCaT by geniposidic acid quantitatively, I used qRT-PCR method. I mixed 0.2 μM of primers, 20 mM of Tris/HCl in a pH of 8.4, 50 mM KCl, 0.8 mM of dNTP, 3 mM of MgCl$_2$, 0.5 U Extaq DNA polymerase, and 1× SYBR green (Invitrogen) in PCR tube to manufacture reaction solution and used Linegene K (BioER, Zhejiang, China). After denaturation with temperature at 94 °C for 3 min, I performed denaturation (94 °C, 30 s), annealing (58 °C, 30 s), and polymerization (72 °C, 30 s) for 40 cycles and proceeded PCR. With melting curve, I verified the effectiveness of PCR, and by standardizing expression of *β-actin*, I performed the comparative analysis for each gene expression, and the primer used in the experiment is shown as Table 1.

DPPH radical scavenging activity assay

I injected the geniposidic acid diluent of each density into 96-well plate, added 50 μL of 0.2 mM of 1,1-diphenyl-2-picrylhydrazyl (DPPH), and settled it for 30 min. Using a microplate reader (Bio-Rad), I estimated the absorbance in the scale of 514 nm and repeated this estimation three times. I derived the average value and standard deviation of absorbance.

ABTS$^+$ radical scavenging assay

I mixed 7.4 nm of 2,2-azino-bis-3-ethylbenzthiazoline-6-sulfonic acid (ABTS) and 2.6 mM of potassium persulfate in the final density, reacted in dark room at room temperature for 12 h, and formed ABTS$^+$, and then, I made the value of the absorbance to be 0.706 (± 0.01) in the scale of 732 nm. After adding 100 μL of ABTS$^+$ into 100 μL geniposidic acid in 96-well plate and neglecting for 7 min, I estimated the absorbance in the scale of 732 nm. I repeated this estimation three times and derived the average value and standard deviation of the absorbance.

Caspase-3 activity

Caspase-3 which induces apoptosis is affiliated with cysteine proteinase family, and I used Apoalert caspase-3 colorimetric assay kit (Clontech, Mountain View, CA, USA) as method to estimate pNA (p-nitroanilide) action using its character to decompose Ac-DEVD-pNA (*N*-acetyl-Asp-Glu-Val-Asp p-nitroanilide) which is a substrate complex. I separated the cells treated by sample from culture dish, centrifuged it at 1500 rpm for 5 min, and added cold cell lysis buffer into cell pellet whose culture medium was removed, and then, I settled it under the condition of the ice for 10 min and centrifuged it at 15000 rpm with temperature at 4 °C for 3 min to separate supernatant only. With regard to the separated supernatant, I used bradford assay to quantify only total 50 μg of protein and apply to caspase-3 activity reaction. I put suspension which I finished protein quantification into 96-well plate, added reaction buffer, and cultured it with temperature at 37 °C for 30 min. Then, I added caspase-3 substrate, cultured with temperature at 37 °C for 1 h, and used microplate reader (Bio-Rad) to estimate the absorbance in the scale of 405 nm.

Table 1 List of primers

Gene	Forward primer	Reverse primer
β-actin	GGATTCCTATGTGGGCGACGA	CGCTCGGTGAGGATCTTCATG
P21	GTCCAGCGACCTTCCTCATCCA	CCATAGCCTCTACTGCCACCATC
GADD45a	GAGAGCAGAAGACCGAAAGGA	CACAACACCACGTTATCGGG
SOD1	GGGAGATGGCCCAACTACTG	CCAGTTGACATGCAACCGTT
SOD2	GCCCTGGAACCTCACATCAA	GGTACTTCTCCTCGGTGACGTT
PCNA	TAACAGTTCCTGCATGGGCGGC	CGTGCAAATTCACCAGAAGGC
XPC	AGCAGCTTCCCACCTGTTC	GTGGGTGCCCCTCTAGTG

Comet assay (single-cell gel electrophoresis)

I used CometAssay® Reagent Kits (Trevigen, Gaithesburg, MD, USA) and melted LMAgarose (low melting agarose) completely for 5 min, and then, I covered it with cab, cooled in water bath whose temperature was at 37 °C for 20 min, and mixed 1×10^5 cells/mL of cell with melted LMAgarose (at 37 °C) at the ratio of 1 to 10 (v/v). Afterward, I poured 50 μL of mixed liquor onto Comet slide and kept in slide in the refrigerator with temperature at 4 °C for 10 min, and then, I immersed the slide in alkaline solution at room temperature for 20 min. After I immersed the slide in alkaline electrophoresis solution and covered, I electrophoresed it with voltages at 21 V for 30 min, and after finishing electrophoresis, I immersed it twice in distilled water for 4 min to remove electrophoresis solution and immersed in 70% ethanol for 5 min. I dried it with temperature at 37 °C, put dried agarose gel into 100 μL of SYBR® gold nuclei acid gel stain (Invitrogen), and dyed it in the dark room for 30 min. I rinsed it with water simply to remove dyeing reagent and observed agarose gel which I dried it completely with temperature at 37 °C through fluorescence microscope.

MDA assay

I used colorimetric method to estimate malondialdehyde (MDA) level and used Lipid Peroxidation (MDA) Assay Kit (Abcam, Cambridge, UK). First, I inoculated 1×10^7 cells/well of HaCaT in 6-well plate and pretreated it with reagent, and then, I tested the UV and cultured it for 48 h. I used a microplate reader (Bio-Rad) to estimate in the scale of 586 nm and used the principle that oxidated lipid (MDA) reacts with TBA (thiobarbituric acid) within kit and detects through colorimetric method.

Statistical process

In this research, I performed every experiment more than three times separately under the same condition and obtained experimental result, and used Student's t test for each experiment and found p value. When p value in every experimental result is less than 0.05, I analyzed that it is statistically significant.

Results

Cell viability analysis

To find out cytotoxicity which geniposidic acid influences on HaCaT, I performed the cell viability assay. I treated the HaCaT keratinocytes with geniposidic acid of each density of 5, 10, 20, 30, and 40 μM respectively. As the result of testing cytotoxicity, it did not influence on viability till 20 μM. When geniposidic acid was 20 μM, the viability was 87%, and when geniposidic acid was 30 μM, it was 73%, and when geniposidic acid was 40 μM, it was 66%, so the cell viability appeared as decreasing (Fig. 1a). To find out whether geniposidic acid has an effect to preserve HaCaT keratinocytes against UVB irradiation, I pretreated the HaCaT keratinocytes with geniposidic acid of each density of 10, 20, and 30 μM respectively and tested UVB of 40 mJ/cm² to find out changing of cell viability. As the result, when I did not treat HaCaT keratinocytes with geniposidic acid but tested UVB only, cell viability decreased to 72%, but at the case of pretreatment with geniposidic acid of 10 μM, it was 75%; at the case of pretreatment with 20 μM, it was 81%; at the case of pretreatment with 30 μM, it was 87%, and 88% at 40 μM pretreatment. Therefore, I found out that cell viability of HaCaT keratinocytes restores dependently on density of geniposidic acid (Fig. 1b).

Analysis of cell cycle distribution and apoptotic cell death

To find out through what mechanism geniposidic acid works with regard to the effect to preserve against cytotoxicity caused by UVB dependently on density, I performed cell cycle analysis. I dyed HaCaT with PI and used flow cytometer for untreated control group, treatment group with UVB of 40 mJ/cm², and treatment group with both UVB 40 mJ/cm² and geniposidic acid of each density of 10, 20, and 30 μM respectively to estimate cell cycle progress. As the result of examining changing of cell cycle distribution, it was shown as Fig. 2a

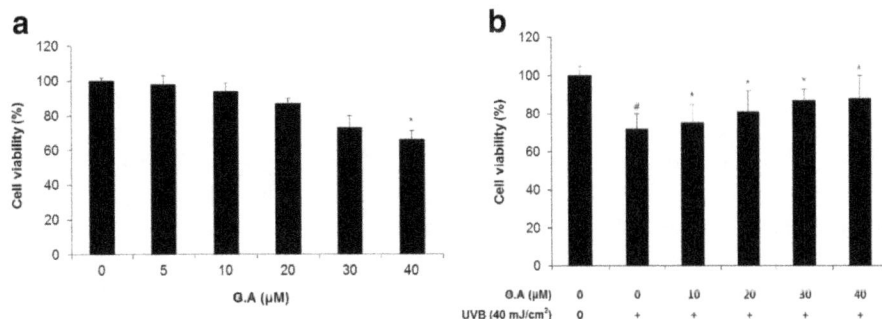

Fig. 1 Cell viability on geniposidic acid in HaCaT keratinocytes. **a** Cell cytotoxicity of geniposidic acid on HaCaT keratinocytes. **b** Protective effect of geniposidic acid on UVB-induced damages in HaCaT cells (*$p < 0.05$)

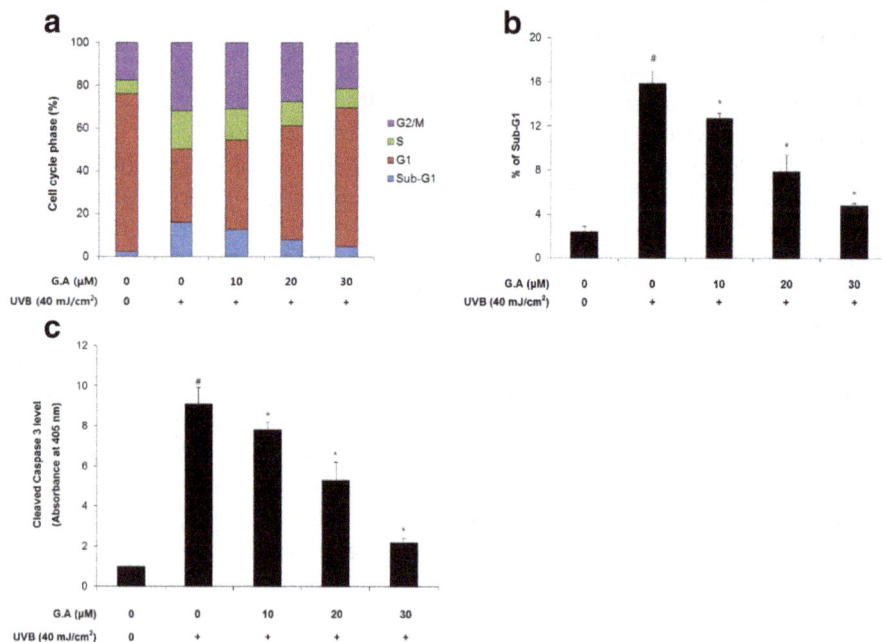

Fig. 2 Cell cycle and sub-G1 analysis of geniposidic acid-treated HaCaT, damaged by UVB. **a** Cell cycle distribution of geniposidic acid-treated HaCaT, damaged by UVB. **b** Effect of geniposidic acid on UVB-induced sub-G1 population in HaCaT. **c** Effect of geniposidic acid on UVB-induced cleaved caspase-3 level in HaCaT ($*p < 0.05$)

in which G1 value of treatment group with UVB of 40 mJ/cm^2 reduces 39.2 to 34.4% while G1 value of control group is 73.6%, so it was shown that UVB causes G1 cell cycle arrest to suppress cell growth. When with geniposidic acid of each density of 10, 20, and 30 μM, I treated the treatment group with UVB of 40 mJ/cm^2 respectively, G1 value increased to 41.8, 53.4, and 64.9% individually. It is considered that G1 cell cycle arrest caused by UVB is suppressed by geniposidic acid (Fig. 2a).

I found out the effect of geniposidic acid on sub-G1 of HaCaT irradiated with UVB. Sub-G1 value of untreated control group increased from 2.4 to 15.9% by UVB; however, it was shown that the value decreases dependently on density of geniposidic acid, so at the case of treatment with 10 μM of geniposidic acid, the value was 12.7%; at the case of 20 μM, it was 7.9%; and at the case of 30 μM, it was 4.8%. It is considered that UVB causes increasement in cell population of sub-G1 and apoptosis increases, but geniposidic acid reduces sub-G1 similar to control group to suppress apoptosis (Fig. 2b).

As the result of searching relative value of cleaved caspase-3 of HaCaT cell treated with geniposidic acid, the amount of cleaved caspase-3 increased to 9.1 at the case of treatment with UVB 40 mJ/cm^2, when the amount of cleaved caspase-3 of untreated control group was 1. It is found that UVB induces apoptosis, and when with geniposidic acid of each density of 10, 20, and 30 μM, I treated the treatment group with UVB 40 mJ/

cm^2 respectively, the amount of cleaved caspase-3 decreased to 7.8, 5.3, and 2.2 individually. It is considered that UVB causes an increase in the amount of cleaved caspase-3 and apoptosis increases, but geniposidic acid suppresses apoptosis, and so geniposidic acid has an effect to preserve cells (Fig. 2c).

Incitation of DNA damage protection and repair mechanism

I found out cell preservation effect of geniposidic acid on DNA damage through comet assay. As the result about changing of DNA damage in HaCaT which was treated with UVB and again with geniposidic acid, DNA tail increased to 67% after treating with UVB of 40 mJ/cm^2, while it was 3% at the case of untreated control group of HaCaT cells. It is considered that UVB causes DNA damage, and when with geniposidic acid of each density of 10, 20, and 30 μM, I treated the treatment group with UVB 40 mJ/cm^2 respectively, DNA tail decreased to 61, 44, and 19% individually. It is considered that UVB causes increase of tailed DNA and DNA damage, but geniposidic acid reduces it to preserve DNA, and that geniposidic acid has an effect to preserve cells (Fig. 3a). To find out what effects on damaged DNA caused by UV geniposidic acid have, I studied changing of CPD, and the result showed that CPD increases to 100% after treating with UVB 40 mJ/cm^2, while it is 1% at the case of untreated control group of HaCaT. It is considered that UVB causes DNA damage and CPD increases, and when with geniposidic acid of each density of

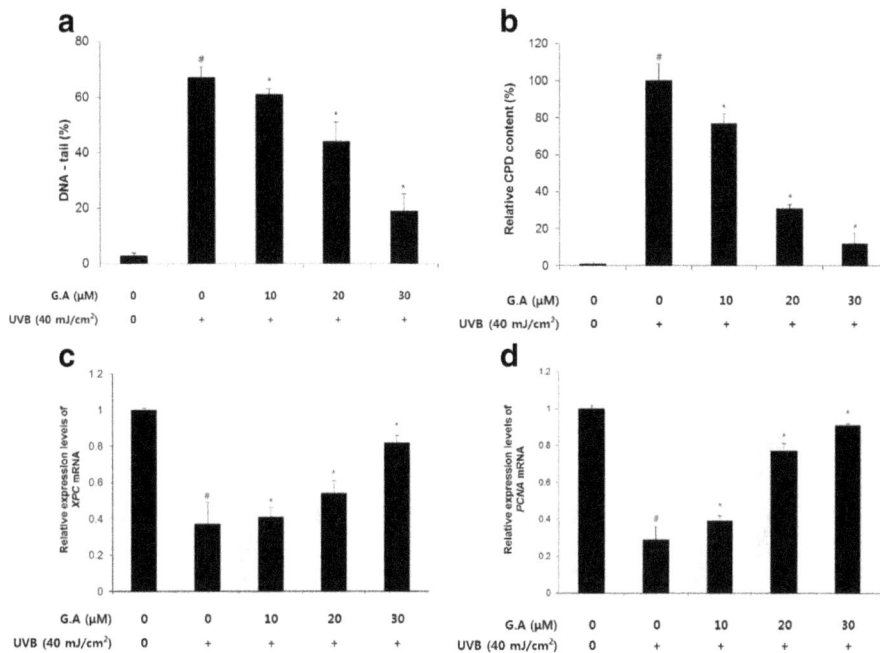

Fig. 3 Analysis of DNA damage protection activity of geniposidic acid on UVB-irradiated HaCaT. **a** Effect of geniposidic acid on UVB-induced DNA damage in HaCaT. **b** Effect of geniposidic acid on UVB-induced CPD formation in HaCaT. **c** Effect of geniposidic acid on UVB-induced *XPC* gene expression in HaCaT. **d** Effect of geniposidic acid on UVB-induced *PCNA* gene expression in HaCaT ($*p < 0.05$)

10, 20, and 30 μM, I treated the treatment group with UVB 40 mJ/cm^2 respectively, CPD decreased to 77, 31, and 12% individually. It is considered that UVB causes increasement in CPD and DNA damage increases, but geniposidic acid preserves cells, and that geniposidic acid has an effect to preserve cells (Fig. 3b). To examine changing of *XPC* expression, the DNA repair gene within HaCaT, caused by geniposidic acid, I performed qRT-PCR. *XPC* expression decreased to 0.37 at the case of treatment with 40 mJ/cm^2 of UVB as compared with the value of untreated control group which was 1. It is expected that UVB causes DNA damage, and I found that when with geniposidic acid of each density of 10, 20, and 30 μM, I treated the treatment group with UVB of 40 mJ/cm^2 respectively, *XPC* expression which was decreased due to UVB irradiation increased to 0.41, 0.54, and 0.82 individually as dose-dependent manner of geniposidic acid (Fig. 3c). It is considered that geniposidic acid has an effect on DNA damage caused by UVB to protect DNA. PCNA is a nucleoprotein of 36 kDa which is called as cyclin, and it increases all over the cell cycle from the end of G1 to S period. This is a secondary protein of DNA polymerase delta, and it has been reported that it has an important role in the beginning of cell proliferation (Jung and Jeong 1997). To examine changing of expression of *PCNA*, the DNA repair gene within HaCaT, I performed qRT-PCR. *PCNA* expression decreased to 0.29 at the case of treatment with UVB of 40 mJ/cm^2 as compared with the value of untreated control group which was 1. It is expected that UVB causes DNA damage, and I found that when with

geniposidic acid of each density of 10, 20, and 30 μM with irradiation of UVB at 40 mJ/cm^2 respectively, the expression which has decreased by UVB increased significantly to 0.39, 0.77, and 0.91 individually and dependently on density (Fig. 3d). It is considered that geniposidic acid has an effect on DNA damage repair caused by UVB.

Anti-oxidant properties analysis

DPPH is a water-soluble substance which has chemically stable free radical and has its maximum absorbance at the scale of 515–520 nm. When it meets with substances which show anti-oxidant action, it gives an electron and its radical becomes extinct to change its color. DPPH radical scavenging ability is a method to estimate the degree of anti-oxidation through the course of reacting with anti-oxidant substance to accept hydrogen atom and suppress oxidation. As the result of examining the anti-oxidation effect of geniposidic acid, I found that when I treated it with geniposidic acid of each density of 10, 20, 30, and 40 μM, its anti-oxidation effect was respectively about 18, 25, 65, and 80% dependently on density and similar to L-ascorbic acid, the positive control group (Fig. 4a).

ABTS reacts with potassium persulfate to form ABTS$^+$ of blue/green. It is the method to evaluate anti-oxidation action through analysis on the degree of decoloration by anti-oxidant. As the result of examining the anti-oxidation effect of geniposidic acid, I found that when I

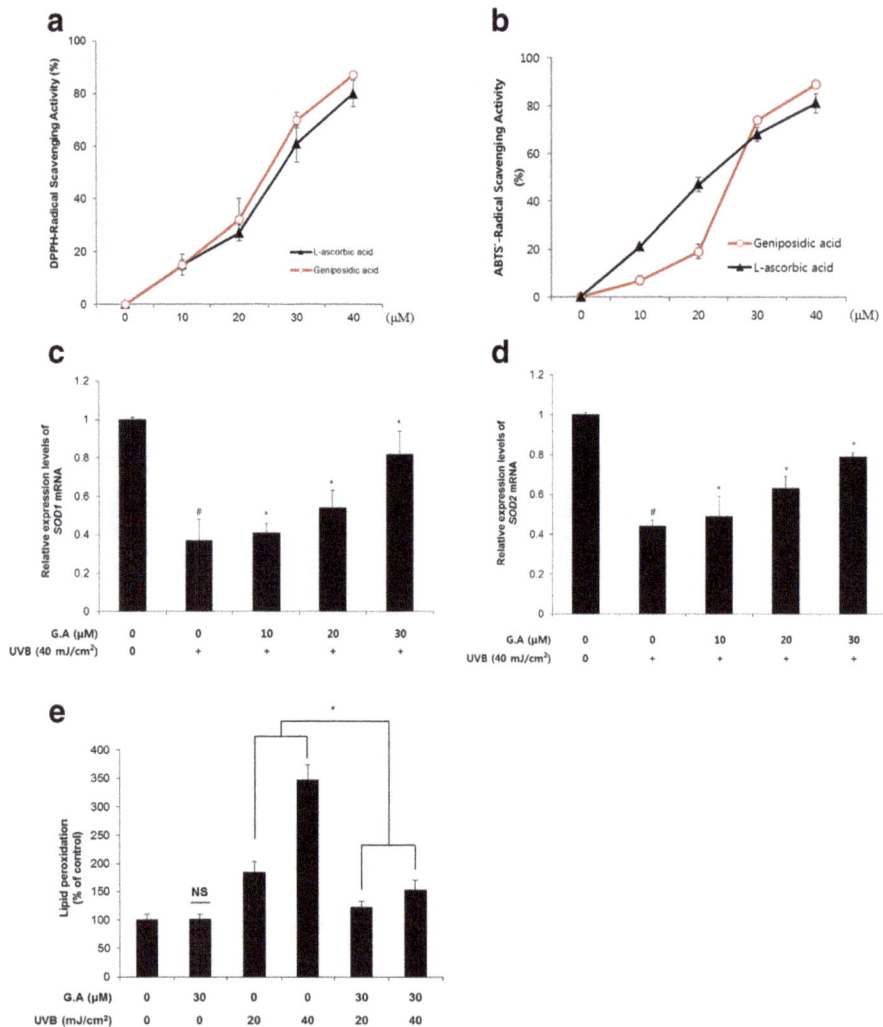

Fig. 4 Anti-oxidant effect of geniposidic acid on HaCaT. **a** Effect of geniposidic acid on DPPH radical scavenging activity. **b** Effect of geniposidic acid on ABTS radical scavenging activity. **c** Effect of geniposidic acid on UVB-induced *SOD1* gene expression in HaCaT. **d** Effect of geniposidic acid on UVB-induced *SOD2* gene expression in HaCaT. **e** Effect of geniposidic acid on UVB-induced lipid peroxidation in HaCaT (*$p < 0.05$)

treated it with geniposidic acid of each density of 10, 20, 30, and 40 µM respectively, the anti-oxidation effect was about 8, 20, 80, and 95% dependently on density and similar to L-ascorbic acid, the positive control group (Fig. 4b). Within the human body, there is a representative anti-oxidation enzyme, SOD which can protect itself against damages by reactive oxygen and has a role to transform the reactive oxygen radical (O_2^-) into H_2O and H_2O_2 to reduce the density of reactive oxygen in the body (McCord and Fridovich 1969; Fridovich 1995). Among this SOD enzyme, there are SOD1 existing in the cytoplasm, SOD2 existing in mitochondria, and SOD3 existing in the outside of cell (Huang et al. 1999), and SOD1 is the representative anti-oxidation enzyme of all SOD enzymes, contains cytoplasm, and has a role to decrease ROS with regard to all tissues in which oxygen exists (Crapo et al. 1992).

To examine what effects on changing of *SOD1* expression geniposidic acid have, I performed qRT-PCR. It was shown that while *SOD1* expression in HaCaT decreases 0.37 times by irradiation with UVB of 40 mJ/cm^2, the amount of expression increases dependently on density of geniposidic acid, so at the case of treatment with 10 µM, the amount increases 0.41 times; at the case of 20 µM, it increases 0.54 times; and at the case of 30 µM, it increases 0.82 times (Fig. 4c). It is considered that geniposidic acid induces increase in *SOD1* expression to reduce reactive oxygen and suppress cellular senescence. To examine what effects on changing of mRNA expression of *SOD2* which is anti-oxidant enzyme existing within mitochondria geniposidic acid have, I used qRT-PCR. It was shown that while *SOD2* expression in HaCaT decreases 0.44 times by treatment with UVB of 40 mJ/cm^2, the amount of expression increases dependently on density of geniposidic acid, so at the case of treatment with 10 μM, the amount increases 0.49 times; at the case of 20 μM, it increases 0.63 times; and at the case of 30 μM, it increases 0.79 times (Fig. 4d). Next, I searched what effects on changing of lipid peroxidation geniposidic acid have. When I treated it with UVB of 20 mJ/cm^2, lipid peroxidation increased to 184%, and at the case of treatment with UVB of 40 mJ/cm^2, it increased to 347%. It is considered that UVB causes oxidative stress and lipid peroxidation increases. With geniposidic acid of 30 μM, I treated both treatment group with UVB 20 and 40 mJ/cm^2 respectively, and I found that lipid peroxidation decreases to 122% at the case of treatment group with UVB 20 mJ/cm^2 and decreases to 153% at the case of treatment group with UVB 40 mJ/cm^2 (Fig. 4e).

Discussion

Cell preservation effects of geniposidic acid on HaCaT against UVB

DNA damage caused by UV results in increase in *p53* gene expression, and *p53*, the transcriptional factor, controls more than 100 genes which are induced by DNA damage (Latonen et al. 2001; Jin et al. 2000). *p53* is a representative transcriptional factor which induces cell cycle arrest, suppression of cell growth, and promotion of apoptosis (Yoon 2013), and cell cycle arrest occurs in G1/S or G2 period of cell cycle depending on the condition of *p53* action. Also, when UV causes DNA damage, *p53* induces *p21* gene expression, and expressed *p21* causes cell cycle arrest through activity of cyclin-dependent kinase (CDK) to hinder cell growth (Smits and Medema 2001; Yoon 2013; Gewirtz et al. 2008). According to recent papers, it has been reported that *p53* expression is suppressed in order to stop the promotion of senescence of normal tissue in adult mouse as the result of analysis on *p53* mouse model (Gannon et al. 2011).

In this research, I found out what effects on cell damage caused by UVB geniposidic acid have, when I treated human keratinocytes with geniposidic acid. When I pre-treated HaCaT keratinocytes with geniposidic acid of each density of 10, 20, and 30 μM respectively and tested with UVB of 40 mJ/cm^2, I found that the cell viability restores dependently on density (Fig. 1b). I could know that geniposidic acid increases in the number of cells during G1 period although UVB causes G1 cell cycle arrest (Fig. 2a), and I could find that sub-G1 decreases as the density of geniposidic acid increases (Fig. 2b). Therefore, it is considered that geniposidic acid has effects on cell damage caused by UVB to suppress apoptosis and preserve cells.

Caspase-3 amplifies initial signal to caspase-8 and caspase-9, and it is known that it is directly related with apoptosis (Kennedy et al. 2001), and it has been recognized that it induces DNA fragmentation and pycnosis to cause apoptosis (Soldani and Scovassi 2002).

As the result of examining changing of caspase-3 action in this research, the amount of cleaved caspase-3 expression increased by UVB, but I could find that the amount of cleaved caspase-3 expression decreases by treatment with geniposidic acid of each density (Fig. 2c). Therefore, it is judged that geniposidic acid has effects on cell damage caused by UVB to suppress apoptosis and preserve cells.

DNA repair effect of geniposidic acid on HaCaT against UVB

As the result of examining cell preservation effects of geniposidic acid on DNA damage, I could know that UVB increases in tailed DNA, but it reduces by treatment with geniposidic acid as indicated concentration (Fig. 3a). Also, I studied changing of CPD formation to find what effects on damaged DNA by UVB have, and I could know that UVB causes increase in CPD and DNA damage and find that CPD reduces as the density of geniposidic acid increases (Fig. 3b). Therefore, it is judged that geniposidic acid has effects to protect DNA and preserve cells. Finally, it is considered that geniposidic acid would have important roles to control expression of hypostatic genes of p53 caused by UVB, to normalize cell cycle, and to suppress dermal cellular senescence.

P53 is activated by UV, oxidative stress or DNA damage, etc. (Miliani de Marval and Zhang 2011; Lee et al. 2016), and it controls expression of genes related with various senescence such as *p21* (cyclin-dependent kinase inhibitor 1A), *14–3-σ* and *GADD45α* (growth arrest and DNA-damage-inducible, alpha) which are subordinate targets (Brown et al. 1997; Kortlever et al. 2006). P21 arrests cell cycle and hinders cell growth through the activity of CDK (Smits and Medema 2001; Gewirtz et al. 2008). GADD45α controls superordinate stage of transmission system of Cdc2 protein kinase, PCNA, p21Waf1/Cip1 protein, core histone protein, MTK/MEKK4, and JNK/SAPK, and it is concerned with suppression of cell cycle and DNA repair through protein and signal transmission system within various cells, and it has an important role to prevent DNA damage. XPC is known that it reacts first for recognition of damaged DNA. As the result of examining changing of expression of *XPC* which is one of DNA repair genes, I found that *XPC* expression significantly increases dependently on density of geniposidic acid while it reduces by UVB (Fig. 3c). Therefore, it is considered that geniposidic acid has an effect on DNA damage to repair DNA. It has been reported that PCNA is a nucleoprotein of 36 kDa which is called as cyclin and increases all over the cell cycle from the end of G1 to S period, and it is also secondary protein of DNA polymerase delta and has an important role in the beginning of cell proliferation (Jung and Jeong 1997). As the result of examining changing of expression of *PCNA*, the DNA repair gene, I could know that *PCNA* expression increases dependently on density of geniposidic acid while it reduces by UVB (Fig. 3d). Therefore, it is judged that geniposidic acid has an effect on damaged DNA by UVB to repair DNA.

Anti-oxidation effects of geniposidic acid on HaCaT against UVB

ROS which has been increased within cells causes intracellular damages such as DNA damage, mitochondria damage, protein oxidation, and disorder of energy metabolism, and intracellular damage caused by oxidative stress can result in cell cycle arrest, cellular senescence, and apoptosis (Cerella et al. 2009).

As shown in Fig. 4a, b, with regard to anti-oxidation effects, I found that geniposidic acid has an anti-oxidation effect similar to L-ascorbic acid which is known as anti-oxidation standard substance through DPPH assay and ABTS$^+$ assay with treatment of geniposidic acid. Its function to remove reactive oxygen works effectively at normal time to continue homeostasis in our human body, but it can have harmful effects on cells when it loses its balance to incline toward promotion of oxidation, and this harmful activity is called as oxidative stress. To examine what effects on changing of *SOD1* and *SOD2* expression geniposidic acid have, I performed qRT-PCR in this research. As shown in Fig. 4c, d, I could know that the amount of *SOD1* and *SOD2* expression increases dependently on density of geniposidic acid while it decreases by UVB which is one of oxidative stress. Therefore, it is considered that geniposidic acid increases *SOD1* and *SOD2* expression to reduce reactive oxygen and suppress cellular senescence, and it is judged that geniposidic acid has an anti-oxidation effect. To examine anti-oxidation effects of geniposidic acid, I used lipid peroxidation which is an indicator to estimate oxidative stress and observed its changing. As the result of this experiment, I found that lipid peroxidation reduces at the case of treatment with geniposidic acid of 30 μM while the oxidative stress caused by UVB increases in lipid peroxidation (Fig. 4e). It is considered that with particular density of 30 μM, geniposidic acid has an anti-oxidation effect.

Finally, it is considered that the study on the effectiveness of geniposidic acid on the mechanism controlling expression of factors which promote senescence through damage of dermal cells caused by UVB can help evaluating whether geniposidic acid is a natural functional cosmetic material which is helpful to

preserve dermal cells and delay their senescence against UVB.

Conclusions

This paper used a natural compound, geniposidic acid, affiliated with iridoid glycoside which is known as effective for anti-oxidation, anti-inflammation, anticancer, anti-stress, and improvement of immune system to study about such effects as cell preservation, anti-oxidation, and DNA repair on human keratinocyte damaged by UVB.

I found that at the case of testing HaCaT with UVB of 40 mJ/cm^2, cell viability reduces to 26% and cell proliferation is suppressed, but at the case of testing with the same UVB of 40 mJ/cm^2 after pretreating with geniposidic acid of each density of 10, 20, and 30 μM respectively for 3 h, the cell viability restores dependently on density (Fig. 1b).

I performed cell cycle analysis and found that geniposidic acid has an effect to increase in G1 to prevent G1 cell cycle arrest caused by UVB (Fig. 2a) and that UVB causes increasement in cell population of sub-G1 and apoptosis increases, but sub-G1 reduces as the density of geniposidic acid increases. From these results, I could know that geniposidic acid has effects to suppress apoptosis and preserve cells (Fig. 2b). As the result of examining changing of caspase-3 action, I found that the amount of cleaved caspase-3 decreases to 7.8, 5.3, and 2.2 respectively when with geniposidic acid of each density of 10, 20, and 30 μM, I treated treatment group with UVB of 40 mJ/cm^2 individually. I could know that UVB causes increasement in the amount of cleaved caspase-3 expression and apoptosis increases, and it decreases at the case of treatment with geniposidic acid of each density, and so geniposidic acid has effects to suppress apoptosis and preserve cells (Fig. 2c). Through single-cell gel electrophoresis, I found cell preservation effect of geniposidic acid on DNA damage. I found that when with geniposidic acid of each density of 10, 20, and 30 μM, I treated treatment group with UVB of 40 mJ/cm^2 respectively, DNA tail decreases to 61, 44, and 19% individually, and I could know that UVB causes increasement in DNA tail and DNA damage increases, and it decreases as I treated it with geniposidic acid of each density, and so geniposidic acid has a cell preservation effect (Fig. 3a). To find out what effects on damaged DNA by UVB geniposidic acid have, I studied changing of CPD. As the result of this experiment, I found that CPD increases to 100% when I treated HaCaT with UVB of 40 mJ/cm^2, and at the case of treatment with geniposidic acid of each density of 10, 20, and 30 μM respectively, CPD decreases to 77, 31, and 12% individually. I found that UVB causes increasement in CPD and DNA damage increases, and I could know that CPD decreases at the case of treatment with geniposidic acid of each density, and so geniposidic acid has effects to protect DNA and preserve cells (Fig. 3b).

By using qRT-PCR, I analyzed the effect of geniposidic acid on gene expression in HaCaT which was treated with UVB. I found that *XPC*, the DNA repair gene, decreases in its expression by UVB, but *XPC* expression significantly increases dependently on density of geniposidic acid, and I could find that geniposidic acid has a DNA repair effect on DNA damage caused by UVB (Fig. 3c). I found that *PCNA*, the DNA repair gene, decreases in its expression by UVB, but *PCNA* expression significantly increases dependently on density of geniposidic acid, and I could find that geniposidic acid has a DNA repair effect on DNA damage caused by UVB (Fig. 3d).

To examine an anti-oxidation effect of geniposidic acid, I used DPPH radical scavenging activity. As the result of analysis, I found that when I treated it with geniposidic acid of each density of 10, 20, 30 and 40 μM, its anti-oxidation effect appears as about 18, 25, 65, and 80% dependently on density, and so geniposidic acid has a similar anti-oxidation effect to L-ascorbic acid which is the positive control group (Fig. 4a). Also, as the result of examining the anti-oxidation effect of geniposidic acid through ABTS radical scavenging activity, I found that when I treated it with geniposidic acid of each density of 10, 20, 30, and 40 μM respectively, its anti-oxidation effect appears as about 8, 20, 80, and 95% dependently on density, and so geniposidic acid has a similar anti-oxidation effect to L-ascorbic acid which is the positive control group (Fig. 4b). To find out what effects on changing of expression of *SOD* which is an anti-oxidation enzyme existing in our human body have, I performed qRT-PCR. Among *SOD* enzyme, I found that *SOD1* which exists in cytoplasm increases in its amount of expression dependently on density of geniposidic acid and that this increase in *SOD1* expression reduces reactive oxygen within cytoplasm, and so geniposidic acid has an anti-oxidation effect (Fig. 4c). Also, I found that *SOD2* which exists in mitochondria increases in its expression dependently on density of geniposidic acid and that increase in *SOD2* expression reduces reactive oxygen within mitochondria, and so geniposidic acid has an anti-oxidation effect and cellular senescence suppression effect (Fig. 4d). Finally, I examined what effects on changing of lipid peroxidation geniposidic acid have. As the result, I found that lipid peroxidation increases in accordance with the amount of UVB but decreases as I treated it with geniposidic acid of particular density, and from this, I could find that geniposidic acid shows an effective anti oxidative activity against the oxidative stress caused by UVB (Fig. 4e).

In this research, I found that geniposidic acid has such effects as cell preservation, anti-oxidation, and DNA repair in HaCaT damaged by UVB and I assure that this result proves sufficient value of geniposidic acid as a natural cosmetic material which effectively preserves cells and delays dermal cellular senescence against damage caused by UVB.

Abbreviations
ABTS: 2,2-Azino-bis-3-ethylbenzoline-6-sulphonic acid; Ac-DEVD-pNA: *N*-Acetyl-Asp-Glu-Val-Asp p-nitroanilide; ATM: Ataxia-telangiectasia mutated; ATR: ATM- and Rad3-related; CDK: Cyclin-dependent kinase; CPD: Cyclobutane pyrimidine dimer; DMEM: Dulbecco's modified Eagle's medium; DMSO: Dimethyl sulfoxide; DPPH: 1,1-Diphenyl-2-picrylhydrazyl; FACS: Fluorescence-activated cell sorting; FBS: Fetal bovine serum; G.A: Geniposidic acid; GADD45α: Growth arrest and DNA-damage-inducible, alpha; HaCaT: Human keratinocyte; LMAgarose: Low melting agarose; MDA: Malondialdehyde; P21: Cyclin-dependent kinase inhibitor 1A; PBS: Phosphate-buffered saline; PCNA: Proliferating cell nuclear antigen; PI: Propidium iodide; pNA: p-nitroanilide; qRT-PCR: Quantitative real-time polymerase chain reaction; ROS: Reactive oxygen species; SOD1: Superoxide dismutase 1; SOD2: Superoxide dismutase 2; TBA: Thiobarbituric acid; UV: Ultraviolet; WST: Water-soluble tetrazolium salts; XPC: XPC complex subunit, DNA damage recognition, and repair factor

Acknowledgements
Not applicable

Funding
Not applicable

Competing interests
The author declares no competing interests.

References
Brown JP, Wei W, Sedivy JM. Bypass of senescence after disruption of p21CIP1/WAF1 gene in normal diploid human fibroblasts. Science. 1997;277:831–4.

Cerella C, Coppola S, Maresca V, De Nicola M, Radogna F, Ghibelli L. Multiple mechanisms for hydrogen peroxide-induced apoptosis. Ann N Y Acad Sci. 2009;1171:559–63.

Chang YC, Tseng TH, Lee MJ, Hsu JD, Wang CJ. Induction of apoptosis by penta-acetyl geniposide in rat C6 glioma cells. Chem Biol Interact. 2002;141:243–57.

Choi YH, Seo JH, Kim JS, Heor J, Kim SK, Choi SU, et al. Inhibitory effects of the stem bark extract of *Eucommia ulmoides* on the proliferation of human tumor cell lines. Kor J Pharmacogn. 2003;34:308–13.

Crapo JD, Qury T, Rabouille C, Slot JW, Chang LY. Cooper, zinc superoxide dismutase is primarily a cytosolic protein human cells. Pro Natl Acad Sci U S A. 1992;89:10405–9.

Deng Y, Guan M, Xie X, Yang X, Xiang H, Li H, et al. Geniposide inhibits airway inflammation and hyperresponsiveness in a mouse model of asthma. Int Immunopharmacol. 2013;17:561–7.

Fridovich I. Superoxide radical and superoxide dismutase. Annu Rev Biochem. 1995;64:97–112.

Gannon HS, Donehower LA, Lyle S, Jones SN. Mdm2-p53 signaling regulates epidermal stem cell senescence and premature aging phenotypes in mouse skin. Dev Biol. 2011;353:1–9.

Gewirtz DA, Holt SE, Elmore LW. Accelerated senescence: an emerging role in tumor cell response to chemotherapy and radiation. Biochem Pharmacol. 2008;76:947–57.

Guan L, Feng H, Gong D, Zhao X, Cai L, Wu Q, et al. Genipin ameliorates age-related insulin resistance through inhibiting hepatic oxidative stress and mitochondrial dysfunction. Exp Gerontol. 2013;48:1387–94.

Hong YJ, Yang KS. Anti-inflammatory activities of crocetin derivatives from processed Gardenia jasminoides. Arch Pharm Res. 2013;36:933–40.

Hsu HY, Yang JJ, Lin SY, Lin CC. Comparisons of geniposidic acid and geniposide on antitumor and radioprotection after sublethal irradiation. Cancer Lett. 1997;113:31–7.

Huang TT, Carlson EJ, Raineri I, Grillespie AM, Kozy H, Epstein CJ. The use of transgenic and mutant mice to study oxygen free radical metabolism. Ann N Y Acad Sci. 1999;893:95–112.

Jenkins G. Molecular mechanisms of skin aging. Mech Ageing Dev. 2002;123:801–10.

Jin S, Antinore MJ, Lung FD, Dong X, Zhao H, Fan F, et al. The GADD45 inhibition of Cdc2 kinase correlates with GADD45-mediated growth suppression. J Biol Chem. 2000;275:16602–8.

Jung SI, Jeong GB. P53 and PCNA protein expression on the colorectal cancer tissue. Chungbuk Med J. 1997;7:223–36.

Kennedy DO, Kojima A, Yano Y, Hasuma T, Otani S, Matsui-Yuasa I. Growth inhibitory effect of green tea extract in Ehrlich ascites tumor cells involves cytochrome c release and caspase activation. Cancer Lett. 2001;166:9–15.

Kortlever RM, Higgins PJ, Bernards R. Plasminogen activator inhibitor-1 is a critical downstream target of p53 in the induction of replicative senescence. Nat Cell Biol. 2006;8:877–84.

Kulms D, Zeise E, Pöppelmann B, Schwarz T. DNA damage, death receptor activation and reactive oxygen species contribute to ultraviolet radiation-induced apoptosis in an essential and independent way. Oncogene. 2002;21:5844–51.

Latonen L, Taya Y, Laiho M. UV-radiation induces dose-dependent regulation of p53 response and modulates p53-HDM2 interaction in human fibroblasts. Oncogene. 2001;20:6784–93.

Lee S, Han HS, An IS, Ahn KJ. Effects of amentoflavone on anti-inflammation and cytoprotection. Asian J Beauty Cosmetol. 2016;14:201–11.

Lee YR, Noh EM, Han JH, Kim JM, Hwang JK, Hwang BM, et al. Brazilin inhibits UVB-induced MMP-1/3 expressions and secretions by suppressing the NF-κB pathway in human dermal fibroblasts. Eur J Pharmacol. 2012;674:80–6.

McCord JM, Fridovich I. The utility of superoxide dismutase in studying free radical reactions. I. Radicals generated by the interaction of sulfite, dimethyl sulfoxide and oxygen. J Biol Chem. 1969;244:6056–63.

Miliani de Marval PL, Zhang Y. The RP-Mdm2-p53 pathway and tumorigenesis. Oncotarget. 2011;2:234–8.

Park SD, Kim GW. Experimental studies of eucommiae cortex according to processing. The Journal of Dong Guk Oriental Medicine. 1992;1:81–107.

Smits VA, Medema RH. Checking out the G(2)/M transition. Biochim Biophys Acta. 2001;1519:1–12.

Soldani C, Scovassi AI. Poly(ADP-ribose) polymerase-1 cleavage during apoptosis: an update. Apoptosis. 2002;7:321–8.

Yoon YM. Gene expression profiling in protection mechanism of silibinin against damage to human dermal fibroblasts caused by UVB. Asian J Beauty Cosmetol. 2013;11:93–102.

10

A brief review of pemphigus vulgaris

William J. Sanders[1,2]

Abstract

Pemphigus vulgaris is an autoimmune disorder which presents with painful mucocutaneous blisters and erosions. On the skin, they are flaccid bullae or erosions, and on the mucosa, they present as erosions. This disease is rare but is devastating to those who have it; it also is related—perhaps genetically—to other autoimmune conditions. This is to say that a patient can develop pemphigus vulgaris if they have thyroiditis or diabetes mellitus. Biopsy is needed to obtain histopathological evidence of the breakdown of intercellular connections due to the autoimmune attack on components of desmosomes, which are responsible for intercellular integrity above the basement membrane. When these desmosomes are attacked, loss of connection ensues, and the cells break apart at these connections; this leads to fluid buildup, seen grossly as bullae. Treatment of the disease is difficult and sometimes unsafe. For decades, the mainstay of treatment has been glucocorticoids followed by other drugs. Unfortunately, these drugs are systemically absorbed, and the side effect profile can be unfavorable. In the past several years however, more innovative treatments have emerged that may help ease the cost and safety burden to patients. This review highlights the major points about pemphigus vulgaris, its pathophysiology, and its treatment.

Keywords: Pemphigus vulgaris, Autoimmune, Acantholysis, Mucosal, Skin, Erosion, Bullae

Background

Pemphigus vulgaris (PV) is a debilitating dermatologic condition that is autoimmune in nature. It can be life threatening and can have a mortality rate between 5 and 15% (Razzaque Ahmed and Moy 1982). Usually, mortality has been associated with skin infections or pneumonias as a result of the structural damage caused by PV. It can present with lesions on the mucosal and skin surfaces (Mustafa et al. 2015). Usually, the oral mucosa will be the first to present with lesions. The reason PV is so devastating is that often times the treatment for it causes further medical problems and conditions. However, as in all of medicine, the treatment protocol is becoming more streamlined and advanced as we learn more about the disease. There are emerging options for treatment that will benefit patients with the disease while decreasing the likelihood of creating or exacerbating a new medical condition concomitant to that of PV.

Main text
Epidemiology

PV has an average age of onset of 40–60 years (Joly and Litrowski 2011). It has a prevalence of around 30,000 cases in the USA and an incidence of 1–10 new cases per 1 million people (Pemphigus. Pemphigus Pemphigoid Foundation (IPPF) 2014). It is a rare disease—especially in the pediatric population, but it needs no less study because it does affect patients and also does affect certain groups of people more than others. Ashkenazi Jews and people from India and the Middle East have higher rates of the disease (Pisanti et al. 1974). It is equally distributed among genders.

Clinical presentation

Patients can present with painful ulcerations of especially the buccal or palatine mucosa, but it can also present in the nose, genitals, anus, esophagus, and conjunctiva (Kavala et al. 2015; Kavala et al. 2011). In the skin, the bullae have a tendency to rupture, because the cellular interconnections are weakened by the autoimmune attack on desmogleins 1 and 3 (Stanley and Amagai 2006). Figure 1 shows PV of the oral mucosa as well as on the skin. The clinician can reproduce this rupturing or sloughing of the epidermis by putting

Correspondence: Williamsan@pcom.edu
[1]Georgia Campus-Philadelphia College of Osteopathic Medicine (GA-PCOM), Suwanee, GA 30024, USA
[2]Houston Medical Center, Warner Robins, GA 31088, USA

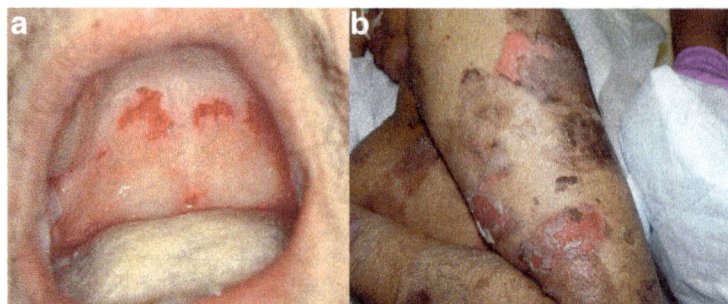

Fig. 1 PV on oral/skin mucosa. **a**: Pemphigus of the soft palate due to erosive disconnection of intraepidermal desmosomes. **b**: These are Pemphigus lesions of flaccid bullae that have ruptures on the upper arm. Loss of connections between keratinocytes due to autoantibodies against desmosome components render fluid buildup between these cells. They can rupture and slough away with time or manual pressure, such as seen in Nikolsky's sign

lateral pressure or traction on the bullae. When these slough off, it is referred to as a positive Nikolsky's sign (Venugopal and Murrell 2011). Because patients can have oral erosions, the pain can come with chewing and swallowing. This may lead to an avoidance of food and long-term nutritional deficiencies, which cause their own problems.

Pathophysiology

PV, as noted above, is an autoimmune disease. There are cell surface components known as desmoglein proteins which are components of the desmosomes in between keratinocytes. Keratinocytes are the cells which make up the layers of the epidermis. Particularly, in the stratum spinosum (called spinosum (Beutner and Jordon 1964) because the "spines"—which are desmosomes—can be seen between conjoining cells in this epidermal layer), desmosomes contribute to mechanical strength and integrity of and between cells, as well as cellular differentiation (Garrod and Chidgey 2008). The stratum spinosum also produces the keratin seen in the corny layer. This integrity of the cellular structure is part of the reason why skin is waterproof and tough. Antibodies to the two most common desmogleins—1 and 3—attack the epitope structure of these desmosomes and cause damage. Particularly, the immunoglobulin subclass of these autoantibodies is IgG4 (Ding et al. 1999; Bhol et al. 1995). Essentially, a type 2 hypersensitivity reaction takes place in which antibodies attach and destroy cell surface receptors. This leads to loss of integrity between keratinocytes in the stratum spinosum and loss of intercellular connectivity; this is referred to as acantholysis (Kumaran et al. 2013).

PV, like other autoimmune diseases, is related to major histocompatibility complex (MHC) variation. MHC is a structure located on certain immune cells like macrophages and B cells which carry out immunologic functions, such as presenting to T cells and recognizing host and foreign antigens. Human leukocyte antigen (HLA) genes encode the MHC so that different variations in these genes cause a different immunologic function downstream (Janeway 1999). Particularly, PV is associated with HLA-DR4. This may explain why there is a positive association between type 1 diabetes mellitus, Hashimoto's thyroiditis, and rheumatoid arthritis (Parameswaran et al. 2015). However, HLA-DRB1 0402 is mostly associated with those of Ashkenazi Jewish descent (Kwon et al. 2001).

Diagnosis

There are other less common and less severe forms of pemphigus under the pemphigus umbrella, so weaving through the differential diagnosis involves a keen clinical acumen as well as the laboratory. To help confirm the diagnosis, other tests are run. After punch biopsy and histopathologic preparation, PV displays a particular cellular pattern. Because the problem is in between cells and not under the basal aspect of the cell, there is no space between the cell and the basement membrane. This leaves an intact, bottom layer of cells connected to the basement membrane. There is intraepidermal acantholysis seen (Bystryn and Rudolph 2005). If there was an autoimmune attack against hemidesmosomes on the basal side of the cell, there would be a loss of connection of the basal keratinocyte to the basement membrane, yielding a different and clinically less severe condition known as bullous pemphigoid. In the case of PV, the new pathologic space is in between the cells; this causes fluid to build up in places with lower intercellular integrity. Because the intercellular connections are lost—like a zipper, where the unzipped part is the damaged intercellular piece—and yet the cells are still intact on the basement membrane, they are said to have a tombstone pattern on histopathology (Baum et al. 2014). Figure 2 shows acantholysis and the "row of

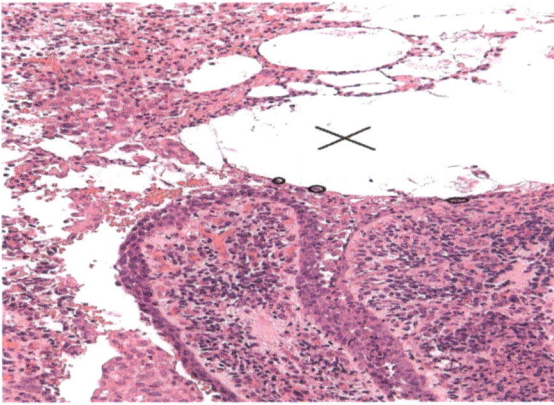

Fig. 2 PV histopathology. The "x" represents edema buildup between intraepidermal keratinocytes-also known as acantholysis- due to loss of adhesion between cells. Fluid will build up in these potential spaces when the chance arises. The bottom layer of cells (some have been circled) located underneath the edema are left intact and have been said to have a tombstone appearance. They represent the intact basal layer.

tombstones" pattern in PV. An increase in eosinophils can also be seen in the dermis.

Upon direct immunofluorescence of the skin or mucosal lesion, IgG can be seen as a "net-like" or reticular pattern where the IgG autoantibodies to desmogleins have been bound (Morrison 2001). This can be seen below in Fig. 3. An ELISA can be done to find autoantibodies to desmogleins 1 and 3 in the serum as well (Joly and Litrowski 2011). These can actually be tracked to assess remission and control of the disease (Abasq et al. 2009; Amagai et al. 1999).

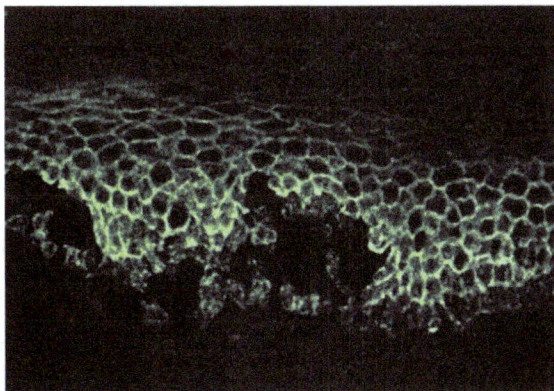

Fig. 3 PV direct immunofluorescence. IgG deposits intercellularly, along with intraepidermal acantholysis. The IgG deposition is represented by the hyperintense, brighter color distributed in a net-like or reticular pattern in between cells. The dark spaces nearby represent the fluid buildup that ensues as a result of loss of intercellular connection because of the IgG deposition. Courtesy of Wikipedia user: Emmanuelm

Management

Management of acute attacks and original management of the disease is with systemic glucocorticoids such as prednisolone, 1–1.5 mg/kg PO per day (Chams-Davatchi et al. 2007). The idea is to bring the patient into remission of their disease with steroids, using the smallest dosage possible; the reason for the smallest possible dosages is to avoid the possible comorbidities, such as Cushing's disease, osteoporosis, hypertension, and diabetes to name a few (Schacke 2002). As the patient begins to take systemic glucocorticoids, they can also be prescribed an adjunct treatment protocol with nonsteroidal but immunosuppressant drugs such as azathioprine and mycophenolate (Bystryn 1996). These are the same drugs used in many chemotherapy regimens for different cancers and other autoimmune conditions.

Being in remission is usually considered when the patient has been free of lesions for several weeks and with a negative Nikolsky's sign. At such a point, the systemic glucocorticoids are tapered down to a gradually decreasing dose. When the steroids can be stopped and the patient kept in remission, the other aforementioned adjunct drugs can begin to be tapered.

However, some of these drugs have potentially fatal side effects and do require monitoring. Azathioprine inhibits purine formation and can lead to myelosuppression. This requires quite frequent blood checkups and monitoring of kidney and liver function bi-weekly for the first 3 months and again periodically subsequently (Meggitt et al. 2011). Also because azathioprine is metabolized in the body by thiopurine methyltransferase (TPMT), the levels of this enzyme will need to be obtained upon initiating treatment (Jackson et al. 1997). Too little TPMT activity could result in gross overdosing of azathioprine and increased risk of adverse events such as myelosuppression. Mycophenolate has a safer side effect profile—aside from some gastrointestinal issues—than azathioprine, but it was found in randomized trials to have a lesser glucocorticoid-sparing effect than azathioprine (Martin et al. 2011); this means that patients who use azathioprine as an adjunct to glucocorticoids needed to use less glucocorticoids due to azathioprine's superior glucocorticoid-sparing effect. Therefore, these drugs both have pros and cons, but each patient needs to be treated in a fashion that caters to his or her specific needs and pre-existing conditions.

Many patients go on to have recalcitrant PV after long periods of successful treatment with the aforementioned medications. A large majority do in fact achieve remission for at least 6 months if they have been treated with glucocorticoids and adjunct medications for close to 10 years; however, around 20–40% of patients do not ever go into remission and are considered refractory (Herbst and Bystryn 2000). PV can be a deadly disease, so enhanced treatment in these refractory patients is absolutely necessary. Rituximab has a place in treatment for PV based on the premise that a disease of antibodies is a disease of B cells. Being an antibody against the CD 20 antigen expressed on B cells. Rituximab can curb the disease, especially in refractory cases. Several case studies have shown rituximab to be efficacious (Hertl et al. 2008; Arin et al. 2005). Cyclophosphamide is also used in refractory cases, but it has an unsafe side effect profile (Saha et al. 2009). It can cause hemorrhagic cystitis. Because of its safety profile, it requires regular monitoring by the patient, which is an inconvenience. Plasmapheresis is also used occasionally by non-specifically removing proteins from the blood, but it is costly and has its own unfavorable side effects, depending on the patient's condition. IVIG can also be used to dilute the autoantibodies with regular immunoglobulin.

The main reason that these interventions are used for recalcitrant disease instead of first line is simply their cost. Rituximab treatment can cost $16,000 (Bomm et al. 2013). Patients may benefit by switching to a more practical, safer, and cheaper alternative. New advances in treatment of PV have emerged, specifically by way of innovative therapies such as subcutaneous veltuzumab injections. It has the same mechanism of action as rituximab, but it is cheaper and not as systemically absorbed. Some studies have shown that it can induce remission in patients after just two injections, 2 weeks apart (Ellebrecht et al. 2014). This drug may need more long-term controlled trials to further evaluate the efficacy for sustained remission, but it has been shown clinically to induce remission for patients who are refractory in their condition. With no monitoring and it being a cheaper, safer alternative, this could provide a new road for those suffering from recalcitrant disease.

Conclusions

PV, while rare, is very distressing and painful for those who have it. The disease is not always isolated; many people also have concomitant chronic diseases to go along with it. This fact makes it urgent that PV be treated in a specific, patient-centered manner. We would not want someone who has diabetes mellitus and PV to take long-term glucocorticoids. The treatment plan should be tailored to the specific individual patient, following evidence-based recommendations mentioned herein. We can use the first-line drugs and a large majority of patients will be treated successfully; for the 20–40% of patients who are recalcitrant despite first-line and adjunctive agents, they must be treated with an innovative protocol. The use of new topical drugs and subcutaneous injections like veltuzumab has created a protocol whereby refractory PV patients can safely and

effectively try a new, promising method of treatment. More numerous and long-term studies need to be done to evaluate the long-term benefits of these less systemic therapies. Perhaps one day, these drugs will be backed by enough evidence demonstrating their favorable safety profile and lower cost that they will be the first line of treatment instead of glucocorticoids. Until then, new randomized controlled trials will add power to an ever-growing body of evidence that there will always be newer, better therapies for those who suffer from PV.

Abbreviations
IVIG: Intravenous immunoglobulin G; PV: Pemphigus vulgaris; TPMT: Thiopurine methyltransferase

Acknowledgements
Not applicable.

Funding
There was no funding for this review.

Author's contributions
WS worked on this review and did all of the researching groundwork as well as typing and formatting the work.

Author's information
William Sanders is a third year medical student at Georgia Campus-Philadelphia College of Osteopathic Medicine (PCOM). His interests include Dermatology and Internal Medicine.

Competing interests
The author declares that he has no competing interests.

References
Abasq C, Mouquet H, Gilbert D, Tron F, Grassi V, Musette P, et al. ELISA Testing of Anti–Desmoglein 1 and 3 Antibodies in the Management of Pemphigus. Arch Dermatol. 2009;145(5):529–35.

Amagai M, Komai A, Hashimoto T, Shirakata Y, Hashimoto K, Yamada T, et al. Usefulness of enzyme-linked immunosorbent assay using recombinant desmogleins 1 and 3 for serodiagnosis of pemphigus. Br J Dermatol. 1999;140(2):351–7.

Arin M, Engert A, Krieg T, Hunzelmann N. Anti-CD20 monoclonal antibody (rituximab) in the treatment of pemphigus. Br J Dermatol. 2005;153(3):620–5.

Baum S, Sakka N, Artsi O, Trau H, Barzilai A. Diagnosis and classification of autoimmune blistering diseases. Autoimmun Rev. 2014;13(4–5):482–9.

Beutner E, Jordon R. Demonstration of Skin Antibodies in Sera of Pemphigus Vulgaris Patients by Indirect Immunofluorescent Staining. Exp Biol Med. 1964;117(2):505–10.

Bhol K, Natarajan K, Nagarwalla N, Mohimen A, Aoki V, Ahmed A. Correlation of peptide specificity and IgG subclass with pathogenic and nonpathogenic autoantibodies in pemphigus vulgaris: a model for autoimmunity. Proc Natl Acad Sci. 1995;92(11):5239–43.

Bomm L, Fracaroli T, Sodré J, Bressan A, Gripp A. Off-label use of rituximab in dermatology: pemphigus treatment. An Bras Dermatol. 2013;88(4):676–8.

Bystryn J. The adjuvant therapy of pemphigus. Arch Derm. 1996;132(2):203–12.

Bystryn J, Rudolph J. Pemphigus. Lancet. 2005;366(9479):61–73.

Chams-Davatchi C, Esmaili N, Daneshpazhooh M, Valikhani M, Balighi K, Hallaji Z, et al. Randomized controlled open-label trial of four treatment regimens for pemphigus vulgaris. J Am Acad Dermatol. 2007;57(4):622–8.

Ding X, Diaz L, Fairley J, Giudice G, Liu Z. The Anti-Desmoglein 1 Autoantibodies in Pemphigus Vulgaris Sera are Pathogenic. J Investig Dermatol. 1999;112(5):739–43.

Ellebrecht C, Choi E, Allman D, Tsai D, Wegener W, Goldenberg D, et al. Subcutaneous Veltuzumab, a Humanized Anti-CD20 Antibody, in the

Treatment of Refractory Pemphigus Vulgaris. JAMA Dermatology. 2014;150(12):1331.

Garrod D, Chidgey M. Desmosome structure, composition and function. Biochim Biophys Acta Biomembr. 2008;1778(3):572–87.

Herbst A, Bystryn J. Patterns of remission in pemphigus vulgaris. J Am Acad Dermatol. 2000;42(3):422–7.

Hertl M, Zillikens D, Borradori L, Bruckner-Tuderman L, Burckhard H, Eming R, et al. Recommendations for the use of rituximab (anti-CD20 antibody) in the treatment of autoimmune bullous skin diseases. J Dtsch Dermatol Ges. 2008;6(5):366–73.

Jackson A, Hall A, McLelland J. Thiopurine methyltransferase levels should be measured before commening patients on azathioprine. Br J Dermatol. 1997;136(1):133–4.

Janeway C. Immunobiology: The Immune System in Heath and Disease. 5th ed. London: Harcourt Brace and Company; 1999.

Joly P, Litrowski N. Pemphigus group (vulgaris, vegetans, foliaceus, herpetiformis, brasiliensis). Clin Dermatol. 2011;29(4):432–6.

Kavala M, Altıntaş S, Kocatürk E, Zindancı İ, Can B, Ruhi Ç, et al. Ear, nose and throat involvement in patients with pemphigus vulgaris: correlation with severity, phenotype and disease activity. J Eur Acad Dermatol Venereol. 2011;25(11):1324–7.

Kavala M, Topaloğlu Demir F, Zindanci I, Can B, Turkoğlu Z, Zemheri E, et al. Genital involvement in pemphigus vulgaris (PV): Correlation with clinical and cervicovaginal Pap smear findings. J Am Acad Dermatol. 2015;73(4):655–9.

Kumaran M, Kanwar A, Seshadri D. Acantholysis revisited: Back to basics. Indian J Dermatol Venereol Leprol. 2013;79(1):120.

Kwon O, Brautbar C, Weintrob N, Sprecher E, Saphirman C, Bloch K, et al. Immunogenetics of HLA class II in Israeli Ashkenazi Jewish, Israeli non-Ashkenazi Jewish, and in Israeli Arab IDDM patients. Hum Immunol. 2001;62(1):85–91.

Martin L, Werth V, Villaneuva E, Murrell D. A systematic review of randomized controlled trials for pemphigus vulgaris and pemphigus foliaceus. J Am Acad Dermatol. 2011;64(5):903–8.

Meggitt S, Anstey A, Mohd Mustapa M, Reynolds N, Wakelin S. British Association of Dermatologists' guidelines for the safe and effective prescribing of azathioprine 2011. Br J Dermatol. 2011;165(4):711–34.

Morrison L. Direct immunofluorescence microscopy in the diagnosis of autoimmune bullous dermatoses. Clin Dermatol. 2001;19(5):607–13.

Mustafa M, Porter S, Smoller B, Sitaru C. Oral mucosal manifestations of autoimmune skin diseases. Autoimmun Rev. 2015;14(10):930–51.

Parameswaran A, Attwood K, Sato R, Seiffert-Sinha K, Sinha A. Identification of a new disease cluster of pemphigus vulgaris with autoimmune thyroid disease, rheumatoid arthritis and type I diabetes. Br J Dermatol. 2015;172(3):729–38.

Pemphigus. Pemphigus Pemphigoid Foundation (IPPF) 2014. http://www.pemphigus.org/research/clinically-speaking/pemphigus/. Accessed 11 Feb 2017.

Pisanti S, Sharav Y, Kaufman E, Posner L. Pemphigus vulgaris: Incidence in Jews of different ethnic groups, according to age, sex, and initial lesion. Oral Surg Oral Med Oral Pathol. 1974;38(3):382–7.

Razzaque Ahmed A, Moy R. Death in pemphigus. J Am Acad Dermatol. 1982;7(2):221–8.

Saha M, Powell A, Bhogal B, Black M, Groves R. Pulsed intravenous cyclophosphamide and methylprednisolone therapy in refractory pemphigus. Br J Dermatol. 2009;162(4):790–7.

Schacke H. Mechanisms involved in the side effects of glucocorticoids. Pharmacol Ther. 2002;96(1):23–43.

Stanley J, Amagai M. Pemphigus, Bullous Impetigo, and the Staphylococcal Scalded-Skin Syndrome. N Engl J Med. 2006;355(17):1800–10.

Venugopal S, Murrell D. Diagnosis and Clinical Features of Pemphigus Vulgaris. Dermatol Clin. 2011;29(3):373–80.

11

Characterization of adipose-derived stem cells freshly isolated from liposuction aspirates performed with Prolipostem®

Antonella Savoia[1], Angelica Perna[2], Basso Di Pasquale[1], Nicoletta Onori[3], Antonio De Luca[2], Angela Lucariello[2] and Alfonso Baldi[4*] (iD)

Abstract

Background: Lipofilling is a cosmetic surgical procedure that consists in the withdrawal of a small quantity of fat tissue from a suitable anatomic area and the reimplantation of this tissue in another corporeal district in the same individual, so as to obtain a filling effect. Recently, adipose-derived stem cells (ADSCs) have been isolated in the aspirates. These are pluripotent mesenchymal stem cells that are able to differentiate in mature adipose cells or other adult mesenchymal cells after paracrine or autocrine hormonal stimulations, thus favoring a longer survival of the implanted tissues.

Methods: In this article, we have defined a new method for liposuction (Prolipostem®), where the ADSCs are recovered and mixed with the suctioned adipose tissue derived from the abdominal fat, before the reimplantation.

Results: We have demonstrated by immunocytochemistry the presence of ADSCs in the adipose tissue taken with Prolipostem® from the abdominal fat and the ability of these ADSCs to differentiate in mature adipose cells in vitro.

Conclusions: The possibility to enrich the tissue to be implanted with ADSCs would assure a longer survival of the cells implanted and a regeneration of the host tissue thanks to growth and angiogenic stimuli induced by the ADSCs.

Keywords: Adipose-derived stem cells (ADSCs), Diaminobenzidine (DAB), Dulbecco's modified Eagle's medium (DMEM), Fetal bovine serum (FBS), Phosphate-buffered saline (PBS)

Background

Lipofilling is a very popular cosmetic surgical procedure. It finds several indications both in reconstructive surgery and esthetic surgery for the body remodeling (Sinno et al. 2016; Kasem et al. 2015). The technique consists in the withdrawal of a small quantity of fat tissue from a suitable anatomic area (abdomen, sides, thighs, knees) and the reimplantation of this tissue in another corporeal district in the same individual, so as to obtain a filling effect (Joyce et al. 2015; Savoia et al. 2014; Savoia et al. 2013). Therefore, the adipose tissue is taken and reimplanted in security in the same patient setting up an autologous transplant.

After implantation, the adipose tissue can undergo various transformations: (a) it can be quickly degraded by the organism itself if there is not adequate hematic contribution; (b) it can be encapsulated if the plan of implantation is not correct; (c) it can be calcified (above all in the mammary gland) if the amount of tissue implanted is big (Yoshimura et al. 2006). It is therefore clear that, if the fat is injected in large quantities, not all fat cells will be in contact with vascularized tissues and they will subsequently undergo apoptosis, necrosis, and resorption.

Recently, adipose-derived stem cells (ADSCs) have been isolated in the aspirates (Sterodimas et al. 2011). These are pluripotent mesenchymal stem cells that are similar to bone marrow-derived mesenchymal stem cells (Sterodimas et al. 2011; Tiryaki et al. 2011; Park et al. 2008). Indeed, ADSCs are able to differentiate in mature adipose cells or other adult mesenchymal cells after

* Correspondence: alfonsobaldi@tiscali.it
[4]Department of Environmental, Biological and Pharmaceutical Sciences and Technologies, Università degli Studi della Campania "L. Vanvitelli", Caserta, Italy
Full list of author information is available at the end of the article

paracrine or autocrine hormonal stimulations (Yang et al. 2010; Takeda et al. 2015; Wang et al. 2015; Salibian et al. 2013). This characteristic of ADSCs would allow the regeneration and, therefore, a longer survival of the implanted tissues (Ryu et al. 2013; Ellenbogen et al. 2005). Unfortunately, with the standard techniques for liposuction, the vast majority of ADSCs are lost during the procedure (Sterodimas et al. 2011). In fact, suctioned adipose tissue by means of centrifugation and vacuum pressure is divided in two portions: a fatty portion that consists of shredded adipose tissue and a fluid portion composed by the saline solution pre-injected into the site of suction, peripheral blood and cells derived from adipose tissue (Sterodimas et al. 2011; Tiryaki et al. 2011). Among these cells, there are also ADSCs, as clearly demonstrated (Sterodimas et al. 2011). The liquid portion of the suction, indeed, is generally discarded and not included in the material that is implanted.

To overcome this problem, our research group has defined a new method for liposuction (Prolipostem®), where the ADSCs are recovered and mixed with the suctioned adipose tissue before the reimplantation. The possibility to enrich the tissue to be implanted with ADSCs would assure a longer survival of the cells implanted and a regeneration of the host tissue thanks to growth and angiogenic stimuli induced by the ADSCs. Goal of this work is to demonstrate the presence of ADSCs in the adipose tissue taken with Prolipostem® and the ability of these ADSCs to, eventually, differentiate in mature adipose cells in vitro.

Methods

Patients
Five female patients aged between 37 and 50 years old have participated in the study. All the procedures have been performed in anti-aging centers of PROMOITALIA (Pozzuoli, Italy). All the patients had typical aging signs and required a lipofilling. All patients were carefully informed about the procedures and all signed an informed consent.

Liposuction protocol
Local anesthesia, was done with Lidocain at 1–2%, diluted Epinefrin 1/200,000 and the addition of NaHCO3 diluted 1/9 cc. Liposuction from the abdominal fat was performed with the Prolipostem® kit. Two liposuctions for a total of 40 ml of adipose tissue were accomplished for each patient. The kit uses a special syringe with a controlled vacuum that allows the fat aspiration without the necessity of a pneumatic pump and a distinct chamber for the collection of the adipose tissue (Promobarell®). This chamber was, then, centrifuged at 3000 rpm for 7 min. At the end of the centrifugation, a fatty and a fluid portion were clearly visible in the chambers (Fig. 1). The

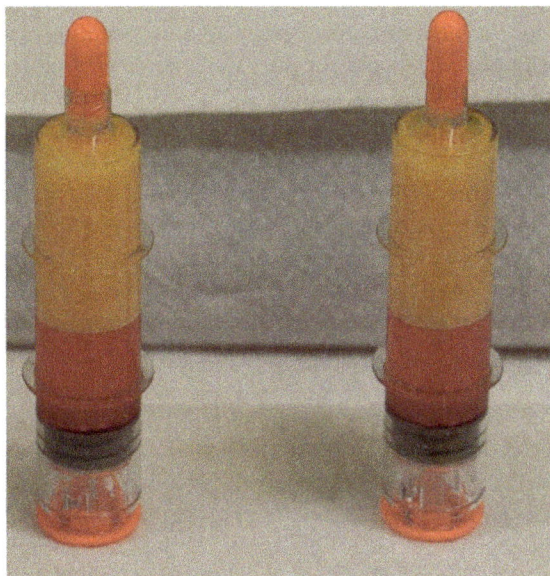

Fig. 1 Isolation of ADSCs from liposuction aspirates. At the end of the centrifugation, a fatty and a fluid portion are clearly visible in the chambers

upper portion was fatty and consisted of the suctioned adipose tissue and an oily component coming from the damaged adipose tissue; the lower portion was fluid and consisted of physiological solution mixed with anesthetics, peripheral blood, stromal tissue and ADSCs. By the use of a special nut runner, the oil component together with peripheral blood and the physiological solution were removed and the adipose tissue was mixed with the staminal cell and with the stromal component.

Cell isolation
The sample obtained from the liposuction with the Prolipostem® kit was washed with phosphate-buffered saline (PBS) containing 5% penicillin/streptomycin in order to remove debris and the local anesthetic present after liposuction. For the tissue digestion, a 0.075% solution of collagenase I was used at a temperature of 37 °C under stirring for 30 min. After 30 min, a culture medium DMEM (Dulbecco's modified Eagle's medium) containing a 10% fetal bovine serum (FBS) was added to neutralize collagenase I. After centrifuging samples at a speed of 1300 rpm for a time of 10 min, a pellet containing ADSCs was obtained. The pellet was resuspended with a solution containing ammonium chloride (0.16 M NH_4Cl) for the lysis of erythrocytes for 10 min and then centrifuged at a speed of 1300 rpm for 10 min. The pellet then was resuspended in complete culture medium (DMEM supplemented with 10% FBS and 1% antibiotic/antimycotic) and the cells plated at a density of 1×10^6 cells per dish.

Cell culture

Freshly isolated ADSCs were plated in medium at a density of 1×10^6 cells per dish. Cells were cultured with standard protocol as previously described (Lucariello et al. 2015; Lucariello et al. 2013). Briefly, cells were cultured at 37 °C, 5% CO_2, in humid air. The culture medium was DMEM supplemented with 10% FBS and 1% antibiotic/antimycotic. Primary cells were cultured for 7 days and were defined as "Passage 0." The medium was replaced every 3 days, and cells were passaged every week. After primary culture for 7 days, attached cells were passaged by trypsinization and plated in the same medium at a density of 2000 cells/cm^2.

Induced differentiation

Differentiation was performed with standard protocol as previously described (Manente et al. 2012; Esposito et al. 2013; Esposito et al. 2012a). Briefly, 7 days after seeding ADSCs at Passage 3–5, cell differentiation was initiated by replacing the DMEM culture medium. Cells cultured in control medium were used as negative controls. For adipogenic differentiation, confluent cultures were incubated for 14 days either in a medium without FBS and supplemented with platelets and calcium gluconate 5%, or in a medium containing a "lipogenic solution" made up with an insulin-like peptide, glucose 5%, hyaluronic acid 0.5%, and calcium gluconate 1%. The media were replaced every 3 days, and at 0–7–14 days of treatment, cells were stained with Oil Red O in order to highlight the lipid droplets.

Oil Red O

Oil Red O was performed to visualize lipid droplets. Briefly, as previously described (Esposito et al. 2009; Esposito et al. 2012b; Esposito et al. 2015), cells were fixed with 4% paraformaldehyde for 10 min, after they were washed with 60% isopropanol and incubated for 15 min to visualize lipid droplets. Cells were then washed with isopropanol and counterstained with hematoxylin. Plates were observed by a phase contrast microscope. Lipids appeared red and the nuclei appeared blue.

Immunocytochemistry

Immunocytochemistry was performed as previously described (Signorile and Baldi 2015; Spugnini et al. 2013). Briefly, fixed cells on microscope slides (4% paraformaldehyde for 10 min) were washed with PBS, then immunocytochemical analysis were made in order to confirm the presence of stem cells. For this analysis, a specific antibody for β1-integrin (Sigma) has been used at a dilution of 1:100 for 1 h at room temperature. Negative controls for each tissue section were prepared by leaving out the primary antibody. After washing with triphosphate-buffered saline (TBS), sections were incubated with biotinylated goat anti-mouse\anti-rabbit immuno-globulin G (Dako A\S, Denmark) for 10 min, then washed with TBS, treated with streptoavidin-peroxydase reagent (Dako A\S, Denmark) for 10 min and washed again with TBS. Finally, cells were incubated in diaminobenzidine (DAB) for 5 min, followed by hematoxylin counterstaining. Negative controls were performed by leaving out the primary antibody.

Results

ADSCs are present in the adipose tissue taken with Prolipostem®

It is well known that ADSCs express several markers (Zhu et al. 2010). To investigate the possibility that among the cells extracted from the tissue sample obtained from the liposuction with the Prolipostem® procedure there were also ADSCs, we performed immunocytochemical analysis for β1-integrin essentially as described in the "Materials and methods" section. ADSCs, once isolated from the adipose tissue, have been propagated in suitable flasks and the cultivation medium has been renewed every 2 or 3 days in order to remove the left cells in suspension. After three passages, cells were fixed and analyzed by immunohistochemistry as described in the "Materials and methods" section. Indeed, several cells were positive for integrin as shown in Fig. 2.

ADSCs are able to differentiate in adult adipocytes

ADSCs in culture, under adequate stimulus, are able to differentiate in osteoblasts, adipocytes, and chondro-cytes. In this work we have induced the differentiation in adipocytes using different medium with various induc-tion factors. Cells have been treated by 14 days, period during which they have been monitored and stained to verify any changes.

At day 0, a first Oil Red staining has been made to exclude the presence of adipocytes in the culture (Fig. 3a). At day 7, a second Oil Red staining has been made on the cells treated with the two differentiation medium. Indeed, we observed the total absence of lipid droplets in the cytoplasm of the cells treated with the first differentiation medium (Fig. 3c, d), while they were already visible in the cells treated with the second differ-entiation medium (Fig. 3e).

At the day 14 (end of the treatment), another Oil Red staining was performed and lipidic droplets in the cell cytoplasm were visible in all treatments (Fig. 3g–i). A negative staining with Oil Red in control cells is depicted in Fig. 3f.

Discussion

Autologous fat transplantation is an ideal treatment for facial rejuvenation and soft tissue augmentations provid-ing "like for like" tissue material; however, the success of

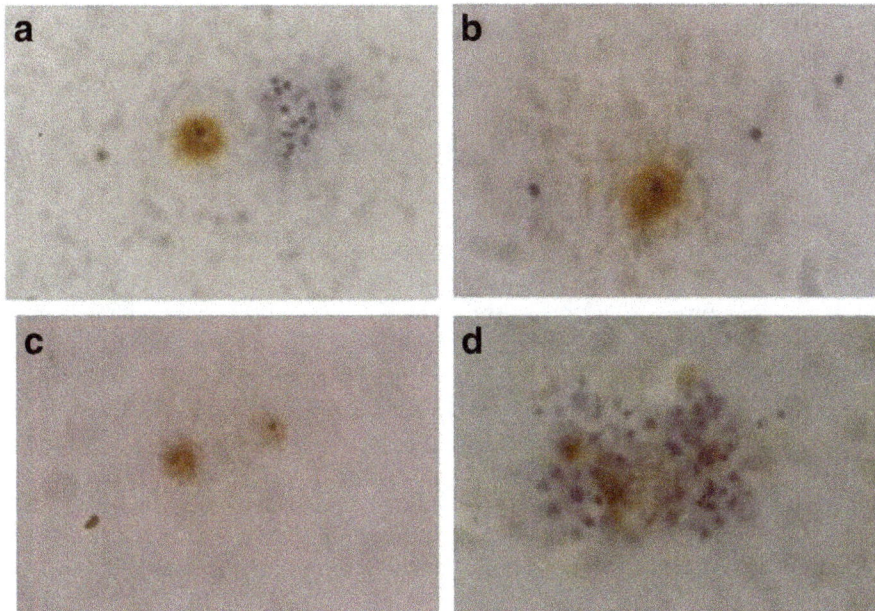

Fig. 2 Expression of β1-integrin on the ADSCs isolated from the liposuction aspirates (**a–c**, original magnification ×40). **a** β1-integrin expression in an ADSC demonstrated by immunohistochemistry. **b** β1-integrin expression in an ADSC demonstrated by immunohistochemistry. **c** β1-integrin expression in two ADSCs demonstrated by immunohistochemistry. **d** A cluster of cells containing also ADSCs expressing β1-integrin demonstrated by immunohistochemistry

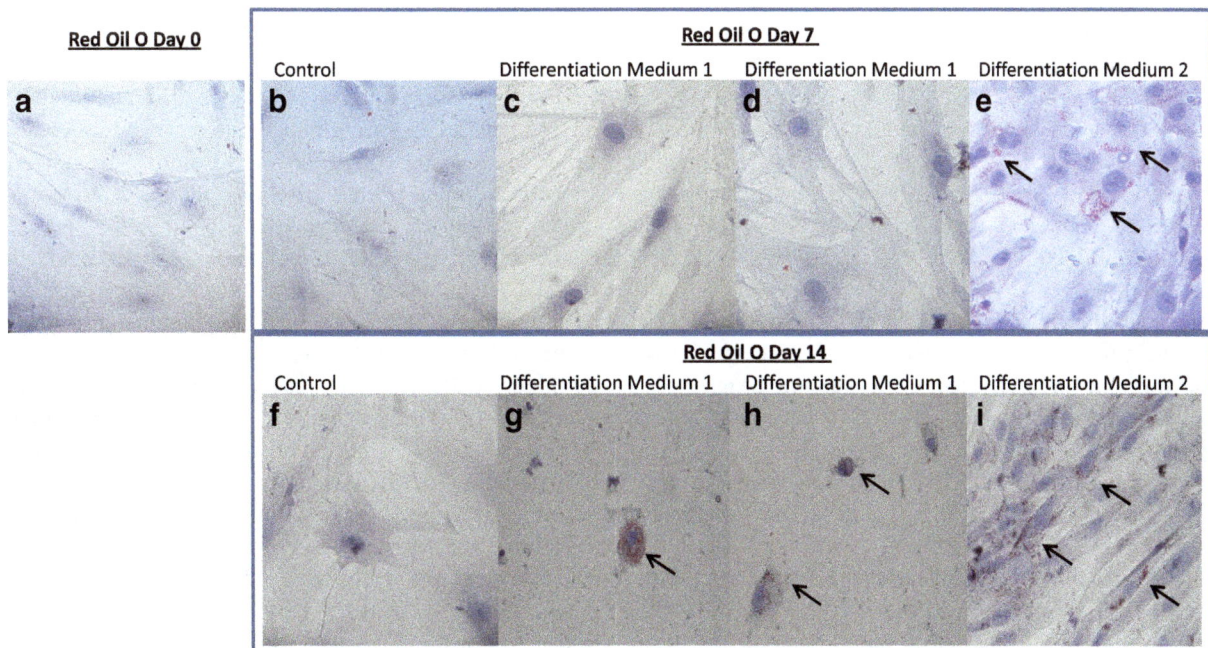

Fig. 3 Effect of treatment with the two media used for the differentiation of ADSCs in adipocytes. **a** Oil Red O staining on cells before starting differentiation treatment. **b** Oil Red O staining on control cells. **c, d** Oil Red O staining of cells treated with medium 1 after 7 days of treatment. **e** Oil Red O staining on cells treated with medium 2 after 7 days of treatment. **f** Oil Red O staining on control cells after 14 days of treatment. **g, h** Oil Red O staining on cells treated with medium 1 after 14 days of treatment. **i** Oil Red O staining on cells treated with medium 2 after 14 days of treatment. Arrows indicate lipid red drops present in differentiated cells

traditional fat grafting has been unpredictable and often unsatisfactory. The persistent clinical confusion associated with the viability and predictability of fat grafting is related to the mechanism of fat survival in the recipient area (Zhu et al. 2010). For large-volume fat transfers or relocations into a hostile recipient bed, the beneficiary area vascularity might be insufficient for the ischemic graft, leading to graft necrosis (Sinno et al. 2016; Kasem et al. 2015). This may be particularly true for injections into areas where the circulation and wound-healing capacity is impaired by previous fibrosis due to surgery, injections, radiotherapy, or any other acquired pathology (Kasem et al. 2015; Yoshimura et al. 2006). One recent innovation to deal with such problems is the enrichment of the transplant with autologous regenerative cells (Yoshimura et al. 2010; Yoshimura et al. 2008). For example, Yoshimura et al. (Yoshimura et al. 2008) described a cell-assisted lipo-transfer (CAL) method to graft large amounts of fat for breast augmentation and breast reconstruction.

Autologous regenerative cells can be obtained from the processing of either lipo-suctioned or excised fat (Sterodimas et al. 2011). This tissue is ease to harvest and the volume of tissue obtainable from liposuction contains 100–1000 times more pluripotent cells per cubic centimeter than bone marrow (Strem et al. 2005). According to the literature, it is possible to harvest up to 200×10^6 regenerative cells from 500 cc of lipo-aspirate, which makes cell culture unnecessary (Aust et al. 2004). This leads to higher safety and efficacy in clinical setting, since cells are minimally manipulated. These regenerative cells contain several types of cells, including ADSCs, vessel-forming cells, and progenitor cells, from which a variety of mesodermal cell types (bone, cartilage, blood) can be generated (Ryu et al. 2013). In detail, the ratio of adipocytes to ADSCs is constant in humans and it is independent of age and body mass index (van Harmelen et al. 2003).

Although the exact mechanism of ADSCs is unknown, it is thought that staminal cells contribute to graft survival through proangiogenic, anti-apoptotic, and pro-adipogenic effects (Yoshimura et al. 2010). Indeed, these cells have been shown to promote adipose cell replication, incorporate into vessel walls, and decrease the local inflammatory response (Rehman et al. 2004). Potentially, they produce a series of autocrine factors, that affect the cell itself, and paracrine, that have an effect on neighboring cells (Yang et al. 2010; Takeda et al. 2015; Wang et al. 2015). Moreover, they may contribute to neo-angiogenesis in the acute phase by secreting angiogenic factors and by acting as endothelial progenitor cells (Tiryaki et al. 2011). Thanks to their ability to differentiate into adipocytes and to induce neo-angiogenesis, when they are transplanted together with the adipose tissue, qualitatively and quantitatively improve the adipocytes increasing the possibilities for the adipose tissue to engraft (Sterodimas et al. 2011). Indeed, several clinical evidences have been published, confirming the potential role of ADSCs in either reconstructive surgery or esthetic surgery for the body remodeling (Zhu et al. 2010; Yoshimura et al. 2010; Yoshimura et al. 2008; Strem et al. 2005).

Leaving from this background, the goal of our project was to define an original and efficacious method to isolate ADSCs from liposuction aspirates. First point was the selection of the most suitable anatomical area for the liposuction. In a recent study, no statistical differences were demonstrable in adipocyte viability among thigh fat, flank fat, abdominal fat, or knee fat donor sites (Ullmann et al. 2005). Nevertheless, the abdominal area seems to be preferable for harvesting adipose tissue in which the stromal vascular fraction is well represented (Jurgens et al. 2008); therefore, in our experimental setting, the abdominal fat was chosen as an ideal source of ADSCs.

Second point was to define an experimental protocol where mechanical or chemical insults are greatly reduced to avoid damages to the tissue architecture that could cause the necrosis of the injected fat tissue (Pereira and Sterodimas 2010). Recent reports have shown that mechanical centrifugation does not appear to enhance immediate fat tissue viability before implantation (Rohrich et al. 2004). Centrifugation, however, is able to increase the concentration of the stromal vascular fraction and of ADSCs, although disproportionate centrifugation can damage adipocytes as well as ADSCs. The degree of adipocyte destruction differs among patients, but only minor differences in percentage of cell destruction have been shown among the different centrifugal forces, while a great variability is demonstrated among patients (Kurita et al. 2008). In our setting, we used centrifugation conditions comparable to that considered optimal for obtaining good results in adipose transplantation (Kim et al. 2009). To further overcome the mechanical injury of fat tissue, the Prolipostem® kit was equipped with a special vacuum syringe that allows the aspiration of fat without the use of pneumatic pumps. Moreover, a special tissue fat collection chamber, defined Promobarell®, was designed to efficiently recover from the lower portion the stromal tissue and ADSCs at the end of the centrifugation.

The first end-point of the study was to determine the presence of ADSCs in the fatty and fluid portions of the liposuction aspirate treated with the Prolipostem® kit. It is well known that ADSCs express, among the other superficial markers, β1-integrin (Quisenberry et al. 2016; Lu et al. 2014). To this end, an immunocytochemical approach was used to demonstrate the expression of β1-integrin on the surface of the ADSCs recovered.

The second end-point of the study was to demonstrate the ability of ADSCs to differentiate in adipocytes using different mediums. Indeed, in our in vitro experimental conditions, ADSCs were able to completely differentiate into mature adipocytes, as morphologically demonstrated by Oil Red staining. The stimulation of stem cells was determined not only by biomimetic peptide but also by the other reagents, including hyaluronic acid and calcium gluconate. Interestingly, the use of platelets resulted in a more toxic effect.

Indeed, previous experiences have led to the reflection that lipogenic glucose solutions enriched with 0.5% hyaluronic acid and calcium gluconate 1% are able to induce further engraftment and differentiation of ADSCs in the host tissue (Ceccarelli and García 2010). In detail, the dermal implantation of adipose tissue is able to induce also a fibroblast differentiation of stem cells that extend and enhance the regenerative effects of the implant (Ceccarelli and García 2010). It is possible to hypothesize that the addition of lipogenic solutions to the fat tissue enriched with ADSCs in the site of implant would increase the number of mature adipocytes. This, in turn, would increase the percentage of success of the implant. This phenomenon has been named liposowing (Ceccarelli and Garcia 2011).

Conclusions

In conclusion, treatment of the abdominal fat derived from liposuction aspirates with the Proplipostem® kit is capable to isolate ADSCs that are able to differentiate in mature adipocytes in vitro thanks also to the action of lipogenetic factors that are able to amplify the phenomenon. Therefore, by combining traditional fat grafting with ADSCs, obtained by Proplipostem® kit, it could be possible to overcome the problems associated with autologous fat transfer into areas with an impaired environment for fat graft survival. Additional studies are ongoing to confirm the clinical relevance of these results.

Abbreviations
ADSCs: Adipose-derived stem cell; DAB: Diaminobenzidine; DMEM: Dulbecco's modified Eagle's medium; FBS: Fetal bovine serum; PBS: Phosphate-buffered saline

Acknowledgements
None

Funding
None to acknowledge.

Authors' contributions
AS performed the liposuction with BDP; AP performed the in vitro experiments; NO and AL performed the immunohistochemical staining; and ADL together with AB and AS conceived the work, analyzed the data and wrote the paper. All authors read and approved the final manuscript.

Competing interests
AS, BDP, and AB are scientific advisors of Promoitalia Group S.p.A.

Author details
[1]Promoitalia Group S.p.A, Pozzuoli, Naples, Italy. [2]Department of Mental and Physical Health and Preventive Medicine, Section of Human Anatomy, Università degli Studi della Campania "L. Vanvitelli", Caserta, Italy. [3]San Giovanni Addolorata Hospital, Rome, Italy. [4]Department of Environmental, Biological and Pharmaceutical Sciences and Technologies, Università degli Studi della Campania "L. Vanvitelli", Caserta, Italy.

References
Aust L, Devlin B, Foster SJ, Halvorsen YD, Hicok K, du Laney T, Sen A, Willingmyre GD, Gimble JM. Yield of human adipose-derived adult stem cells from liposuction aspirates. Cytotherapy. 2004;6:7–14.

Ceccarelli M, García JV. The medical face lift: face tissue regeneration. The Medical Letter Physiological. 2010;1:1–15.

Ceccarelli, M., Garcia, J.V.: Stem cell enriched fat transfer, advanced techniques in liposuction and fat transfer, Prof. NIkolay Serdev (Ed.), ISBN: 978-953-307-668-3, InTech, (2011).

Ellenbogen R, Motykie G, Youn A, Svehlak S, Yamini D. Facial reshaping using less invasive methods. Aesthet Surg J. 2005;25:144–52.

Esposito M, Lucariello A, Costanzo C, Fiumarella A, Giannini A, Riccardi G, Riccio I. Differentiation of human umbilical cord-derived mesenchymal stem cells, WJ-MSCs, into chondrogenic cells in the presence of pulsed electromagnetic fields. In Vivo. 2013;27:495–500.

Esposito M, Lucariello A, Riccio I, Riccio V, Esposito V, Riccardi G. Differentiation of human osteoprogenitor cells increases after treatment with pulsed electromagnetic fields. In Vivo. 2012a;26:299–304.

Esposito V, Manente L, Lucariello A, Perna A, Viglietti R, Gargiulo M, Parrella R, Parrella G, Baldi A, De Luca A, Chirianni A. Role of FAP48 in HIV-associated lipodystrophy. J Cell Biochem. 2012b;113:3446–54.

Esposito V, Manente L, Perna A, Gargiulo M, Viglietti R, Sangiovanni V, Doula N, Liuzzi G, Baldi A, De Luca A, Chirianni A. Role of NEDD8 in HIV-associated lipodystrophy. Differentiation. 2009;77:148–53.

Esposito V, Perna A, Lucariello A, Carleo MA, Viglietti R, Sangiovanni V, Guerra G, De Luca A, Chirianni A. Different impact of antiretroviral drugs on bone differentiation in an in vitro model. J Cell Biochem. 2015;116:2188–94.

Joyce, C.W., Joyce, K.M., Rahmani, G., Walsh, S.R., Carroll, S.M., Hussey, A.J., Kelly, J. L: Fat grafting: a citation analysis of the seminal articles. Plast Reconstr Surg Glob Open 3, e295 (2015).

Jurgens WJ, Oedayrajsingh-Varma MJ, Helder MN, Zandiehdoulabi B, Schouten TE, Kuik DJ, Ritt MJ, van Milligen FJ. Effect of tissue-harvesting site on yield of stem cells derived from adipose tissue: implications for cell-based therapies. Cell Tissue Res. 2008;332:415–26.

Kasem A, Wazir U, Headon H, Mokbel K. Breast lipofilling: a review of current practice. Arch Plast Surg. 2015;42:126–30.

Kim IH, Yang JD, Lee DG, Chung HY, Cho BC. Evaluation of centrifugation technique and effect of epinephrine on fat cell viability in autologous fat injection. Aesthet Surg J. 2009;29:35–9.

Kurita M, Matsumoto D, Shigeura T, Sato K, Gonda K, Harii K, Yoshimura K. Influences of centrifugation on cells and tissues in liposuction aspirates: optimized centrifugation for lipotransfer and cell isolation. Plast Reconstr Surg. 2008;121:1033–41.

Lu T, Xiong H, Wang K, Wang S, Ma Y, Guan W. Isolation and characterization of adipose-derived mesenchymal stem cells (ADSCs) from cattle. Appl Biochem Biotechnol. 2014;174:719–28.

Lucariello A, Trabucco E, Boccia O, Perna A, Sellitto C, Castaldi MA, De Falco M, De Luca A, Cobellis L. Small leucine rich proteoglycans are differently distributed in normal and pathological endometrium. In Vivo. 2015;29:217–22.

Lucariello A, Trabucco E, Sellitto C, Perna A, Costanzo C, Manzo F, Laforgia V, Cobellis L, De Luca A, De Falco M. Localization and modulation of NEDD8 protein in the human placenta. In Vivo. 2013;27:501–6.

Manente L, Lucariello A, Costanzo C, Viglietti R, Parrella G, Parrella R, Gargiulo M, De Luca A, Chirianni A, Esposito V. Suppression of pre adipocyte differentiation and promotion of adipocyte death by anti-HIV drugs. In Vivo. 2012;26:287–91.

Park BS, Jang KA, Sung JH, Park JS, Kwon YH, Kim KJ, Kim WS. Adipose-derived stem cells and their secretory factors as a promising therapy for skin aging. Dermatol Surg. 2008;34:1323–6.

Pereira LH, Sterodimas A. Long-term fate of transplanted autologous fat in the face. J Plast Reconstr Aesthet Surg. 2010;63:e68–9.

Quisenberry CR, Nazempour A, Van Wie BJ, Abu-Lail NI. Evaluation of β1-integrin expression on chondrogenically differentiating human adipose-derived stem cells using atomic force microscopy. Biointerphases. 2016;11:021005.

Rehman J, Traktuev D, Li J, Merfeld-Clauss S, Temm-Grove CJ, Bovenkerk JE, Pell CL, Johnstone BH, Considine RV, March KL. Secretion of angiogenic and antiapoptotic factors by human adipose stromal cells. Circulation. 2004;109:1292–8.

Rohrich RJ, Sorokin ES, Brown SA. In search of improved fat transfer viability: a quantitative analysis of the role of centrifugation and harvest site. Plast Reconstr Surg. 2004;113:391–5.

Ryu YJ, Cho TJ, Lee DS, Choi JY, Cho J. Phenotypic characterization and in vivo localization of human adipose-derived mesenchymal stem cells. Mol Cells. 2013;35:557–64.

Salibian AA, Widgerow AD, Abrouk M, Evans GR. Stem cells in plastic surgery: a review of current clinical and translational applications. Arch Plast Surg. 2013; 40:666–75.

Savoia A, Accardo C, Vannini F, Di Pasquale B, Baldi A. Outcomes in thread lift for facial rejuvenation: a study performed with happy lift™ revitalizing. Dermatol Ther. 2014;4:103–14.

Savoia A, Landi S, Baldi A. A new minimally invasive mesotherapy technique for facial rejuvenation. Dermatol Ther. 2013;3:83–93.

Signorile PG, Baldi A. A tissue specific magnetic resonance contrast agent, Gd-AMH, for diagnosis of stromal endometriosis lesions: a phase I study. J Cell Physiol. 2015;230:1270–5.

Sinno S, Wilson S, Brownstone N, Levine SM. Current thoughts on fat grafting: using the evidence to determine fact or fiction. Plast Reconstr Surg. 2016;137:818–24.

Spugnini EP, Di Tosto G, Salemme S, Pecchia L, Fanciulli M, Baldi A. Electrochemotherapy for the treatment of recurring aponeurotic fibromatosis in a dog. Can Vet J. 2013;54:606–9.

Sterodimas A, de Faria J, Nicaretta B, Boriani F. Autologous fat transplantation versus adipose-derived stem cell-enriched lipografts: a study. Aesthet Surg J. 2011;31:682–93.

Strem BM, Hicok KC, Zhu M, Wulur I, Alfonso Z, Schreiber RE, Fraser JK, Hedrick MH. Multipotential differentiation of adipose tissue-derived stem cells. Keio J Med. 2005;54:132–41.

Takeda K, Sowa Y, Nishino K, Itoh K, Fushiki S. Adipose-derived stem cells promote proliferation, migration, and tube formation of lymphatic endothelial cells in vitro by secreting lymphangiogenic factors. Ann Plast Surg. 2015;74:728–36.

Tiryaki T, Findikli N, Tiryaki D. Staged stem cell-enriched tissue (SET) injections for soft tissue augmentation in hostile recipient areas: a preliminary report. Aesthet Plast Surg. 2011;35:965–71.

Ullmann Y, Shoshani O, Fodor A, Ramon Y, Carmi N, Eldor L, Gilhar A. Searching for the favorable donor site for fat injection: in vivo study using the nude mice model. Dermatol Surg. 2005;31:1304–7.

van Harmelen V, Skurk T, Röhrig K, Lee YM, Halbleib M, Aprath-Husmann I, Hauner H. Effect of BMI and age on adipose tissue cellularity and differentiation capacity in women. Int J Obes Relat Metab Disord. 2003;27:889–95.

Wang T, Guo S, Liu X, Xu N, Zhang S. Protective effects of adipose-derived stem cells secretome on human dermal fibroblasts from ageing damages. Int J Clin Exp Pathol. 2015;8:15739–48.

Yang JA, Chung HM, Won CH, Sung JH. Potential application of adipose-derived stem cells and their secretory factor to skin: discussion from both clinical and industrial viewpoints. Expert Opin Biol Ther. 2010;10:495–503.

Yoshimura A, Aoi N, Kurita M, Oshima Y, Sato K, Inoue K, Suga H, Eto H, Kato H, Harii K. Progenitor-enriched adipose tissue transplantation as rescue for breast implant complications. Breast J. 2010;16:169–75.

Yoshimura K, Sato K, Aoi N, Kurita M, Hirohi T, Harii K. Cell-assisted lipotransfer for cosmetic breast augmentation: supportive use of adipose-derived stem/stromal cells. Aesthet Plast Surg. 2008;32:48–55.

Yoshimura K, Shigeura T, Matsumoto D, Sato T, Takaki Y, Aiba-Kojima E, Sato K, Inoue K, Nagase T, Koshima I, Gonda K. Characterization of freshly isolated and cultured cells derived from the fatty and fluid portions of liposuction aspirates. J Cell Physiol. 2006;208:64–76.

Zhu M, Zhou Z, Chen Y, Schreiber R, Ransom JT, Fraser JK, Hedrick MH, Pinkernell K, Kuo HC. Supplementation of fat grafts with adipose-derived regenerative cells (ADRCs) improves long-term graft retention. Ann Plast Surg. 2010;64:222–8.

12

Epigallocatechin-3-gallate inhibits paclitaxel-induced apoptosis through the alteration of microRNA expression in human dermal papilla cells

Shang Hun Shin[1,2], Hwa Jun Cha[3], Karam Kim[2], In-Sook An[2], Kyung-Yun Kim[4], Jung-Eun Ku[5], Sun-Hee Jeong[6] and Sungkwan An[1*] [iD]

Abstract

Background: Paclitaxel well known as anti-cancer drug has been shown to cause alopecia in chemotherapy. The paclitaxel chemotherapy-mediated alopecia is induced by apoptotic damage in human dermal papilla (HDP) cells. Epigallocatechin-3-gallate (EGCG) inhibits apoptosis against anti-cancer drug such as cisplatin. EGCG, one of the green tea extract ingredients, has been reported to enhance cell viability and to inhibit apoptosis. However, it is unclear that EGCG enhances cell viability and inhibits apoptosis against paclitaxel-induced apoptotic damage in HDP cells.

Methods: We show cell viability, cell cycle, and microRNA (miRNA) expression in EGCG-mediated rescue cell to paclitaxel-mediated cell death and growth arrest.

Results: EGCG promotes cell survival and cell death inhibitory effects and alteration of miRNA expression in paclitaxel-exposed HDP cells were investigated. Firstly, paclitaxel increases apoptosis and EGCG promotes cell survival and represses paclitaxel-induced apoptosis in a dose-dependent manner. Fluorescence-activated cell sorting (FACS) analysis showed that EGCG protects apoptosis in paclitaxel-exposed HDP cells. miRNA microarray analysis was performed and 48 miRNAs changed by EGCG in paclitaxel-exposed HDP cells were identified. In gene ontology analysis in silico, miRNAs regulate apoptosis and cell proliferation-regulated genes, such as BCL2L1, BCL2L2, BBC3, and MDM2. In Kyoto Encyclopedia of Genes and Genomes (KEGG) pathway analysis, miRNAs are related to mitogen-activated protein kinase (MAPK) signaling pathway and Wnt signaling pathway, which regulate apoptosis and cell proliferation.

Conclusions: EGCG inhibits apoptosis through regulating miRNA expression related to apoptosis and cell proliferation in paclitaxel-treated HDP cells.

Keywords: Epigallocatechin-3-gallate, Paclitaxel, Human dermal papilla cell, MicroRNA

Background

Paclitaxel, taxane-based anticancer drugs, purified in bark of *Taxus brevifolia* regulates microtubule dynamics by binding with β-tubulin (Manfredi and Horwitz 1984; Amos and Löwe 1999). Paclitaxel-mediated regulation repressed mitotic activity and then induces apoptosis. Thus, it is generally used in therapy of metastatic breast cancer, ovarian cancer, and non-small cell lung cancer (Khanna et al. 2015; Chen et al. 2011; Jordan and Wilson 2004).

In anticancer chemotherapy, the risk of potential side effects is one of the important features (Macdonald et al. 2015; Balagula et al. 2011). In the case of paclitaxel, a known side effects include leukopenia, thrombocytopenia, anemia, muscle pain, and hair loss symptoms. Especially, hair loss is the major side effects of paclitaxel (Ozcelik et al. 2010; Shapiro and Recht 2001). Paclitaxel-mediated hair loss is resulted by apoptotic damage of dermal papilla

* Correspondence: ansungkwan@konkuk.ac.kr
[1]Department of Cosmetics Engineering, Konkuk University, 120 Neungdong-ro, Gwangjin-gu, Seoul 05029, Republic of Korea
Full list of author information is available at the end of the article

cells (Chen et al. 2011; McElwee et al. 2003; Yang and Cotsarelis 2010). However, it has not been identified the detailed mechanism of paclitaxel-mediated apoptotic damage of dermal papilla cells.

Hair is grown by a repetitive cycle consisted of anagen, catagen and telogen, which is regulated by HDP cells in normal and abnormal condition, such as hair loss (Inui et al. 2003; Stenn and Paus 2001). Since the HDP cells can significantly affect the hair growth, HDP cell-regulating factor is implicated in therapy of hair loss (Kwon et al. 2007; Aljuffali et al. 2015).

Recently, miRNA is studied as a factor affecting the function of the dermal papilla cells. miRNA is a non-coding small nucleotide consisted of 18–24 nucleotides and interfere translation of target genes by binding to a 3′-untranslated region (UTR) of the mRNA in the gene expression process (Bartel 2004; Bartel 2009; Carrington and Ambros 2003). miRNA is known to play a role in apoptosis, cell proliferation, and differentiation and recently has been reported that miR-31 is highly expressed in hair growth phase, which regulated the expression of Krt16, Krt17, Dlx3, and Fgf10. In addition, miR-24 is implicated in hair follicle formation through regulating known as stemness regulator of human keratinocytes role (Wan et al. 2011; Mardaryev et al. 2010; Amelio et al. 2013).

EGCG, a major compound of green tea that contained polyphenols, is effective in anti-cancer and antioxidant (Hsu 2005; Wang and Bachrach 2002; Katiyar and Elmets 2001). In addition, EGCG induced cell growth and is prevented against UV-mediated cell death in keratinocytes and HDP cells, which regulate hair growth (Kwon et al. 2007; Yang and Landau 2000; Katiyar et al. 1995; Chung et al. 2003).

In our study, we show protection activity of EGCG to paclitaxel-induced HDP cell death. Moreover, we demonstrate a cellular signaling mechanism of EGCG-mediated paclitaxel protection mechanism through analyzing alteration miRNA expression profile.

Methods

Cell culture and materials
HDP cells were maintained using Dulbecco's modified Eagle's medium (DMEM; Hyclone, Logan, UT, USA) with 1% penicillin/streptomycin (10,000 units/mL penicillin G sodium, 10,000 μg/mL streptomycin; Gibco-BRL/Invitrogen Life Technologies, Gaithersburg, MD, USA) and 10% fetal bovine serum (FBS; Hyclone) and incubated at 5% CO_2 at 37 °C. Paclitaxel was purchased from Sigma-Aldrich (St. Louis, MO, USA).

Cell viability assay
HDP cells were seeded in 96-well plates at 2×10^3 cells/well and then incubated for 24 h. After 24 h, EGCG and paclitaxel was treated with indicated concentrations for 24 h. Water-soluble tetrazolium-1 (WST-1) solution was added and incubated for 20 min. Optical density of each well was measured at 450 nm using a iMark™ microplate reader (Bio-Rad, Hercules, CA, USA). And the value was calibrated by measuring a reference absorbance at 650 nm.

Cell cycle assay
HDP cells were incubated with EGCG and paclitaxel for 24 h. Cells were harvested and washed with phosphate-buffered saline (PBS; sodium chloride 137 mM, phosphate buffer 10 mM, potassium chloride 2.7 mM, all from BioPure (Canada). After washing, cells were fixed by 70% ethanol and then stained with propidium iodide (PI) staining buffer (PI 50 μg/mL, RNase 0.1 mg/mL, 0.05% Triton X-100). Fluorescence intensity was measured by FACS Calibur (BD Biosciences, San Jose, CA, USA). And Sub-G1, G0/G1, S, and G2/M were measured by Cell Quest software (BD Biosciences).

miRNA microarray
To analyze miRNA expression profile, HDP cells were seeded and treated with EGCG and paclitaxel. After 24 h, total RNA was extracted using TRIzol reagent (Sigma-Aldrich) according to the manufacturer's instructions. Total RNA was stained with Cy3 using Agilent miRNA Labeling kit (Agilent Technologies, Santa Clara, CA, USA). Labeled RNAs were hybridized using a Sure-Print G3 Human v16 miRNA 8x60K microarray (Agilent Technologies) at 65 °C for 20 h. The miRNA expression profile was analyzed using Feature Extraction version 10.7 software (Agilent Technologies) and GeneSpring GX software, version 11.5 (Agilent Technologies).

miRNA target and ontology analysis
Target genes were predicted using seed sequence-based miRNA target prediction database, TargetScan (Target scan human 2017) and miRbase (miRbase 2017). Additionally, to categorize hair follicle development, apoptosis, and cell proliferation, gene ontology of predicted target genes of miRNA was analyzed by DAVID Bioinformatics Resources 6.7 (National Institute of Allergy and Infectious Diseases 2017).

Results

Protective effects of EGCG to paclitaxel-mediated growth arrest in HDP cells
To demonstrate protection effects of EGCG in paclitaxel-mediated growth arrest, we co-treated it with paclitaxel and EGCG. As shown in Fig. 1, 5 μM EGCG decreased 1 μM paclitaxel-induced growth arrest (62%) to 84%. Furthermore, in cell cycle analysis, 1 μM paclitaxel induced cell death fraction (sub-G1) in the same

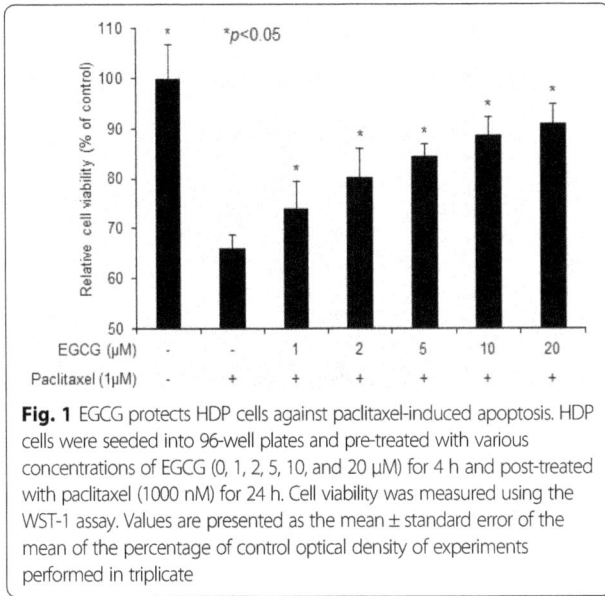

Fig. 1 EGCG protects HDP cells against paclitaxel-induced apoptosis. HDP cells were seeded into 96-well plates and pre-treated with various concentrations of EGCG (0, 1, 2, 5, 10, and 20 μM) for 4 h and post-treated with paclitaxel (1000 nM) for 24 h. Cell viability was measured using the WST-1 assay. Values are presented as the mean ± standard error of the mean of the percentage of control optical density of experiments performed in triplicate

condition. However, co-treatment with 10 μM EGCG reduced paclitaxel-mediated cell death in HDP cells (Fig. 2).

EGCG-mediated alteration of miRNA profile in paclitaxel-exposed HDP cells

We showed EGCG-mediated alteration of miRNA profile in paclitaxel-exposed HDP cells. As shown in Fig. 3, EGCG upregulated 20 miRNAs and downregulated 28 miRNAs in paclitaxel-exposed HDP cells. Among 48 miRNAs, miR-3663-3p, miR-1181, miR-3613-3p, miR-1281, and miR-1539 had increased by 293.52-fold, 241.98-fold, 188.91-fold, 177.18-fold, and 169.23-fold, respectively. Additionally, miR-221-5p, miR-374b, miR-590-5p, miR-4306, and miR-500a-5p had decreased by 132.32-fold, 124.96-fold, 122.52-fold, 116.09-fold, and 105.14-fold, respectively (Table 1).

Bioinformatic analysis of EGCG-regulated miRNAs in paclitaxel-exposed HDP cells

To analyze relation between growth arrest and cell death and EGCG-regulated miRNAs, we predicted target genes of EGCG-regulated miRNAs using TargetScan (Target scan human 2017) and miRbase (miRbase 2017). And

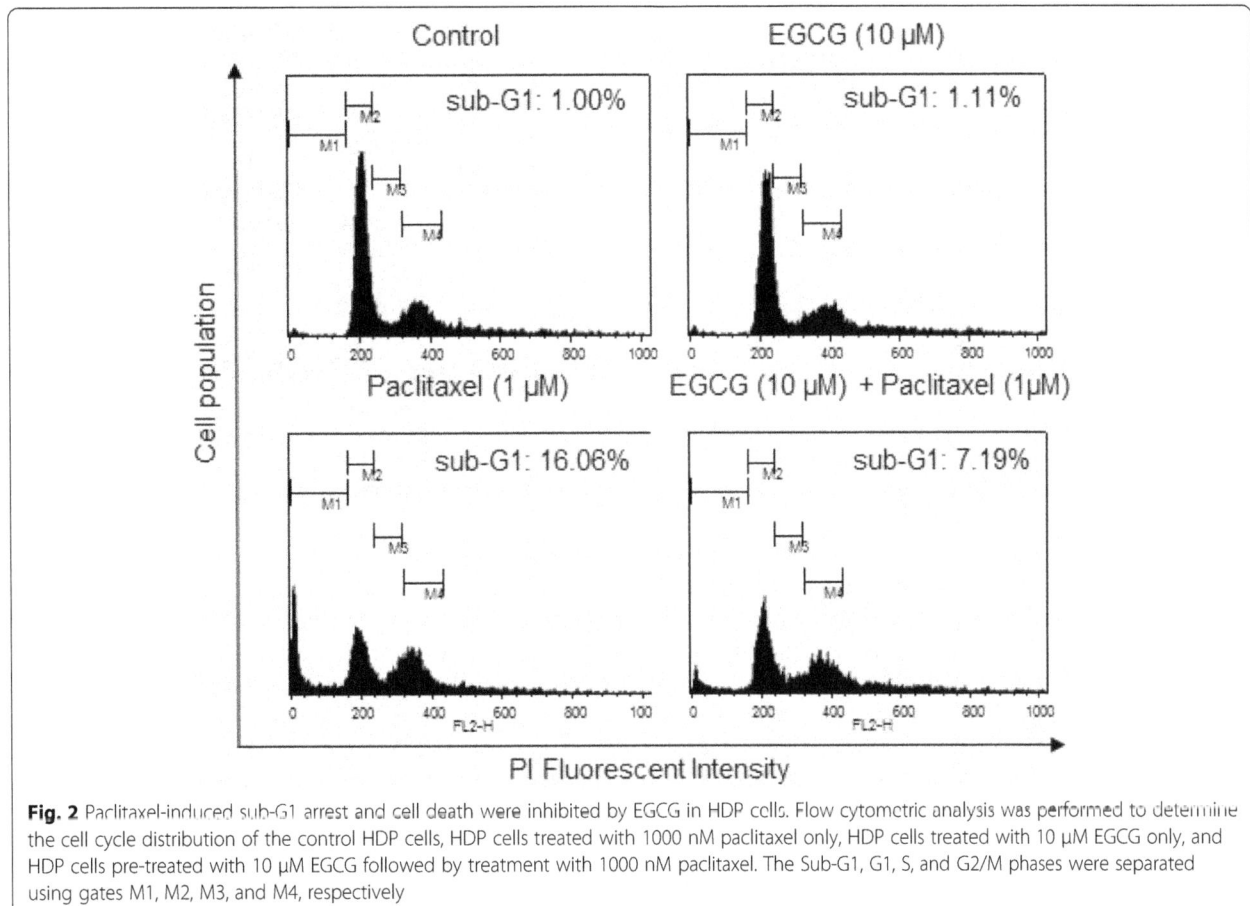

Fig. 2 Paclitaxel-induced sub-G1 arrest and cell death were inhibited by EGCG in HDP cells. Flow cytometric analysis was performed to determine the cell cycle distribution of the control HDP cells, HDP cells treated with 1000 nM paclitaxel only, HDP cells treated with 10 μM EGCG only, and HDP cells pre-treated with 10 μM EGCG followed by treatment with 1000 nM paclitaxel. The Sub-G1, G1, S, and G2/M phases were separated using gates M1, M2, M3, and M4, respectively

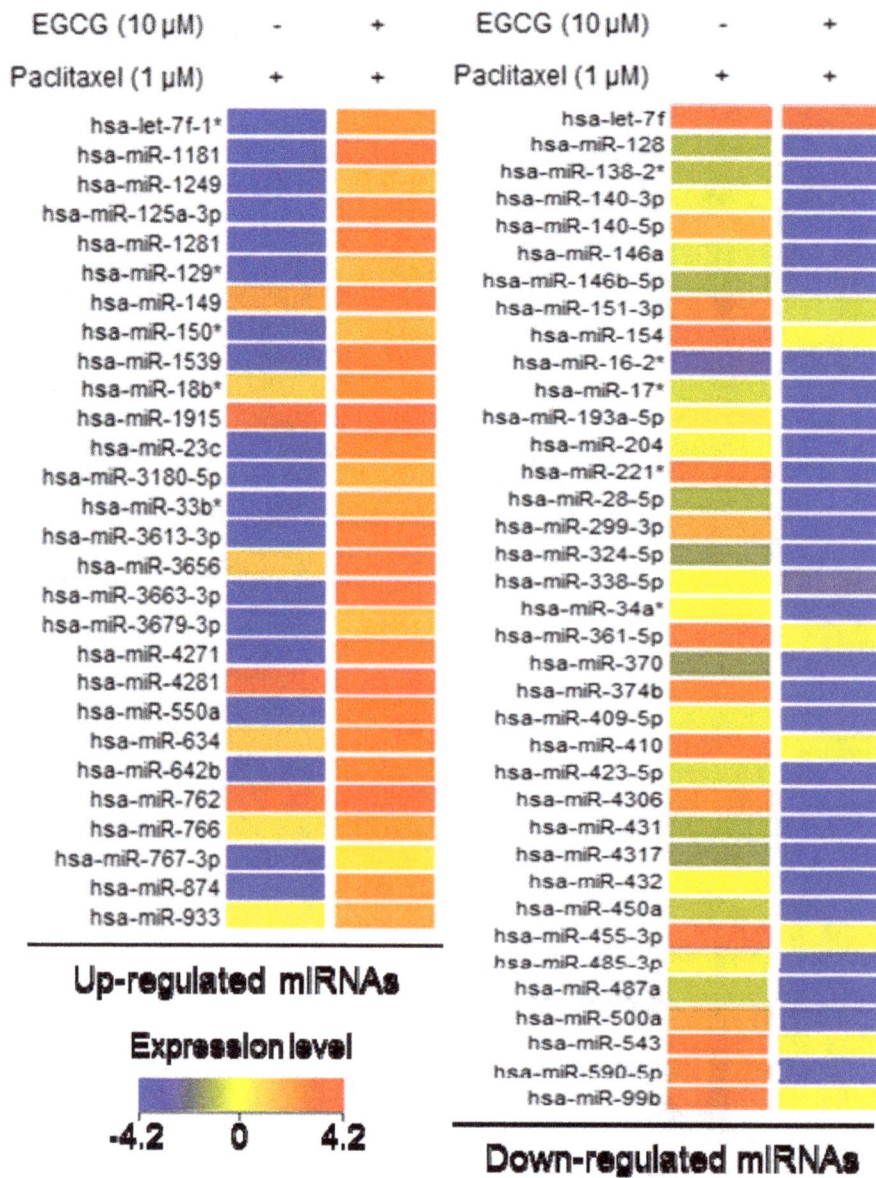

Fig. 3 EGCG alters miRNA expression profiles in paclitaxel-treated HDP cells. Heat map analysis of miRNAs upregulated and downregulated with a ≥ 2-fold change in expression in paclitaxel-treated HDP cells. HDP cells were seeded in 60-mm culture dishes and pre-incubated with 10 μM EGCG for 4 h. Following pre-treatment, the HDP cells were treated with 10 μM EGCG and 1000 nM paclitaxel and incubated for 24 h. miRNA expression was determined using the SurePrint G3 Human v16 miRNA 8x60K Microarray Kit. The color bars displaying fluorescence intensity correspond to each miRNA expression. Expression levels are indicated in the legend bar

then, in Additional file 1: Table S1 and Table S2, we categorized functions of target genes using their functions, apoptosis, cell proliferation, and hair follicle development, using DAVID (National Institute of Allergy and Infectious Diseases 2017). Additionally, to demonstrate relation between target genes of EGCG-regulated miRNAs and identified signal pathways, we analyzed signal pathway using KEGG pathway database. As shown in Additional file 1: Table S3 and Table S4, at in silico analysis, EGCG-upregulated miRNAs regulated various KEGG pathways, such as MAPK signaling pathway, pathways in cancer, neurotrophin signaling pathway, long-term depression, pancreatic cancer, chronic myeloid leukemia, colorectal cancer, ECM-receptor interaction, vibrio cholera infection, glycerolipid metabolism, lysine degradation, cell adhesion molecules (CAMs), glioma, melanoma, endocytosis, focal adhesion, ubiquitin-mediated proteolysis, ErbB signaling pathway, tight junction, Jak-STAT signaling pathway, renal cell carcinoma, adherens junction, Fc gamma R-mediated phagocytosis, epithelial cell signaling in *Helicobacter pylori* infection, p53 signaling pathway, long-term potentiation,

Table 1 miRNAs showing > 3-fold expression change following treatment with EGCG in paclitaxel-exposed HDP cells

miRNA	Change relative to controls	Direction of regulation	chr.	miRNA	Change relative to controls	Direction of regulation	chr.
hsa-miR-3663-3p	293.53	Up	chr10	hsa-miR-500a-5p	105.14	Down	chrX
hsa-miR-1181	241.98	Up	chr19	hsa-miR-299-3p	102.72	Down	chr14
hsa-miR-3613-3p	188.92	Up	chr13	hsa-miR-140-5p	97.50	Down	chr16
hsa-miR-1281	177.19	Up	chr22	hsa-miR-193a-5p	73.05	Down	chr17
hsa-miR-1539	169.23	Up	chr18	hsa-miR-34a-3p	61.13	Down	chr1
hsa-miR-125a-3p	159.16	Up	chr19	hsa-miR-432-5p	60.05	Down	chr14
hsa-miR-4271	158.48	Up	chr3	hsa-miR-204-5p	56.88	Down	chr9
hsa-miR-550a-5p	156.32	Up	chr7	hsa-miR-485-3p	55.67	Down	chr14
hsa-miR-642b-3p	142.71	Up	chr19	hsa-miR-140-3p	55.23	Down	chr16
hsa-miR-23c	134.49	Up	chrX	hsa-miR-409-5p	54.21	Down	chr14
hsa-let-7f-1-3p	108.08	Up	chr9	hsa-miR-146a-5p	52.69	Down	chr5
hsa-miR-874	96.40	Up	chr5	hsa-miR-423-5p	50.69	Down	chr17
hsa-miR-33b-3p	88.74	Up	chr17	hsa-miR-17-3p	50.49	Down	chr13
hsa-miR-3180-5p	76.65	Up	chr16	hsa-miR-487a	47.24	Down	chr14
hsa-miR-150-3p	65.94	Up	chr19	hsa-miR-450a-5p	47.14	Down	chrX
hsa-miR-129-1-3p	64.80	Up	chr7	hsa-miR-138-2-3p	45.41	Down	chr16
hsa-miR-1249	63.67	Up	chr22	hsa-miR-128	44.19	Down	chr2
hsa-miR-3679-3p	60.74	Up	chr2	hsa-miR-28-5p	43.34	Down	chr3
hsa-miR-767-3p	34.07	Up	chrX	hsa-miR-431-5p	43.33	Down	chr14
hsa-miR-3656	3.60	Up	chr11	hsa-miR-146b-5p	43.22	Down	chr10
hsa-miR-221-5p	132.32	Down	chrX	hsa-miR-4317	38.84	Down	chr18
hsa-miR-374b	124.96	Down	chrX	hsa-miR-324-5p	38.47	Down	chr17
hsa-miR-590-5p	122.52	Down	chr7	hsa-miR-370	37.81	Down	chr14
hsa-miR-4306	116.09	Down	chr13	hsa-miR-16-2-3p	22.41	Down	chr3

Chr. chromosome

phosphatidylinositol signaling system, non-small cell lung cancer, aldosterone-regulated sodium reabsorption, Wnt signaling pathway, regulation of actin cytoskeleton, axon guidance, TGF-beta signaling pathway, melanogenesis, basal cell carcinoma, arrhythmogenic right ventricular cardiomyopathy (ARVC), pathogenic *Escherichia coli* infection, circadian rhythm, T cell receptor signaling pathway, B cell receptor signaling pathway, glycosphingolipid biosynthesis, valine, leucine and isoleucine degradation, insulin signaling pathway, Hedgehog signaling pathway, mTOR signaling pathway, RNA degradation, heparan sulfate biosynthesis, one carbon pool by folate, prostate cancer, cell cycle, spliceosome, apoptosis, small cell lung cancer, acute myeloid leukemia, adipocytokine signaling pathway, endometrial cancer, inositol phosphate metabolism, and sphingolipid metabolism in paclitaxel-treated HDP cells, and EGCG-downregulated miRNAs regulated Fc gamma R-mediated phagocytosis, pathways in cancer, MAPK signaling pathway, focal adhesion, regulation of actin cytoskeleton, Wnt signaling pathway, chemokine signaling pathway, axon guidance, TGF-beta signaling pathway, renal cell carcinoma, melanoma, melanogenesis, basal cell carcinoma, ErbB signaling pathway, prostate cancer, Hedgehog signaling pathway, p53 signaling pathway, notch signaling pathway, cytokine-cytokine receptor interaction, Jak-STAT signaling pathway, calcium signaling pathway, T cell receptor signaling pathway, dilated cardiomyopathy, amino sugar and nucleotide sugar metabolism, ubiquitin-mediated proteolysis, pathogenic *Escherichia coli* infection, small cell lung cancer, valine, leucine and iso-leucine degradation, purine metabolism, gap junction, glycerolipid metabolism, Huntington's disease, *N*-glycan biosynthesis, fatty acid metabolism, butanoate metabolism, glioma, long-term depression, cysteine and methionine metabolism, neurotrophin signaling pathway, adherens junction, vascular smooth muscle contraction, insulin signaling pathway, progesterone-mediated oocyte maturation, oocyte meiosis, non-small cell lung cancer, chronic myeloid leukemia, dorso-ventral axis formation, mTOR signaling pathway, phosphatidylinositol signaling system, CAMs, endocytosis, splicesome, endometrial cancer, tight junction, chondroitin sulfate biosynthesis, inositol phosphate metabolism, colorectal cancer, GnRH signaling pathway, ECM-receptor interaction, Fc epsilon RI signaling pathway, ABC transporters, neuroactive ligand-receptor interaction, aldosterone-regulated sodium reabsorption, propanoate metabolism, natural killer cell-mediated cytotoxicity, B cell receptor signaling pathway, vascular endothelial growth factor (VEGF) signaling pathway, and pyrimidine metabolism in paclitaxel-treated HDP cells.

Discussion

Therapeutic effect of paclitaxel on tumor cells is reported in many different cancers (Sunters et al. 2003; Millenbaugh et al. 1998; Ettinger 1993). However, paclitaxel also affects other normal cell and then occurs a lot of side effects (Chon et al. 2012). Especially, paclitaxel-induced hair loss, one of the paclitaxel side effects, is caused by the apoptotic damage in HDP cells, one of the key players to form hair follicle and grow hair (Chen et al. 2011). EGCG extracted from green tea has been shown as effective anti-cancer agent and antioxidation agent in normal cells (Hsu 2005; Wang and Bachrach 2002; Hsu et al. 2003). In addition, EGCG is attenuated in cisplatin-mediated HDP cell death (Hsu et al. 2003). Thus, we showed effects of EGCG in paclitaxel-mediated HDP cell death. In this study, to determine regulation of miRNAs by EGCG in paclitaxel-exposed HDP cells, we showed the EGCG-mediated alteration of miRNA profile in HDP cells treated with paclitaxel.

Firstly, we showed that EGCG repressed paclitaxel-mediated growth arrest and cell death in HDP cells (Figs. 1 and 2). In the same condition, we analyzed miRNA profile, since, in recent study, HDP cells regulate cellular signal pathway, such as survival, death, and cell cycle arrest (Kim et al. 2014; Cha et al. 2014). As shown in Figs. 1 and 3, 48 miRNAs have confirmed the EGCG-mediated upregulation or downregulation in paclitaxel-treated HDP cells. In significantly up- and downregulated miRNA, miR-129-1-3p (64.8-fold upregulation) is reported as repressor of PDCD2 which is overexpressed

in proliferation of human gastric cancer (Du et al. 2014) and miR-128 (44.19-fold downregulation) was reported to inhibit cell growth, when overexpressed in head and neck squamous cell carcinoma (Hauser et al. 2015). Additionally, EGCG-regulated miRNAs targeted *FOXO1*, *BCL2L1*, *BCL2L2*, *PTEN*, *BBC3*, and *MDM2* which are the regulator genes against cell growth, proliferation, and cell death. When FOXO1 is overexpressed, cell proliferation and growth is inhibited by upregulating caspase-3 and caspase-9 and inducing G2/M arrest and (Yang et al. 2015). BCL2L1 and BCL2L2, BCL2 family, are pro-oncogene and repress intrinsic pathway-mediated cell death (Denoyelle et al. 2014; Zhang et al. 2015). Other genes, PTEN, BBC3, and MDM2, also rescue cell death and induce proliferation (Fortunato et al. 2014; Zhang et al. 2010).

In KEGG pathway analysis against target genes, we find upregulated miRNA-related 58 KEGG pathways and downregulated miRNA-related 68 KEGG pathways. Among these KEGG pathway, Wnt signaling pathway, pathways in cancer, MAPK signaling pathway, and basal cell carcinoma, adherens junction is highly related with upregulated miRNA. And MAPK signaling pathway, neurotrophin signaling pathway, melanogenesis, axon guidance, Wnt signaling pathway are most related to downregulated miRNAs. MAPK signaling pathway and Wnt signaling pathway related to both up- and downregulated miRNAs are involved in cell survival and apoptosis (Zhang et al. 2010; Shang et al. 2015). Thus, we suggest that EGCG-mediated miRNA expression change regulates cell survival and apoptosis through MAPK signaling pathway and Wnt signaling pathway.

Following our results, we demonstrate that EGCG-regulated alteration of miRNA expression increase proliferation and decrease cell death in paclitaxel-treated HDP cells. Additionally, these results suggest that EGCG reduced paclitaxel-mediated hair loss by alteration of miRNA profile.

Conclusions

This is the first study to address positive effects of EGCG in paclitaxel-mediated hair loss. The study demonstrated that EGCG increases proliferation, decreases cell death by alteration of miRNA profile in HDP cells, and sequentially affects paclitaxel-mediated hair loss.

Abbreviations

ARVC: Arrhythmogenic right ventricular cardiomyopathy; CAMs: Cell adhesion molecules; DMEM: Dulbecco's modified Eagle's medium; EGCG: Epigallocatechin-3-gallate; FACS: Fluorescence-activated cell sorting; FBS: Fetal bovine serum; HDP: Human dermal papilla; KEGG: Kyoto Encyclopedia of Genes and Genomes; MAPK: Mitogen-activated protein kinase; miRNA: MicroRNA; PBS: Phosphate-buffered saline; PI: Propidium iodide; UTR: Untranslated region; VEGF: Vascular endothelial growth factor; WST-1: Water-soluble tetrazolium-1

Acknowledgements
Not applicable

Funding
This work was supported by a grant from the Korean Health Technology R&D Project (Grant No. HN13C0075), Ministry of Health and Welfare, Republic of Korea.

Authors' contributions
SHS, HJC, and KK conducted the study and drafted the manuscript. All authors analyzed the data and reviewed the literatures. SHS and SA wrote the manuscript. All authors read and approved the final manuscript.

Competing interests
The authors declare that they have no competing interests.

Author details
[1]Department of Cosmetics Engineering, Konkuk University, 120 Neungdong-ro, Gwangjin-gu, Seoul 05029, Republic of Korea. [2]Korea Institute of Dermatological Sciences, 6F Tower A, 25, Beobwon-ro 11-gil, Songpa-gu, Seoul 05836, Republic of Korea. [3]Department of Skin Care and Beauty, Osan University, Osan-si, Gyeonggi-do 18119, Republic of Korea. [4]URG Inc., URG Building, Seochogu, Seoul 06753, Republic of Korea. [5]Department of Cosmetology, Kyung-In Women's University, Incheon 21014, Republic of Korea. [6]Department of Beauty Art, Faculty of Art, Suwon Women's University, Suwon-si, Gyeonggi-do 16632, Republic of Korea.

References
Aljuffali IA, Pan TL, Sung CT, Chang SH, Fang JY. Anti-PDGF receptor β antibody-conjugated squarticles loaded with minoxidil for alopecia treatment by targeting hair follicles and dermal papilla cells. Nanomedicine. 2015;11:1321–30.

Amelio I, Lena AM, Bonanno E, Melino G, Candi E. miR-24 affects hair follicle morphogenesis targeting Tcf-3. Cell Death Dis. 2013;4:e992.

Amos LA, Löwe J. How taxol stabilises microtubule structure. Chem Biol. 1999;6: R65–9.

Balagula Y, Rosen ST, Lacouture ME. The emergence of supportive oncodermatology: the study of dermatologic adverse events to cancer therapies. J Am Acad Dermatol. 2011;65:624–35.

Bartel DP. MicroRNAs: genomics, biogenesis, mechanism, and function. Cell. 2004; 116:281–97.

Bartel DP. MicroRNAs: target recognition and regulatory functions. Cell. 2009; 136:215–33.

Carrington JC, Ambros V. Role of microRNAs in plant and animal development. Science. 2003;301:336–8.

Cha HJ, Lee KS, Lee GT, Lee KK, Hong JT, Lee SN, et al. Altered miRNA expression profiles are involved in the protective effects of troxerutin against ultraviolet B radiation in normal human dermal fibroblasts. Int J Mol Med. 2014;33:957–63.

Chen PH, Wang CY, Hsia CW, Ho MY, Chen A, Tseng MJ, et al. Impact of taxol on dermal papilla cells—a proteomics and bioinformatics analysis. J Proteonics. 2011;74:2760–73.

Chon SY, Champion RW, Geddes ER, Rashid RM. Chemotherapy-induced alopecia. J Am Acad Dermatol. 2012;67:e37–47.

Chung JH, Han JH, Hwang EJ, Seo JY, Cho KH, Kim KH, et al. Dual mechanisms of green tea extract (EGCG)-induced cell survival in human epidermal keratinocytes. FASEB J. 2003;17:1913–5.

Denoyelle C, Lambert B, Meryet-Figuière M, Vigneron N, Brotin E, Lecerf C, et al. miR-491-5p-induced apoptosis in ovarian carcinoma depends on the direct inhibition of both BCL-XL and EGFR leading to BIM activation. Cell Death Dis. 2014;5:e1445.

Du Y, Wang D, Luo L, Guo J. miR-129-1-3p promote BGC-823 cell proliferation by targeting PDCD2. Anat Rec (Hoboken). 2014;297:2273–9.

Ettinger DS. Taxol in the treatment of lung cancer. J Natl Cancer Inst Monogr. 1993;15:177–9.

Fortunato O, Boeri M, Moro M, Verri C, Mensah M, Conte D, et al. Mir-660 is downregulated in lung cancer patients and its replacement inhibits lung tumorigenesis by targeting MDM2-p53 interaction. Cell Death Dis. 2014;5:e1564.

Hauser B, Zhao Y, Pang X, Ling Z, Myers E, Wang P, et al. Functions of MiRNA-128 on the regulation of head and neck squamous cell carcinoma growth and apoptosis. PLoS One. 2015;10:e0116321.

Hsu S. Green tea and the skin. J Am Acad Dermatol. 2005;52:1049–59.

Hsu S, Bollag WB, Lewis J, Huang Q, Singh B, Sharawy M, et al. Green tea polyphenols induce differentiation and proliferation in epidermal keratinocytes. J Pharmacol Exp Ther. 2003;306:29–34.

Inui S, Fukuzato Y, Nakajima T, Yoshikawa K, Itami S. Identification of androgen-inducible TGF-beta1 derived from dermal papilla cells as a key mediator in androgenetic alopecia. J Invest Dermatol Symp Proc. 2003;8:69–71.

Jordan MA, Wilson L. Microtubules as a target for anticancer drugs. Nat Rev Cancer. 2004;4:253–65.

Katiyar SK, Elmets CA. Green tea polyphenolic antioxidants and skin photoprotection (review). Int J Oncol. 2001;18:1307–13.

Katiyar SK, Elmets CA, Agarwal R, Mukhtar H. Protection against ultraviolet-B radiation-induced local and systemic suppression of contact hypersensitivity and edema responses in C3H/HeN mice by green tea polyphenols. Photochem Photobiol. 1995;62:855–61.

Khanna C, Rosenberg M, Vail DM. A review of paclitaxel and novel formulations including those suitable for use in dogs. J Vet Intern Med. 2015;29:1006–12.

Kim OY, Cha HJ, Ahn KJ, An IS, An S, Bae S. Identification of microRNAs involved in growth arrest and cell death in hydrogen peroxide-treated human dermal papilla cells. Mol Med Rep. 2014;10:145–54.

Kwon OS, Han JH, Yoo HG, Chung JH, Cho KH, Eun HC, et al. Human hair growth enhancement in vitro by green tea epigallocatechin-3-gallate (EGCG). Phytomedicine. 2007;14:551–5.

Macdonald JB, Macdonald B, Golitz LE, LoRusso P, Sekulic A. Cutaneous adverse effects of targeted therapies: part I: inhibitors of the cellular membrane. J Am Acad Dermatol. 2015;72:203–18.

Manfredi JJ, Horwitz SB. Taxol: an antimitotic agent with a new mechanism of action. Pharmacol Ther. 1984;25:83–125.

Mardaryev AN, Ahmed MI, Vlahov NV, Fessing MY, Gill JH, Sharov AA, et al. Micro-RNA-31 controls hair cycle-associated changes in gene expression programs of the skin and hair follicle. FASEB J. 2010;24:3869–81.

McElwee KJ, Kissling S, Wenzel E, Huth A, Hoffmann R. Cultured peribulbar dermal sheath cells can induce hair follicle development and contribute to the dermal sheath and dermal papilla. J Invest Dermatol. 2003;121:1267–75.

Millenbaugh NJ, Gan Y, Au JL. Cytostatic and apoptotic effects of paclitaxel in human ovarian tumors. Pharm Res. 1998;15:122–7.

National Institute of Allergy and Infectious Diseases: DAVID bioinformatics resources 6.7 (2017). https://david-d.ncifcrf.gov. Accessed 20 Jun 2017.

Ozcelik B, Turkyilmaz C, Ozgun MT, Serin IS, Batukan C, Ozdamar S, et al. Prevention of paclitaxel and cisplatin induced ovarian damage in rats by a gonadotropin-releasing hormone agonist. Fertil Steril. 2010;93:1609–14.

miRBase. (2017). http://www.mirbase.org. Accessed 22 May 2017.

Shang Y, Wang LQ, Guo QY, Shi TL. MicroRNA-196a overexpression promotes cell proliferation and inhibits cell apoptosis through PTEN/Akt/FOXO1 pathway. Int J Clin Exp Pathol. 2015;8:2461–12.

Shapiro CL, Recht A. Side effects of adjuvant treatment of breast cancer. N Engl J Med. 2001;344:1997–2008.

Stenn KS, Paus R. Controls of hair follicle cycling. Physiol Rev. 2001;81:449–94.

Sunters A, Fernández de Mattos S, Stahl M, Brosens JJ, Zoumpoulidou G, Saunders CA, et al. FoxO3a transcriptional regulation of Bim controls apoptosis in paclitaxel-treated breast cancer cell lines. J Biol Chem. 2003;278: 49795–805.

Target scan human. (2017). www.targetscan.org. Accessed 21 May 2017.

Wan G, Mathur R, Hu X, Zhang X, Lu X. miRNA response to DNA damage. Trends Biochem Sci. 2011;36:478–84.

Wang YC, Bachrach U. The specific anti-cancer activity of green tea (−)-epigallocatechin-3-gallate (EGCG). Amino Acids. 2002;22:131–43.

Yang CC, Cotsarelis G. Review of hair follicle dermal cells. J Dermatol Sci. 2010;57:2–11.

Yang CS, Landau JM. Effects of tea consumption on nutrition and health. J Nutr. 2000;130:2409–12.

Yang T, Thakur A, Chen T, Yang L, Lei G, Liang Y, et al. MicroRNA-15a induces cell

13

Neem-silicone lotion and ultrasound nit comb: a randomised, controlled clinical trial treating head louse infestation

Ian F. Burgess[*], Elizabeth R. Brunton, Nazma A. Burgess and Mark N. Burgess

Abstract

Background: A neem-based conditioner lotion (ONC) used against head lice was previously tested clinically and shown to be relatively ineffective. To improve the activity against lice and their eggs, it was reformulated into a silicone vehicle (NNC) as part of a project to improve pediculicidal medical devices. An ultrasound nit comb was also developed to be used in conjunction with the neem lotion to remove louse eggs from the hair.

Methods: A single-centre, parallel group, randomised, controlled, open-label community-based clinical study was set up to test the NNC lotion in comparison with a marketed product based on isopropyl myristate and cyclomethicone (IPM/C) with two treatments 7 days apart. In parallel, the lubrication effects of the NNC and ONC lotions were compared in use with the ultrasound comb.

Results: For 134 randomised participants (50 NNC, 53 IPM/C, 17 NNC plus comb, and 14 ONC plus comb), the cure rate was 72.0% for NNC and 69.8% for IPM/C (OR 1.112, 95% CI, 0.47 to 2.61). Additional combing gave 82.4% cure using NNC and 28.6% using ONC (OR 11.67; 95% CI 2.13 to 64.04). No difference in efficacy of nit removal was detected although combing with conditioner was physically easier.

Conclusions: One percent neem oil in silicone (NNC) is as effective to eliminate head lice as other silicone products. Nit combing is easier using a conditioner lubricant to facilitate sliding of the eggshells along hairs.

Trial registration: Current Controlled Trials Registry ISRCTN77673809

Keywords: Pediculosis capitis, Treatment, Silicone, Neem oil, Nit combing, Ultrasound

Background

Consumer preference to use natural treatments to eliminate head lice has increased with the spread of resistance to insecticides. Apart from essential oils (Grieve et al. 2007; Burgess et al. 2010; Barker and Altman 2010), few plant products have undergone clinical trials. The most widely used is oil from the neem tree, *Azadirachta indica* A. Juss (Meliaceae), which contains a number of putatively pharmacologically active triterpenoids. One shampoo from Germany based on a concentrated extract has undergone investigations in villages in Egypt and Arabia (Heukelbach et al. 2006; Abdel-Ghaffar and Semmler 2007; Schmahl et al. 2010; Mehlhorn et al. 2011; Abdel-Ghaffar et al. 2012) with

reported high efficacy following a single application. In contrast, an alcohol-based Australian product, containing 6% neem oil and 16% eucalyptus, required two applications plus combing in a Thai study (Thawornchaisit et al. 2012). However, both results contrast strongly with our earlier low success using a neem oil-based conditioner plus combing (Brown and Burgess 2017).

This work formed part of a European Commission Sixth Framework Craft project to develop new medical devices to treat head louse infestation. Previously, we described a laboratory evaluation of the ultrasound comb, developed as part of this investigation, for facilitation of nit removal (Burgess et al. 2016). In parallel, the neem oil-based lotion was reformulated to improve the activity against both lice and their eggs. It was hoped the changes would also improve the lubrication characteristics for nit removal.

* Correspondence: ian@insectresearch.com
Medical Entomology Centre, Insect Research & Development Limited, 6 Quy Court, Colliers Lane, Stow-cum-Quy, Cambridge CB25 9AU, UK

These newly developed class I medical devices were investigated in a randomised controlled clinical study.

Methods

Setting

This randomised, controlled comparison of two pediculicide treatments and two combing plus combing-aid treatments was a single-site study conducted in and around Cambridge, UK. Participants were recruited through local advertising. Each household received an information booklet, and an investigator arranged a domiciliary visit. All household members were screened for lice using a plastic detection comb and followed eligibility criteria used in previous studies (Burgess et al. 2007). Exclusions were treatment for lice within 2 weeks; sensitivity to treatment components or long-term scalp conditions other than lice; using hair bleach, dyes, or permanent waves; or treatments with trimethoprim products within 4 weeks. We also excluded pregnant and breast feeding females, previous participation in this study, or other studies within 4 weeks. Age eligibility ranged from 2 years with no upper limit. Infested non-participants were offered a standard of care treatment (4% dimeticone lotion) to minimise reinfestation of participants. No payment was offered for participation.

Enrolment was planned at 176 participants across four treatment groups: 66 using reformulated Nice 'n Clear lotion (NNC), 66 50:50 isopropyl myristate in cyclomethicone (IPM/C) (Full Marks solution), 22 original formulation Nice 'n Clear head lice lotion (ONC) plus combing using the ClearBrush® ultrasound nit comb (CB), and 22 NNC plus the ClearBrush® ultrasonic nit comb. Following manufacturing difficulties for the ultrasound comb, the study was terminated early to comply with European Commission deadline rules for project completion. At premature termination, 134 participants had been treated and followed up: 50 NNC, 53 IPM/C, 14 ONC plus ClearBrush®, and 17 NNC plus ClearBrush®.

A total of 136 people from 75 households (112 children and 24 adults) were consented between 13 September 2007 and 25 March 2008. Other household members and four other families were screened but had no lice, and two consenting participants were eliminated from analyses for a protocol violation before the first treatment. There were two withdrawals from each lotion group (Fig. 1); seven others missed one or more assessments. Therefore, the intention to treat (ITT) population analysed was 134 and the per-protocol (PP) population 125.

Treatments

All treatments were given on day 0 and repeated on day 7. Four treatment products were used:

1. Investigative product: a new formulation containing 1% neem seed oil, dimeticone PEG-PPG co-polymer,

and cyclomethicone-5 (reformulated Nice 'n Clear lotion or "New Nice 'n Clear" lotion (NNC), Nelsons, Wimbledon, UK)
2. Comparator product: a 50:50 mixture of isopropyl myristate with cyclomethicone (Full Marks solution (IPM/C), Reckitt Benckiser, Slough, UK)
3. Combing aid: the original 1% neem oil conditioner rinse (original formulation Nice 'n Clear head lice lotion (ONC), Nelsons, Wimbledon, UK) containing 1% neem seed oil, tea tree oil, lavender oil, and other herbal extracts
4. Nit comb: a newly designed comb activated by ultrasound (ClearBrush®, Nelsons, Wimbledon, UK) (Burgess et al. 2016), which was the primary development objective of the whole project

NNC and IPM/C were compared for efficacy against head lice when applied to dry hair until saturated. NNC was left in place overnight and then washed off with shampoo. IPM/C was applied for 10 min before washing off with shampoo. All participants used the same shampoo, supplied by the investigators.

The lubricant effects of NNC and ONC were compared during nit removal using the ClearBrush®. This device (Fig. 2) delivered ultrasound to the comb teeth through two piezoelectric actuators, as described previously (Burgess et al. 2016). A fresh standard comb tooth unit (Innomed™ comb, Hogil Pharmaceutical Corp., White Plains, NY, USA) was fitted for each participant to eliminate any risk of cross-contamination. Before the clinical work, the two lubricants were compared in the laboratory for their effect on loosening louse eggs (peak force) and sliding them along hair (average force), using a slip-peel tester (SP-2000, IMASS, Inc., Accord, MA, USA) as described previously (Burgess et al. 2016; Burgess 2010).

NNC was applied to dry hair but ONC to pre-washed and towel-dried hair. After thorough application, the hair was combed systematically using the ClearBrush® comb with ultrasound switched on. Louse eggs and nits removed during combing were recovered for later examination and counting in the laboratory. The use of other nit combs or treatment products was not permitted during the course of the study.

Outcome measures

Follow-up assessments were made in all groups on days 2, 6, 9, and 14 using a plastic detection comb ("PDC" comb, KSL Consulting ApS, Helsinge, Denmark). Any lice recovered were fixed into the case documentation as a permanent record. The primary outcome measure was the elimination of infestation after completing treatment, i.e. no lice at days 9 and 14. Outcomes were classified as cure, reinfestation after cure, or treatment failure.

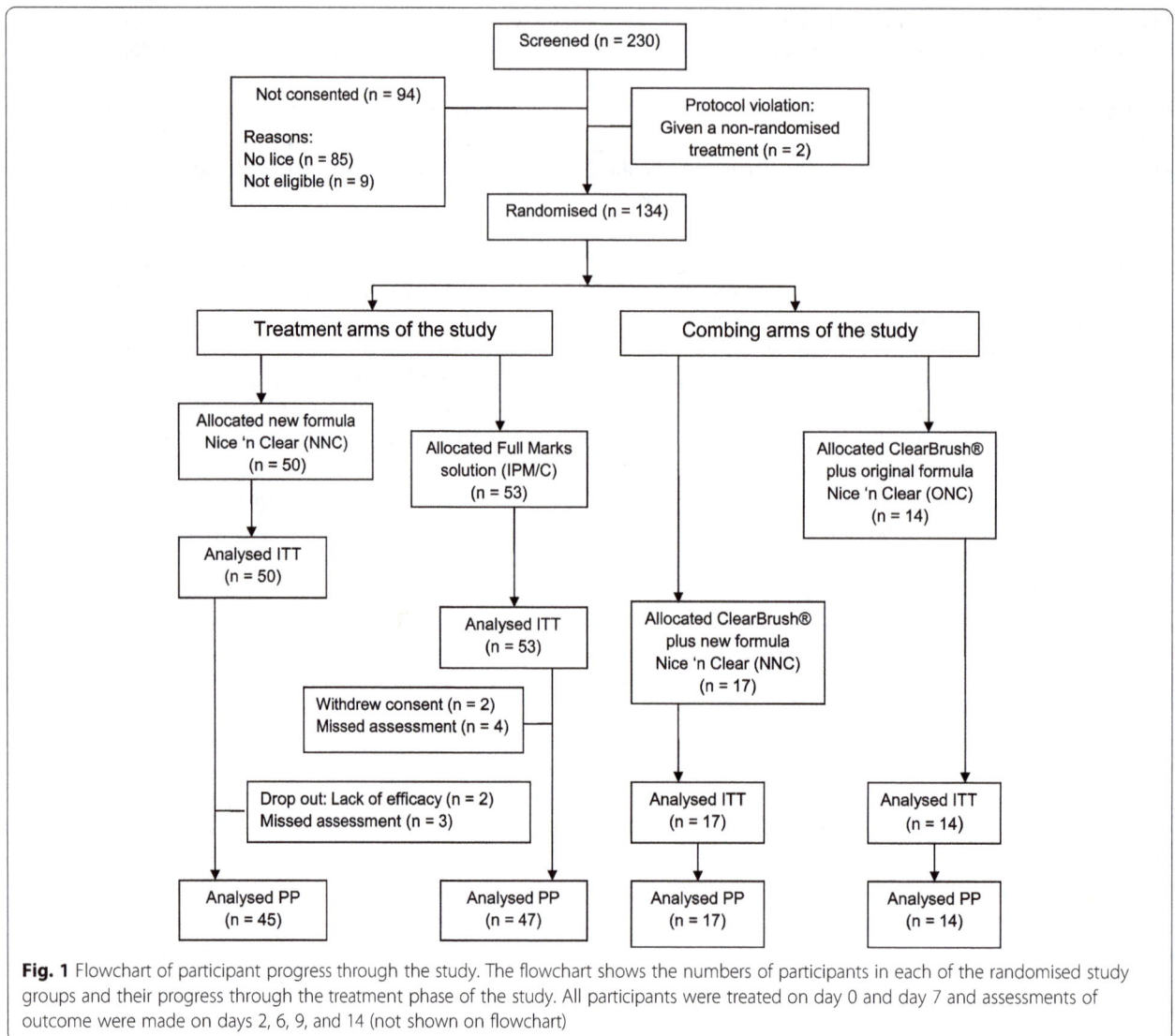

Fig. 1 Flowchart of participant progress through the study. The flowchart shows the numbers of participants in each of the randomised study groups and their progress through the treatment phase of the study. All participants were treated on day 0 and day 7 and assessments of outcome were made on days 2, 6, 9, and 14 (not shown on flowchart)

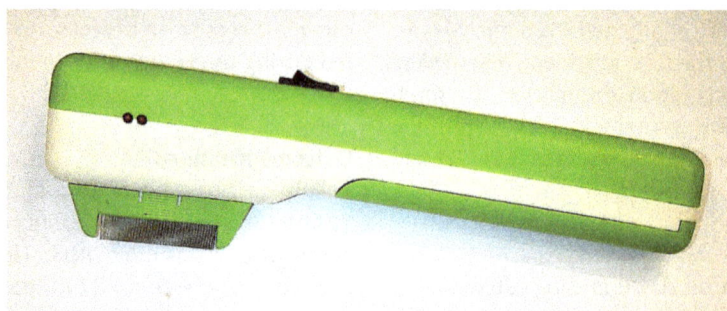

Fig. 2 Production prototype ClearBrush® comb for use in the clinical investigation. This device consists of a long handle to house the batteries to power the ultrasound actuators. The combing head has a detachable section for changing the steel comb tooth units and has tell-tale lights for ultrasound generation and battery power, actuated by an on/off switch. The comb head is angled relative to the handle by 16.5°

Sample size

It was estimated that equivalence for the lotions to within 25% could be identified using 132 participants (66 treated with NNC and 66 with IPM/C) with 90% power and 95% confidence, assuming an underlying success rate for NNC of 75% based on ex vivo data. The premature termination and lower efficacy outcomes reduced the power of the study for identification of 25% equivalence with 95% confidence to 75%.

For the comparison of lubricants using the Clear-Brush® ultrasound comb to remove nits, we could make no clear estimation of the required number of participants based on expectations of outcome because there were no appropriate prior data to work from comparing different combs or combing techniques. Only one broadly similar investigation was found, which used 22 participants per group, so the study was structured on that basis (de Souza et al. 2001).

Randomisation and blinding

Treatment instructions in sealed, opaque, numbered envelopes randomised using an online computer generated list (Dallal 2007) were distributed to investigators in balanced blocks of eight. Participants were allocated treatment using the next available numbered envelope held by the investigator. Post-treatment assessments were performed by different investigators from those involved in treatment so that they remained blind to the treatment allocation.

It became necessary to generate a two-stage randomisation because usable models of the ClearBrush® could not be manufactured in time for the study initiation. Initially, half of the participants were randomised only between the two lotion treatments (NNC and IPM/C). As soon as the ClearBrush® combs became available, the randomisation sequence was recalculated to include all four treatment groups.

Statistical analysis

We conducted analyses based on both the ITT and PP populations. Differences in success rates were measured by the 95% confidence interval calculated using a normal approximation to the binomial distribution. Comparison of groups in baseline characteristics, safety, acceptability, and efficacy were tested using Fisher's exact test for yes/no variables and the Mann-Whitney U test for ranked variables.

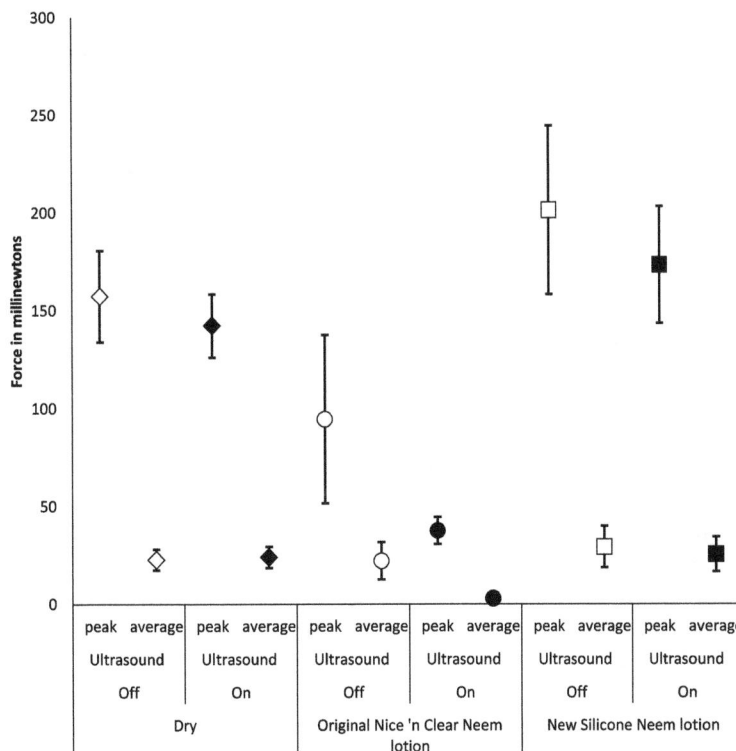

Fig. 3 Comparison of peak and average force required to remove louse eggs using the NNC and ONC products as lubricants using a slip-peel tester to measure forces. White symbols indicate the forces generated when no ultrasound was applied; black symbols show the same forces under the influence of ultrasound. Each dataset was generated using a minimum of 20 louse eggs on human hairs

Table 1 Demographic characteristics of the intention to treat population at baseline

Characteristic		NNC lotion	IPM/C lotion	NNC + CB	ONC + CB	Total
Number of participants		50	53	17	14	134
Age	2–6	12 (24.0%)	11 (20.8%)	4 (23.5%)	2 (14.3%)	29 (21.6%)
	7–9	19 (38.0%)	15 (28.9%)	4 (23.5%)	7 (50.0%)	45 (33.6%)
	10–16	8 (16.0%)	16 (30.2%)	7 (41.2%)	5 (35.7%)	36 (26.9%)
	>17	11 (22.0%)	11 (20.8%)	2 (11.8%)	0 (0.0%)	24 (17.9%)
	Median	9	10	10	9	9
Sex	Female	38 (76.0%)	43 (81.1%)	12 (70.6%)	9 (64.3%)	102 (76.1%)
Infestation	Light	33 (66.0%)	31 (58.5%)	10 (58.8%)	10 (71.4%)	84 (62.7%)
	Heavy	4 (8.0%)	8 (15.1%)	1 (5.9%)	0 (0.0%)	13 (9.7%)
Hair characteristics						
Length	Above ears	12 (24.0%)	8 (15.1%)	3 (17.7%)	4 (28.6%)	27 (20.2%)
	Below shoulders	27 (54.0%)	32 (60.4%)	10 (58.8%)	8 (57.1%)	77 (57.5%)
Thickness	Fine/medium	36 (72.0%)	28 (52.8%)	11 (64.7%)	11 (78.6%)	86 (64.2%)
	Thick	14 (28.0%)	25 (47.2%)	6 (35.3%)	3 (21.4%)	48 (35.8%)
Curl	Straight	31 (62.0%)	38 (71.7%)	14 (82.4%)	5 (35.7%)	88 (65.7%)
	Wavy/curly	19 (38.0%)	15 (28.3%)	3 (17.7%)	9 (64.3%)	46 (34.3%)
Type	Normal	49 (98.0%)	51 (96.2%)	17 (100%)	14 (100%)	131 (97.8%)
Other family member in study		40 (80.0%)	44 (83.0%)	14 (82.4%)	12 (85.7%)	110 (82.1%)

Results

Laboratory combing comparison

The laboratory comparison of the two neem-based lubricants plus the ClearBrush® ultrasound comb found the silicone-based NNC was a less-effective lubricant than the conditioner-based ONC, irrespective of the use of ultrasound. Ultrasound reduced both peak force and average force for all evaluations, but removing eggs treated with NNC was more difficult than removing eggs from dry, untreated hair (Fig. 3). In contrast, the conditioner-based ONC showed a trend for reduction of both forces.

Participants

At day 0, we recorded baseline characteristics for all participants (Table 1). Most commonly, household sizes were 4 (57 participants), 6 (27 participants), and > 8 (16 participants), with households ranging from 2 to 12 members. For 110/134 (82.1%) participants, one or more other family members took part, two families having six participants and one family five. In most households with multiple family members, there were participants in different treatment groups. The distribution of household size was similar between the groups (but was not tested statistically due to the non-independence of the data).

Outcomes

Of the 136 participants who gave consent, two, randomised to NNC, were mistakenly given ONC, withdrawn, and excluded from ITT analysis. There were two withdrawals each from the NNC group, for lack of efficacy of the treatment, and the IPM/C group because of an unrelated adverse event. Each of these was included in the ITT analysis but excluded from the per-protocol (PP) analysis.

Comparison of the lotion products

In the comparison of lotion products, there were 103 evaluable participants, 50 treated using NNC and 53

Table 2 Comparison of the two lotion groups for the presence of lice and mean numbers of lice recovered

Endpoint	Group	Day			
		2	6	9	14
Presence of lice	NNC	38.5%	42.3%	32.7%	23.1%
	IPM/C	41.5%	56.6%	21.2%	18.9%
Total lice	NNC	2.09	3.25	0.90	1.04
	IPM/C	2.34	4.11	0.42	0.42
Adult males	NNC	0.12	0.14	0.10	0.15
	IPM/C	0.15	0.06	0.01	0.04
Adult females	NNC	1.25	0.37	0.08	0.35
	IPM/C	0.26	0.15	0.00	0.19
Stage 3 nymphs	NNC	0.40	0.37	0.31	0.10
	IPM/C	0.40	0.30	0.09	0.09
Stage 2 nymphs	NNC	0.21	1.10	0.27	0.29
	IPM/C	0.47	1.21	0.13	0.09
Stage 1 nymphs	NNC	1.12	1.29	0.15	0.15
	IPM/C	1.06	2.40	0.19	0.02

There were no significant differences between the treatments with regard to numbers of lice found at any assessment day using IPM/C (Table 1). Analyses of the presence, number, and stages of lice from each assessment (Table 2) found no significant differences ($p < 0.05$) between the groups at any time point other than significantly ($p < 0.05$) more stage 1 nymphs in the NNC group at day 14. Fewer lice were found following the second treatment, but an increase occurred by day 14 from failure to kill all louse eggs.

The main analysis, the comparison of rates of cure, or cure followed by reinfestation, in the ITT population, found success in 36/50 (72.0%) of those using NNC and 37/53 (69.8%) treated with IPM/C. This difference was estimated as 2.2% (95% confidence interval (CI), −15.4 to 19.7%; odds ratio (OR) 1.112, 95% CI, 0.47 to 2.61). There was no significant ($p < 0.05$) difference between the two treatments. Five cases of re-infestation after cure were found: four treated with NNC and one with IPM/C. Of the 33 treatment failures (14 NNC vs. 16 IPM/C), two from each group had only stage 1 nymphs indicating ovicidal failure. For this analysis, the four dropouts were counted as treatment failures.

After the elimination of dropouts and participants failing to attend one of the post-treatment visits, the PP population was 94, with successful treatments for 35/45 (77.8%) in the NNC group and 33/47 (70.2%) in the IMP/C group (OR 1.4848, 95% CI, 0.58 to 3.80).

Analyses of demographic subsets found no difference in the success rate in any of the subgroups analysed (Table 3). There was an overall non-significant trend for decreased efficacy on participants with heavier infestations, the exception being the within group difference in the rate of success for IPM/C where a light infestation was significantly ($p = 0.01$) more likely to be cured than a medium infestation. Cure rates also decreased slightly in both groups with increasing hair length.

Opinions of cosmetic characteristics were contradictory. Most (31/50, 62.0%) thought NNC had a moderate/strong odour, compared with 11/53 (20.8%) using IPM/C. Similar numbers, eight vs. seven respectively, reported the odour unpleasant, although 41/53 IPM/C users could not detect any odour, whereas NNC always

Table 3 Success rate for NNC and IPM/C by demographic characteristics subgroup

Subgroup		NNC		IPM/C		
		n/N	%	n/N	%	p value
All participants		36/50	72.0	37/53	69.8	NS
Sex	Males	10/12	83.3	6/10	60.0	NS
	Females	26/38	68.4	31/43	72.1	NS
Age	2 to 6	7/12	58.3	9/11	81.8	NS
	7 to 9	11/19	57.9	11/15	73.3	NS
	10 to 16	7/8	87.5	10/16	62.5	NS
	> 16	11/11	100	9/11	81.8	NS
Infestation[a]	Light	26/33	78.8	27/31	87.1[b]	NS
	Moderate	6/10	60.0	5/11	45.5[b]	NS
	Heavy	2/4	50.0	5/8	62.5	NS
Hair length	Close cut	1/1	100.0	2/2	100	NS
	Above ears	9/11	81.8	4/6	66.7	NS
	Ears to shoulders	7/11	63.6	10/13	76.9	NS
	Below shoulders	19/27	70.4	22/32	68.8	NS
Hair thickness	Fine	6/7	85.7	7/9	77.8	NS
	Medium	21/29	72.4	17/19	89.5	NS
	Thick	9/14	64.3	14/25	65.0	NS
Hair curl	Straight	21/31	67.7	21/38	55.3	NS
	Wavy or curly	15/19	78.9	13/15	86.7	NS
Hair type	Normal	34/49	69.4	37/51	72.6	NS
	Dry or oily	0/1	0.0	1/2	50.0	NS
Other family member in study	No	8/10	80.0	7/9	77.8	NS
	Yes	26/40	65.0	30/44	68.2	NS

[a]Data missing from three participants in each of the treatment groups
[b]There was a significant difference in efficacy rates between "light" and "moderate" infestations given this treatment

developed a strong onion-like odour as it dried. Significantly, more (34/53, 64.2%) ($p < 0.015$) found IPM/C left the hair greasy after washing compared with 20/50 (40.0%) using NNC.

Comparison of treatments using ClearBrush®

ClearBrush® combing with ultrasound examined 17 people treated with NNC and 14 with ONC. On days 0 and 7, the outcomes were analysed for the presence of lice and louse eggs/nits, but for each of days 2, 6, 9, and 14, the analysis was for the presence of live lice only. The Clearbrush® did not remove lice or nits from two participants using ONC and one using NNC, but all other assessment data were complete. Table 4 shows the percentage of participants with lice and mean number of each development stage, and any significant differences, at each of the 6 days.

The ClearBrush®-treated groups showed significantly ($p \leq 0.05$) more stage 1 and 2 nymphs on ONC users at day 6 and stage 3 nymphs at days 6 and 14. The ONC group had significantly ($p < 0.05$) more lice in total at day 9, becoming highly significant ($p < 0.005$) by day 14. Although ONC removed more than 13 times as many nits on day 0 and over six times the

number on day 7, this difference was not significant, due partly to the small group sizes but also the skewed distribution of nits on a few people.

The overall efficacy comparison between NNC and ONC showed a significant ($p < 0.01$) pediculicidal advantage for the neem-in-silicone treatment (NNC), although the group sizes were too small for firm conclusions. NNC was successful for 14/17 (82.4%) compared with 4/14 (28.6%) cures for ONC (OR 11.67; 95% CI 2.13 to 64.04). No differences were found for efficiency of removing nits because so many cases had few nits present, but NNC plus ClearBrush® showed a slight non-significant trend ($p = 0.53$) in favour of using the comb as an adjunct to treatment.

Adverse events

There were seven reported adverse events in five people. None was linked with treatment, although one cough was possibly exacerbated by the odour of neem. All but one of the events, back pain, were associated with seasonal respiratory tract infections. One girl in the IPM/C group experienced two adverse events, one of which was an asthma attack requiring a visit to hospital for nebulisation,

Table 4 Comparison of the two ultrasound comb-treated groups for the presence of lice, presence of louse egg/nits, and mean numbers of lice and louse eggs/nits recovered

Endpoint	Treatment	Day of study					
	Lotion	0	2	6	7	9	14
Presence of live lice	NNC	94.1%	35.3%	41.2%	32.7%	11.8%	17.7%
	ONC	85.7%	64.3%	71.4%	21.2%	50.0%	71.4%*
Total lice	NNC	20.9	2.12	2.06	0.90	0.12	0.35
	ONC	28.4	4.93	11.86	0.42	1.79**	5.93
Adult males	NNC	1.69	0.53	0.06	0.38	0.0	0.06
	ONC	2.25	0.29	0.79	0.33	0.07	0.86
Adult females	NNC	2.69	0.65	0.18	0.06	0.0	0.18
	ONC	3.50	0.86	1.21	0.75	0.14	1.79
Stage 3 nymphs	NNC	3.31	0.59	0.18	0.13	0.0	0.12
	ONC	3.33	0.29	1.71**	1.67	0.29	1.00**
Stage 2 nymphs	NNC	6.00	0.18	0.59	1.81	0.06	0.0
	ONC	4.33	1.14	3.07**	6.17	1.00	1.21
Stage 1 nymphs	NNC	7.25	0.18	1.06	5.94	0.06	0.0
	ONC	13.7	2.36	5.07***	12.8	0.29	1.07
Presence of eggs/nits	NNC	94.1%	–	–	82.4%	–	–
	ONC	71.4%	–	–	78.6%	–	–
Number of eggs/nits	NNC	13.25	–	–	19.80	–	–
	ONC	181.83	–	–	124.20	–	–

Mean figures should only be taken as indicative due to the skew distribution of the data
Day 0 and Day 7 treatment days, Days 2, 6, 9, and 14 assessment days only
***Significant difference at $p < 0.005$, **significant difference at $p < 0.05$, *near significant difference at $p = 0.05$

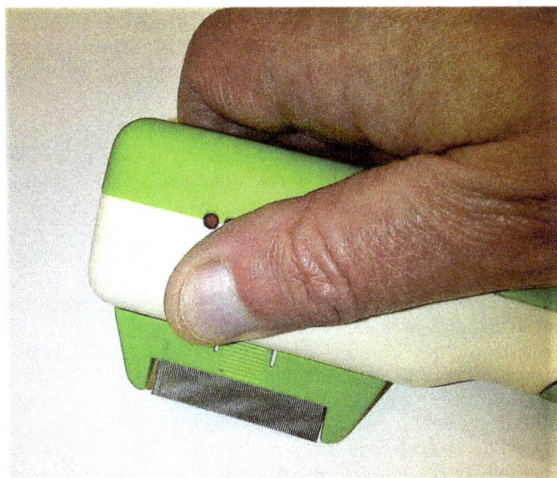

Fig. 4 Hand position taken up by investigators, close to the tooth unit, in order to retain a firm grip whilst combing. Moving the hand to this position largely eliminated the angle of the combing head, which had previously been shown to improve louse egg removal. Consequently, this would have resulted in some of the extra combing efficiency delivered through the ultrasound actuation being lost in practice

resulted in her dropping out to avoid further possible stress despite no evidence of a link between treatment on day 0 and the attack on day 5. There was no difference between groups in respect of frequency, outcome, action taken, relationship to study treatment, or severity.

Discussion

This clinical investigation showed that a silicone fluid formulated with a heavy plant oil, in this case neem seed oil, can be a pediculicide as effective as other lipid and silicone mixes. However, we detected no activity from the neem oil apart from physical occlusion effects. The activity of the solvent showed in the relative performance of the silicone-based lotion (74.6% success overall) and original Nice 'n Clear head lice lotion (28.6%

success), which was equally ineffective in an earlier study (Brown and Burgess 2017).

Irrespective of activity, the natural oil presents a number of practical problems. Neem seed oil is often cloudy, difficult to clarify by filtration, becomes gelatinous at cool room temperatures, and hard to formulate in any dosage form other than an emulsion, trapping the oil in micelles. In the silicone base, only one of several apparently similar PEG/PPG-dimeticone copolymer formulation aids allowed the mix to remain physically stable. A major problem was the recurrence of turbidity, apparently due to oxidative interactions with the air. It was difficult to wash out from hair requiring two or three shampoo washes, although the isopropyl myristate in IPM/C was even more difficult to remove, especially from fine hair. However, the most important drawback was the pungent odour, which is was not masked by addition of a citronella fragrance.

Clinically, the neem-silicone lotion (NNC) with the ultrasound generating ClearBrush® was non-significantly better than lotion alone but less successful at removing nits than the comb with the original lotion (ONC), although the skew distribution of eggs among relatively few participants meant the results were inconclusive. The benefits of using a comb with an angled head were demonstrated in laboratory tests (Burgess et al. 2016) but not replicated clinically. The prototype was not ergonomic with a long, thick handle to accommodate batteries, which required effort to pull it through the hair. Consequently, to retain a firm grip, investigators often held it around the tooth unit (Fig. 4), which negated the angle of the combing head. A design change would be required to address the problem.

In some ways, using the ultrasound comb was less physically demanding because the cavitation effects predicted to facilitate penetration of fluid into the spaces between the egg glue and the hairs themselves (Fig. 5) made sliding easier, especially with the ONC conditioner

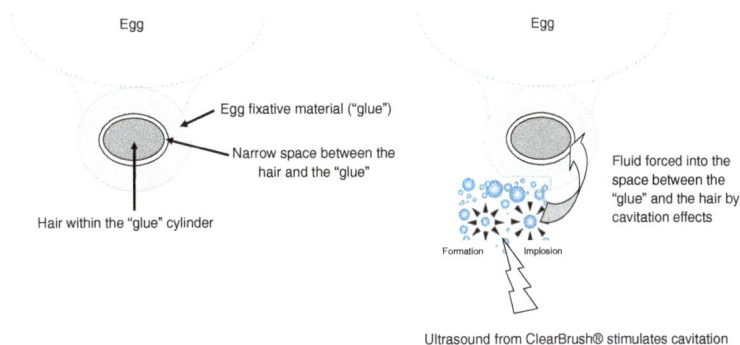

Fig. 5 Diagrammatic representation of the putative effect of ultrasound to produce cavitation effects in fluids resulting in increased flow into the space between the hair and the fixative "glue" binding the louse egg to the hair

lotion. In contrast, when using the silicone-based lotion, the comb scraped over the eggshells, which were not removed as efficiently.

Conclusions

As previously (Brown and Burgess 2017), this project could not identify any specific activity for neem in either formulation. The ClearBrush® device concept has also not been confirmed clinically and not exploited commercially, requiring a more compact power unit to make the device small enough to fit into the hand. Nevertheless, this project has demonstrated scope for improvement in treating head louse infestation and nit removal suggesting further investigation of the principles could prove beneficial.

Abbreviations
CB: ClearBrush® ultrasonic nit comb; CI: Confidence interval; IPM/C: 50:50 isopropyl myristate in cyclomethicone; ITT: Intention to treat; n: Number of participants with a particular characteristic; N: Total number of participants in a particular cohort group; NNC: Reformulated Nice 'n Clear head louse lotion; ONC: Original formulation Nice 'n Clear head lice lotion; OR: Odds ratio; PEG/PPG: Polyethylene glycol/polypropylene glycol; PP: Per-protocol

Acknowledgements
The project co-ordinator was A Nelson & Co Ltd. (UK). Other SME partners involved were Denman International Ltd. (UK) and Innowacja Polska Sp. z.o.o. (Poland). Thanks are due to the following individuals for their contributions: Ulli Jonsson and Peter Palmer (Nelsons—coordinators), Andrew Harrower and Marcus McCay (Denman—prototype comb design and production), and Marcin Opoka and Leonard Płonka (Innowacja Polska—ultrasound unit design and technical co-ordination). Sample size calculations were performed on behalf of the sponsor by PN Lee Statistics and Computing Ltd., an independent statistical consultancy. In addition to the authors, treatments and/or assessments were performed by Audrey Pepperman, Christine Sullivan, Geraldine Matlock, Gillian Clarke, and Ian M Jones. Dr. Paul Silverston was the research physician and evaluated the adverse events. The documents and conduct of Good Clinical Practice were monitored by Ulli Jonsson on behalf of A Nelson & Co Ltd.

Funding
This project was part of a co-operative research project initiated under the Sixth Framework Programme of the European Commission, project number COOP-CT-2005-017916, with the title "A novel integrated ultrasonic brush and sonically activated lotion to provide a full system approach to the eradication of the European head louse menace". The project co-ordinator was A Nelson & Co Ltd. (UK) who played no role in the study design, its execution, interpretation of the data, decision to publish, or the preparation of the manuscript.

Authors' contributions
IFB, ERB, and NAB collectively conceived and designed the clinical investigation, organised the study, performed the treatments, and collected the raw data. IFB performed the analyses of the data and wrote the draft manuscript. MNB designed and performed the laboratory experiments for evaluation of the ClearBrush®. All authors read and approved the final manuscript.

Competing interests
IFB has been a consultant to various makers of pharmaceutical products, medical devices, and combs for treating infestations of head lice and their eggs. The other authors declare that they have no competing interests.

References
Abdel-Ghaffar F, Al-Quraishy S, Al-Rasheid KA, Mehlhorn H. Efficacy of a single treatment of head lice with a neem seed extract: an in vivo and in vitro study on nits and motile stages. Parasitol Res. 2012;110:277–80.

Abdel-Ghaffar F, Semmler M. Efficacy of neem seed extract shampoo on head lice of naturally infected humans in Egypt. Parasitol Res. 2007;100:329–32.

Barker SC, Altman PM. A randomised, assessor blind, parallel group comparative efficacy trial of three products for the treatment of head lice in children—melaleuca oil and lavender oil, pyrethrins and piperonyl butoxide, and a "suffocation" product. BMC Dermatol. 2010;10:6.

Brown CM, Burgess IF. Can neem oil help eliminate lice? Randomised controlled trial with and without louse combing. Adv Pediatr Res. 2017;4:9.

Burgess IF. Do nit removal formulations and other treatments loosen head louse eggs and nits from hair? Med Vet Entomol. 2010;24:55–61.

Burgess IF, Brunton ER, Burgess NA. Clinical trial showing superiority of a coconut and anise spray over permethrin 0.43% lotion for head louse infestation, ISRCTN9646978. Eur J Pediatr. 2010;169:55–62.

Burgess IF, Lee PN, Matlock G. Randomised, controlled, assessor blind trial comparing 4% dimeticone lotion with 0.5% malathion liquid for head louse infestation. PLoS One. 2007;2:11.

Burgess MN, Brunton ER, Burgess IF. A novel concept nit comb using ultrasound actuation: pre-clinical evaluation. J Med Entomol. 2016;53:152–6.

Dallal GE. Randomization.com. 2007. http://www.randomization.com. Accessed 11 Sept 2007.

de Souza BV, de Oliveira GL, de Oliveira NJ, da Silva Ribeiro DC. Estudo comparativo da eficiência de três diferentes pentes finos na retirada de piolhos e lêndeas. Rev Bras Med. 2001;58:398–402.

Grieve KA, Altman PM, Rowe SJ, Staton JA, Oppenheim VMJ. A randomised, double-blind, comparative efficacy trial of three head lice treatment options: malathion, pyrethrins with piperonyl butoxide and MOOV head lice solution. Aust Pharmacist. 2007;26:738–43.

Heukelbach J, Oliveira FA, Speare R. A new shampoo based on neem (Azadirachta indica) is highly effective against head lice in vitro. Parasitol Res. 2006;99:353–6.

Mehlhorn H, Abdel-Ghaffar F, Al-Rasheid KA, Schmidt J, Semmler M. Ovicidal effects of a neem seed extract preparation on eggs of body and head lice. Parasitol Res. 2011;109:1299–302.

Schmahl G, Al-Rasheid KA, Abdel-Ghaffar F, Klimpel S, Mehlhorn H. The efficacy of neem seed extracts (Tre-san®, MiteStop®) on a broad spectrum of pests and parasites. Parasitol Res. 2010;107:261–9.

Thawornchaisit P, Amornsak W, Mahannop P, Buddhirakkul P, Pandii W, Connellan P, et al. Combined neem oil 6% w/w and eucalyptus oil 16% w/w lotion for treating head lice: in vitro and in vivo efficacy studies. J Pharm Pract Res. 2012;42:189–92.

14

In vitro and in vivo anti-allergic effects of an extract of a traditional Chinese medicine preparation

Li Li[1], Xiao-yue Wang[1], Hong Meng[1], Guang-rong Liu[2], Chang Liu[1] and Yin-Mao Dong[1*]

Abstract

Background: The present research was conducted to investigate the in vivo and in vitro anti-allergic activity of a traditional Chinese medicine formulation comprising *Ampelopsis grossedentata*, *Saposhnikovia divaricata*, *Sophora flavescens*, *Angelica sinensis*, *Ophiopogon japonicus*, and *Cornus officinalis*.

Methods: The hyaluronidase inhibitory activity of an active extract of this formulation (AEF) was evaluated in vitro. In vivo studies were conducted to explore its effects on pruritus, the anti-dinitrophenyl (DNP) IgE-induced passive cutaneous anaphylaxis (PCA) reaction, and skin repair, in order to investigate the therapeutic effects of AEF in allergic skin reactions. The inhibitory effects of the main active ingredient of AEF (dihydromyricetin (DMY)) on the pro-inflammatory cytokines, interleukin (IL)-6 and IL-8 in phorbol-12-myristate 13-acetate plus the calcium ionophore A23187 (PMACI)-stimulated KU812 cells, were measured using enzyme-linked immunosorbent assays.

Results: An in vivo test showed that AEF produced significant inhibition of pruritus, PCA reaction, and skin barrier dysfunction. The main chemical DMY significantly decreased the PMACI-induced increase in pro-inflammatory cytokines, including IL-6 and IL-8 in KU812 cells. The in vivo anti-allergy effects on the skin may have resulted from reduced levels of IL-6 and IL-8.

Conclusions: These findings indicated that the formulation and one of its constituents, DMY, may exert excellent anti-inflammatory effects, with applications in the treatment of skin allergic reactions including pruritus, diffuse redness, and swelling.

Keywords: Anti-allergic activity, Traditional Chinese medicine formulation, Dihydromyricetin, KU812 cells, Interleukin-6, Interleukin-8

Background

In recent years, increased air pollution and dietary changes have increased the prevalence of sensitive skin, associated with allergic reactions and inflammation. This problem affects human health worldwide (Farage et al. 2013; Xu et al. 2012). Pharmacological options for the treatment of allergic diseases are sometimes associated with side effects and drug resistance (Liu et al. 2014). Research into naturally occurring anti-allergy agents present in plants and traditional Chinese medicine (TCM) formulations is therefore currently underway,

with the aim of identifying effective treatments with fewer side effects (Jung et al. 2012).

The stems and leaves of *Ampelopsis grossedentata* provide a traditional Chinese herbal tea named Rattan, which was considered to be cool and sweet and was used to clear heat and dredge meridians. Modern pharmacological studies have shown that *A. grossedentata* has antioxidant, anti-inflammatory, and antibacterial activities (Kou and Chen 2012). The main chemical constituent of *A. grossedentata*, dihydromyricetin (DMY), is known to have a broad range of biological functions including hypoglycemic, antioxidant, anti-inflammatory, antitumor, hepatoprotective, and neuroprotective effects. These reported effects have led to increased research into the bioactivity of DMY over the last decade, leading

* Correspondence: ymdong2008@163.com
[1]Beijing Key Laboratory of Plant Resources Research and Development, Beijing Technology and Business University, Beijing 100048, People's Republic of China
Full list of author information is available at the end of the article

to improved understanding of its pharmacological effects and their underlying mechanisms (Kou and Chen 2012).

We previously screened out *A. grossedentata*, *Saposhnikovia divaricata*, *Sophora flavescens*, *Angelica sinensis*, *Ophiopogon japonicus*, and *Cornus officinalis* from a large number of herbs used in TCMs, including for hyaluronidase inhibition, antioxidant effects (radical scavenging test using 1,1-diphenyl-2-picrylhydrazyl (DPPH)), and antibacterial activities. In order to obtain a formulation with better anti-allergic properties, the ratios of the six herbs and its extraction method were further optimized by the single factor and response surface methodology (Lin and Ji 2013) directed by hyaluronidase inhibition test. An active extract obtained from the formulation (AEF) was used to do further anti-allergic evaluation in vitro and in vivo.

In the present study, the effects on pruritus, antidinitrophenyl (DNP) IgE-induced passive cutaneous anaphylaxis (PCA), and skin repair of AEF were evaluated in vivo. Human leukemia KU812 cells stimulated with phorbol 12-myristate 13-acetate (PMA) and the calcium ionophore, A23187, were exposed to DMY in order to evaluate the effects of this compound on levels of the pro-inflammatory cytokines, interleukin (IL)-6 and IL-8. The KU812 myeloid precursor cell line, which was originally established from a patient with chronic myelogenous leukemia, has been shown to be a suitable model for studying the activation and degranulation of human mast cells (Rasheed et al. 2009). These studies indicated that *A. grossedentata* and related TCM formulations have the potential to provide raw materials for the production of anti-allergy medicines and cosmetics.

Methods

Chemicals and reagents

Anti-DNP IgE, DNP-human serum albumin (HSA), Evans blue, histamine phosphate, hyaluronidase, *p*-dimethylaminobenzaldehyde, fluocinonide ointment, disodium cromoglycate (DSCG), A23187, and PMA were purchased from Sigma (St. Louis, MO, USA). KU812 cells were purchased from the Shanghai Institute cell library. Iscove's Modified Dulbecco's Medium (IMDM), penicillin, and streptomycin were purchased from Gibco (Invitrogen Corporation, Carlsbad, CA, USA). Fetal bovine serum (FBS) was purchased from HyClone (Logan, UT, USA). Cytokine-specific enzyme-linked immunosorbent assay (ELISA) kits were purchased from R&D Systems (USA). DMY was purchased from Shanghai Tauto Biotech. Co., Ltd. (Shanghai, China), and was determined to be greater than 98% pure by high-performance liquid chromatography (HPLC) analysis. Other reagents used were of analytical grade.

Sample preparation

A. grossedentata, *S. divaricata*, *S. flavescens*, *A. sinensis*, *O. japonicus*, and *C. officinalis* were purchased from the Beijing Tongrentang Co., Ltd. (Beijing, China). All herbs were authenticated by Professor Y. Peng, a medical botanist at the Institute of Medicinal Plant Development (IMPLAD), Chinese Academy of Medical Science (CAMS), Beijing, China. The optimized ratio of the herbs was determined to be 3:2:2:1.7:1.2:1.2, using a Design-Expert regression model directed by hyaluronidase inhibitory activity. The formulation (100 g) was extracted by thermal recycling with 70% ethanol (1:13) for 140 min at 68 °C and filtered. The AEF was concentrated in a rotary vacuum evaporator, lyophilized, and stored at $-$ 20 °C until use.

The AEF was standardized based on its DMY content. Chromatographic separation was carried out on an Agilent 1260 LC series system (Agilent Technologies, Palo Alto, CA, USA) equipped with online vacuum degasser, quaternary pump, autosampler, temperature-controlled column compartment, and a diode array detector. Agilent Technologies ChemStation software for LC (B.02.01) was used. Chromatographic separation was achieved on an Agilent RP C18 (150 mm × 4.6 mm, 5 µm) using a mobile phase consisting of water to acetic acid (99.8:0.1, *v/v*) (A) and methanol (B). The gradient program consisted of 60% (B) for 0–30 min. The flow rate was 0.5 mL/min, and the column temperature was set to 25 °C. The detection wavelength was 290 nm. DMY was detected at around 5.6 min in this system. The DMY content of the AEF was 10.25 ± 0.83 mg/g ($n = 3$).

Cell culture

KU812 cells were grown in IMDM culture medium supplemented with 10% heat-inactivated FBS and 1% penicillin-streptomycin at 37 °C in 5% CO_2. KU812 cells were pre-treated with the AEF (50, 200, or 300 µg/mL) for 2 h prior to stimulation with 40 nM PMA and 1 µM A23187 for different periods of time. The AEF was diluted in nuclease-free double-filtered distilled water, whereas PMA and A23187 were dissolved in DMSO.

Animals

Hartley guinea pigs (250 ± 10 g) and Sprague-Dawley rats (200–250 g) were obtained from the Vital River Laboratory Animal Technology Co. Ltd. (Beijing, China). These animals were housed under standard conditions with a 12/12-h light/dark cycle at a temperature of 22 ± 1 °C with $55 \pm 10\%$ humidity and were given standard laboratory feed (Beijing Jinmuyang Laboratory Animals, Inc., Beijing, China) and water ad libitum. The animal certification number was SCXK (Jing) 2010-0001. Animal protocols were developed in accordance with the institution's guidelines for the care and use of laboratory animals and were approved by the local Animal Care and Use Committee.

Inhibition of hyaluronidase activity

Hyaluronidase inhibition was determined by measuring the amount of β-N-acetylglucosamine formed from sodium hyaluronate, using a spectrophotometer (Kakegawa 1992). Bovine hyaluronidase (500 µL of 7420 units/mL in 0.1 M acetate buffer; pH 5.6) was mixed with 100 µL calcium chloride (0.25 mM) and then incubated in a water bath at 37 °C for 20 min. The indicated test sample was added in a volume of 500 µL, and the mixture was incubated in a water bath at 37 °C for 20 min, after which sodium hyaluronate (500 µL of 0.5 mg/mL in 0.1 M acetate buffer; pH 5.6) was added. After a 30-min incubation in a water bath at 37 °C, 100 µL of 0.4 M sodium hydroxide was added to stop the reaction, and the mixture was placed in an ice-water bath for 5 min. Next, 500 µL acetylacetone was added, and the mixture was incubated in boiling water for 30 min to produce a chromogenic reaction. After cooling to 25 °C, 1.0 mL of p-dimethylaminobenzaldehyde solution was added to the reaction mixture for 20 min at 25 °C. The optical density of the reaction mixture was measured at 555 nm using a microplate reader (RT-6000; Leidu, Shenzhen, China). All determinations were performed in triplicate.

Measurement of pruritus

Hartley guinea pigs (250 ± 10 g) were randomly divided into four groups with eight animals/group; these groups consist of model control group (physiological saline, 100 mg/cm2), positive control group (DSCG, 100 mg/cm^2), low dosage experimental group (AEF, 50 mg/cm^2), middle dosage experimental group (AEF, 100 mg/cm^2) and high dosage experimental group (AEF, 150 mg/cm^2) applied to shaved dorsal skin sites (2 cm^2) on their back right feet for 2 days. On the third day, the samples were applied to the shaved sites for 10 min, followed by 0.05 mL of increasing concentrations of histamine phosphate (0.01, 0.02, 0.03, 0.04, 0.05, 0.06, 0.07, 0.08, 0.09, or 0.1%), each of which was dripped onto the test site for 3 min. The scratching behavior induced by histamine phosphate was recorded, and the itch threshold was the level required to produce itching (Hu and Zhong 2013).

Induction of the PCA reaction

Sprague-Dawley rats (200–250 g) were divided into six groups with eight rats/group: the untreated control group, the model group (distilled water, 100 mg/cm^2), the positive control group (fluocinonide ointment, 50 mg/cm^2), and the high AEF (100 mg/cm^2), middle AEF (50 mg/cm^2), and low AEF (25 mg/cm^2) dose groups. Each group had the appropriate treatment

applied to the skin at three dorsal skin injection sites, which were outlined with a water-insoluble red marker. One hour later, the PCA reaction was generated by sensitizing the skin with an intradermal injection of 0.5 µg anti-DNP IgE into each of the sites. After 48 h, this was followed by a tail vein injection of 100 µg DNP-HSA in phosphate-buffered saline containing 4% Evans blue. The rats were sacrificed 30 min after the administration of DNP-HSA. The skin at the injection site was removed for measurement of the pigment area. The amount of dye was determined by colorimetry after extraction using a 1:1 mixture of acetone and physiological saline (Shin et al. 2004). The absorbance of the skin extract was measured at 620 nm in a microplate reader (RT-6000; Leidu), and the amount of dye was calculated using an Evans blue calibration curve.

Evaluation of skin repair activity

Hartley guinea pigs (250 ± 10 g) were randomly divided into five groups with eight animals/group: a blank control group (physiological saline), a model control group, and groups exposed to different dosages of AEF. The hair on the back of the neck of each guinea pig was shaved the day before the experiment to expose about 2 cm^2 skin. Each group (except for the blank control group) had 150 µL acetone to ether (1:1) solution dripped onto the shaved skin. Test samples (0.1 mL/cm^2) were smeared onto the shaved skin; 0.1 mL/cm^2 distilled water was applied to the model control group. Treatments were administered twice daily for five consecutive days. On the fifth day, the skin moisture loss of the shaved skin was tested 20 min after sample administration. Protection rates (%) were calculated for each study group.

Cytokine ELISAs

Levels of IL-6 and IL-8 in the culture medium were quantified by specific sandwich ELISAs. Briefly, KU812 cells were stimulated with PMA (40 nM) plus A23187 (1 µM) for 12 h, with or without pre-treatment with AEF (Rasheed et al. 2009). The ELISAs were performed using the culture supernatants, in accordance with the manufacturer's instructions (R&D Systems). Plates were read at 450 nm using the RT-6000 microplate reader (Leidu).

Statistical methods

The results were expressed as mean ± standard error of the mean (S.E.M.). The statistical significance of the differences between the treated and control groups were calculated using Student's t test. Results with $P < 0.05$ were considered statistically significant.

Results and discussion

Hyaluronidase inhibition activity

In vitro hyaluronidase inhibition activity was used to evaluate the anti-allergic activity of DMY, *A. grossedentata*, and AEF. The results (Fig. 1) showed that AEF inhibited hyaluronidase activity more effectively than DMY or *A. grossedentata*. It was concluded that different constituents of the TCM formulation had synergistic interactions, which led to an obvious improvement in anti-allergic activity.

Effect on histamine phosphate-induced pruritus

AEF significantly increased the histamine phosphate itching threshold in guinea pigs in a dose-dependent manner (Table 1). Allergen-induced itching is sometimes caused by the release of vasoactive substances, such as histamine, from mast cells and basophils. These results showed that AEF had a protective function when applied to the skin, and this could relieve the itching and discomfort associated with sensitive skin.

The PCA reaction in rats

The anti-IgE antibody-induced PCA has been established as a typical model for a mast cell-dependent immediate-type allergic reaction (Shin et al. 2004). We examined the anti-allergic effects of AEF using a rat PCA model. Local extravasation was induced by a local injection of anti-DNP IgE, followed by an antigenic challenge (Lu et al. 2012). PCA was best visualized by the extravasation of dye. Administration of a high dosage of AEF 1 h prior to antigen injection significantly suppressed the PCA reaction (Table 2). PCA reaction-induced capillary permeability leads to skin inflammation and infiltration, diffuse skin redness, and swelling. AEF produced significant protection from skin allergic and inflammatory injury through inhibition of the PCA reaction.

Table 1 The effects of samples on the pruritus response induced by histamine ($x \pm s$, $n = 8$)

Groups	Dosage (mg/cm^2)	Itching threshold(μg)	Inhibition (%)
Model control group	–	31.67 ± 2.58	
DSCG	100	73.21 ± 12.49**	131.17
Low dosage	50	62.50 ± 13.69**	97.37
Middle dosage	100	85.00 ± 15.49**	168.42
High dosage	150	90.00 ± 16.43**	184.21

Tips: compared with model control group, **$P < 0.01$

Skin-repairing activity

When the skin was scratched by acetone to ether (1:1) solution, the moisture loss was increased to 19.99% in the model group. High, moderate, and low dosages of AEF significantly decreased this moisture loss and significantly protected the scratched parts of the skin (Table 3). The barrier function of the skin has three elements: the stratum corneum (air-liquid barrier), tight junctions (liquid-liquid barrier), and the Langerhans cell network (immunological barrier) (Kubo et al. 2012). The barrier function is often impaired in sensitive skin, which leads to moisture loss, drying, and itching. The findings of the present study indicated that AEF could contribute to a restoration of skin barrier integrity, thus relieving sensitivity.

Inhibition of IL-6 and IL-8

DMY was the main chemical constituent of *A. grossedentata* and of AEF (10.25 ± 0.83 mg/g). It was reported to inhibit nitric oxide (NO) production in lipopolysaccharide-stimulated RAW264.7 macrophages and to reduce carrageenan-induced acute inflammation in vivo (Kou and Chen 2012). In the present study, basophilic KU812 cells were stimulated with PMA and the calcium ionophore, A23187. The levels of the pro-inflammatory cytokines, IL-6 and IL-8, in stimulated KU812 cells were measured by ELISA. DMY produced a significant dose-dependent reduction in the levels of IL-6 and IL-8 in media conditioned by this cell line (Table 4).

Table 2 Influence of PCA reaction

Groups	Dosage (mg/cm^2)	Amount of dye (μg/mL)	Inhibition (%)
Blank control group	–	3.65 ± 0.46	–
Model control group	100	144.32 ± 7.74##	–
Fluocinonide ointment	50	130.25 ± 5.14*	9.75
Low dosage	25	139.97 ± 7.22	3.02
Middle dosage	50	137.18 ± 4.98	4.95
High dosage	100	128.61 ± 12.34*	10.89

Tips: compared with blank control group, ##$P < 0.01$; compared with model control group, *$P < 0.05$

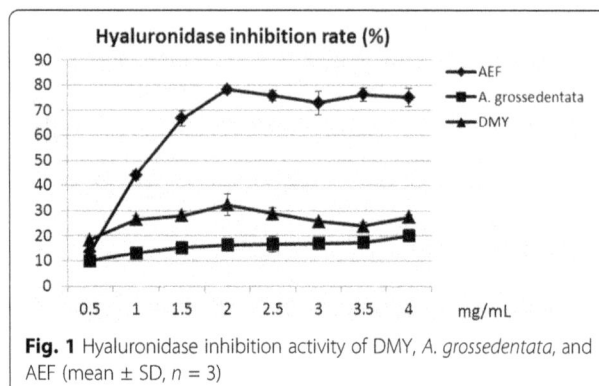

Fig. 1 Hyaluronidase inhibition activity of DMY, *A. grossedentata*, and AEF (mean ± SD, $n = 3$)

Table 3 The skin repairing effects of samples ($x \pm s$, $n = 8$)

Groups	Dose (mg/cm²)	Moisture loss	Protection rate (%)
Blank control group	–	39.08 ± 6.51	–
Model control group	100	19.25 ± 3.14##	–
Low dosage	50	16.04 ± 0.61**	19.79
Moderate dosage	100	14.22 ± 0.67**	28.90
High dosage	150	13.87 ± 0.47**	30.62

Tips: compared with blank control group, ##$P < 0.01$; compared with model control group, **$P < 0.01$

Mast cells and basophils are known to play a central role in inflammatory, allergic, and immune events (Galli 1993). Activation of these cells results in degranulation, accompanied by the production of chemical mediators, such as histamine, proteases, metabolites of arachidonic acid, and several inflammatory and chemotactic cytokines, including IL-6, IL-8, IL-1β, and tumor necrosis factor (TNF)-α. These molecules act on the vasculature and skin, resulting in the recruitment of activated immune and inflammatory cells to the site of inflammatory lesions, thereby amplifying and sustaining the inflammatory condition (Nigrovic and Lee 2005). In various studies, pro-inflammatory cytokines IL-6 and IL-8 released during KU812 cell activation were shown to act on the blood vessels and skin, amplifying the inflammatory and allergic response (Choi et al. 2012).

IL-6 is produced by T cells, monocytes, macrophages, and synovial fibroblasts. It promotes the immune response by increasing IgE production and by increasing IL-8 expression. IL-6 is also produced by mast cells and basophils, accumulates locally in the skin, and is associated with delayed hypersensitivity. In type I allergies, antigens such as foods, dust mites, medicines, pollen, and cosmetics were bound to toll receptors on basophils, leading to IL-6, IL-4, and IL-10 release. These cytokines activate immediate hypersensitivity, increasing IgE generation and producing pro-inflammatory effects. IL-8 has potent chemoattractant activity for neutrophils and T cells. The IL-8 protein is normally secreted at very low levels from non-induced cells, but its production is rapidly induced by a very wide range of stimuli,

encompassing pro-inflammatory cytokines such as TNF-α or IL-1, IL-6, bacterial or viral products, and cellular stress (Hoffmann et al. 2002). The chemoattractant activity of IL-8 aggravated local inflammation and extended the development of skin allergy (Rasheed et al. 2009). The results of the present study therefore suggested that DMY and AEF produced protective effects on the acute phase of hypersensitivity, through inhibition of IL-6, and on delayed hypersensitivity, through inhibition of IL-8.

Conclusions

The TCM formulation comprising *A. grossedentata*, *S. divaricata*, *S. flavescens*, *A. sinensis*, *O. japonicus*, and *C. officinalis* (3:2:2:1.7:1.2:1.2) has significant potential for the treatment of sensitive skin. The AEF could relieve pruritus of scratched skin, repair diffuse skin redness, and restore the skin barrier function. The anti-allergic activity of AEF may be associated with inhibition of the pro-inflammatory cytokines, IL-6 and IL-8. These results provided an evidence base for the traditional use of *A. grossedentata* and related TCM formulations for the protection of sensitive skin.

Abbreviations
AEF: An active extract of this formulation; CAMS: Chinese Academy of Medical Science; DMSO: Dimethyl sulfoxide; DMY: Dihydromyricetin; DNP: Dinitrophenyl; DPPH: 1,1-Diphenyl-2-picrylhydrazyl; DSCG: Disodium cromoglycate; ELISA: Enzyme-linked immune sorbent assay; FBS: Fetal bovine serum; HPLC: High-performance liquid chromatography; HSA: Human serum albumin; IL: Interleukin; IMDM: Iscove's Modified Dulbecco's Medium; IMPLAD: Institute of Medicinal Plant Development; NO: Nitric oxide; PCA: Passive cutaneous anaphylaxis; PMA: Phorbol 12-myristate 13-acetate; PMACI: Phorbol-12-myristate 13-acetate plus the calcium ionophore A23187; TCM: Traditional Chinese medicine; TNF: Tumor necrosis factor

Acknowledgements
Not applicable.

Funding
This work was supported by the National Natural Science Foundation of China (31501402).

Authors' contributions
HM performed the animal experiment. LL did the cell experiment. XW was a major contributor in writing the manuscript. GL carried out additional analyses and finalized this paper. CL did the extraction experiment. YD designed the experiment. All authors read and approved the final manuscript.

Competing interests
The authors declare that they have no competing interests.

Author details
¹Beijing Key Laboratory of Plant Resources Research and Development, Beijing Technology and Business University, Beijing 100048, People's Republic of China. ²Infinitus (China) Company Ltd., Guangzhou 510665, China.

Table 4 IL-6 and IL-8 inhibition results of DMY in KU812 cells

Groups	Dose (μg/mL)	IL-6	Inhibition (%)	IL-8	Inhibition (%)
Blank control group		–		37.0 ± 0.8	
Model control group		38.5 ± 5.2	–	207.0 ± 40.9	–
Low dosage	50	32.0 ± 6.4	11.7	182.8 ± 24.1	16.9
Moderate dosage	200	29.8 ± 2.5	28	149.1 ± 25.0	22.6
High dosage	300	15.5 ± 1.6**	50.6	102.2 ± 13.9**	59.7

Tips: compared with model control group, **$P < 0.01$

References

Choi SJ, Tai BH, Cuong NM, Kim YH, Jang HD. Antioxidative and anti-inflammatory effect of quercetin and its glycosides isolated from mampat (*Cratoxylum formosum*). Food Sci Biotechnol. 2012;21(2):587–95.

Farage MA, Miller KW, Wippel AM, Misery L, Mailbach H. Sensitive skin in the United States: survey of regional differences. Fam Med Medic Sci Res. 2013; 112(2):2.

Galli JG. New concepts about the mast cell. N Engl J Med. 1993;328:257–65.

Hoffmann E, Dittrich-Breiholz O, Holtmann H, Kracht M. Multiple control of interleukin-8 gene expression. J Leukoc Biol. 2002;72:847–55.

Hu YM, Zhong ZD. Study on effect of Ma Chi Xian extract for the rat foot itch threshold induced by histamine phosphate. Chin J Ethnomed Ethnopharm. 2013;6:34–5.

Jung HS, Kim MH, Gwak NG, Im YS, Lee K, Sohn Y, Choi H, Yang WM. Antiallergic effects of *Scutellaria baicalensis* on inflammation in vivo and in vitro. J Ethnopharmacol. 2012;141:345–9.

Kakegawa H. Inhibitory effects of some natural products on the activation of hyaluronidase and their antiallrgic actions. Chen Pharm. 1992;40(6):1439–42.

Kou X, Chen N. Pharmacological potential of ampelopsin in Rattan tea. Food Sci Human Wellness. 2012;1:14–8.

Kubo A, Nagao K, Amagai M. Epidermal barrier dysfunction and cutaneous sensitization in atopic diseases. J Clin Invest. 2012;122(2):440–7.

Lin JY, Ji LH. Optimization of flavonoids from Ginkgo Biloba using response surface analysis. J Chin Inst Food Sci Technol. 2013;13(2):83–90.

Liu XY, Deng W, Li L, Meng H, Ren HK, Dong YM. Skin allergy causes, solution way, and development trend of anti-allergic cosmetics. China Cosmet. 2014; 7:72–7.

Lu Y, Li Y, Jin M, Yang JH, Li X, Chao GH, Park HH, Park YN, Son JK, Lee E, Chang HW. Inula japonica extract inhibits mast cell-mediated allergic reaction and mast cell activation. J Ethnopharmacol. 2012;43(1):151–7.

Nigrovic PA, Lee DM. Mast cells in inflammatory arthritis. Arthritis Res Ther. 2005; 7:1–11.

Rasheed Z, Akhtar N, Anbazhagan AN, Ramamurthy S, Shukla M, Haqqi TM. Polyphenol-rich pomegranate fruit extract (POMx) suppresses PMACI-induced expression of pro-inflammatory cytokines by inhibiting the activation of MAP Kinases and NF-κB in human KU812 cells. J Inflamm. 2009;6:1–12.

Shin HY, Na HJ, Moon PD, Shin T, Shin TY, Kim SH, Hong SH, Kim HM. Inhibition of mast cell-dependent immediate-type hypersensitivity reactions by purple bamboo salt. J Ethnopharmacol. 2004;91:153–7.

Xu F, Yan S, Wu M, Li F, Sun Q, Lai W, Shen X, Rahhali N, Taieb C, Xu J. Self-declared sensitive skin in China: a community-based study in three top metropolises. J Eur Acad Dermatol Venereol. 2012;27(3):370–5.

15

Anti-inflammatory effects of prunin on UVB-irradiated human keratinocytes

Eun Ju Na[1] and Ji Young Ryu[2*]

Abstract

Background: The flavonoid prunin is a flavanone glycoside found in cherry trees, including the flowering cherry *Prunus yedoensis Matsumura* (Rosacea). Although this compound has been studied for its antioxidant, anti-bacterial, and blood-sugar-lowering effects, no studies address its use in cosmetics. This study investigates whether prunin exhibits anti-inflammatory effects in cells exposed to ultraviolet B (UVB) radiation.

Methods: The effects of prunin were assessed by measuring cell viability using the water-soluble tetrazolium salt-1 assay and free radical damage using the dichlorofluorescein diacetate assay as well as by quantitative real-time PCR.

Results: UVB-induced decrease in cell viability diminished by pretreatment with prunin in a concentration-dependent manner. Intracellular reactive oxygen species (ROS) quantitative analysis revealed that the expression of nuclear factor kappa-light-chain-enhancer of activated B cells (NF-κB), which is associated with the inflammatory response, and mRNA expression of interleukin-6 (*IL-6*), interleukin-8 (*IL-8*), cyclooxygenase-2 (*COX2*), tumor necrosis factor-alpha (*TNF-α*), and protease-activated receptor (*PAR2*) decreased with prunin pretreatment in a concentration-dependent manner.

Conclusions: Prunin increased the survival rate of UVB-treated human keratinocyte HaCaT cells. Prunin protected the HaCaT cells, eliminated ROS, and demonstrated anti-inflammatory effects. Thus, prunin is worthy of investigation for use as a cosmetic ingredient that protects the skin and has anti-inflammatory effects.

Keywords: Prunin, HaCaT keratinocyte, Anti-inflammation, Reactive oxygen species, Ultraviolet B

Background

The skin is put under oxidative stress when UV radiation induces the formation of reactive oxygen species (ROS), which damage DNA, lipids, and proteins (Devasagayam and Kamat 1994). Ultraviolet light acts as an external stress-stimulating factor, which increases the expression and activity of 11β-hydroxysteroid ehydrogenase type 1 (11β-HSD1), an enzyme that converts ROS and inactive cortisone to active cortisol in keratinocytes (Itoi et al. 2013).

Increased oxidative stress in the skin leads to inflammatory responses such as erythema, edema, and fever. These responses attempt to restore and regenerate wounds caused by chemical, physical, and bacterial assaults (Greaves and Sondergaard 1970; Hruza and Pentland 1993). During an inflammatory response, immune cells such as monocytes and macrophages are stimulated to express inflammation-related genes through the activation of transcription factors. Macrophages express the transcription factor nuclear factor kappa-light-chain-enhancer of activated B cells (NF-κB) in response to stimuli such as lipopolysaccharide and interferon-γ. NF-κB induces inflammatory responses by producing nitric oxide synthase, nitric oxide, prostaglandins, and cyclooxygenase-2 (COX2) (Nathan 1987). NF-κB is usually bound to inhibitor kappa B (IκB), which maintains the inactive state. When exposed to external stimuli such as UV light, IκB is rapidly phosphorylated and degraded (Maziere et al. 1999; Nomoto et al. 2001; Gomez-Nicola et al. 2010; Baeuerle and Henkel 1994). After NF-κB separates from IκB and becomes activated, it migrates to the nucleus, where it increases the expression of genes that induce inflammatory responses, including interleukin-6 (*IL-6*), interleukin-8 (*IL-8*), tumor necrosis factor-alpha (*TNF-α*), and *COX2* (Baeuerle and Baltimore 1988). In addition, a variety of proteases are expressed in the skin. These proteases are involved in

* Correspondence: ji02ji2@naver.com
[2]Halla University, 28, Halladae-gil, Heungeop-myeon, Wonju-si, Gangwon-do 25404, Republic of Korea
Full list of author information is available at the end of the article

maintaining homeostasis through immune response, inflammation, cytokine expression, vascular function, tissue recovery, host defense, and apoptosis (Sharlow et al. 2000).

Protease-activated receptor 2 (PAR2) plays an important role in inflammation. In 1995, we observed PAR-2 expression in Santulli in vitro. D 'Andrea observed PAR-2 expression and formed surface, superficial, and granular layers. PAR-2 and PAR-4 indicate that trypsin activates mast cell tryptase PAR-2 (Santulli et al. 1995; Coughlin 1999; D'Andrea et al. 1998). In addition, trypsin, a mast cell tryptase or SLGRL-NH2 (synthetic peptide) also activates PAR-2 and causes extensive inflammation (Kong et al. 1997).

Prunin is a flavonoid, which is a family of polyphenolic compounds with its name derived from the Greek word flavus that means yellow. This plant pigment possesses flavone as its basic structure. Found in relatively small amounts in animals, prunin is mainly present in vegetables, fruits, flowers, leaves, stems, roots, and fruits (Middleton et al. 2000). Prunin is a flavanone glycoside with the molecular formula $C_{21}H_{22}O_{10}$ and a molecular weight of 434.39. Prunin was isolated from *P. davidiana* Fr. (Rosacea) stems (Jung et al. 2017). The stems of *P. davidiana* Fr. (Rosacea) are used in Korean traditional medicine for treating neuritis and rheumatism (Choi et al. 1991). These stems contain antiviral agents and a variety of flavonoids that possess antioxidant, anti-inflammatory, hypocholesterolemic, and cardioprotective properties, and the DNA-binding activity (Jung et al. 2003; Yousuf et al. 2013; Zhang et al. 2008). Previous studies on prunin report that it has antioxidant and anti-inflammation properties, decreases blood glucose and insulin levels, and improves blood circulation (Céliz et al. 2013; Céliz et al. 2010; Céliz et al. 2011; Choi et al. 2006; Kimihisa et al. 2010). In this study, we investigated the effects of prunin treatment on ultraviolet (UVB)-induced cell damage and inflammation.

Methods

Cell culture

The human keratinocyte HaCaT cells used in this experiment were purchased from ATCC (USA). To incubate HaCaT cell strains, Dulbecco's Modified Eagle Medium (Hyclone, USA) containing 10% fetal bovine serum (Hyclone) and 1% penicillin/streptomycin (penicillin 100 IU/ml, streptomycin 100 µg/ml; Invitrogen, USA) was used. The cells were incubated at 37 °C with 5% CO_2.

Sample treatment

Prunin was purchased from Sigma-Aldrich (USA) in purified (> 95%) powder, which was dissolved in dimethyl sulfoxide (Sigma-Aldrich) at an appropriate concentration for the experiment. HaCaT (1×10^6cell/well) was incubated in the culture dish for 24 h, and prunin was subsequently added at an appropriate concentration and preprocessed for 6 additional hours. A UVB lamp (UVP, USA) was used to irradiate the cells with UVB. The wavelength of UVB irradiation was measured with a fiberoptic Spectrometer System USB2000 (Ocean Optics, USA). After the irradiation, PBS was removed, and a new medium was added, followed by additional incubation of 24 h prior to use in the experiment.

Cell viability estimation

The principles of the WST-1 assay were used for the experiment on cell survival. Overall, 100 µL HaCaT (3×10^3cells/well) was inoculated on a 96-well plate and incubated for 24 h. Afterward, prunin was added at 1, 5, 10, 20, and 40 µM and 40 mJ/cm^2 and UVB was irradiated to these cells, which were subsequently incubated for additional 24 h. In addition, 10 µL of EZ-Cytox cell viability assay kit reagent (ITSBio, Korea) was added to the incubated cells for 1 h, and the absorbance was measured using a microplate reader (Bio-Rad, USA) at 490 nm.

Quantitative analysis of intracellular ROS

In total, 10 µM dichlorofluorescein diacetate was added as a dye to measure intracellular ROS. The cells were harvested after incubation for 30 min. After adding PBS to release the cells, a flow cytometer (BD Biosciences, USA) was used to measure the changes in ROS. To verify the removal effects of prunin on ROS, N-acetyl-L-cysteine (NAC) was used as a positive control group that acts as a ROS scavenger and measured after the same treatment as prunin.

Quantitative real-time PCR

The cells obtained from the cell culture were extracted with Trizol reagent (Invitrogen, USA). The extracted RNA was quantified using a Nanodrop (Maestrogen, USA), and only RNA with a purity of 260 nm/280 nm (ratio 1.8) was used for the experiment.

In total, 10 µl of DNA was prepared by adding 1 µg RNA, 0.5 ng oligo dT18, and DEPC water in a PCR tube and processing it for 10 min at 70 °C to induce RNA denaturation. Subsequently, M-MLV reverse transcriptase (Enzynomics, Korea) was used to induce a reaction at 37 °C for 1 h to synthesize cDNA.

For qRT-PCR, 0.2 µM primers, 50 mM KCl, 20 mM Tris/HCl pH 8.4, 0.8 mM dNTP, 0.5 U Extaq DNA polymerase, 3 MgCl2, and 1X SYBR green (Invitrogen) were mixed in a PCR tube to produce a reagent. PCR was performed with Linegene K (BioER, China) through

Table 1 List of primers used in this study

Gene	Forward primer	Reverse primer
β-actin	GGATTCCTATGTGGGCGACGA	CGCTCGGTGAGGATCTTCATG
TNF-α	CCCAGGGACCTCTCTCTAATC	GGTTTGCTACAACATGGGCTACA
IL-6	TAACAGTTCCTGCATGGGCGGC	AGGACAGGCACAAACACGCACC
IL-8	CTCTCTTGGCAGCCTTCC	CTC AATCACTCTCAGTTCTTTG
COX2	CGCGGATCCGCGGTGAGAAC CGTTTAC	GCGAGGAAGCGGAAGAGTCT AGAGTCGACC
PAR-2	GGGTTTGCCAAGTAACGGC	GGGAACCAGATGACAGAGAGG

40 cycles (3 min per cycle) of denaturation, denaturation (94 °C, 30 s), annealing (58 °C, 30 s), and polymerization (72 °C, 30 s) at 94 °C. The significance of PCR was validated using a melting curve. The gene expressions were compared for analysis by normalizing the β-actin expression. The primers used for this experiment are shown in Table 1.

Statistical analysis

Each experiment in this study was performed three times or more under the same conditions, and the results are expressed as mean and standard deviation. For each experiment, the Student's t test was used to analyze all findings, with a p value of 0.05 or below considered as statistically significant.

Results

Cytotoxic and protective effects of prunin

The water-soluble tetrazolium salt-1 assay was performed to determine the cytotoxicity of prunin in human keratinocyte HaCaT cells. Treatment of the cells with prunin at concentrations of 1, 5, 10, 20, and 40 μM revealed the following survival rates: 1 μM, 100%; 5 μM, 102%; 10 μM, 102%; 20 μM 93%, and 40 μM, 75%. These results suggest that prunin is cytotoxic at concentrations ≥ 40 μM (Fig. 1a). To examine the cytoprotective effects of prunin, damaged HaCaT cells were treated with

prunin (5 or 10 μM) and irradiated with 40 mJ/cm^2 UVB. Compared to the cell survival rate of 53% in the control group, the survival rate of prunin-treated cells increased to 71% (5 μM) and 96% (10 μM). The cell survival rate was increased by prunin treatment in a concentration-dependent manner (Fig. 1b).

ROS elimination effect of prunin in HaCaT cells irradiated with UVB

The cell-permeable reagent 2′,7′-dichlorofluorescin diacetate was used to investigate the effect of prunin on ROS in UVB-irradiated HaCaT cells. This reagent fluorescent stains intracellular ROS, which were then analyzed by flow cytometry. ROS increased from 1 to 7.28 in cells exposed to 40 mJ/cm^2 UVB. Treatment of cells with prunin at concentrations of 5 and 10 μM before irradiation resulted in a decrease in ROS to 4.32 and 1.57, respectively. As a positive control, treatment with 10 mM NAC resulted in a decrease to 1.35, a result similar to that after treatment with 10 μM prunin (Fig. 2).

Anti-inflammatory effect of prunin on UVB-irradiated HaCaT cells

The expression level of IL-6, IL-8, COX2, TNF-α, and PAR2 was confirmed by quantitative real-time PCR to assess the effect of prunin on UVB-induced inflammation in HaCaT cells. First, we examined the effect of prunin on the UVB-induced increase in IL-6 mRNA (5.17). Cells treated with prunin at concentrations of 5 and 10 μM before UVB exposure exhibited a decrease in IL-6 mRNA to 3.55 and 1.40, respectively. Prunin treatment decreased IL-6 mRNA expression in a concentration-dependent manner (Fig. 3a). The IL-8 mRNA expression of 3.17 after UVB exposure decreased to 2.43 and 1.78 with prunin treatment at 5 and 10 μM, respectively. Prunin decreased IL-8 mRNA expression in a concentration-dependent manner (Fig. 3b). COX2 mRNA, encoding a protein that induces inflammation,

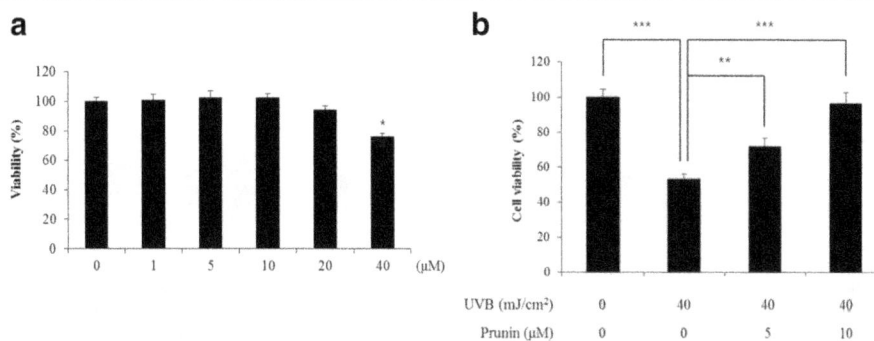

Fig. 1 Cell viability on prunin in HaCaT keratinocytes. **a** The cellular toxicity of prunin on HaCaT keratinocytes (*p < .05). **b** The effect of prunin on cell viability in UVB-irradiated HaCaT keratinocytes (**p < .01, ***p < .001)

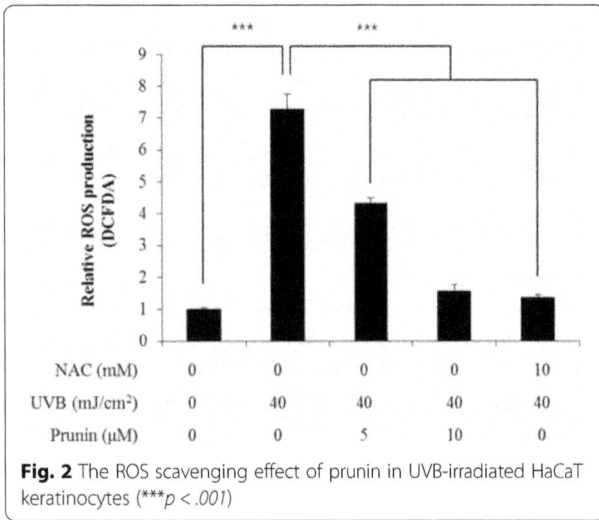

Fig. 2 The ROS scavenging effect of prunin in UVB-irradiated HaCaT keratinocytes (***$p < .001$)

Pretreatment with 5 or 10 µM prunin resulted in a decrease in *PAR2* mRNA expression to 1.83 and 1.06, respectively. Prunin decreased *PAR2* mRNA expression in a concentration-dependent manner (Fig. 3e).

Discussion

Intracellular damage by oxidative stress causes cell cycle arrest and cellular aging and increases the production of ROS (Cerella et al. 2009). Intracellular ROS can damage DNA and mitochondria, resulting in abnormalities in energy metabolism along with protein oxidation (Lang et al. 2018). In addition, ROS activates NF-κB, which promotes the expression of genes that induce inflammatory responses (Nathan 1987; Baeuerle and Baltimore 1988).

We observed here that exposing HaCaT cells to 40 mJ/cm^2 UVB leads to an increase in ROS. Figure 2 shows that prunin inhibits this UVB-induced increase in ROS in HaCaT cells in a concentration-dependent manner, inhibits the increased cellular aging caused by UVB, and is effective for ROS elimination. In addition, we observed that exposure of these cells to 40 mJ/cm^2 UVB causes a rapid increase in the activity of NF-κB, a proinflammatory transcription factor. Prunin pretreatment inhibited this increase in activity in a concentration-dependent manner. In other words, prunin inhibits the activation of NF-κB in the nucleus, thereby decreasing the expression of several inflammation-related substances. In particular, the expression levels of *IL-8*, *IL-6*, *COX2*, *TNF-α*, and

increased to 8.14 after UVB exposure. Pretreatment with 5 or 10 µM prunin decreased *COX2* mRNA expression to 4.55 and 1.23, respectively. Prunin decreased *COX2* mRNA expression in a concentration-dependent manner (Fig. 3c). *TNF-α* mRNA expression increased to 5.04 after UVB exposure. Pretreatment with 5 or 10 µM prunin decreased *TNF-α* mRNA expression to 3.26 and 1.26, respectively. Prunin decreased *TNF-α* mRNA expression in a concentration-dependent manner (Fig. 3d). *PAR2* mRNA increased to 3.80 upon UVB exposure.

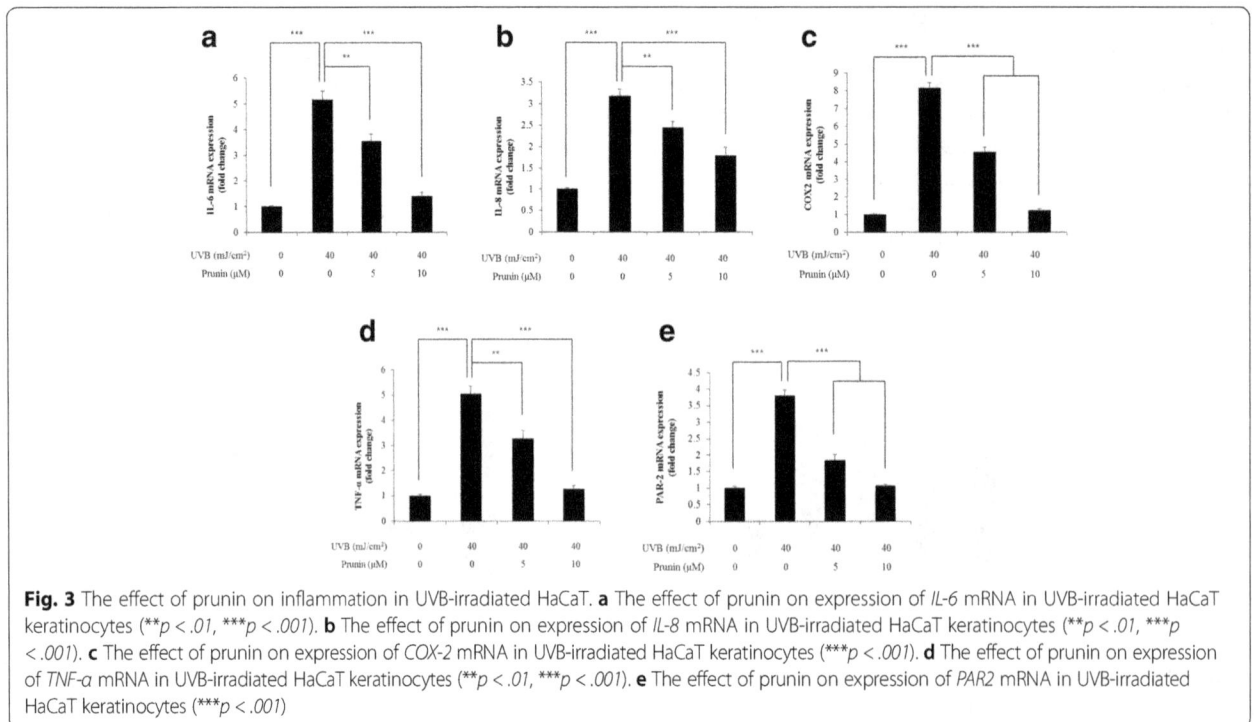

Fig. 3 The effect of prunin on inflammation in UVB-irradiated HaCaT. **a** The effect of prunin on expression of *IL-6* mRNA in UVB-irradiated HaCaT keratinocytes (**$p < .01$, ***$p < .001$). **b** The effect of prunin on expression of *IL-8* mRNA in UVB-irradiated HaCaT keratinocytes (**$p < .01$, ***$p < .001$). **c** The effect of prunin on expression of *COX-2* mRNA in UVB-irradiated HaCaT keratinocytes (***$p < .001$). **d** The effect of prunin on expression of *TNF-α* mRNA in UVB-irradiated HaCaT keratinocytes (**$p < .01$, ***$p < .001$). **e** The effect of prunin on expression of *PAR2* mRNA in UVB-irradiated HaCaT keratinocytes (***$p < .001$)

$PAR2$, which are induced upon activation of NF-κB, decreased with increasing concentrations of prunin. These results suggest that prunin inhibits UVB-induced inflammation in HaCaT cells and therefore is effective for anti-inflammatory skin.

Conclusions

Prunin pretreatment protects HaCaT cells against UVB-induced damage by preventing the generation of ROS and decreasing the expression of IL-6, IL-8, $COX2$, TNF-α, and $PAR2$ in a concentration-dependent manner. Prunin improves the survival rate of UVB-damaged HaCaT cells and blocks the NF-κB pathway through ROS elimination, thereby inhibiting inflammatory responses. In summary, prunin has cytoprotective and anti-inflammatory effects in HaCaT cells.

Abbreviations
11β-HSD1: 11β-hydroxysteroid ehydrogenase type 1; COX2: Cyclooxygenase-2; IL-6: Interleukin-6; IL-8: Interleukin-8; IκB: Inhibitor kappa B; NAC: N-acetyl-L-cysteine; NF-κB: Nuclear factor kappa-light-chain-enhancer of activated B cells; PAR2: Protease-activated receptor 2; ROS: Reactive oxygen species; TNF-α: Tumor necrosis factor-alpha; UVB: Ultraviolet

Acknowledgements
Not applicable

Funding
Not applicable

Authors' contributions
EJN and JYR did all of research background such as experiments, data collecting, and statistical analysis as well as draft manuscript. Both authors read and approved the final manuscript.

Competing interests
The authors declare that they have no competing interests.

Author details
[1]Department of Biological Engineering, Konkuk University, 120 Neungdong-ro, Gwangjin-gu, Seoul 05029, Republic of Korea. [2]Halla University, 28, Halladae-gil, Heungeop-myeon, Wonju-si, Gangwon-do 25404, Republic of Korea.

References
Baeuerle PA, Baltimore D. I kappa B: a specific inhibitor of the NF-kappa B transcription factor. Science. 1988;242(4878):540–6.

Baeuerle PA, Henkel T. Function and activation of NF-kappa B in the immune system. Annu Rev Immunol. 1994;12(1):41–79.

Céliz G, Audisio MC, Daz M. Antimicrobial properties of prunin, a citric flavanone glucoside, and its prunin 6″-O-lauroyl ester. J Appl Microbiol. 2010;109(4):1450–7.

Céliz G, Daz M, Audisio MC. Antibacterial activity of naringin derivatives against pathogenic strains. J Appl Microbiol. 2011;111(3):731–8.

Céliz G, Alfaro FF, Cecilia C, Daz M, Verstraeten SV. Prunin- and hesperetin glucoside-alkyl (C4-C18) esters interaction with Jurkat cells plasma membrane: consequences on membrane physical properties and antioxidant capacity. Food Chem Toxicol. 2013;55:411–23.

Cerella C, Coppola S, Maresca V, De Nicola M, Radogna F, Ghibelli L. Multiple mechanisms for hydrogen peroxide-induced apoptosis. Ann N Y Acad Sci. 2009;1171:559–63.

Choi JS, Yokozawa T, Oura H. Antihyperlipidemic effect of flavonoids from Prunus davidiana. J Nat Prod. 1991;54(1):218–24.

Choi JS, Yokozawa T, Oura H. Improvement of hyperglycemia and hyperlipemia in streptozotocin-diabetic rats by a methanolic extract of Prunus davidiana stems and its main component, prunin. Planta Med. 2006;57(3):208–19.

Coughlin SR. How the protease thromgin talks to cells. Proc Natl Acad Sci U S A. 1999;96(20):11023–7.

D'Andrea MR, Derian CK, Leturcq D, Baker SM, Grunmark A, Ling P. Characterization of protease-activatedreceptor-2 immunoreactivity in normal human tissues. J Histochem Cytochem. 1998;46:157–64.

Devasagayam TP, Kamat JP. Biological significance of oxygen. Indian J Exp Biol. 1994;67:319–25.

Gomez-Nicola D, Valle-Argos B, Nieto-Sampedro M. Blockade of IL-15 activity inhibits microglial activation through the NF-kappaB, p38, and ERK1/2 pathways, reducing cytokine and chemokine release. Glia. 2010;58(3):264–76.

Greaves MW, Sondergaard J. Pharmacological agents released in ultraviolet inflammation studies by continuous skin perfusion. J Invest Dermatol. 1970;54:365–7.

Hruza L, Pentland AP. Mechanisms of UV-induced inflammation. J Invest Dermatol. 1993;100:35–41.

Itoi S, Terao M, Murota H, Katayama. 11β-Hydroxysteroid dehydrogenase 1 contributes to the pro-inflammatory response of keratinocytes. Biochem Biophys Res Commun. 2013;440(2):265.

Jung HA, Jung MJ, Kim JY, Chung HY, Choi JS. Inhibitory activity of flavonoids from Prunus davidiana and other flavonoids on total ROS and hydroxyl radical generation. Arch Pharm Res. 2003;26(10):809–15.

Jung HA, Ali MY, Bhakta HK, Min B-S, Choi JS. Prunin is a highly potent flavonoid from Prunus davidiana stems that inhibits protein tyrosine phosphatase 1B and stimulates glucose uptake in insulin-resistant HepG2 cells. Arch Pharm Res. 2017;40:37–48.

Kimihisa I, Megumi M, Shunsuke N, Kazuya M, Hideaki M. Effects of unripe Citrus hassaku fruits extract and its flavanone glycosides on blood fluidity. Biol Pharm Bull. 2010;33(4):659–64.

Kong W, Mcconalogue K, Khitin LM, Hollenberg MD, Payan DG, Bohm SK, Bunnett NW. Luminal trypsin may regulate enterocytes through proteinase-activated receptor-2. Proc Natl Acad Sci U S A. 1997;94:8884–9.

Lang JY, Ma K, Guo JX, Sun H. Oxidative stress induces B lymphocyte DNA damage and apoptosis by upregulating p66shc. Eur Rev Med Pharmacol Sci. 2018;22:1051–60.

Maziere C, Conte MA, Degonville J, Ali D, Maziere JC. Cellular enrichment with polyunsaturated fatty acids induces an oxidative stressand activates the transcription factors AP-1 and NF-kappaB. Biochem Biophys Res Commun. 1999;265(1):116–22.

Middleton E, Kandaswami C, Theoharides TC. The effects of plant flavonoids on mammalian cells: implications for inflammation, heart disease, and cancer. Pharmacol Reu. 2000;52(4):673–751.

Nathan CF. Secretory products of macrophages. J Clin Invest. 1987;79:319–26.

Nomoto Y, Yamamoto M, Fukushima T, Kimura H, Ohshima K, Tomonaga M. Expression of nuclear factor kappaB and tumor necrosis factoralpha in the mouse brain after experimental thermal ablation injury. Neurosurgery. 2001;48:158–66.

Santulli RJ, Derian CK, Darrow AL, Tomko KA, Eckardt AJ, Seiberg M. Evidence for the presence of a protease-activated receptor distinct from the thrombin receptor in human keratinocytes. Proc Natl Acad Sci U S A. 1995;92:9151–5.

Sharlow ER, Paine CS, Babiarz L, Eisinger M, Shapiro S, Seiberg M. The protease-activated receptor-2 upregulates keratinocyte phagocytosis. J Cell Sci. 2000;113:3093–101.

Yousuf S, Sudha N, Murugesan G, Enoch IVMV. Isolation of prunin from the fruit shell of Bixa orellana and the effect of bcyclodextrin on its binding with calf thymus DNA. Carbohydr Res. 2013;365:46–51.

Zhang L, Liu W, Hu T, Du L, Luo C, Chen K, Shen X, Jiang H. Structural basis for catalytic and inhibitory mechanisms of beta-hydroxyacyl-acyl carrier protein dehydratase (FabZ). J Biol Chem. 2008;283(9):5370–9.

16

Coptis chinensis inhibits melanogenesis increasing miR-340-mediated suppression of microphathalmia-associated transcription factor

Hyun Kyung Lee[1], Seonghee Jeong[1], Shang Hun Shin[1], Dahye Joo[1], Seong Jin Choi[1], Karam Kim[1], In-Sook An[1], Kyung-Yun Kim[2], Jung-Eun Ku[3], Sun-Hee Jeong[4] and Hwa Jun Cha[5,6*]

Abstract

Background: Coptis chinensis (C. chinensis) contains various antioxidants, including berberine, epiberberlin, ferulic acid, magnoflorine, palmatine, and worenine, which have antibacterial, anti-inflammatory, haemostatic, hypotensive, and anticancer effects. In the present study, the melanogenesis-inhibiting effects of C. chinensis were investigated and the molecular mechanisms were elucidated.

Methods: The melanogenesis-inhibiting effect of C. chinensis was verified by measuring melanin contents, melanogenesis-related tyrosinase activities, and mRNA and protein expression levels of tyrosinase and microphthalmia-associated transcription factor (MITF). In addition, changes in miR-340 expression by C. chinensis were verified, and the activity of the miR-340 binding site of the target MITF gene was determined using luciferase reporter assays.

Results: Assays of melanin contents showed that C. chinensis had a skin-whitening effect and controlled mRNA and protein expression levels of tyrosinase. However, C. chinensis controlled protein levels of MITF without affecting mRNA levels. Determinations of miR-340 expression, which directly influences MITF translation, showed increased miR-340 mRNA levels in the presence of C. chinensis. Finally, luciferase reporter assays of the binding site on MITF showed that C. chinensis inhibits melanogenesis by directly controlling the miR-340–MITF axis.

Conclusions: The results of the present study verified the skin-whitening effect of C. chinensis and its molecular mechanisms and indicated that C. chinensis has high potential as an ingredient in skin-whitening cosmetics.

Keywords: Coptis chinensis, Tyrosinase, Melanogenesis, Melanin contents, MITF, miR-340, Skin-whitening effect

Background

Melanin is synthesized in melanosomes of melanocytes from basal layers of the epidermis and is transported to epidermal keratinocytes through dendrites to provide skin pigmentation and protection from ultraviolet light and external stimuli (Fajuyigbe and Young 2016; Fitzpatrick et al. 1967). However, excessive melanogenesis and abnormal melanin distribution may lead to the formation of melasmas and freckles or may cause abnormal hyperpigmentation, such as spots during aging (Amaro-Ortiz et al. 2014). Melanogenesis is triggered by the conversion of tyrosine to dopaquinone by tyrosinase (Pillaiyar et al. 2017). Dopaquinone is then converted to dopachrome in the presence of thiol groups, and this metabolite is then converted by a tyrosinase-related protein (TRP)-2 into 5,6-dihydroxyindole-2-carboxylic acid, which is in turn converted by TRP-1 to indole-5,6-quinone-2-carboxylic acid to produce melanin (Tsukamoto et al. 1992; Boissy et al. 1998). The cyclic monophosphate/protein kinase A (cAMP/PKA) pathway is the main mode of signal transduction for melanin production, wherein cAMP, through PKA and cAMP-responsive element-

* Correspondence: hjcha@osan.ac.kr
[5]Department of Skin Care and Beauty, Osan University, Osan-si, Gyeonggi-do 18119, Republic of Korea
[6]Department of Skin Care and Cosmetics, Osan University, Osan-si45 Cheonghak-roGyeonggi-do 18119, Republic of Korea
Full list of author information is available at the end of the article

binding protein 1 (CREB1), enhances the expression of microphthalmia-associated transcription factor (MITF) (D'Mello et al. 2016). MITF is a critical transcription factor for melanogenesis and is known to enhance the transcription of tyrosinase and its related proteins TRP-1 and TRP-2 (Buscà and Ballotti 2000; Saha et al. 2006). The cAMP-derived α-melanocyte-stimulating hormone (α-MSH) is a neuropeptide from proopiomelanocortin (POMC) that is produced in the hypophysis and in various other organs including the skin. In the skin, α-MSH is produced by melanocytes, Langerhans cells, fibroblasts, and endotheliocytes and, particularly, in keratinocytes following exposure to ultraviolet light (Chakraborty et al. 1996). In addition, α-MSH induces melanogenesis by increasing intracellular cAMP levels and membrane expression of the melanocortin-1 receptor (MC1R) (Videira et al. 2013). Therefore, modulation of intracellular signal transduction by α-MSH is recognized as an important target for the control of melanogenesis (Nasti and Timares 2015). Multiple studies report effective skin-whitening effects of treatments that modulate MITF expression, and although the melanogenic gene tyrosinases, TRP-1 and TRP-2, have been implicated, control of tyrosinase activity and expression did not affect melanogenesis in isolation.

Coptis chinensis (*C. chinensis*) is a perennial plant of the Ranunculaceae family. *C. chinensis* produces the active ingredient of berberine, which is an isoquinoline alkaloid, and other substances such as coptisine, epiberberlin, ferulic acid, magnoflorine, palmatine, and worenine. Berberine reportedly has excellent antibacterial, anti-inflammatory, haemostatic, hypotensive, and anticancer activities and has been used to inhibit the central nervous system activity to treat nephritis and induce bronchial smooth muscle expansion (Tang et al. 2016; Lee et al. 2003). Previous studies of the anti-inflammatory effects of *C. chinensis* extracts showed inhibition of lipopolysaccharide (LPS)-induced inducible nitric oxide synthase (iNOS), cyclooxygenase (COX)-2, and tumor necrosis factor (TNF)-α production in peritoneal macrophages, inhibition of apoptosis in pancreatic cells, TNF-α production in keratinocytes, and improvements in memory disorders (Kim et al. 2007; Enk et al. 2007; Wang et al. 2005). In the present study, the signalling mechanisms of the *C. chinensis* extracts were investigated to confirm skin-whitening effects.

Materials and methods
Cell line and culture
B16F10 cells were supplied by the Department of Dermatology of the College of Medicine at Seoul National University (Korea). Cells were subcultured in Dulbecco's modified Eagle's medium (DMEM; Welgene Inc., Korea) containing 10% fetal bovine serum (FBS) (*v/v*), 1 mM glutamine, 100 units/mL penicillin, and 50 μg/mL streptomycin in 100-mm

cell culture dishes in a 37 °C incubator containing 5% CO_2.

Extraction of *C. chinensis*
C. chinensis (100 g) plant samples were sonicated for 2 h in round flasks containing 1 L of 70% ethanol. The resulting extracts were decompressed and concentrated using a rotary evaporator (Eyela, Japan) and then dried using a freezing dryer for use in experiments.

Cytotoxicity
Cell growth inhibitory effects of *C. chinensis* extracts were determined using 3-(4,5-dimethylthiazol-2-yl)-2,5-diphenyl-tetrazolium bromide (MTT; Sigma-Aldrich, USA) assays. In these experiments, cells were seeded into 96 wells at 2×10^3 cells/well and then cultured for 24 h at 37 °C in an incubator containing 5% CO_2. Cells were then cultured with 0–120 μg/mL *C. chinensis* extracts for 24 h. Following treatments, cells were cultured with MTT for 4 h to allow formation of formazan crystals. The culture medium was then removed, the formazan crystals were dissolved by adding dimethyl sulphoxide (DMSO; Biopure, Canada), and cell survival rates were determined by measuring absorbance at 540 nm using a Microplate Reader (Bio-Rad, USA).

Assays of melanin contents
B16F10 cells were seeded into six-well plates at 5×10^4 cells/well and then cultured for 24 h at 37 °C in 5% CO_2. Cells were then treated with 200 nM α-MSH (Sigma-Aldrich) for 48 h to induce melanogenesis. Subsequently, numbers of harvested cells were counted, and absorption was measured at 400 nm after lysing cells with 1 N NaOH.

qRT-PCR analysis
To determine changes in the expression of α-MSH mRNA following treatments with *C. chinensis* extracts, B16F10 cells were cultured in six-well plates at 5×10^4 cells/well. The cells were then treated with 200 nM α-MSH for 48 h to induce melanogenesis. The cells were then harvested, and extracted RNA was used to synthesize cDNA using Moloney murine leukaemia virus (M-MLV) reverse transcriptase (Enzynomics, Korea) at 37 °C for 1 h. Quantitative real-time PCR (qRT-PCR) was then performed using cDNA as a template, and gene expression levels in *C. chinensis*-treated cells were compared with those in untreated controls. Reaction mixes contained HOT FIREPol EvaGreen PCR Mix Plus (Solis BioDyne, Estonia), 1 pmol of forward primer and reverse primers (Table 1) and 10 ng of cDNA, and qRT-PCR was performed using a LincGene K (BioER, China) instrument with initial denaturation at 94 °C for 3 min, followed by 40 cycles of denaturation (94 °C, 30 s), annealing (58 °C, 30 s), and polymerization (72 °C, 30 s).

Table 1 Primers used in the qRT-PCR analyses

Gene	Forward primer (5′ → 3′)	Reverse primer (5′ → 3′)
MITF	GGAACAGCAACGAGCTAAGG	TGATGATCCGATTCACCAGA
Tyrosinase	CAAGTACAGGGATCGGCCAAC	GGTGCATTGGCTTCTGGGTAA
β-actin	CCCTGTATGCCTCTGGTC	GTCTTTACGGATGTCAACG

PCRs were validated using melting curves, and gene expression levels were normalized to that of β-actin. The expression of miR-340 was determined using PCR according to the instructions of the miScript SYBR® Green PCR Kit (Qiagen, Germany) and a LineGene K instrument (BioER). Expression levels were normalized to that of U6 miRNA.

miRNA transfection

To determine whether miR-340 regulates MITF expression in B16F10 cells following treatment with *C. chinensis* extracts, we transformed cells with anti-miR-340 (Bioneer, Korea) using RNAi max (Invitrogen, USA) and negative scramble miRNA as a control.

Western blotting analysis

B16F10 cells were seeded into six-well plates at 5×10^4 cells/well and then cultured for 24 h. Subsequently, the cells were treated with *C. chinensis* extracts and 200 nM α-MSH and then cultured for an additional 48 h. The cells were lysed and centrifuged in radioimmunoprecipitation assay (RIPA) buffer, and supernatants were subjected to sodium dodecyl sulphate-polyacrylamide gel electrophoresis on 10% gels. Proteins were then transferred to nitrocellulose membranes (Bio-Rad), blocked for 1 h in Tris-buffered saline/Tween 20 (TBS/T) buffer containing 5% skimmed milk and incubated with primary monoclonal antibodies against MITF, tyrosinase, and β-actin. Protein bands were detected using appropriate secondary antibody Immobilon Western Chemiluminescent HRP substrate (Thermo Scientific, USA), and images were developed using ChemiDoc (Bio-Rad).

Luciferase assays

B16F10 cells were transfected with reporter plasmid (pGL3-MITF-3′UTR, 1 μg) and normalization plasmid (pCMV-β-gal, 0.2 μg) using Lipofectamine 2000 (Invitrogen). The cells were cultured for 24 h under appropriate conditions and then treated with reagents for 24 h. The cells were then harvested in 100 μL of ×1 luciferase lysis buffer (Promega, USA) at 4 °C for 10 min and then centrifuged at 12,000 rpm for 10 min. Luciferase assays were then performed in the resulting supernatants using luciferase reagent (Promega) and a Luminometer (Veritas, USA). Luciferase activities were normalized to β-galactosidase, as determined using O-nitrophenyl-β-D-galactopyranoside assays.

Statistical analysis

All experiments were independently performed in triplicate. Data are expressed as means ± standard deviations. Statistical analyses were performed using Microsoft Excel, and differences were considered significant when $p < 0.05$.

Results

Regulation of melanogenesis by *C. chinensis* extracts

Cytotoxic activities of *C. chinensis* extracts in mouse melanoma cells were determined using MTT assays, and effective concentration ranges were calculated. B16F10 melanoma cell survival rates were 90% or higher in the presence of up to 15 μg/mL *C. chinensis* extracts (Fig. 1a). Melanin contents in the mouse melanoma cells were then measured to assess skin-whitening effects of *C. chinensis* extracts. Under these conditions, α-MSH-mediated melanogenesis was inhibited by treatments with *C. chinensis* extracts (Fig. 1b).

C. chinensis extracts also inhibited tyrosinase activities by more than 50% at 15 μg/mL (Fig. 2a), which was related to concomitant decreases in tyrosinase expression (Fig. 2b, d). In subsequent qRT-PCR and Western blotting analyses, decreases in melanogenesis were

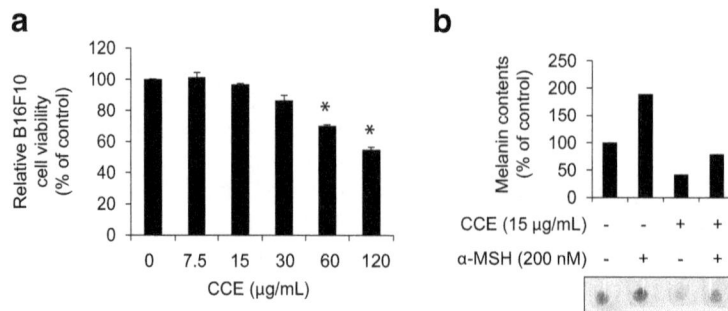

Fig. 1 *C. chinensis* extracts decreased α-MSH-mediated melanogenesis in B16F10 cells. **a** Cytotoxicity of *C. chinensis* extracts. **b** Melanin contents in *C. chinensis*-treated B16F10 mouse melanoma cells. Statistically significant differences are indicated with an asterisk for $p < 0.05$

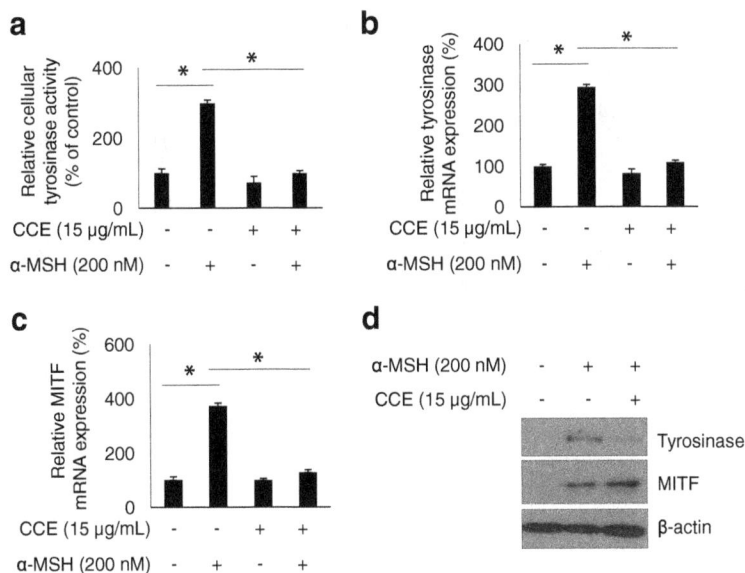

Fig. 2 *C. chinensis* extracts decrease the expression and activity of melanogenesis-related genes. **a** *C. chinensis*-mediated changes in tyrosinase activity. **b** Tyrosinase mRNA expression. **c** MITF mRNA expression. **d** Melanogenesis-related protein expression. Statistically significant differences are indicated with an asterisk for $p < 0.05$

correlated with tyrosinase mRNA and protein expression levels and with MITF protein expression (Fig. 2c, d).

Regulation of miR-340 expression by *C. chinensis* extracts

Previous studies showed that MITF translation is regulated by miR-340. Accordingly, treatments of the present B16F10 melanoma cells with *C. chinensis* extracts at 0, 7.5, and 15 μg/mL increased miR-340 expression in a concentration-dependent manner (Fig. 3).

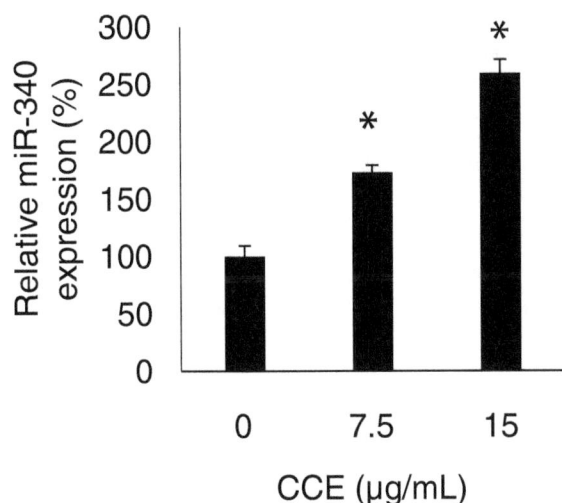

Fig. 3 Regulation of miR-340 expression by *C. chinensis* extracts. *C. chinensis* extracts increased miR-340 expression in a concentration-dependent manner. Statistically significant differences are indicated with an asterisk for $p < 0.05$

Regulation of MITF by *C. chinensis* extracts is mediated by miR-340

To confirm the roles of the miR-340–MITF axis in the regulation of melanogenesis by *C. chinensis* extracts, we performed reporter assays of the miR-340 target on the MITF promoter. In these experiments (Fig. 4), luciferase activity was decreased following treatments with *C. chinensis* extracts but was recovered following transfection with anti-miR-340.

Discussion

During melanogenesis, melanin is produced from L-tyrosine by the key enzyme tyrosinase (Pillaiyar et al. 2017; Kwon et al. 2014; D'Mello et al. 2016), and various skin-whitening raw materials have been developed to inhibit the expression and activity of tyrosinases (Gunia-Krzyżak et al. 2016; Lee et al. 2016; Choi et al. 1998). The present study shows that *C. chinensis* extracts inhibit melanogenesis by decreasing tyrosinase activity (Fig. 2a) and expression (Fig. 2b, d). Moreover, we investigated the roles of α-MSH and MITF in tyrosinase-mediated melanogenesis and showed that MITF protein but not mRNA expression was decreased in the presence of *C. chinensis*, suggesting regulation by post-transcriptional mechanisms. Among potential regulators, miRNAs of 16 to 29 nucleotides are known to regulate protein expression by inhibiting translation (Bartel 2004; Murchison and Hannon 2004). Previous studies showed that miR-340 regulates melanogenesis by directly inhibiting MITF (Goswami et al. 2015). In agreement, miR-340 expression was increased and luciferase activity of the

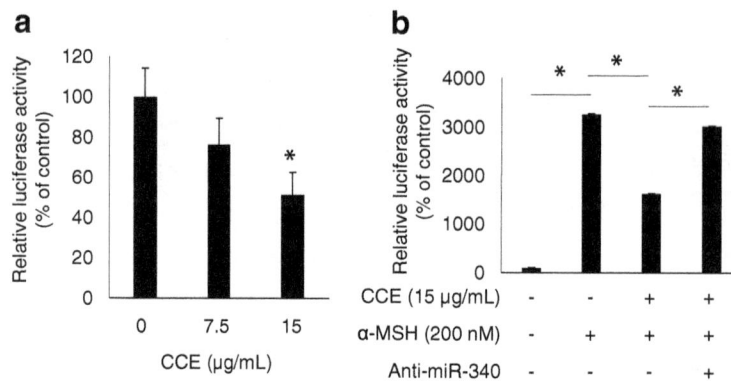

Fig. 4 *C. chinensis* extracts regulated melanogenesis via the miR-340–MITF axis. **a** *C. chinensis*-mediated changes in luciferase activity of the miR-340 target sequence. **b** miR-340-mediated blockade of *C. chinensis*-induced luciferase activity of the miR-340 target sequence. Statistically significant differences are indicated with an asterisk for $p < 0.05$

MITF reporter sequence was decreased following the present treatments with *C. chinensis* extracts (Fig. 4). Moreover, transfection with anti-miR-340 restored MITF protein levels under these conditions, confirming that miR-340 inhibits translation of MITF in the presence of *C. chinensis* extracts. Taken together, the present data show that *C. chinensis* extracts inhibit MITF translation by increasing miR-340 expression, leading to decreased tyrosinase protein and mRNA expression and reduced melanogenesis.

Conclusions

To investigate the potential of *C. chinensis* extracts as a raw material for skin-whitening cosmetics, we initially determined changes in tyrosinase activities in B16F10 melanoma cells and showed that *C. chinensis* extracts inhibit melanogenesis in a concentration-dependent manner. Subsequent Western blotting experiments showed that tyrosinase and MITF protein expression levels were decreased by *C. chinensis* extracts, whereas only tyrosinase mRNA levels were affected under these conditions, indicating that MITF is regulated at the protein level. Accordingly, the known MITF translation regulator miR-340 was induced following treatments with *C. chinensis* extracts, and the resulting suppression of MITF was mitigated by an anti-miR-340 antibody. The results of the present study confirm the skin-whitening effects of *C. chinensis* extracts and demonstrate that miR-340-mediated inhibition of MITF translation leads to decreased tyrosinase expression and melanin synthesis.

Abbreviations

C. chinensis: *Coptis chinensis*; cAMP/PKA: Cyclic monophosphate/protein kinase A; CCE: *C. chinensis* extracts; COX: Cyclooxygenase; CREB1: cAMP-responsive element-binding protein 1; DMEM: Dulbecco's modified Eagle's medium; DMSO: Dimethyl sulphoxide; FBS: Fetal bovine serum; iNOS: Inducible nitric oxide synthase; LPS: Lipopolysaccharide; MC1R: Melanocortin-1 receptor; MITF: Microphthalmia-associated transcription factor; M-MLV: Moloney murine leukaemia virus; MTT: 3-(4,5-Dimethylthiazol-2-yl)-2,5-diphenyltetrazolium bromide; POMC: Proopiomelanocortin; qRT-PCR: Quantitative real-time PCR; RIPA: Radioimmunoprecipitation assay; TBS/T: Tris-buffered saline/Tween 20; TNF: Tumor necrosis factor; TRP: Tyrosinase-related protein; α-MSH: α-Melanocyte-stimulating hormone

Acknowledgements

This work was supported by a grant from the Korean Health Technology R&D Project (Grant No. HN13C0075), Ministry of Health & Welfare, Republic of Korea.

Funding

This work was supported by a grant from the Korean Health Technology R&D Project (Grant No. HN13C0075), Ministry of Health & Welfare, Republic of Korea.

Authors' contributions

HKL, SJ, SHS, DJ, SJC, and KK performed the experiments. KYK, JEK, SHJ, and HJC were involved in experimental design and advising. HKL, ISA, and HJC analysed the data and wrote the manuscript. All authors have read and approved the final manuscript.

Competing interests

The authors declare that they have no competing interests.

Author details

[1]Korea Institute of Dermatological Sciences, Cheongju-si, Chungcheongbuk-do 28160, Republic of Korea. [2]URG Inc., URG Building, Seochogu, Seoul 06753, Republic of Korea. [3]Department of Cosmetology, Kyung-In Women's University, Incheon 21014, Republic of Korea. [4]Department of Beauty Art, Faculty of Art, Suwon Women's University, Suwon-si, Gyeonggi-do 16632, Republic of Korea. [5]Department of Skin Care and Beauty, Osan University, Osan-si, Gyeonggi-do 18119, Republic of Korea. [6]Department of Skin Care and Cosmetics, Osan University, Osan-si45 Cheonghak-roGyeonggi-do 18119, Republic of Korea.

References

Amaro-Ortiz A, Yan B, D'Orazio JA. Ultraviolet radiation, aging and the skin: prevention of damage by topical cAMP manipulation. Molecules. 2014;19:6202–19.

Bartel DP. MicroRNAs: genomics, biogenesis, mechanism, and function. Cell. 2004;116:281–97.

Boissy RE, Sakai C, Zhao H, Kobayashi T, Hearing VJ. Human tyrosinase related protein-1 (TRP-1) does not function as a DHICA oxidase activity in contrast to murine TRP-1. Exp Dermatol. 1998;7:198–204.

Buscà R, Ballotti R. Cyclic AMP a key messenger in the regulation of skin pigmentation. Pigment Cell Res. 2000;13:60–9.

Chakraborty AK, Funasaka Y, Slominski A, Ermak G, Hwang J, Pawelek JM, et al. Production and release of proopiomelanocortin (POMC) derived peptides by human melanocytes and keratinocytes in culture: regulation by ultraviolet B. Biochim Biophys Acta. 1996;1313:130–8.

Choi BW, Lee BH, Kang KJ, Lee ES, Lee NH. Screening of the tyrosinase inhibitors from marine algae and medicinal plants. Kor J Pharmacogn. 1998;29:237–42.

D'Mello SA, Finlay GJ, Baguley BC, Askarian-Amiri ME. Signaling pathways in melanogenesis. Int J Mol Sci. 2016;17:1144.

Enk R, Ehehalt R, Graham JE, Bierhaus A, Remppis A, Greten HJ. Differential effect of *Rhizoma coptidis* and its main alkaloid compound berberine on TNF-α induced NFκB translocation in human keratinocytes. J Ethnopharmacol. 2007;109:170–5.

Fajuyigbe D, Young AR. The impact of skin colour on human photobiological responses. Pigment Cell Melanoma Res. 2016;29:607–18.

Fitzpatrick TB, Miyamoto M, Ishikawa K. The evolution of concepts of melanin biology. Arch Dermatol. 1967;96:305–23.

Goswami S, Tarapore RS, Poenitzsch Strong AM, TeSlaa JJ, Grinblat Y, Setaluri V, et al. MicroRNA-340-mediated degradation of microphthalmia-associated transcription factor (MITF) mRNA is inhibited by coding region determinant-binding protein (CRD-BP). J Biol Chem. 2015;290:384–95.

Gunia-Krzyżak A, Popiol J, Marona H. Melanogenesis inhibitors: strategies for searching for and evaluation of active compounds. Curr Med Chem. 2016;23:3548–74.

Kim EK, Kwon KB, Han MJ, Song MY, Lee JH, Lv N, et al. *Coptis chinensis* extract protects against cytokine-induced death of pancreatic β-cells through suppression of NF-κB activation. Exp Mol Med. 2007;39:149–59.

Kwon KJ, Bae S, Kim K, An IS, Ahn KJ, An S, Cha HJ. Asiaticoside, a component of Centella asiatica, inhibits melanogenesis in B16F10 mouse melanoma. Mol Med Rep. 2014;10:503–7.

Lee DU, Kang YJ, Park MK, Lee YS, Seo HG, Kim TS, et al. Effects of 13-alkyl-substituted berberine alkaloids on the expression of COX-II, TNF-alpha, iNOS and IL-12 production in LPS-stimulated macrophages. Life Science. 2003;73:1401–12.

Lee SY, Baek N, Nam TG. Natural, semisynthetic and synthetic tyrosinase inhibitors. J Enzyme Inhib Med Chem. 2016;31:1–13.

Murchison EP, Hannon GJ. miRNAs on the move: miRNA biogenesis and the RNAi machinery. Curr Opin Cell Biol. 2004;16:223–9.

Nasti TH, Timares L. MC1R, eumelanin and pheomelanin: their role in determining the susceptibility to skin cancer. Photochem Photobiol. 2015;91:188–200.

Pillaiyar T, Manickam M, Namasivayam V. Skin whitening agents: medicinal chemistry perspective of tyrosinase inhibitors. J Enzyme Inhib Med Chem. 2017;32:403–25.

Saha B, Singh SK, Sarkar C, Bera R, Ratha J, Tobin DJ, Bhadra R. Activation of the Mitf promoter by lipid-stimulated activation of p38-stress signalling to CREB. Pigment Cell Res. 2006;19:595–605.

Tang C, Wu XD, Yu YM, Duan H, Zhou J, Xu L. Cell extraction combined with off-line HPLC for screening active compounds from *Coptis chinensis*. Biomed Chromatogr. 2016;30:658–62.

Tsukamoto K, Jackson IJ, Urabe K, Montague PM, Hearing VJ. A second tyrosinase-related protein, TRP-2, is a melanogenic enzyme termed DOPAchrome tautomerase. EMBO J. 1992;11:519–26.

Videira IF, Moura DF, Magina S. Mechanisms regulating melanogenesis. An Bras Dermatol. 2013;88:76–83.

Wang X, Xing D, Wang W, Su H, Tao J, Du L. Pharmacokinetics of berberine in rat thalamus after intravenous administration of *Coptidis rhizoma* extract. Am J Chin Med. 2005;33:935–43.

17

Assessment of bacterial carriage on the hands of primary school children in Calabar municipality, Nigeria

Ofonime M. Ogba[*], Patience E. Asukwo[†] and Iquo B. Otu-Bassey[†]

Abstract

Background: Hand washing with soap and water is a good hand hygiene practice which reduces the chance of infection transmission through hand contact. This study was designed to determine the microbial hand carriage among nursery and primary school children in Calabar Metropolis and to assess the effect of hand washing in the reduction of bacterial hand carriage among these children.

Methods: A total of 150 pupils aged 2–13 years were enrolled in the study from both private and public nursery and primary schools. Ethical approval was obtained from the Cross River State Ministry of Health, before the collection of the samples. Informed consent was obtained from the management of the schools and the parents and guardian of the children. A structured questionnaire was administered to the pupils for information on demography, hand hygiene practice, and their awareness on the importance of hand washing. Hand swabs were obtained from the pupils before and after hand washing respectively. Samples were subjected to culture, microscopy, and biochemical analysis. Data obtained in the study were analyzed by Epi-Info CDC, 2012 package.

Results: Males had the highest occurrence of the isolates 82 (62.1%) than females 50 (37.8%). This study recorded 88.0% prevalence of bacterial hand carriage among school children. *Staphylococcus aureus* was the most common isolate (68.9%) recovered before hand washing followed by *Escherichia coli* (25.0%). *Proteus vulgaris* and *Pseudomonas aeruginosa* were not found on the pupils' hands after hand washing. There was a significant difference in the bacterial carriage after hand washing between the two soap types ($x^2 = 19.9$, $p = 0.001$) with Dettol soap subjects having a lower bacterial carriage (31.2%) than Tetmosol soap subjects (68.8%).

Conclusion: The isolated bacteria were potential pathogens in humans. There was a significant reduction in bacterial carriage after hand washing with antibacterial soaps. School children should be educated on the need to wash hands with clean water and soap and dry with clean towels as this will reduce the risk of transmission of pathogenic bacteria orally or into open wounds.

Keywords: Bacterial carriage, Hand hygiene, Children, Soaps

Background

Hand hygiene has been recognized as an important public health measure, but the use of soap to remove pathogens from hands has not been concluded. Soap usage for hand hygiene has not been unanimously recommended in low-income settings (Ejemot et al., 2008).

The primary mode of transmission of many infectious diseases is the hand, especially among people working in close proximity to one another such as in schools. Contaminated hands serve as vehicles of transmission of infectious diseases (Ogba et al., 2016) which may increase infection rates among children. Hand washing is the most effective and simple method of preventing the spread of communicable diseases (Burton et al., 2011).

Lack of compliance to basic hand washing practice in the school environments due to time constraints and lack of water and sinks in most classrooms has been

* Correspondence: ofonimemark@yahoo.com
†Equal contributors
Department of Medical Laboratory Science, Faculty of Allied Medical Sciences, University of Calabar, Calabar, Nigeria

reported as a contributor to disease outbreaks by the World Health Organization (World Health Organization guidelines on hand hygiene in health care, 2013).

Infection transmission through contaminated hands of school children is a common pattern seen in most nursery and primary schools. Failure to perform appropriate hand hygiene practice has been recognized as a significant contributor to outbreaks of infectious diseases by the World Health Organization (World Health Organization guidelines on hand hygiene in health care, 2013). This study was designed to determine the microbial hand carriage among nursery and primary school children in Calabar Metropolis and to evaluate the effect of hand washing in the reduction of bacterial hand carriage among these children.

Methods
Study design/setting
The study was a prospective cross-sectional study carried out in three primary and nursery schools in Calabar Metropolis of Cross River State, Nigeria.

Study population
The study population comprised of pupils in both private and public nursery and primary schools, aged 2–11 years.

Inclusion and exclusion criteria
Pupils and teachers who did not give consent were excluded from the study while those who gave consent were recruited into the study.

Sample collection
A structured questionnaire was administered to the Head teacher and children for information on hand hygiene practice and awareness of the importance of hand washing. A total of 300 hand swabs were obtained from all the pupils. One hundred and fifty swabs were obtained before hand washing and 150 after hand washing respectively. Sterile cotton swabs dampened in sterile 0.85% saline were used to obtain samples from the fingers, between the fingers, and from the palm of the school children (De Alwis et al., 2012). The swab sticks were transported to the Microbiology Laboratory, University of Calabar Teaching Hospital (UCTH), for processing. The samples were transported in an Amies transport medium.

Indicated soaps for the study and product formulation
The indicated soaps for the study were Dettol and Tetmosol soaps.

Dettol soap
Dettol is an antiseptic cleaning agent with 4.8% w/v chloroxylenol as the active ingredient. The other

ingredients include isopropyl alcohol, pine oil, castor oil, caramel, and water. These ingredients make Dettol an effective antiseptic-disinfectant that kills bacteria. Chloroxylenol is the antibacterial in Dettol that acts to kill germs and reduce inflammation (Chew, 2015). Chloroxylenol has good activity against gram-positive bacteria but poor activity against gram-negative bacteria, enveloped viruses, mycobacteria, and fungi. It has doubtful activity against non-enveloped viruses and no activity against bacterial spores (Mathur, 2011; Kampf & Kramer, 2004). Chloroxylenol activity is minimally affected in the presence of organic materials but neutralized by non-ionic surfactants. It is well tolerated when absorbed through the skin (Mathur, 2011; Kampf & Kramer, 2004).

Tetmosol soap
Tetmosol soap is an antibacterial and antigermicidal soap. It is composed of monosulfiram 5% w/w as the active ingredient. The other constituent of Tetmosol is 75% total fatty matter (TFM). Monosulfiram is active against the skin mite *Sarcoptes scabei* which causes scabies (Piramal Healthcare, 2016).

Training for hand washing
The training of hand washing was conducted before the experiment. It was carried out according to WHO guidelines (Guide to implementation of the WHO multimodal hand hygiene improvement strategy, 2010; WHO Guidelines on Hand Hygiene in Health Care, 2010). All the pupils enrolled in the study and the teachers that washed the younger pupils were trained 2 days before the sample collection.

Grouping method for the two soaps
The random assignment principle was followed for grouping the school children between the two soap types provided for them to wash hands. Dettol and Tetmosol were printed on paper, wrapped, and put in a basket for them to pick. Whatever soap the pupils picked was provided for them to wash with. Out of the 150 subjects enrolled in the study, 75 (50.0%) washed with Dettol while the other 75 (50.0%) washed with Tetmosol. Out of the 85 female children, 43 (50.6%) washed with Dettol soap while 42 (49.4%) washed with Tetmosol soap. A total of 65 male subjects were enrolled in the study, 32 (49.2%) washed with Dettol soap while 33 (50.8%) washed with Tetmosol soap.

Pre-wash and hand washing procedure
The procedure is done as follows: Remove jewelries and rinse hands under running water. Lather with soap and using friction, cover all surfaces of hands and fingers. Rub your left hand's dorsum with your

Table 1 The demography of subjects in selected schools

	Females No. (%) enrolled	Males No. (%) enrolled	Total
Age (years)			
2–4	15(17.6)	10(15.4)	25(16.7)
5–7	35(41.2)	28(43.1)	63(42.0)
8–10	20(23.5)	17(26.2)	37(24.7)
11 and above	15(17.7)	10(15.4)	25(16.7)
Total	85(56.7)	65(43.3)	150
Class in school			
Nursery	15(17.7)	10(15.4)	25(16.7)
Primary	70(82.4)	55(84.6)	125(83.3)

right hand and your right hand's dorsum with the left hand. Rub your palms and clean your fingers. Clean hand dorsa by rubbing them to your palms. Rub your two thumbs with your other hand. Clean finger tips, rinse hands with water, and dry with disposable paper towel. The paper towel is used to turn off the faucet and trashed after the process without touching the trash (Cevizci et al., 2015).

Culture

The samples collected were cultured on chocolate agar, cysteine lactose electrolyte-deficient (CLED) agar, and blood agar. Plates were incubated at 37 °C in a canister with 5–10% CO_2 but CLED were incubated aerobically at 37 °C respectively for 24–48 h.

Identification of isolates

Plates were examined for growth and isolates were identified morphologically, physiologically, and biochemically. The tests carried out on the isolates include gram staining technique, oxidase test, coagulase test, catalase test, urease test, indole test, motility, citrate test, and sugar fermentation tests.

Statistical analysis

Data were analyzed using Epi Info 2010 (CDC, Atlanta, Georgia, USA) statistical software. Descriptive statistics were carried out. Frequencies were calculated for

categorical variables. Interactions between specific categorical clinical variables were tested for significance using the χ^2 test. A p value of ≤ 0.05 was considered statistically significant.

Results

Table 1 shows the demography of the subjects. Out of 150 pupils enrolled in the study, 85 (56.7%) were females while 65 (43.3%) were males with a mean age of 7.17 ± 2.73. The mean age for females was 6.7 ± 2.9, while the mean age for boys was 7.6 ± 2.2. The minimum age among the subjects was 2.0 years while the maximum age was 13 years. Subjects were aged 2–13 years. Most of the subjects enrolled (42.0%) were aged 5–7 years. More pupils were also enrolled from the primary sections 125 (83.3%) than from the nursery classes 25 (16.7%).

Figure 1 shows the different reasons for hand washing as given by the school children. Most of the pupils (45.3%) responded that they washed hands to remove germs and dirt, while others (38.6%) said the exercise was to keep their hands clean. Only 16.0% said it was to avoid infection from germs.

Figure 2 shows the water availability in schools for hand hygiene practice. Most of the pupils (52.0%) responded that they were provided a tap with running water for washing hands after playing and using toilets in the school and 32.6% said they had sinks in their classroom with running water, while 15.3% said a basin of water was provided in the class for hand washing

Out of the 150 pupils enrolled in the study, 67 (33.1%) said hand washing does not take a long time while 83 (66.9%) said it was time wasting. Also, 105 (70.0%) said they felt dirty after using the toilet but only 94 (62.7%) remember to wash their hands after using the toilet. Of the 150 pupils, only 48 (32.0%) washed hands after playing in the school (Table 2).

Figure 3 shows the distribution of bacterial isolates among subjects by gender. Males had the highest occurrence of the isolates 82 (62.1%) than females 50 (37.8%).

Table 3 shows the bacterial hand carriage by age of subjects. Those aged 5–7 years had the highest bacterial carriage rate 52 (39.4%) followed by those aged

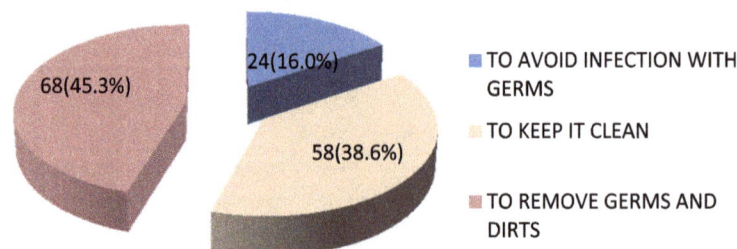

Fig. 1 Reasons for hand washing by school children

- TO AVOID INFECTION WITH GERMS
- TO KEEP IT CLEAN
- TO REMOVE GERMS AND DIRTS

24(16.0%) 58(38.6%) 68(45.3%)

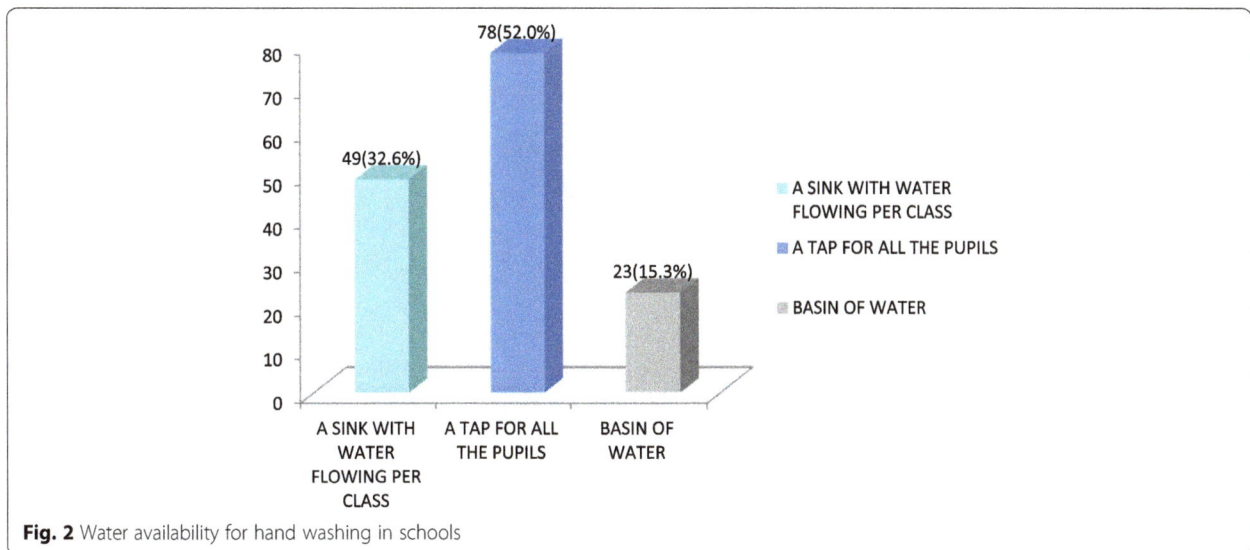

Fig. 2 Water availability for hand washing in schools

8-10 years 41 (31.1%). The lowest bacterial carriage rate 13 (9.9%) was recorded among children aged 11 years and above.

Table 4 shows the distribution of bacterial isolates before and after hand washing among pupils by soap types. More isolates were recovered from the subjects before hand washing 132 (88.0%) than after hand washing 32 (21.3%). *Staphylococcus aureus* was the most common isolate (68.9%) recovered before hand washing followed by *Escherichia coli* (25.0%). *Staphylococcus aureus* was also the most common isolate (81.3%) recovered after hand washing followed by *E. coli* (18.7%). *Proteus vulgaris* and *Pseudomonas aeruginosa* were not found on the pupils' hands after hand washing.

Out of the 150 pupils enrolled in the study, 75 washed with Tetmosol and the other 75 washed with Dettol soap respectively. Isolate recovery from subjects that washed hands with Tetmosol was higher 22 (68.8%) than those that washed with Dettol soap 10 (31.2%). *Staphylococcus aureus* was the highest recovered isolate 26 (81.3%) from both soaps, followed by *E. coli* 6 (18.8%). *Pseudomonas aeruginosa* and *P. vulgaris* were not recovered after hand washing. There was a significant difference in the bacterial carriage after hand washing between the two soap types

($\chi^2 = 19.9$, $p = 0.001$) with Dettol soap subjects having a lower bacterial carriage 10 (31.2%) than Tetmosol soap subjects 22 (68.8%) (Table 4).

Discussion

The challenges of hand hygiene practice in the school environment include time constraints, lack of sinks in most classrooms, and inadequate supply of pipe-borne water or clean water.

This study recorded a prevalence of 88.0% bacterial hand carriage among school children before hand washing and 21.3% after hand washing. The 88.0% carriage before hand washing is higher than the 81.0% reported by Vivas et al. (2010) while the carriage after hand washing in this study is lower than the 29.0% reported by Vivas et al. (2010). Despite the campaign of hand hygiene practice in schools after the *Ebola* outbreak in Nigeria, bacterial hand carriage among pupils was still high (88.0%). This may be due to lack of availability of water and soap in designated areas in the school premises. Some of the schools provided one washing point for the entire school. The pupils become discouraged because of the crowd at the washing point.

Table 2 Distribution of pupils by their hand hygiene habits

Hand hygiene habits	No. (%) of respondents	
	Yes	No
Does washing hands with water take a long time?	67(33.1)	83(66.9)
Do you feel dirty if you do not wash hands after using the toilet?	105(70)	45(30)
Do you always remember to wash hands with soap and water after using the toilet?	94(62.7)	56(37.3)
Do you wash hands after playing?	48 (32.0)	102(68.0)

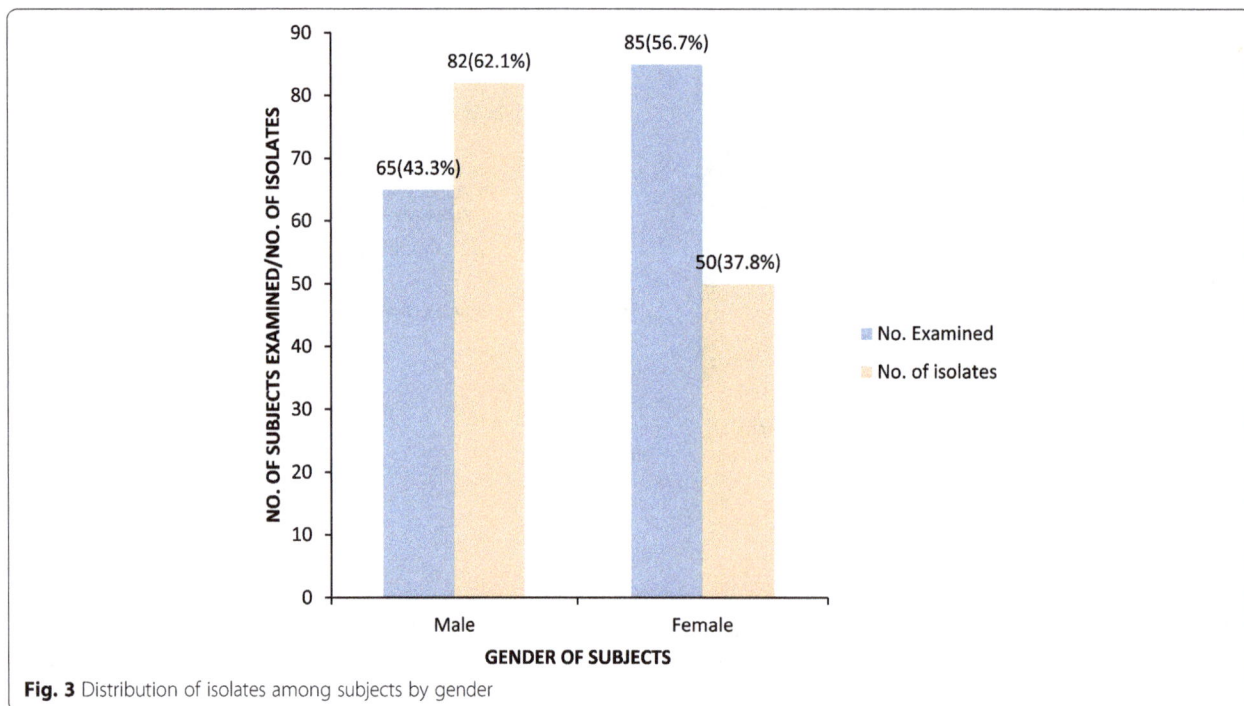

Fig. 3 Distribution of isolates among subjects by gender

The lower recovery rate of 21.3% after hand washing with the provided soap and water compared to the 29.0% reported by Vivas et al. (2010) points to the fact that the medicated soaps provided may have substantially reduced the bacterial load compared to the toilet soap provided by Vivas et al. (2010).

Although more females 85 (56.7%) were recruited than males 65 (43.3%) in the study, most of the isolates 82 (62.1%) were recovered from males. This is in agreement with the report of Cruz et al. (2015) that females had a higher knowledge and positive attitude towards hand hygiene than males.

Subjects aged 5–7 years had the highest carriage rate (39.3%) followed by subjects aged 8–10 years (31.1%). This may be due to the fact that majority of the subjects were in this age group 93 (70.4%). However, a recovery rate of 19.7% was recorded for 25 pupils aged 2–4 years. This was rather surprising because the younger pupils who crawl and play on the floor should pick up more bacteria on their hands but the reverse was the case. The bacterial contamination may have been minimal among this group because their teachers and care givers clean them up after using the toilet, thus minimizing fecal contamination on their hands compared to the older children who are not given such attention. The floor on which they play may have been washed with disinfectant frequently thus minimizing the rate of contamination in this group.

All the bacteria isolated from our subjects were potential pathogens in humans. *Staphylococcus aureus* 91 (68.9%) was the most isolated bacteria before hand washing. Chen et al. (2011) reported that children are at a higher risk of colonization by *S. aureus*. Also, *S. aureus* and *E. coli* were the only recovered isolates after hand washing with the medicated soaps. Although the effect of the soaps on the isolates was not investigated, *P. vulgaris* and *P. aeruginosa* were not found on the pupils' hands after hand washing. This reveals the susceptibility of the two isolates to the medicated soaps. The soaps may have killed or inhibited their growth therefore preventing their recovery.

Table 3 Bacterial hand carriage before hand washing by age of pupils

Age (years)	No. examined	No. (%) of isolates				
		Staphylococcus aureus	*Escherichia coli*	*Pseudomonas aeruginosa*	*Proteus vulgaris*	Total
2–4	25	17(18.7)	9(27.2)	0(0.0)	0(0.0)	26(19.7)
5–7	65	37(40.7)	11(33.3)	3(60.0)	1(33.3)	52(39.3)
8–10	45	28(30.7)	9(27.2)	2(40.0)	2(66.7)	41(31.1)
≥ 11	15	9(9.9)	4(12.1)	0(0.0)	0(0.0)	13(9.9)
Total	150	91(68.9)	33(25.0)	5(3.8)	3(2.3)	132

Table 4 Bacterial hand carriage before and after hand washing by types of soap

	Types of soap/no. (%) of isolates		Total	
	Tetmosol ($n = 75$)	Dettol soap ($n = 75$)		Statistics
Bacterial isolates present before hand washing				
Staphylococcus aureus	42(46.1)	49(53.9)	91(68.9)	$\chi^2 = 8.6$ $p = 0.07$
Escherichia coli	13(39.3)	20(60.0)	33(25.0)	
Pseudomonas aeruginosa	4(80.0)	1(20.0)	5(3.7)	
Proteus vulgaris	0(0.0)	3(100)	3(2.3)	
Total	59(44.7)	73(55.3)	132(88.0)	
Bacterial isolates present after hand washing				
Staphylococcus aureus	17(77.3)	9(90.0)	26(81.3)	$\chi^2 = 19.9$
Escherichia coli	5(22.7)	1(10.0)	6(18.7)	$p = 0.001$
Pseudomonas aeruginosa	0(0.0)	0(0.0)	0(0.0)	
Proteus vulgaris	0(0.0)	0(0.0)	0(0.0)	
Total	22(68.8)	10(31.2)	32	

n number of subjects examined

Although there was a higher bacterial carriage (55.3%) among subjects grouped to washed with Dettol soap than their Tetmosol soap counterparts (44.7%) before hand washing, there was a significant difference in the bacterial carriage after hand washing between the two soap types ($\chi^2 = 19.9$, $p = 0.001$) with Dettol soap subjects having a lower bacterial carriage (31.2%) than Tetmosol soap subjects (68.8%). This is in agreement with the work of Feroze et al. (2014) who reported that Dettol soap has inhibitory effects against *E. coli*, *S. aureus*, and *P. aeruginosa*. In a similar work, Nwambete and Lyombe (2011) reported that Dettol and Tetmosol had inhibitory activities against *E. coli* and *S. aureus*.

The antibacterial soaps used in the study showed significant reduction in bacterial hand carriage which may have resulted from inhibition of bacterial growth alongside the transient removal of these organisms. These may lead to acquisition of resistance genes by the organism. Burton et al. (2011) in London, UK, reported that hand washing with plain non-bacterial soap resulted in a significant reduction in bacterial hand carriage. In this study, the antibacterial soaps gave more significant results as some of the isolates were completely eliminated. However, toilet soap was not tested in this study because of limitation of funds; this may be better for hand washing in children in order to prevent resistance to the active ingredients and skin irritation.

Conclusion

The study recorded bacterial hand carriage rates of 88.0 and 21.3% before and after hand washing respectively. The isolated bacteria were potential pathogens in humans. There was a significant reduction in bacterial carriage after hand washing with antibacterial soaps.

Acknowledgements
We acknowledge Mr. Ben Solomon of the University of Calabar Teaching Hospital for his assistance with the sample analysis. We also acknowledge the University of Calabar for creating an enabling environment for research.

Funding
None.

Authors' contributions
OO conceived the study; PE and IO contributed to the design of the study; OO and PE performed the laboratory studies. All authors analyzed the data, drafted the manuscript, and read and approved the final version. OO is the guarantor of the paper.

Competing interests
The authors declare that they have no competing interests.

References
Burton M, Cobb E, Donachie P, Judah G, Curtis V, Schmidt WP. The effect of Handwashing with water or soap on bacterial contamination of hands. Int J Environ Res Public Health. 2011;8:97–104. https://doi.org/10.3390/ijerph8010097.

Cevizci S, Uludag A, Topaloglu N, Babaoglu UT, Celik M, Bakar C. Developing students' hand hygiene behaviors in a primary school from Turkey: a schoolbased health education study. Int J Med Sci Public Health. 2015;4:155–61.

Chen YC, Sheng WH, Wang JT, Chang SC, Lin HC, Tien KL. Effectiveness and limitations of hand hygiene promotion on decreasing healthcare-associated infections. PLoS One. 2011;6(11):e27163.

Chew, N. (2015). Dettol antiseptic ingredients. http://wwwlivestrongcom/article/166094-dettol-antiseptic-ingredients/ Last Updated: 23 Apr 2015.

Cruz JP, Cruz CP, Al-Otaibi ASD. Gender differences in hand hygiene among Saudi nursing students. Int J Infect Control. 2015;11(4):1–13.

De Alwis WR, Pakirisamy P, San LW, Xiaofen EC. A study on hand contamination and HandWashing practices amongMedical students. Int Sch Res Network. 2012;2012:Article ID 251483, 5 pages. https://doi.org/10.5402/2012/251483.

Ejemot RI, Ehiri JE, Meremikwu MM, Critchley JA. Hand washing for preventing diarrhoea. Cochrane Database Syst Rev. 2008;1 https://doi.org/10.1002/14651858.

Feroze, K., Elsayed, A and Tarek, T. A (2014) Antimicrobial activity of commercial "antibacterial" handwashes and soaps. Indian Dermatol Online J 5 (3): 344-346.

Guide to implementation of the WHO multimodal hand hygiene improvement strategy. [accessed on 24 Aug 2010]. Available from: http://www.who.int/patientsafety/en/

Kampf G, Kramer A. Epidemiologic background of hand hygiene and evaluation of the most important agents for scrubs and rubs. Clin Microbiol Rev. 2004; 17:863–93.

Mathur P. Hand hygiene: back to the basics of infection control. Indian J Med Res. 2011;134(5):611–20. https://doi.org/10.4103/0971-5916.90985.

Nwambete KD, Lyombe F. Antimicrobial activity of medicated soaps commonly used by dares Salam residents in Tanzania. Indian J Pharm Sci. 2011;73(1):92–8.

Ogba OM, Selekeowei T, Otu-Bassey I. Infection transmission potential of reusable phlebotomy tourniquet in selected health facilities in Calabar, Nigeria. Eur J Pharm Med Res. 2016;3(10):96–100.

Piramal Healthcare (2016). https://www.indiamart.com/proddetail/tetmosol-10568848912.html

Vivas AP, Gelaye B, Aboset N, Kumie A, Berhane Y, Williams MA. Knowledge, attitude and practice of hand hygiene among school children in Angolela. Ethiopia J Prev Med Hygiene. 2010;51:73–9.

WHO Guidelines on Hand Hygiene in Health Care. First Global Patient Safety Challenge. Clean Care is Safer Care. Accessed on 24 Aug 2010]. Available from: http://www.who.int/patientsafety/en/

World health organization guidelines on hand hygiene in health care. Hand washing: step procedure and benefits. Geneva: WHO; 2013.

18

TGFβ family mimetic peptide promotes proliferation of human hair follicle dermal papilla cells and hair growth in C57BL/6 mice

Yeong Min Choi[1], Soo Young Choi[1], Hyonmin Kim[1], Jeongmin Kim[1], Mun Sang Ki[2], In-sook An[1] and Jinhyuk Jung[1*]

Abstract

Background: Hair follicle morphogenesis is orchestrated by bidirectional ectodermal–mesenchymal signaling. In particular, TGFβ (transforming growth factor-beta) family is an important regulator of hair follicle formation and cycling. In this study, we investigated the effect of TGFβ family mimetic peptide (dermal papilla stem cell activator-1, DPS-1) on activation of hair follicle formation.

Methods: Cell viability, cell cycle, and mRNA expression of human dermal papilla (HDP) cells after DPS-1 or vehicle treatment were determined, and histological analysis of hair cycle was performed from the mouse dorsal back skin after DPS-1 or vehicle administration.

Results: DPS-1 promotes proliferation from 3D sphered HDP cells, but not from 2D cultured HDP cells. DPS-1 induces mRNA expression of genes, which are responsible for hair growth from HDP cells. Moreover, topical administrated DPS-1 stimulates hair growth in mice. Subsequently, histological analysis showed that the diameter and depth of hair follicles were remarkably higher in mice that were administered with DPS-1 compared to vehicle control.

Conclusions: DPS-1 promotes proliferation of HDP cells as well as hair growth partly via activation of WNT/β-catenin signaling.

Keywords: TGFβ mimetic peptide, DPS-1, Dermal papilla, Hair follicle development

Background

A hair follicle (HF) is composed of several distinct epithelial and mesenchymal lineages (Schmidt-Ullrich and Paus 2005). Each stage of hair cycle is regulated by signaling between the epithelium and mesenchymal cells that are located at the base of HF (Ehama et al. 2007). Dermal papilla (DP), a specialized mesenchymal population of HF, plays vital roles in HF morphogenesis and cycling (Miranda-Vilela et al. 2014). In particular, growth factors secreted by DP cells directly promote proliferation as well as differentiation of surrounding matrix cells. Consequently, DP cells stimulate hair stem cells to initiate

HF generation and new hair growth cycle (Kang et al. 2010). WNT/β-catenin and bone morphogenetic protein (BMP) pathway are one of the crucial signaling for HF generation (Kishimoto et al. 2000). There are reports that WNT/β-catenin is essential for proliferation and differentiation of hair shaft (Millar et al. 1999; Cotsarelis et al. 1990). Moreover, WNT/β-catenin signaling by DP cells is required to maintain hair inductivity (Soma et al. 2012). Additionally, BMP from transforming growth factor β (TGFβ) superfamily is important for HF development (Millar 2002; Botchkarev and Paus 2003; Rendl et al. 2008). Previous studies showed that WNT/β-catenin and TGFβ family interact to regulate the transcription of a number of genes, which is related with HF formation. Furthermore, there are synergistic effects between WNT/β-catenin and TGFβ signaling pathway in various cellular functions

* Correspondence: Jungjh.lab@gmail.com
[1]Korea Institute for Skin and Clinical Sciences, Gene Cell Pharm Corporation, 6F, Tower A, 25, Beobwon-ro 11-gil, Songpa-gu, Seoul, Republic of Korea
Full list of author information is available at the end of the article

including tumorigenesis and stem cell differentiation (Choi et al. 2017). Because TGFβ family is crucial for HF morphogenesis as well as hair cycle, we developed synthetic peptides which are structurally similar to endogenous human TGFβ family but possess unique sequences, which we named, dermal papilla stem cell activator-1 (DPS-1). To investigate the function of DPS-1 on HF formation and cycle, we determined whether DPS-1 promotes human dermal papilla (HDP) cell proliferation as well as WNT/β-catenin signaling. Moreover, we determined stimulatory effects on hair growth by DPS-1 from C57BL/6 mice.

Materials and methods

Synthesis of TGFβ family mimetic peptide

A synthetic peptide (DPS-1), designed based on original protein sequence of TGFβ family, which is part of receptor-binding sequence, GNCWL. DPS-1 was synthesized using the solid phase peptide synthesis method. Briefly, amino acid (3 equiv), HOBt (3 equiv), and diisopropylcarbodiimide (3 equiv) were added into a DMF solution. After activation, the solution was added to the resin DMF solution and agitated for 4 h. Each gradient coupling reaction in solid phase was repeated until no color change of the resin was monitored in ninhydrin test. After cleavage, the crude peptide was triturated with diethyl ether chilled at − 20 °C and was centrifuged at 3000 rpm for 10 min. Diethyl ether was decanted, and the crude peptide was dried under nitrogen. The purity of crude peptide (< 95%) were confirmed by analytical HPLC with a C18 column using a linear gradient of H_2O and acetonitrile (0–100% acetonitrile) containing 0.1% TFA. The resulting product was purified by prep-HPLC with a C18 column using a water (0.1% TFA)-acetonitrile (0.1% TFA) gradient to give DPS-1. DPS-1 was confirmed by MALDI-TOF Mass (Voyager DE-STR, Applied Biosystems, USA, Cal. mass 1335.70, Obs. mass 1335.70).

Cell culture and materials

Human dermal papilla (HDP) cells were maintained using Dulbecco's modified Eagle medium (DMEM; Hyclone, Logan, UT, USA) with 1% penicillin/streptomycin (10,000 units/ml penicillin G sodium, 10,000 µg/ml streptomycin; Gibco-BRL/Invitrogen Life Technologies, Gaithersburg, MD, USA) and 10% fetal bovine serum (FBS; Hyclone) and incubated at 5% CO_2 and 37 °C. Tofacitinib was purchased from Sigma-Aldrich (St. Louis, MO, USA).

Cell viability assay

2×10^3 of HDP cells were plated in a 96-well plate and then incubated for 24 h. After 24 h, DPS-1 was treated with indicated concentration for 24 h. Water-soluble tetrazolium salt (WST-1) solution was added and incubated for 20 min. Optical density of each wells were measured at 450 nm using a microplate reader iMark (Bio-Rad, Hercules, CA, USA). And the value was calibrated by measuring a reference absorbance at 650 nm.

Quantitative RT-PCR (qRT-PCR)

Total RNA was extracted from HDP spheres using a TRIzol reagent (Thermo Fisher Scientific, Rockford, IL, USA). The RNA was converted into cDNA with M-MLV reverse transcriptase (Thermo Fisher Scientific). qRT-PCR was performed using a SYBR™ green PCR master mix (Thermo Fisher Scientific) with a Step OnePlus Real-Time PCR System (Applied Biosystems-Thermo Fisher Scientific). All the above steps were performed according to the manufacturer's protocol. The sequences of the primers used for qRT-PCR are as follows: WNT family member 5A (WNT5A): 5′-TCCACCTTCCTCTTCACACTGA-3′ (forward) and 5′-CGTGGCCAGCATCACATC)-3′ (reverse); lymphoid enhancer-binding factor-1 (LEF1): 5′-CCCGATGACGGAAAGCAT-3′ (forward) and 5′-TCGAGTAGGAGGGTCCCTTGT-3′ (reverse); WNT inhibitor factor-1 (WIF1): 5′-TGGCATGGAAGACACTGCAA-3′ (forward) and 5′-GGCCTCAGGGCATGTATGA-3′ (reverse); GAPDH: 5′-ATCACCATCTTCCAGGAGCGA-3′ (forward) and 5′-TTCTCCATGGTGGTGAAGACG-3′ (reverse). Each mRNA expression level was calculated using the $2^{-\Delta\Delta Ct}$ method and normalized to the expression level of the GAPDH housekeeping gene (Table 1).

Hair growth activity in mice

Eight-week-old female C57BL mice were purchased from Oriental Bio Co (Seoul, Republic of Korea). After a 7-day acclimation period for being automatically maintained at 21–25 °C and a relative humidity of 45–65% with a controlled light–dark cycle, the animals were divided into three randomized groups ($n = 8$) to investigate hair growth-promoting activity of DPS-1. DPS-1 (250 µg/ml) or tofacitinib (500 µg/ml) was topically applied on dorsal back daily for 15 days. Reagents used for the hair growth test were dissolved in a vehicle containing 150 µl of acetone and 30 µl glycerol. All animals were cared for by using protocols approved by the Institutional Animal Care and Use Committee (Konkuk University, Republic of Korea) no. KU16199.

Table 1 The sequences of the primers used for qRT-PCR

Gene	Forward primers	Reverse primers
WNT5A	5′-TCCACCTTCCTCTTCACACTGA-3′	5′-CGTGGCCAGCATCACATC)-3′
WIF1	5′-TGGCATGGAAGACACTGCAA-3′	5′-GGCCTCAGGGCATGTATGA-3′
LEF1	5′-CCCGATGACGGAAAGCAT-3′	5′-TCGAGTAGGAGGGTCCCTTGT-3′
GAPDH	5′-ATCACCATCTTCCAGGAGCGA-3′	5′-TTCTCCATGGTGGTGAAGACG-3′

Statistical analysis

All data are expressed as mean ± standard deviation (SD) of three independent experiments. Statistical analyses were conducted using GraphPad Prism 6 software (Graphpad software, San Diego, CA, USA). Data were analyzed using two-tailed Student's t test or one-way analysis of variance (ANOVA) followed by Tukey's multiple comparison post test. $p < 0.05$ was considered statistically significant.

Results

Effect of DPS-1 on HDP cell proliferation

Because of previous report that TGFβ family activates hair cycle by promoting HDP activation, we determined whether DPS-1 promotes HDP growth. To test this, we performed proliferation analysis using WST-1 assay after culture with or without DPS-1. Because of recent report that 3D spheroid culture of HDP enhances hair inductivity as well as cycle compared to conventional 2D culture, 3D spheroid culture is regarded as relevant culture method for HF formation (Guo et al. 2008). Thus, we tested HDP proliferation by DPS-1 on both conventional 2D and 3D spheroid culture. Although DPS-1 does not promote HDP proliferation on conventional 2D (Fig. 1a), 3D spheroid cultured HDP proliferation was promoted by DPS-1 treatment (Fig. 1b). Tofacitinib, which has been reported to promote hair growth, was used as a positive control (Harel et al. 2015). These results indicate that DPS-1 has a proliferative effect on 3D spheroid cultured HDP cells.

Effect of DPS-1 on HDP sphere formation

We next determined whether DPS-1 increases the sphere size of HDP cells, which is related with hair inductivity.

To test this, microscopic analysis was performed. Self-assembly as well as size of DPS-1-treated HDP spheroids were increased compared to vehicle-treated HDP spheroids (Fig. 2a). We confirmed this result by performing three independent replicate experiments (Fig. 2b). These results demonstrate that DPS-1 promotes the formation of HDP spheroids, which enhances hair growth inductivity.

Effect of DPS-1 on hair growth-related gene expression from HDP cells

We determined whether DPS-1 regulates mRNA expression including *WNT5A*, *WIF1*, and *LEF1*, which were reported as hair growth-related signature genes (Ohyama et al. 2010; Yang and Cotsarelis 2010), using a quantitative reverse transcriptase PCR (RT-PCR). As a result, DPS-1 increased expression levels of *WNT5A* (Fig. 3a), *WIF1* (Fig. 3b), and *LEF1* (Fig. 3c) from 3D spheroid cultured HDP cells. These data indicated that DPS-1 increases spheroid size as well as signature genes of HDP, which is related with HF.

DPS-1 stimulates hair growth in mice

Finally, we investigated whether DPS-1 stimulates hair growth in mice. To test this, the dorsal back of 8.5-week C57BL/6 mice was shaved and vehicle or DPS-1 topically treated for 15 days. Tofacitinib was used as the positive control, which was previously reported to stimulate hair growth by promoting telogen to anagen transition (Harel et al. 2015). As expected, the entry into anagen was evident within 7 days of treatment with tofacitinib, whereas vehicle-treated mice remained in telogen.

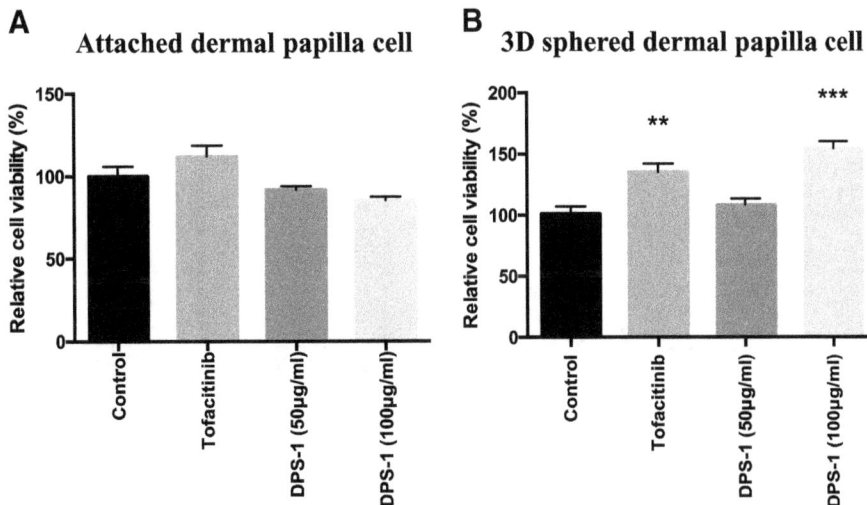

Fig. 1 Effect of DPS-1 on HDP cell proliferation. Effect of DPS-1 treatment on the viability of 2D monolayer cultured (**a**) and 3D spheroid cultured HDP cells (**b**). HDP cells were seeded into 96-well plates and pre-treated with various concentrations of DPS-1 (0, 50, 100 µg/ml) or tofacitinib (200 nM) for 24 h. Cell viability was measured using WST-1 assay. Data are presented as the mean ± SD of results from three independent experiments. HDP human dermal papilla, WST-1 water-soluble tetrazolium salt. $p < 0.01$ is present as ** and $p < 0.005$ is present as ***

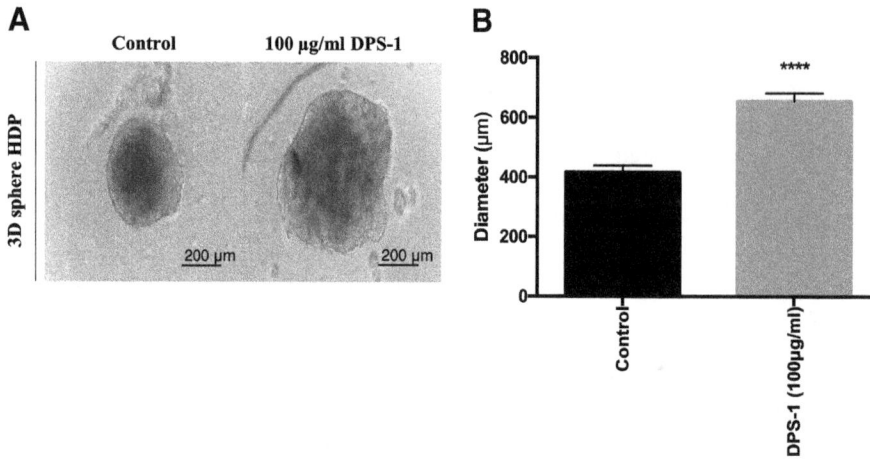

Fig. 2 Effect of DPS-1 on HDP sphere formation. Comparison of spheroid formation of control and DPS-1-treated HDP cells. **a** Phase images of spheroid of control and DPS-1-treated HDP cells. Images were analyzed after 24 h of DPS-1 treatment. **b** The diameter of spheroid was quantified. Data are presented as the mean ± SD of results from three independent experiments. $p < 0.001$ is present as ****

Interestingly, DPS-1 promoted rapid and intense hair growth in mice with kinetics similar to the tofacitinib (Fig. 4). Histological analysis of the mouse dorsal back skin showed that the diameter and depth of HF were remarkably higher from DPS-1-treated mice compared to the vehicle control.

Discussion

HF morphogenesis relies on bidirectional signaling events of dermal papilla (DP)—keratinocyte stem cells. Cyclical periods of growth (anagen), regression (catagen), and rest (telogen) are present during HF development (Paus and Cotsarelis 1999). Each hair cycle is tightly regulated by secreted proteins from DP. A recent report shows that

TGFβ superfamily is involved in HF formation by activating DP through WNT signaling pathway. Thus, we hypothesized TGFβ mimetic peptide, may serve function as a HF morphogen, could reinforce HF formation.

We observed that DPS-1 increased the viability and spheroid formation of 3D cultured HDP. Indeed, recent studies have shown that hair inductivity of HDP cells are markedly improved in 3D spheroid formation rather than 2D culture (Choi et al. 2017). Therefore, promoting HDP inductivity by DPS-1 may contribute to establish protocol for HF generation in vitro. In addition, DPS-1 induces DP signature genes, which serve critical roles in hair formation. In particular, DPS-1 induces expression of *WNT5A*, *WIF1*, and *LEF1* in HDP spheres. Our data

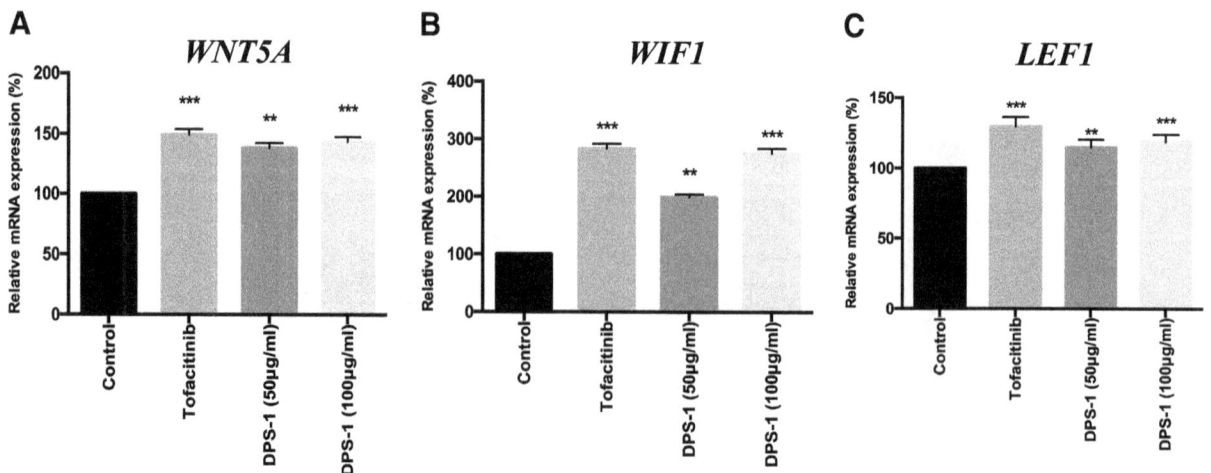

Fig. 3 Effect of DPS-1 on hair growth-related gene expression from HDP cells. HDP cells were seeded into 6-well plates and pre-treated with indicated concentrations of DPS-1 (100 µg/ml) or tofacitinib (200 nM) for 24 h. The gene expression of hair growth-regulating factors, **a** *WNT5A*, **b** *WIF1*, **c** *LEF1*, were measured by quantitative real-time PCR using specific primers in HDP cells. GAPDH was used as an internal control. Data are presented as the mean ± SD of results from three independent experiments. $p < 0.01$ is present as ** and $p < 0.005$ is present as ***

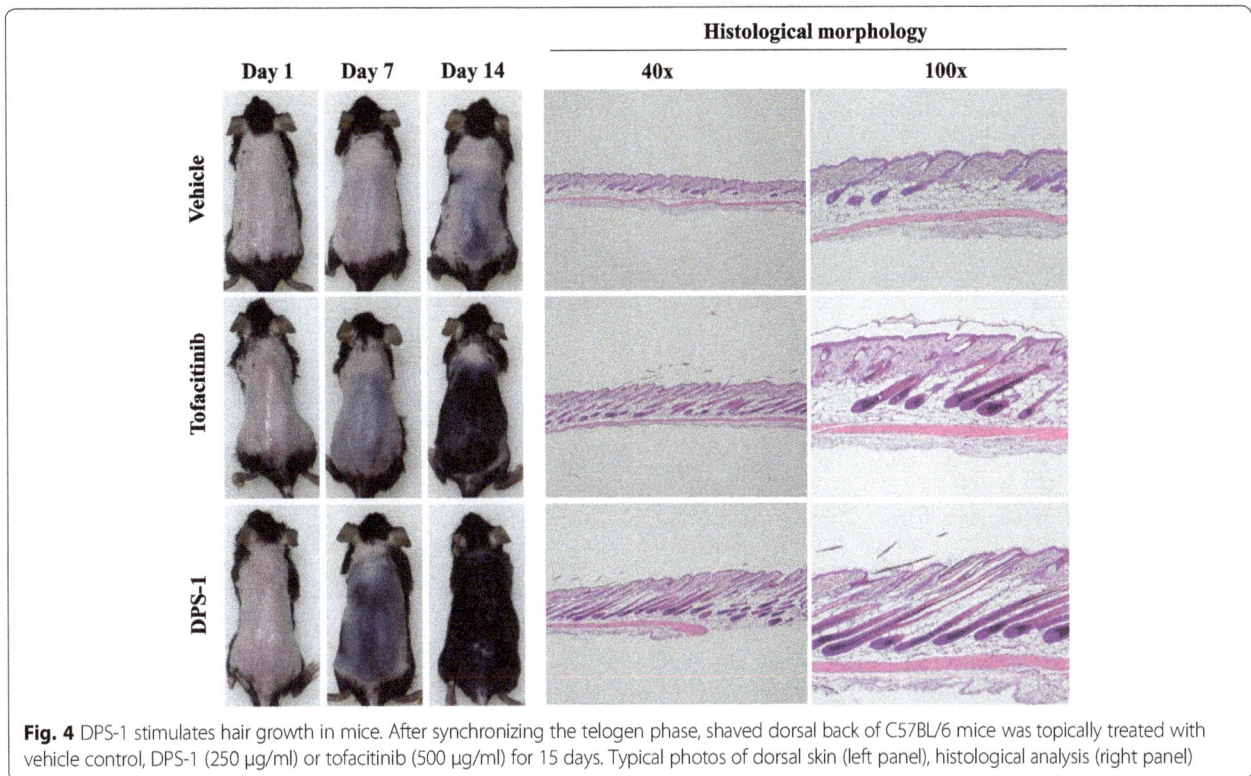

Fig. 4 DPS-1 stimulates hair growth in mice. After synchronizing the telogen phase, shaved dorsal back of C57BL/6 mice was topically treated with vehicle control, DPS-1 (250 μg/ml) or tofacitinib (500 μg/ml) for 15 days. Typical photos of dorsal skin (left panel), histological analysis (right panel)

suggest that DPS-1 may have similar signaling mechanism to TGFβ on the DP inductivity although further experiment about off-target effects of DPS-1 remains unclear. Lastly, we observed that topical treatment of DPS-1 stimulates hair growth than vehicle control. In mice, activation of WNT/β-catenin signaling induces a pro-growth/anti-quiescence signal during telogen (Telerman et al. 2017), thereby allowing reentry into anagen. Anagen reentry after DPS-1 treatment showed when mice are treated in mid-telogen but not in early telogen, suggesting that DPS-1 may not able to override the quiescence-promoting microenvironment in early telogen.

In summary, our data suggest that DPS-1 may reinforce hair formation property by activation of WNT/β-catenin signaling pathway in 3D spheroid cultured HDP cells. And DPS-1 indeed stimulates HF generation in animal model. These data allow us to speculate that DPS-1 treatment may provide novel strategy in treating alopecia in human.

Conclusions

Our study showed that TGFβ family mimetic peptide, DPS-1, activated WNT/β-catenin signaling pathway in spheroid cultured HDP. Moreover, histological analysis by animal model revealed the diameter and depth of the HF in the dermis from DPS-1-treated mice compared to vehicle treated. In conclusion, our study suggests that DPS-1 promotes proliferation of dermal papillae and

stimulates hair growth partly via activation of WNT/β-catenin signaling of hair follicular cells.

Abbreviations

BMP: Bone morphogenetic protein; DP: Dermal papilla; DPS-1: Dermal papilla stem cell activator-1; HDP: Human dermal papilla; HF: Hair follicle; LEF1: Lymphoid enhancer-binding factor-1; qRT-PCR: Quantitative real-time polymerase chain reaction; TGFβ: Transforming growth factor β; WIF1: WNT inhibitor factor-1; WNT5A: WNT family member 5A; WST-1: Water-soluble tetrazolium salt

Acknowledgements

Not applicable

Funding

Not applicable

Authors' contributions

YMC conducted the study and drafted the manuscript. All authors analyzed the data and reviewed the literatures. YMC, SYC, HK, JK, MSK, IA, and JJ wrote the manuscript. All authors read and approved the final manuscript.

Competing interests

The authors declare that they have no competing interests.

Author details

[1]Korea Institute for Skin and Clinical Sciences, Gene Cell Pharm Corporation, 6F, Tower A, 25, Beobwon-ro 11-gil, Songpa-gu, Seoul, Republic of Korea. [2]NB Clinic, Ansan, Republic of Korea.

References

Botchkarev VA, Paus R. Molecular biology of hair morphogenesis: development and cycling. Mol Dev Evol. 2003;298:164–80.

Choi YM, An A, Lee J, Lee JH, Lee JN, Kim YS, Ahn KJ, An IS, Bae S. Titrated extract of Centella asiatica increases hair inductive property through inhibition of STAT signaling pathway in three-dimensional spheroid cultured human dermal papilla cells. Biosci Biotechnol Biochem. 2017;81:2323–9.

Cotsarelis G, Sun TT, Lavker RM. Label-retaining cells reside in the bulge area of pilosebaceous unit: implications for follicular stem cells, hair cycle, and skin carcinogenesis. Cell. 1990;61:1329–37.

Ehama R, Ishimatsu-Tsuji Y, Iriyama S, Ideta R, Soma T, Yano K, Kawasaki C, Suzuki S, Shirakata Y, Hashimoto K. Hair follicle regeneration and human cells using grafted rodent and human cells. J Invest Dermatol. 2007;127:2106–15.

Guo W, Flanagan J, Jasuja R, Kirkland J, Jiang L, Bhasin S. The effects of myostatin on adipogenic differentiation of human bone marrow-derived mesenchymal stem cells are mediated through cross-communication between Smad3 and Wnt/beta-catenin signaling pathway. J Biol Chem. 2008;283:9136–45.

Harel S, Higgins CA, Cerise JE, Dai Z, Chen JC, Clynes R, Christiano AM. Pharmacologic inhibition of JAK-STAT signaling promotes hair growth. Sci Adv. 2015;23:e1500973.

Kang BM, Shin SH, Kwack MH, Shin H, Oh JW, Kim J, Moon C, Moon C, Kim JC, Kim MK, Sung YK. Erythropoietin promotes hair shaft growth in cultured human hair follicles and modulates hair growth in mice. J Dermatol Sci. 2010;59:86–90.

Kishimoto J, Burgeson RE, Morgan BA. Wnt signaling maintains the hair-inducing activity of the dermal papilla. Genes Dev. 2000;14:1181–5.

Millar SE. Molecular mechanisms regulating hair follicle development. J Invest Dermatol. 2002;118:216–25.

Millar SE, Willert K, Salinas PC, Roelink H, Nusse R, Sussman DJ, Barsh GS. WNT signaling in the control of hair growth and structure. Dev Biol. 1999;207:133–49.

Miranda-Vilela AL, Botelho AJ, Muehlmann LA. An overview of chemical straightening of human hair: technical aspects, potential risks to hair fibre and health and legal issues. Int J Cosmet Sci. 2014;36:2–11.

Ohyama M, Zheng Y, Paus R. The mesenchymal component of hair follicle neogenesis: background, methods and molecular characterization. Exp Dermatol. 2010;19:89–99.

Paus R, Cotsarelis G. The biology of hair follicles. N Engl J Med. 1999;341:491–7.

Rendl M, Polak L, Fuchs E. BMP signaling in dermal papilla cells is required for their hair follicle-inductive properties. Genes Dev. 2008;15:543–57.

Schmidt-Ullrich R, Paus R. Molecular principles of hair follicle induction and morphogenesis. BioEssays. 2005;27:247–61.

Soma T, Fujiwara S, Shirakata Y. Hair-inducing ability of human dermal papilla cells cultured under Wnt/beta-catenin signaling activation. Exp Dermatol. 2012;21:307–9.

Telerman SB, Rognoni E, Sequeira I, Pisco AO, Lichtenberger BM, Culley OJ, Viswanathan P, Driskell RR, Watt FM. Dermal Blimp1 acts downstream of epidermal TGFβ and WNT/β-catenin to regulate hair follicle formation and growth. J Invest Dermatol. 2017;137:2270–81.

Yang CC, Cotsarelis G. Review of hair follicle dermal cells. J Dermatol Sci. 2010;57:2–11.

19

Antioxidant and skin protection effect of morin upon UVA exposure

Hee Jung Yong[1] and Jin Jung Ahn[2*]

Abstract

Background: Morin is a family of phenolic compounds and is a bioflavonoid ingredient in fruits and vegetables. Morin exhibits various biological activities, including antioxidant cell protection and antimutagenic and anti-inflammatory effects; these activities safely minimize free radical-mediated damage biologically. However, the photoaging mitigation effect of morin on skin cells remains unknown. To investigate the effect of the morin on cell senescence mitigated against photoaging, cell viability, antioxidation, and anti-inflammation experiments were conducted. As a natural result of oxygen consumption, reactive oxygen species (ROS) in the form of harmful superoxides and hydroxyl radicals are generated through an oxidation reaction involving heavy metal cations such as iron. This adversely affects DNA, lipids, and proteins; therefore, organisms have a self-protective mechanism against oxidative stress via enzymes such as catalase (CAT) and superoxide dismutase (SOD), molecules such as glutathione, and proteins such as thioredoxin. Therefore, in this study, the antioxidative and skin protection functions of morin were examined to investigate the possibility of cosmetics.

Methods: To examine morin-mediated anti-photoaging mechanisms, human dermal fibroblasts (HDFs) were selected as the model cell line and UVA was selected as the stimulus source. The water-soluble tetrazolium salt-1 assay was performed to assess cell viability and cytoxicity in UV-exposed HDFs. To examine the molecular mechanism underlying the antioxidation capacity of morin, genes were analyzed using qRT-PCR, the expressions of several antioxidant enzymes were monitored, and the effect of morin on GPx1, CAT, HO-1, and NRF2 expressions in UV-exposed HDFs was assessed.

Results: The results of the morin toxicity showed the cell viability was above 100% when the concentration of morin was set at 20 and 50 μM. The cytotoxicity test for oxidative stress through UVA showed that the appropriate intensity of UVA 10 J/cm^2 was set as the cell viability reduced by 10 J/cm^2. And the cell survival over 100% rate after the morin treatment was 20 and 50 μM cell. A result of mRNA experiments verified that the expression of the antioxidant enzyme genes *GPx1*, *CAT*, *HO-1*, and *NRF2* increased with morin, in a concentration-dependent manner.

Conclusion: Morin increases the expression of antioxidant enzymes, which facilitates the antioxidant mechanism to respond to oxidative stress associated with exposure to UV and heat, which are considered to be the most harmful factors damaging the skin cells. This results in ROS removal, a byproduct of the natural metabolism of oxygen and the protection of neurons and proteins from toxicity. In conclusion, this study verified the applicability of morin as a cosmetic ingredient for the protection of cells against oxidization and UV.

Keywords: Morin, Fibroblast, UVA, Antioxidant, Cytoprotective effect

* Correspondence: 1THEgirl@swc.ac.kr
This work is part of Jin Jung Ahn's Ph.D. thesis at KonKuk University, Seoul, South Korea.
[2]Department of Cosmetology, Suwon Women's University, Suwon-si, Kyonggi-do, South Korea
Full list of author information is available at the end of the article

Background

As a natural result of oxygen consumption, reactive oxygen species (ROS) in the form of harmful superoxides and hydroxyl radicals are generated through an oxidation reaction involving heavy metal cations such as iron. This adversely affects DNA, lipids, and proteins; therefore, organisms have a self-protective mechanism against oxidative stress, involving enzymes such as catalase (CAT) and superoxide dismutase (SOD), molecules such as glutathione, and proteins such as thioredoxin and glutaredoxin (Cabiscol et al. 2000). ROS created during cellular metabolic processes are by-products of reactions involving oxidase and oxygen lyase. The oxidation state of cells is a major factor that alters gene expression and activity. In particular, imbalanced O_2 generates H_2O_2, which is not precisely defined as a radical but its transformation facilitates quick reaction; SOD contains transition metals (Cu^{2+} and Mn^{3+}) to enable rapid electron exchange. The most abundant peroxidase is glutathione peroxidase (GSH-Px), which is present throughout the cytoplasm and mitochondria. This enzyme contains selenium, a transition metal, at its active site and uses reduced glutathione (GSH) as a substrate to move electrons to H_2O_2 and other peroxides to generate water.

CAT mainly uses iron ions at the active site with peroxisomes to decompose H_2O_2 into water and O_2 (Matés 2000). Therefore, an antioxidant mechanism is activated when insufficient removal of ROS has occurred, and it plays an important role in cytoprotection as a natural biological defense mechanism that protects proteins from oxidative stress. Because molecules that are sensitive to various oxidoreduction reactions participate in numerous cellular reactions such as cell proliferation, cell growth, cell cycle arrest, and cell death, antioxidants and antioxidant enzymes determine the oxidoreduction potential of cells and react with thiol groups to adjust various biological antioxidative activities (Mates et al. 2012). Continuous exposure to UVA causes ROS and DNA oxidization and generates a precursor of melanin that results in pigmentation and erythema. In addition, such exposure depletes cellular antioxidants and generates hydrogen peroxide, superoxide anion, singlet oxygen, hydroxyl radicals, and nitric oxide (NO), which cause free radical-induced inflammatory responses (Ichihashi et al. 2009). ROS may induce immune reactions against infection, but when present in excess levels, it may induce lipid peroxidation and damage proteins and nucleic acids (Castro and Freeman 2001). Therefore, the existence of an antioxidative mechanism is very important for cellular homeostasis.

The antioxidative functions of cells are adjusted by antioxidant enzymes and antioxidants. Antioxidants include glutathione (GSH), thioredoxin (Trx), and melatonin. Antioxidant enzymes include superoxide dismutase (SOD),

glutathione peroxidase (GPx), glutathione reductase (GR), catalase (CAT), and heme oxygenase (HO) (Castro and Freeman 2001; Bhattacharya et al. 2015). Among the major antioxidant mechanisms, Keap1-NRF2 is a major modulator of cytoprotective reactions against oxidation and stress and one of the core signaling proteins; it is a combination of NRF2 and Keap1, transcription factors that combine with antioxidant response element (ARE) along with small Maf protein. Protein 1, which is a repressor protein, promotes protein decomposition via the ubiquitin-proteasome pathway. Keap1 is a protein rich in cysteine, but the details of the mechanism by which it induces NRF2 activity remain unknown. However, it is known that cysteine deformation at the thiol of Keap1 induces the degradation of NRF2 (Kansanen et al. 2013). NRF2 removes carcinogens, ROS, and other DNA-damaging substances as a major modulator involved in cytoprotection. It also inhibits tumors and cancer metastasis. The antioxidant system of Keap1-NRF2 protects proteins and DNA against oxidant damage by ROS by adjusting the important transporters for cell detoxification. As a result, the Keap1-NRF2 system is an important target for treating cancer and neurodegenerative diseases, autoimmune diseases, and inflammatory diseases. The prevention of Keap1 activity and NRF2 induction is effective to promote antioxidant reactions in the battle against disease (Canning et al. 2015).

UVA penetrates indoors even on cloudy days and invades down to the dermal layer of the skin. It is considered a primary cause of skin aging and induces reactions in the immune system. The dermis comprises 80 or 90% of the skin and consists of collagen (70%), elastin, and extracellular matrix originating from the fibroblasts, along with the blood vessels and neurons. The dermis contributes to the skin thickness, and is involved in wrinkle formation, and intervenes in the metabolism, wound healing, and cell repair. Langerhans cells, mast cells, and white blood cells are found in the dermis, which also play an important role in the immune system of the skin. Fibroblasts are directly related to aging because they have receptors for epidermal growth factor and fibroblast growth factor, and they generate collagen, elastin, and extracellular matrix.

This study involves the use of morin as a natural antioxidant to investigate its cytoprotective effects upon a UVA stimulus, which penetrates the dermal fibroblast layer and triggers cell reactions. Morin is a bioflavonoid that is abundant in fruit and vegetables. It shows various biological activities through cytoprotective, antimutation, and anti-inflammatory effects via antioxidative effects (Al-Numair et al. 2014), as an antioxidant that safely and biologically minimizes the damage due to free radicals (Zhang et al. 2009). This study confirms the antioxidant effects and cytoprotective effects of morin for the development of eco-friendly cosmetics and to provide baseline data for cosmeceutical research.

Methods

Cell culture and material treatment

Human dermal fibroblast cells (HDFs; Lonza, Switzerland) were incubated in Dulbecco's modified Eagle medium (DMEM; Hyclone, USA) with 10% fetal bovine serum (FBS; Hyclone), 1% penicillin/streptomycin (penicillin 100 IU/mL, streptomycin 100 μg/mL; Invitrogen, USA) under conditions of 37 °C, and 5% CO_2. The morin sample was purchased from Sigma Aldrich (USA) and 98% purified. It was dissolved in dimethyl sulfoxide (DMSO; Sigma Aldrich) for the experiment. HDFs were incubated at a concentration of 1×10^6 cells/well for 24 h, and the sample was pretreated in the medium for 6 h. Afterward, the cells were stimulated with UVA. The sample was processed for 24 h to measure cell toxicity. The rest of the experiment, including the cell viability measurement, continued after 24 h of UVA irradiation via a UVA lamp (UVP, USA). The wavelength was measured with the Fiberoptic Spectrometer System USB2000 (Ocean Optics, USA). For UV irradiation, the medium was removed from the cell culture tray, which was subsequently cleaned twice with pH 7.4 phosphate-buffered saline (PBS). A total of 1 mL of PBS was poured into the cell culture tray to prevent the cells from drying. The lid was opened, and UVA irradiation was performed, after which PBS was removed from the tray and new medium was added for additional incubation for 24 h.

Cell viability

The water-soluble tetrazolium salt-1 (WST-1) assay was used to test cell viability. Cells were introduced into a 96-well plate at a concentration of 3×10^3 cells/well in 100-μL amounts and incubated for 24 h. Morin was applied at varying concentration and additionally incubated for 24 h. A total of 10 μL of the EZ-Cytox cell viability assay kit reagent (ItsBio, South Korea) was added to the tray to measure the absorbance at 490 nm with a microplate reader (Bio-Rad, USA) after 1 h. The experiment was repeated three times, from which the mean and standard deviation were calculated.

mRNA expression

The quantitative real-time polymerase chain reaction (qRT-PCR) was used to quantitatively analyze the gene expression associated with morin in HDF. In the PCR tube, 0.2 μM primers, 50 mM KCl, 20 mM Tris/HCl pH 8.4, 0.8 mM dNTP, 0.5 U Extaq DNA polymerase, 3 mM $MgCl_2$, and 1× SYBR green (Invitrogen) were mixed to create the reaction solution. Linegene K (BioER, China) was used to perform PCR. Gene expression was measured using SYBR green, which binds to the extracted double-stranded mRNA. PCR was validated with a melting curve. The expression of each gene expression was normalized using the β-actin expression.

Statistical analysis

The statistical analyses were repeated three times for each independent experiment. The mean and standard deviation were calculated for each test result, for which statistical significance was analyzed by nonpaired Student's t test.

Results

Cytotoxicity of morin to HDFs

WST-1 assay was performed to determine the toxicity of morin to cells. In the samples, the morin concentrations were set as 5, 10, 15, 20, and 50 μM. Cell viability was 108% at 10 μM, 115% at 15 μM, 122% at 20 μM, and ≥ 112% at 50 μM. Morin slightly decreased at 50 μM, but the cell viability rate was ≥ 100% (Fig. 1).

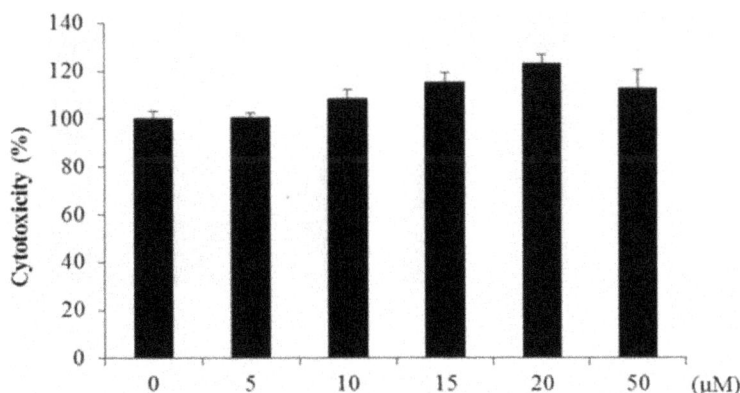

Fig. 1 Analysis of cytotoxic effects of morin on HDFs. Cells were inoculated in 96-well plates at a concentration of 3×10^3 cells/well and incubated for 24 h. Morin was added to the wells and cultured for an additional 24 h. Ten microliters of EZ-Cytox cell viability assay kit reagent (ItsBio, South Korea) was added to the incubated cell culture dish, and the absorbance was measured at 490 nm using a microplate reader (Bio-Rad, USA). The mean and standard deviation of cell viability were determined

Effect of morin on the viability of UVA-irradiated HDFs

HDFs were exposed to oxidative stress through UVA for the cell toxicity test. When the cells were irradiated with 10 J/cm^2 UVA, cell viability was reduced to 50.5%. Consequently, the appropriate strength of UVA was set as 10 J/cm^2. After morin treatment, cell viability increased from 60.2% at 10 μM, to 91.8% at 20 μM, and to 102.8% at 50 μM. As ≥ 70% was considered high for cell viability, this study used 20 and 50 μM morin samples simultaneously (Fig. 2).

GPx1 mRNA expression

Considering that glutathione peroxidase 1 (Gpx1) has a role in making ROS such as hydrogen peroxide and radicals less harmful or to convert them to water molecules with CAT, Gpx1 expression was calculated using qRT-PCR. In terms of the fold change of *GPx1*, it was shown that GPx1 mRNA was decreased to 0.83-fold through UVA irradiation, but increased to 1.01-fold at 20 μM morin and 1.28-fold at 50 μM morin (Fig. 3).

CAT mRNA expression

CAT removes toxins such as hydrogen peroxide and radicals to protect the cells. qRT-PCR was performed to measure CAT mRNA expression, which plays an important role in oxidoreduction reactions. In terms of the *CAT* mRNA fold change, there was a decrease to 0.65-fold under UVA irradiation at 10 J/cm^2, but this was increased by morin to 0.98-fold at 20 μM and 1.28-fold at 50 μM, showing an effect in a concentration-dependent manner (Fig. 4).

HO-1 mRNA expression

qRT-PCR was used to measure *HO-1* mRNA expression, which enables a rapid antioxidative mechanism through heme catabolism. In terms of the *HO-1* mRNA fold change, there was an increase to 1.60-fold through a sensitive reaction even before the sample treatment, and with morin, it was increased to 2.05-fold at 20 μM and 3.21-fold at 50 μM (Fig. 5).

NRF2 mRNA expression

qRT-PCR was performed to measure the nuclear factor (erythroid-derived 2)-like 2 (NRF2) gene, which induces antioxidant enzyme expression. In terms of the *NRF2* mRNA fold change, *NRF2* mRNA decreased to 0.88-fold and increased to 1.24-fold with 20 μM morin and 1.56-fold with 50 μM morin under UVA irradiation (Fig. 6).

Discussion

In this study, UVA-induced cell activity and toxicity of morin were tested. As cell generation was thought to be higher when cell viability is ≥ 70%, a high percentage > 100% may indicate an increase in physiological activity of HDFs and a lack of toxicity of morin. Therefore, it was verified that the concentration-dependent increase of catalase (*CAT*) mRNA in morin induces the increase of *CAT* expression, a strong antioxidant enzyme that causes cell repair in response to cell damage and oxidization by UVA and inhibits or stabilizes hydrogen peroxide generation to inhibit lipid peroxide and protect cells. Through cytoprotective defense mechanisms, heme oxygenase-1 (HO-1) responds to oxidant stressors such as biliverdin, CO, and free iron by inducing enzymes. Therefore, it has anti-inflammatory, antiapoptotic, and antiproliferative effects (Pae et al. 2004). This is because

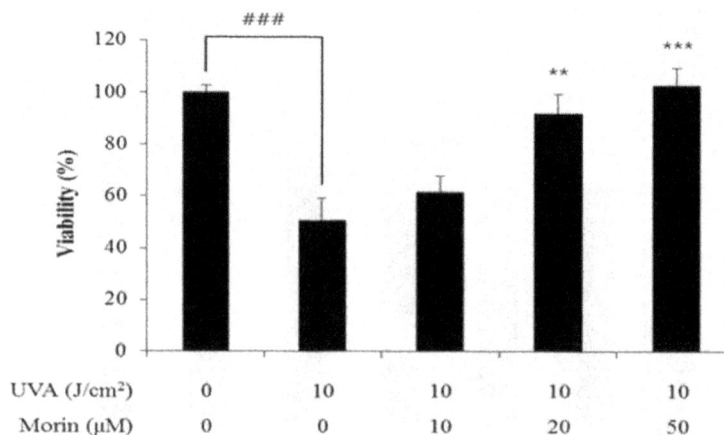

Fig. 2 The effect of morin on cell viability in UVA-irradiated HDFs. HDFs were cultured at 1 × 106 cells/well for 24 h, and then the sample was added to the culture medium and pretreated for 6 h, followed by stimulation with UVA. In the cytotoxicity assay of morin, the cytotoxicity of the sample after treatment for 24 h was confirmed. After the UVA stimulation, 24 h after UVA irradiation, the cell viability and other experiments were performed. The data are expressed as means ± SD (standard deviation) of the relative cell viability in each sample from triplicate experiments. Significantly different from control ($^{###}p < 0.001$, $^{**}p < 0.01$, $^{***}p < 0.001$)

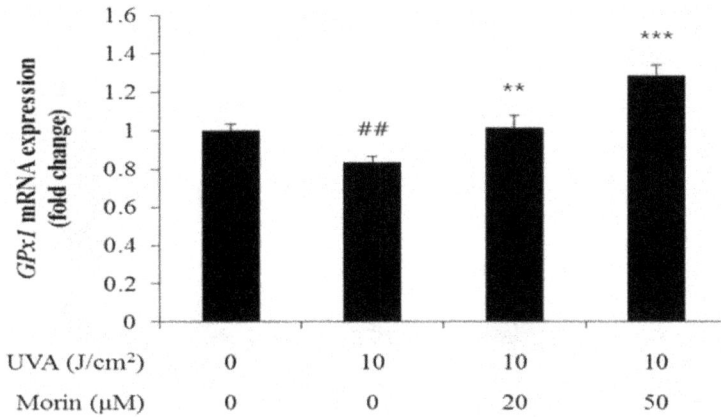

Fig. 3 The effect of morin on GPx1 expression in UVA-irradiated HDFs. Quantitative real-time polymerase chain reaction (qRT-PCR) was used to quantitatively analyze gene expression associated with morin in HDFs. qRT-PCR is a method for quantitatively measuring the level of DNA and the degree of activity of a specific gene. The amount of gene expression was measured using SYBR green in the double strand of extracted mRNA, and the validity of the PCR was confirmed by a melting curve. HDFs (2×10^5) were seeded in a 60-mm culture dish and incubated for 24 h. Prior to UVA exposure, the cells were pretreated with various concentrations of morin. Then, the cells were washed with PBS and irradiated by 10 J/cm2 UVA. After further incubation for 24 h, the expression level of GPx1 mRNA was measured by qRT-PCR. The data are expressed as mean ± SD of the relative cell viability in each sample from triplicate experiments ($^{##}p < 0.01$, $^{**}p < 0.01$, $^{***}p < 0.001$)

the HO-1 promoter induces HO-1 through immediate early gene activation in the activator protein 1 (AP-1 site and degrades the pro-oxidant heme into antioxidant molecules to improve oxidative mechanisms) (Nimura et al. 1996; Wu et al. 1993). Therefore, the concentration-dependent increase of HO-1 mRNA in response to morin causes an increase in the expression of HO-1, which is a powerful antioxidant enzyme. As a result, polymers can be quickly converted to small molecules and ATP (adenosine triphosphate energy) through heme catabolism in order to protect the cells from damage and oxidation due to ultraviolet rays. As *HO-1* increased compared with that before the sample treatment, it was

confirmed that *HO-1* acted as a natural defense mechanism against oxidative stress by UVA. Along with HO-1, *NRF2* is a powerful protein induced by Keap1 to activate antioxidative mechanism through its assistance in antioxidant gene expression, and it usually stays dormant in cells (Ishii et al. 2000). NRF2 is a transcription factor induced by ARE to play an essential role in gene expression for detoxification and oxidative stress. Therefore, the concentration-dependent increase of *NRF2* mRNA verifies that morin increases the expression of *NRF2*, a powerful antioxidant enzyme, to protect cells through its assistance in antioxidant enzyme gene expression against cell damage and oxidization.

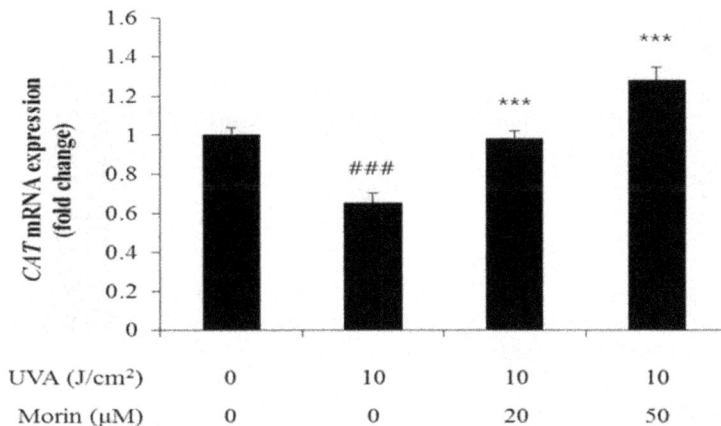

Fig. 4 The effect of morin on CAT mRNA expression in UVA-irradiated HDFs. HDFs (2×10^5) were seeded in a 60-mm culture dish and incubated for 2–4 h. Prior to UVA treatment, cells were pretreated with various concentrations of morin. Then, cells were washed with PBS and irradiated by 10 J/cm2 UVA. After further incubation for 24 h, the expression level of CAT mRNA was measured by qRT-PCR. The data are expressed as mean ± SD of the relative cell viability in each sample from triplicate experiments. Significantly different from control ($^{###}p < 0.001$, $^{***}p < 0.001$)

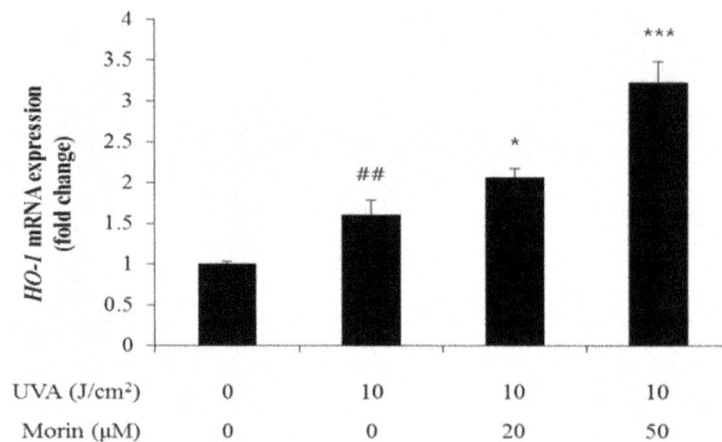

Fig. 5 The effect of morin on the expression of HO-1 mRNA in UVA-irradiated HDFs. HDFs (2×105) were seeded in a 60-mm culture dish and incubated for 24 h. Prior to UVA treatment, cells were pretreated with various concentrations of morin. Then, cells were washed with PBS and irradiated with-10 J/cm2 UVA. After further incubation for 24 h, the expression level of HO-1 mRNA was measured by qRT-PCR. The data are expressed as mean ± SD of the relative cell viability in each sample from triplicate experiments. Significantly different from control ($^{##}p < 0.01$, $^{*}p < 0.5$, $^{***}p < 0.001$)

Conclusions

This study confirmed the applicability of the flavonoid morin as an eco-friendly antioxidative cosmetic ingredient for skin cytoprotective and antioxidant effects against UVA-induced free radicals. This experiment focused on HDFs, which penetrate down into the dermal layer and enable cytoprotection. UVA was selected as a stimulant to test the antioxidant effect and antioxidant enzyme gene expression of morin. In conclusion, the experiment on the UVA-induced antioxidant effect of morin through *GPx1*, *CAT*, *HO-1*, and *NRF2* gene expression under stimulation with 1 J/cm^2 UVA showed that the expression of *GPx1*, *CAT*, *HO-1*, and *NRF2* was increased in a morin concentration-dependent manner.

GPx1 expression increased as a catalyst that converts hydrogen peroxide and free radicals from ROS into less harmful molecules, or water through oxidoreduction reactions, along with *CAT*. Therefore, this study confirmed that *GPx1* and *CAT* protect proteins and eliminate oxidants through a primary cytoprotective effect against acute oxidative stress. *HO-1* increased under UVA irradiation, presumably through sudden induction of antioxidant mechanisms by converting polymers to small molecules and ATP through heme catabolism. In addition, HO-1, which promotes the expression of antioxidant enzymes through immediate early gene activation in response to ultraviolet light, is induced by NRF2, a powerful protein that enables antioxidant mechanisms.

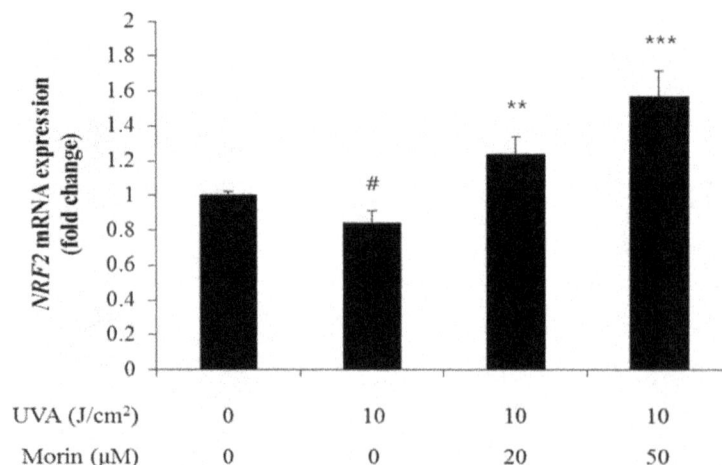

Fig. 6 The effect of morin on the expression of NRF-2 mRNA in UVA-irradiated HDFs. HDFs (2×105) were seeded in a 60-mm culture dish and incubated for 24 h. Prior to UVA treatment, cells were pretreated with various concentrations of Morin. Then, cells were washed with PBS and irradiated by 10 J/cm2 UVA. After further incubation for 24 h, the expression level of NRF2 mRNA was measured by qRT-PCR. The data are expressed as mean ± SD of the relative cell viability in each sample from triplicate experiments. Significantly different from control ($^{#}p < 0.5$, $^{**}p < 0.01$, $^{***}p < 0.001$)

NRF2 is decomposed by oxidative stress from its form in the combined antioxidant network of NRF2-KEAP1 to adjust the expression of various antioxidant factors. Consequently, morin increased *HO-1* and *NRF2* gene expression in a concentration-dependent manner, to enable an oxidoreduction mechanism through photoaging. In summary, morin has been proven to have an antioxidative effect to maintain cellular homeostasis and protect cells through blocking or delaying cell transformation. To conclude, this study verified the applicability of morin as a cosmetic ingredient that protects cells by increasing cytoprotective gene expression, in a concentration-dependent manner. These genes respond to oxidative stress from UVA exposure to remove ROS, a natural by-product of oxygen metabolism, and protect neurons from toxicity. These findings suggest a major role of morin in cell signaling and homeostasis as an applicable cosmetics ingredient.

Abbreviations

AP-1: Activator protein 1; ARE: Antioxidant response element; ATP: Adenosine triphosphate; DNA: Deoxyribonucleic acid; KEAP1: Kelch-like ECH-associated protein 1; Maf: Musculoaponeurotic fibrosarcoma; mRNA: Messenger RNA or messenger ribonucleic acid; NRF2: Nuclear factor (erythroid-derived 2)-like 2; ROS: Reactive oxygen species; UV: Ultraviolet ray; UVA: Ultraviolet absorption

Acknowledgements
Not applicable

Funding
Not applicable

Authors' contributions
HJY and JJA conceived and wrote the editorial. Both authors read and approved the final manuscript.

Competing interests
The authors of this editorial article are members of the Editorial Board of Biomedical Dermatology. Both authors declare that they have no competing interests.

Author details
[1]Beauty People Beauty School, 68 Dolma-ro, Bundang-gu, Seongnam-si 13627, Gyeonggi-do, Republic of Korea. [2]Department of Cosmetology, Suwon Women's University, Suwon-si, Kyonggi-do, South Korea.

References

Al-Numair KS, Chandramohan G, Alsaif MA, Veeramani C, El-Newehy AS. Morin, a flavonoid, on lipid peroxidation and antioxidant status in experimental myocardial ischemic rats. Afr J Tradit Complement Altern Med. 2014;11(3):14–20.

Bhattacharya IS, Woolf DK, Hughes RJ, Shah N, Harrison M, Ostler PJ, Hoskin PJ. Stereotactic body radiotherapy (SBRT) in the management of extracranial oligometastatic (OM) disease. Br J Radiol. 2015;88(1048):1–5.

Cabiscol E, Tamarit J, Ros J. Oxidative stress in bacteria and protein damage by reactive oxygen species. Int Microbiol. 2000;3(1):3–8.

Canning P, Sorrell FJ, Bullock AN. Structural basis of Keap1 interactions with NRF2. Free Radic Biol Med. 2015;88:101–7.

Castro L, Freeman BA. Reactive oxygen species in human health and disease. Nutrition. 2001;17(2):623–6.

Ichihashi M, Ando H, Yoshida M, Niki Y, Matsui M. Photoaging of the skin. Anti-Aging Medicine. 2009;6(6):45–59.

Ishii T, Itoh K, Takahashi S, Sato H, Yanagawa T, Katoh Y, Bannai S, Yamamoto M. Transcription factor NRF2 coordinately regulates a group of oxidative stress-inducible genes in macrophages. J Biol Chem. 2000;275(21):16023–9.

Kansanen E, Kuosmanen SM, Leinonen H, Levonen AL. The Keap1-NRF2 pathway: mechanisms of activation and dysregulation in cancer. Redox Biol. 2013;1(1): 45–9.

Matés JM. Effects of antioxidant enzymes in the molecular control of reactive oxygen species toxicology. Toxicology. 2000;16(153):83–104.

Mates JM, Segura JA, Alonso FJ, Marquez J. Central role of heme oxygenase-1 in cardiovascular protection. Aioxidants & Redox Signaling. 2012;15(7):35–1846.

Nimura T, Weinstein PR, Massa SM, Panter S, Sharp FR. Heme oxygenase-1 (HO-1) protein induction in rat brain following focal ischemia. Mol Brain Res. 1996; 37(1):201–8.

Pae HO, Oh GS, Choi BM, Chae SC, Kim YM, Chung KR, Chung H. Carbon monoxide produced by heme oxygenase-1 suppresses T cell proliferation via inhibition of IL-2 production. The Journal of Immunulogy. 2004;172(8):4744–51.

Wu TW, Zeng LH, Wu J, Fung KP. Morin hydrate is a plant-derived and antioxidant-based hepatoprotector. Life Sci. 1993;53(13):213–8.

Zhang R, Kang KA, Piao MJ, Maeng YH, Lee KH, Chang WY, You HJ, Kim JS, Kang SS, Hyun JW. Cellular protection of morin against the oxidative stress induced by hydrogen peroxide. Chemico-Interactions. 2009;177(1):21–7.

20

Metagenomic approach in study and treatment of various skin diseases

Pragya Nagar and Yasha Hasija[*]

Abstract

Background: Skin is a complex ecosystem hosting a diverse microbial population as well as distinct environmental niches leading to hundreds of skin conditions that affect humans. There is an evident shift towards the metagenomic analysis from less efficient and strenuous culture-based techniques in biomedical research, thus creating a new dimension for dermatological study. A systematic and comprehensive study of skin microbiome appraises the dynamics between species, their interaction with the immune system, and composition in diseases.

Research: Metagenomics include research techniques like next-generation sequencing, sequencing of amplicon-based assays, shotgun metagenomics, gene prediction, metatranscriptomics, and statistical and comparative studies allowing us to access the functional and metabolic diversity of the skin microbiome and their role in host health. In disorders like acne, dandruff, seborrheic dermatitis, and bovine digital dermatitis, metagenomics provides information about the organisms present conferring the condition, inter-microbial interactions, and expression profiles of communities.

Conclusion: We have enriched our understanding of the uncultured world resulting in a better understanding of microbe interaction with each other and their host. Metagenomic analysis provides glimpses into topographical and interpersonal complexity that defines the skin microbiome. It has led to an advanced study of dermatological disorders like acne, dandruff, seborrheic dermatitis, atopic dermatitis, bovine digital dermatitis, and psoriasis, and this knowledge is a breakthrough in dermatology research for creating better therapeutic solutions and personalized treatments.

Keywords: Skin, Metagenomics, Microbiome, Dermatological disorders

Background

Skin is the first outermost layering representing a physical barrier to infections and potential assault by foreign organisms or toxic substances. This complex ecosystem is broadly composed of sebaceous areas (including the face and back); moist areas (including the toe/finger web space and arm pit); dry areas (including the forearm and buttock); sites containing varied densities of hair follicles, skin folds, and skin thicknesses; and characteristic host genetics (Wilantho et al. 2017). This confers to a suitable environment for harboring rich and diverse physiological populations of microorganisms. The microbiome includes bacteria, fungi, viruses, parasites, and microeukaryotes which play significant role in dermatological disorders (Mathieu et al. 2013).

Previously, studies were done using culture-cultivated methods but have proved to be less efficient as less than 1% of bacterial species can be cultivated with standard lab conditions leading to a vast majority of microorganisms gone unnoticed (Chen and Tsao 2013). Hence, for an unbiased identifying and characterizing of skin microbiota and their genetic content, metagenomics and next-generation sequencing techniques are used (Mende et al. 2012). The term metagenome allows for the contribution of all the genes and genetic elements of the microorganisms in and on the host. Metagenomics refers to the structural and functional study of complex microbial communities and their interaction with the host (Virgin and Todd 2011). The

* Correspondence: yashahasija06@gmail.com
Department of Biotechnology, Delhi Technological University, Shahbad Daulatpur, Main Bawana Road, Delhi 110042, India

objective of this study in characterizing the skin microbiome is to define the microbial community and study their consequences for better understanding of the skin diseases. This approach includes amplification, sequencing, and analysis of the hypervariable region of the prokaryotic 16S rRNA gene as a proxy of the full-length gene and other phylogenetic marker genes (Rasheed et al. 2013). Oligonucleotide usage patterns can be utilized for identification of differences across complex microbial communities (Wan et al. 2017).

Metagenomic study permits collection, curation, and extraction of useful information from enormous datasets which is a significant computational challenge. Metagenomics include genomic DNA extraction, library construction, shotgun sequencing, taxonomic composition analysis, statistical analysis, etc (Fig. 1). This development has reframed our knowledge about the skin microbiome and its interactions with the host epithelial and immune system in various dermatological disorders (Kergourlay et al. 2015; Bzhalava et al. 2014; Martín et al. 2014), hence making way for the prevention and treatment of these diseases through diagnostic, prognostic, and therapeutic applications.

For instance, earlier it was believed that diseases like acne and dandruff were caused mainly due to the presence of *Propionibacterium acnes* and Malassezia fungi respectively. But several comprehensive metagenomic study findings have showed that the diseases are rather constituted by involvement of complex microbial communities and are detected by further taxonomic analysis (Barnard et al. 2016; Chng et al. 2016). Dermatological disorders which have been studied and analyzed through metagenomic approaches are acne vulgaris, dandruff, seborrheic dermatitis, atopic dermatitis, bovine digital dermatitis, psoriasis, vitiligo, melanoma, lupus

erythematosus, basal cell carcinoma, erythema, and hidradenitis suppurativa (Table 1) (Actis & Rosina 2013; Horton et al. 2015; Fyhrquist et al. 2016; Guet-Revillet et al. 2017; Kocarnik et al. 2015). This review covers our current knowledge on some of these dermatological disorders and potential aspect of metagenomics in dermatological research.

Skin microbiome

Skin represents a physical barrier to infection as a result of epidermis cohesion, protecting our bodies from potential assault by foreign organisms or toxic substances. There is a delicate balance between host and the skin microbiota including symbiotic bacteria, fungi, parasites, and viruses (Mathieu et al. 2013). Disruptions in the balance on either side can result in skin disorders. These diseases can be studied by characterizing the skin microbiota and analyzing how it interacts with the host (Hannigan and Grice 2013). The surface of the skin is cooler than the core body temperature and is slightly acidic, and squames are continuously shed from the skin surface as a result of terminal differentiation (Fuchs and Raghavan 2002). It mainly consists of sebaceous areas, moist areas, dry areas, and sites containing varied densities of hair follicles, skin folds, and skin thicknesses. Sebaceous glands being relatively anoxic support the growth of facultative anaerobes such as acne causing *Propionibacterium acnes*, which contain lipase-encoding genes that degrade skin lipids of sebum as revealed by full genome sequencing (Liu et al. 2015). Other dominant bacterial genera present in the skin are Staphylococcus and Corynebacterium. The major fungus found on the surface is the Malassezia (formerly known as Pityrosporum) genus which plays role in causing the common skin disease, dandruff, studied and confirmed by 18S

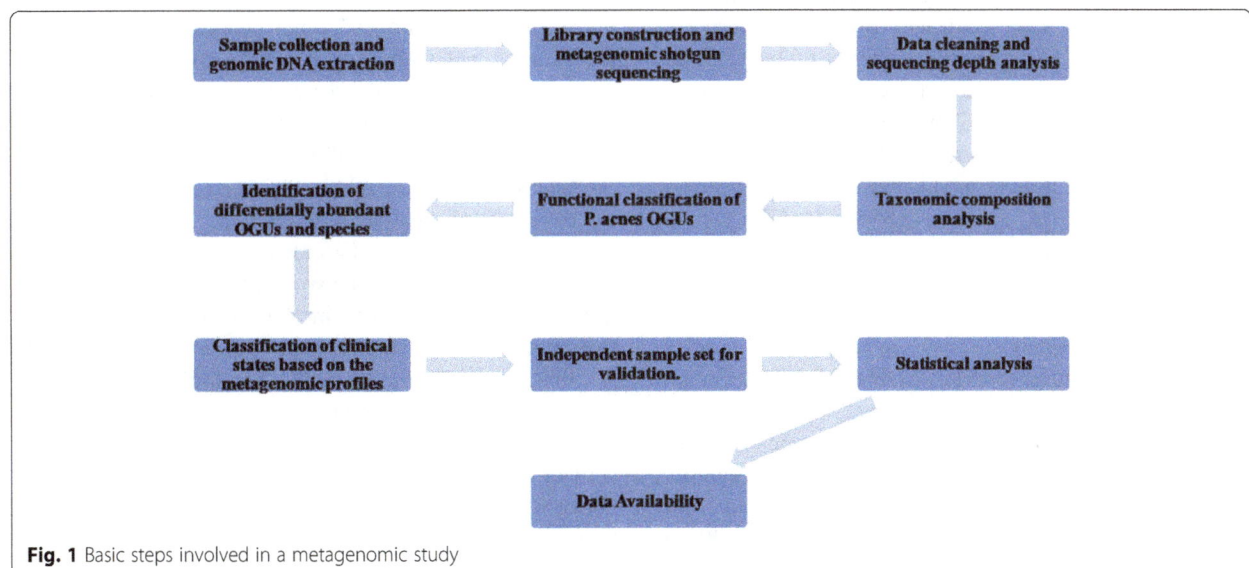

Fig. 1 Basic steps involved in a metagenomic study

Table 1 List of diseases which have been studied using metagenomics

Dermatological diseases in which metagenomic studies have been done successfully	Some common dermatological diseases with potential metagenomic studies
Acne vulgaris	Contact dermatitis
Seborrheic dermatitis	Skin rash
Atopic dermatitis	Wart
Bovine digital dermatitis	Keratosis
Psoriasis	Lichen planus
Vitiligo	Rosacea
Melanoma	Bullous pemphigoid
Lupus erythematosus	Melanocytic nevus
Basal cell carcinoma	Pemphigus
Erythema	Hyperpigmentation
Hidradenitis suppurativa	Ichthyosis

rRNA gene and ITS region sequencing (Tanaka et al. 2016). Whole-genome shotgun metagenomics has made it possible to study the skin viruses, most common being the human papillomavirus (HPV), human polyomaviruses (HPyVs), and circoviruses (Arroyo Mühr et al. 2015; Ma et al. 2014; Tse et al. 2012).

Culture-independent techniques and personalized treatment approaches

Earlier, the information and knowledge regarding the skin-associated microbes were primarily derived by culturing the microorganism and defining its phylogeny and taxonomy through phenotypic, microscopic, and biochemical relationships. But majority of microorganisms are retractile to cultivation or are unable to grow under the specified conditions, and thus, this approach significantly underestimates the complexity of the sample (Hugenholz et al. 1998). Hence, access to metagenomics has extensively fueled the growing segment of research in study and treatment of various dermatological disorders. Metagenomic analysis involves isolating DNA from an environmental sample or component under study, cloning the DNA into a suitable vector, transforming the clones into a host bacterium, and screening the resulting transformants for phylogenetic markers or "anchors," such as 16S rRNA and recA, for expression of certain traits like enzyme activity or antibiotic production, or for finding other conserved genes (Ferretti et al. 2017; Lau et al. 2017; Hannigan et al. 2015; Lane et al. 1985).

Metagenomic study generally includes preparation and sequencing of amplicon-based assays, shotgun metagenomics, primary computational analysis, and statistical and comparative studies (Kim et al. 2017). The shotgun metagenomic method comprises of collection and analysis of total DNA from the community without relying upon marker genes and sequencing directly

(Eisen, 2007). Another approach can be of consequent sequencing of amplified targeted microbial regions usually contained in the 16S Rrna called ribosomal community profiling (Zinicola et al. 2015; Pace et al. 1985). Marker genes used in these techniques enclose both conserved regions, which allow for PCR primer binding and phylogenetic analysis, along with variable regions, whose sequences allow to be used for inferring the taxonomic composition of the community (Grice 2015).

Metatranscriptomics is a useful way to study species present in abundance as instead of DNA, RNA is obtained from a skin sample and then sequenced using next-generation sequencing (Baldrian et al. 2012; Poinar et al. 2006; Schuster, 2007). The transcriptome data provides this information better with the previously amplified RNA. Metatranscriptomic study detects majorly the live microorganisms due to unstable RNA sample as compared to DNA (Urich et al. 2008).

High-throughput sequencing technique does not require cloning of the DNA before sequencing, making the process less strenuous and time-consuming. Accuracy of assemblies obtained can be improved by correcting misassemblies using the paired-end tags by various assembly programs like Phrap assembler or velvet assembler (Chen and Pachter 2005). BLAST is used for rapid search of phylogenetic markers in existing databases used in MEGAN (Wooley et al. 2010). Sequences are binned, a process of association of a particular sequence with an organism, in order to perform comparative analysis of diversity using tools like PhymmBL, AMPHORA, and SLIMM which use individual reference genome to get reliable relative abundance by minimizing the false-positive hits (Kunin et al. 2008). There is an advent of faster and efficient tools like CLARK which can perform taxonomic annotation at extremely high speed than BLAST-based approaches like MG-RAST or MEGAN (Nicola et al. 2012). Comparison of obtained sequences against reference databases like KEGG can give functional comparisons between metagenomes (Mitra et al. 2011). Metagenomic study permits collection, curation, and extraction of useful information from enormous datasets which is a considerable computational challenge, hence leading to the analysis of functional potential of the skin microbiome, improvement of metabolic pathways, about genes encoding virulence and pathogenicity factors, and hence can be used for creating new therapeutic solutions to treat such diseases.

One major application of metagenomics in diseases are personalized medicine, defined as a medical procedure involving molecular profiling, medical imaging, and lifestyle data that separates patients into different groups—with medical decisions, practices, interventions and/or products being tailored to the individual patient based on their predicted response or risk of disease (Afshinnekoo et al. 2017). Thus, we have now the ability to affordably and rapidly generate large datasets which are used to interpret data obtained from microbial community via analytical tools and databases (Wylie et al. 2014). Such advanced study lead to the use of effective and safe probiotics (live microorganisms or their components that confer health benefits) for the use in skin diseases that may be influenced by the gut microbiota along with prebiotics consisting of substrates that promote the growth and/or metabolic activity of beneficial indigenous microbiota for treating skin diseases due to microbial cause (Grice 2015).

Metagenomics in skin disorders

Acne

Acne vulgaris (commonly called acne) is the most common skin disorder characterized by abnormalities of sebum production by the pilosebaceous unit (commonly known as the hair follicle), bacterial proliferation, and inflammation and affects 80–85% of the population (Barnard et al. 2016). This disease is most prevalent in adolescents (85%) and rarely occurs in adults (11%) (White 1998). *Propionibacterium acnes* is said to be an important pathogenic factor accounting for nearly 90% of the microbiota demonstrated by 16SrRNA metagenomic study along with other microbes *Staphylococcus epidermidis, Propionibacterium humerusii,* and *Propionibacterium granulosum* (Fitz-Gibbon et al. 2013).

After examining various healthy and acne patients, it was found that such human diseases are often caused by certain strains of a species, rather than the entire species being pathogenic. *P. acnes* contribute to skin health also by preventing the colonization of opportunistic pathogens as it maintains an acidic pH by converting sebum to free fatty acids (Liu et al. 2015). Thus, only some strains are related to acne and not all. The metagenomic approach in determining disease associations provides

significant result as it is more commanding and less biased than traditional methods.

There was no statistically significant difference in the relative abundance of *P. acnes* found when comparison of acne patients and normal individuals was performed (Wilantho et al. 2017). The examination of differences at the strain level of *P. acnes* by defining each unique 16S rDNA sequence as a 16S rDNA allele type, called a ribotype (RT), was done and hence allowed us to compare the *P. acnes* strain populations in individuals (Barnard et al. 2016). The balance between acne and metagenomic elements determines the virulence and health properties of the skin microbiota in disease and health (Kwon and Suh 2016).

This study provides novel insights into the microbial environment and mechanism of acne pathogenesis and hence can lead to designing of probiotic and phage therapies as potential acne treatments for maintaining a healthy skin.

Dandruff and seborrheic dermatitis (SD)

Dandruff is a prevalent mild chronic inflammatory condition of the scalp characterized by itching and scaling of the skin on the scalp (Soares et al. 2016). Seborrheic dermatitis being considered the more severe form of dandruff affects areas other than the scalp with sebaceous glands like the face and chest. Generally, this includes events like dysbiosis and disruption of skin barrier and epidermal cellular proliferation and differentiation (Soares et al. 2016). This common disease affects approximately half the population of adults worldwide, mainly caused by the Malassezia fungi. But recent research has suggested that the microbial communities present are more complex (Byrd et al. 2017).

Several comprehensive analyses like next-generation sequencing (NGS), performed on healthy and dandruff-suffering scalps, have revealed that Propionibacterium, Staphylococcus, and Corynebacterium are the three most abundant genera in both healthy and dandruff subjects but with the Malassezia sp. being the vast majority of fungi. The most abundant, *M. restricta* along with *M. globosa, M. sympodialis, M. dermatis, M. japonica, M. obtusa, M. pachydermatis, M. sloofiae,* and *M. furfur,* were detected by further taxonomic analysis (Byrd et al. 2017). Metagenomic and molecular studies have shown that *Propionibacterium acnes* is found to be greater in healthy scalps while *Staphylococcus epidermidis* in dandruff scalp along with bacterial genera Pseudomonas, Leptotrichia, Micrococcus, Selenomonas, Erwinia, Enhydrobacter, and Bartonellaceae and fungal genera Candida, Aspergillus, and Filobasidium, and more Malassezia by 26S r RNA molecular analysis (Wan et al. 2017) (Fig. 2). Further studies on scalp and forehead by high-throughput 16S rDNA and ITS1 sequencing, pyrosequencing, and

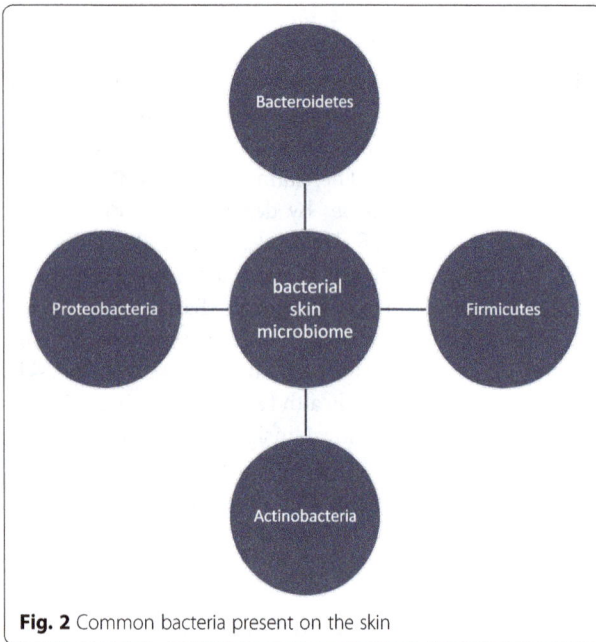

Fig. 2 Common bacteria present on the skin

qPCR (Fig. 3) have shown that both lesional and non-lesional skin sites contain Acinetobacter, Corynebacterium, Staphylococcus, Streptococcus, and Propionibacterium with Propionibacterium being more abundant in non-lesional sites (Wan et al. 2017).

These technological advancements have increased our knowledge of the disease etiology and the role of the microbiome in the symptom development significantly in recent years which could be helpful for redefining the therapeutic approaches.

Atopic dermatitis

Atopic dermatitis (AD) is another frequently studied disease using metagenomics. AD is a chronic, noninfectious, recurring inflammatory disease characterized by itching and xerosis that affects majorly children (approximately 15% children were affected in the USA). Effective treatments of this disease include antibiotics, corticosteroids, and dilute bleach baths (Huang et al. 2009). AD patients have an altered microbial community, and the pathogenesis is mainly associated with skin colonization by *Staphylococcus aureus* and immune hypersensitivity (Song et al. 2016; Weidinger et al. 2006). Filaggrin deficiency also plays role in AD as seen in mouse model with mutation in St14 that regulates filaggrin processing leading to increased Corynebacterium and Streptococcus and decreased Pseudomonas species (Scharschmidt et al. 2009). A 16S-rRNA-based metagenomic study of this disease has shown that both *S. aureus* and *S. epidermidis* increased in AD flares along with changes in abundance of some non-staphylococcal species leading to decreased bacterial diversity (Kong et al. 2012). There is domination of Staphylococcus, Pseudomonas, and Streptococcus in AD with Alcaligenaceae, Sediminibacterium, and Lactococcus being the characteristic of healthy skin, studied by high-throughput pyrosequencing on a Roche 454 GS-FLX

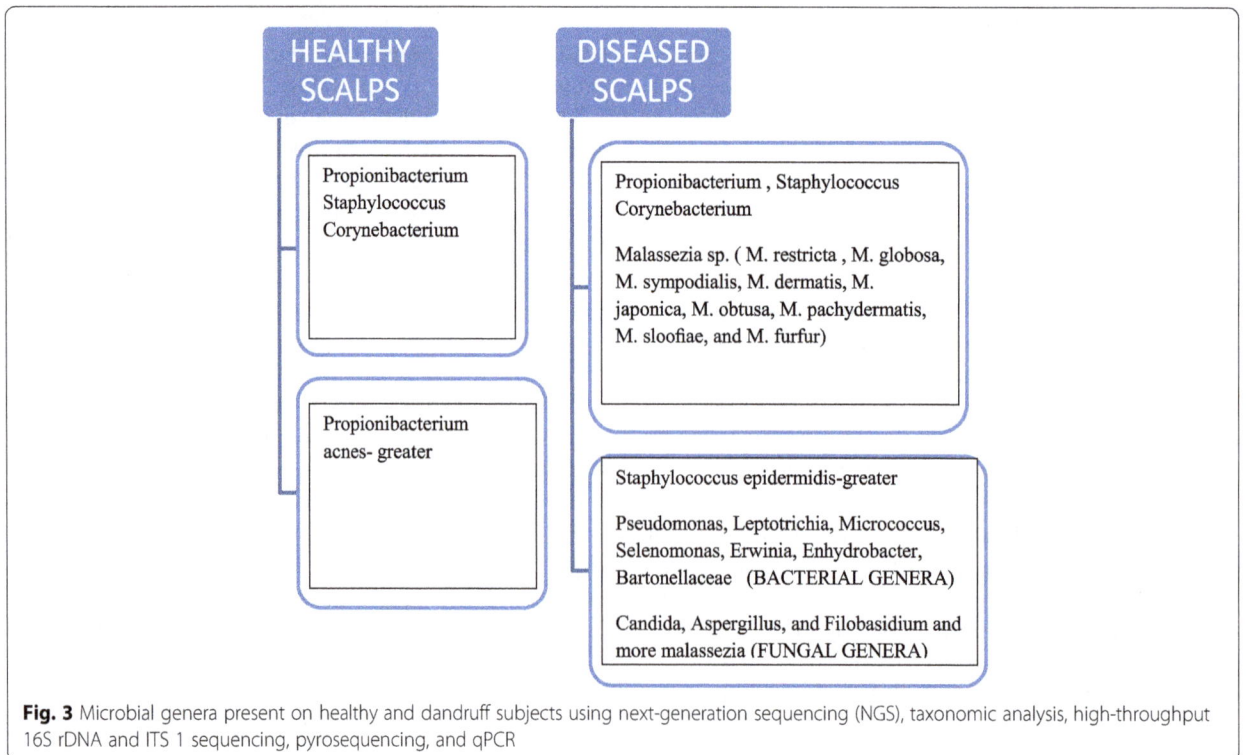

Fig. 3 Microbial genera present on healthy and dandruff subjects using next-generation sequencing (NGS), taxonomic analysis, high-throughput 16S rDNA and ITS 1 sequencing, pyrosequencing, and qPCR

platform (Kim et al. 2017). Hence, metagenomic analysis is important to study the action of these species and their association with the microbiome fluctuations and with one another. This will lead to designing of novel treatments like rebalancing of the skin microbiome.

Psoriasis

Psoriasis is a chronic inflammatory skin disease affecting about 2–3% of the world's population. Plaque psoriasis is the most common form of psoriasis affecting 85–90% of patients (Boehncke and Schon 2015). Although psoriasis is a skin disease, it can lead to development of psoriatic arthritis (PsA), metabolic syndromes, and cardiovascular diseases along with skin lesions (Grozdev et al. 2014). It has been known from the previously performed experiments that the immune system plays a key role in the disease pathogenesis. For PsA prevention in patients, the first step towards future development in therapeutics and early identification involves having the knowledge of the skin microbiome (Andersen et al. 2017; Castelino et al. 2014). Early culture-based studies identified Malassezia, group A and B beta-hemolytic streptococci, *S. aureus*, and *Enterococcus faecalis* being associated with the disease (Tett et al. 2017). 16S rRNA gene compositional analysis reveals that neonatal antibiotic treatment dysregulates skin microbiota and the imbalance is associated with development of experimental psoriasis. High-resolution shotgun metagenomics and finer strain-level analysis revealed decreased diversity and association of psoriasis with increase in Staphylococcus and its heterogeneity colonization and strain-level variability (Zanvit et al. 2015). Metagenomic study has been perceptive in understanding the taxonomic differences associated with psoriasis and hence offers the potential to overcome the limitations of culture-based studies.

Bovine digital dermatitis

It is a highly contagious infectious dermatitis with lesions near the interdigital spaces usually in cattle (Ganju et al. 2016). It causes discomfort and often severe lameness (LAMENESS, ANIMAL). Lesions can be either erosive or proliferative and wart-like with papillary growths and hypertrophied hairs. *Dichelobacter nodosus* and Treponema are the most commonly associated causative agents for this mixed bacterial infection disease (Drago et al. 2016; Krull et al. 2014) (year introduced, 2011).

Conclusions

Skin being the largest body organ leads to hundreds of skin conditions that have a significant impact on several aspects of human health and can lead to various skin disorders. It is vital to understand beneficial and harmful microorganisms and their mechanism. Advances in metagenomics and next-generation sequencing techniques have enhanced our ability to identify and characterize microbial communities colonizing the skin. It includes sensitive and rapid methods of sequencing to diagnose infection by comparing genetic material found in sample to a database of bacteria, viruses, and other pathogens. This field is promising in redefining therapeutic approaches for precision and personalized medicine and might transform management and treatment of dermatological disorders like acne vulgaris, seborrheic dermatitis, atopic dermatitis, psoriasis, and vitiligo by creating a broader view of disease etiology. However, for better diagnostic, prognostic, and therapeutic applications, further research is necessary to expand our understanding of healthy skin microbiota.

Funding

This work was supported by the Department of Biotechnology, Government of India [No. BT/PR5402/BID/7/508/2012].

Authors' contributions

YH conceived and designed the study. PN and YH wrote the manuscript. Both the authors approved the final manuscript.

Competing interests

The authors declare that they have no competing interests.

References

Actis GC, Rosina F. Inflammatory bowel disease: an archetype disorder of outer environment sensor systems. World J Gastrointest Pharmacol Ther. 2013;4(3): 41–6. https://doi.org/10.4292/wjgpt.v4.i3.41. PMID: 23919214

Afshinnekoo E, Chou C, Alexander N, Ahsanuddin S, Schuetz AN, Mason CE. Precision metagenomics: rapid metagenomic analyses for infectious disease diagnostics and public health surveillance. J Biomol Tech. 2017;28(1):40–5. https://doi.org/10.7171/jbt.17-2801-007.

Andersen V, Holmskov U, Sørensen SB, et al. A proposal for a study on treatment selection and lifestyle recommendations in chronic inflammatory diseases: a Danish multidisciplinary collaboration on prognostic factors and personalised medicine. Nutrients. 2017;9(5):499. https://doi.org/10.3390/nu9050499.

Arroyo Mühr LS, Hultin E, Bzhalava D, Eklund C, Lagheden C, Ekström J, Johansson H, Forslund O, Dillner J. Human papillomavirus type 197 is commonly present in skin tumors. Int J Cancer. 2015;136(11):2546–55. https://doi.org/10.1002/ijc.29325. Epub 2014 Nov 25.PMID: 25388227

Baldrian P, Kolarik M, Stursova M, Kopecky J, Valaskova V, Vetrovsky T, et al. Active and total microbial communities in forest soil are largely different and highly stratified during decomposition. ISME J. 2012;6:248–58. [PubMed: 21776033]

Barnard E, Shi B, Kang D, Craft N, Li H. The balance of metagenomic elements shapes the skin microbiome in acne and health. Sci Rep. 2016;6:39491. https://doi.org/10.1038/srep39491. PMID: 28000755

Boehncke WH, Schon MP. Psoriasis. Lancet. 2015; https://doi.org/10.1016/S0140-6736(14) 61909-7.

Byrd AL, Deming C, Cassidy SKB, Harrison OJ, Ng WI, Conlan S, Comparative Sequencing Program NISC, Belkaid Y, Segre JA, Kong HH. Staphylococcus aureus and Staphylococcus epidermidis strain diversity underlying pediatric atopic dermatitis. Sci Transl Med. 2017;9(397) https://doi.org/10.1126/scitranslmed.aal4651. PMID: 28679656

Bzhalava D, Mühr LS, Lagheden C, Ekström J, Forslund O, Dillner J, Hultin E. Deep sequencing extends the diversity of human papillomaviruses in human skin. Sci Rep. 2014;4:5807. https://doi.org/10.1038/srep05807.PMID: 25055967.

Castelino M, Eyre S, Upton M, Ho P, Barton A. The bacterial skin microbiome in psoriatic arthritis, an unexplored link in pathogenesis: challenges and opportunities offered by recent technological advances. Rheumatology (Oxford). 2014;53(5):777–84. https://doi.org/10.1093/rheumatology/ket319. Epub 2013 Sep 24. Review.PMID: 24067887

Chen K, Pachter L. Bioinformatics for whole-genome shotgun sequencing of microbial communities. PLoS Comput Biol. 2005;1(2):e24. https://doi.org/10.1371/journal.pcbi.0010024. PMC 1185649 Freely accessible. PMID 16110337

Chen YE, Tsao H. The skin microbiome: current perspectives and future challenges. J Am Acad Dermatol. 2013;69(1):143–55. https://doi.org/10.1016/j.jaad.2013.01.016. Epub 2013 Mar 13. Review.PMID: 23489584

Chng KR, Tay AS, Li C, Ng AH, Wang J, Suri BK, Matta SA, McGovern N, Janela B, Wong XF, Sio YY, Au BV, Wilm A, De Sessions PF, Lim TC, Tang MB, Ginhoux F, Connolly JE, Lane EB, Chew FT, Common JE, Nagarajan N. Whole metagenome profiling reveals skin microbiome-dependent susceptibility to atopic dermatitis flare. Nat Microbiol. 2016;1(9):16106. https://doi.org/10.1038/nmicrobiol.2016.106. PMID: 27562258

Drago L, De Grandi R, Altomare G, Pigatto P, Rossi O, Toscano M. Skin microbiota of first cousins affected by psoriasis and atopic dermatitis. Clin Mol Allergy. 2016;14:2. https://doi.org/10.1186/s12948-016-0038-z. eCollection 2016.PMID: 26811697

Eisen JA. Environmental shotgun sequencing: its potential and challenges for studying the hidden world of microbes. PLoS Biol. 2007;5(3):e82. https://doi.org/10.1371/journal.pbio.0050082. PMC 1821061 Freely accessible. PMID 17355177

Ferretti P, Farina S, Cristofolini M, Girolomoni G, Tett A, Segata N. Experimental metagenomics and ribosomal profiling of the human skin microbiome. Exp Dermatol. 2017;26(3):211–9. https://doi.org/10.1111/exd.13210. Epub 2017 Jan 20. Review.PMID: 27623553

Fitz-Gibbon S, Tomida S, Chiu BH, Nguyen L, Du C, Liu M, Elashoff D, Erfe MC, Loncaric A, Kim J, Modlin RL, Miller JF, Sodergren E, Craft N, Weinstock GM, Li H. Propionibacterium acnes strain populations in the human skin microbiome associated with acne. J Invest Dermatol. 2013;133(9):2152–60. https://doi.org/10.1038/jid.2013.21. Epub 2013 Jan 21.PMID: 23337890

Fuchs E, Raghavan S. Getting under the skin of epidermal morphogenesis. Nat Rev Genet. 2002;3:199–209. https://doi.org/10.1038/nrg758

Fyhrquist N, Salava A, Auvinen P, Lauerma A. Skin biomes. Curr Allergy Asthma Rep. 2016;16(5):40. https://doi.org/10.1007/s11882-016-0618-5. Review.PMID: 27056560

Ganju P, Nagpal S, Mohammed MH, Nishal Kumar P, Pandey R, Natarajan VT, Mande SS, Gokhale RS. Microbial community profiling shows dysbiosis in the lesional skin of vitiligo subjects. Sci Rep. 2016;6:18761. https://doi.org/10.1038/srep18761. PMID: 26758568

Grice EA. The intersection of microbiome and host at the skin interface: genomic- and metagenomic-based insights. Genome Res. 2015;25(10):1514–20. https://doi.org/10.1101/gr.191320.115. PMID: 26430162

Grozdev I, Korman N, Tsankov N. Psoriasis as a systemic disease. Clin Dermatol. 2014;32:343–50.

Guet-Revillet H, Jais JP, Ungeheuer MN, Coignard-Biehler H, Duchatelet S, Delage M, Lam T, Hovnanian A, Lortholary O, Nassif X, Nassif A, Join-Lambert O. The microbiological landscape of anaerobic infections in hidradenitis suppurativa: a prospective metagenomic study. Clin Infect Dis. 2017;65(2):282–91. https://doi.org/10.1093/cid/cix285. PMID: 28379372

Hannigan GD, Grice EA. Microbial ecology of the skin in the era of metagenomics and molecular microbiology. Cold Spring Harb Perspect Med. 2013;3(12):a015362. https://doi.org/10.1101/cshperspect.a015362. Review. PMID: 24296350

Hannigan GD, Meisel JS, Tyldsley AS, Zheng Q, Hodkinson BP, SanMiguel AJ, Minot S, Bushman FD, Grice EA. The human skin double-stranded DNA virome: topographical and temporal diversity, genetic enrichment, and dynamic associations with the host microbiome. MBio. 2015;6(5):e01578–15. https://doi.org/10.1128/mBio.01578-15. PMID: 26489866

Horton JM, Gao Z, Sullivan DM, Shopsin B, Perez-Perez GI, Blaser MJ. The cutaneous microbiome in outpatients presenting with acute skin abscesses. Horton J Infect Dis. 2015;211(12):1895–904. https://doi.org/10.1093/infdis/jiv003. Epub 2015 Jan 12.PMID: 25583170

Huang JT, Abrams M, Tlougan B, Rademaker A, Paller AS. Treatment of Staphylococcus aureus colonization in atopic dermatitis decreases disease severity. Pediatrics. 2009;123:e808–14. [PubMed: 19403473]

Hugenholz P, Goebel BM, Pace NR. Impact of culture-independent studies on the emerging phylogenetic view of bacterial diversity. J Bacteriol. 1998;180(18):4765–74. PMC 107498 Freely accessible. PMID 9733676

Kergourlay G, Taminiau B, Daube G, Champomier Vergès MC. Metagenomic insights into the dynamics of microbial communities in food. Int J Food Microbiol. 2015;213:31–9. https://doi.org/10.1016/j.ijfoodmicro.2015.09.010. Epub 2015 Sep 16. Review.PMID: 26414193

Kim MH, Rho M, Choi JP, Choi HI, Park HK, Song WJ, Min TK, Cho SH, Cho YJ, Kim YK, Yang S, Pyun BY. A metagenomic analysis provides a culture-independent pathogen detection for atopic dermatitis. Allergy Asthma Immunol Res. 2017;9(5):453–61. https://doi.org/10.4168/aair.2017.9.5.453. PMID: 28677360

Kocarnik JM, Park SL, Han J, Dumitrescu L, Cheng I, Wilkens LR, Schumacher FR, Kolonel L, Carlson CS, Crawford DC, Goodloe RJ, Dilks HH, Baker P, Richardson D, Matise TC, Ambite JL, Song F, Qureshi AA, Zhang M, Duggan D, Hutter C, Hindorff L, Bush WS, Kooperberg C, Le Marchand L, Peters U. Pleiotropic and sex-specific effects of cancer GWAS SNPs on melanoma risk in the population architecture using genomics and epidemiology (PAGE) study. PLoS One. 2015;10(3):e0120491. https://doi.org/10.1371/journal.pone.0120491. eCollection 2015.PMID: 25789475

Kong HH, Oh J, Deming C, Conlan S, Grice EA, Beatson MA, et al. Temporal shifts in the skin microbiome associated with disease flares and treatment in children with atopic dermatitis. Genome Res. 2012;22:850–9. [PubMed: 22310478]

Krull AC, Shearer JK, Gorden PJ, Cooper VL, Phillips GJ, Plummer PJ. Deep sequencing analysis reveals temporal microbiota changes associated with development of bovine digital dermatitis. Infect Immun. 2014;82(8):3359–73. https://doi.org/10.1128/IAI.02077-14. Epub 2014 May 27.PMID: 24866801

Kunin V, Copeland A, Lapidus A, Mavromatis K, Hugenholtz P. A bioinformatician's guide to metagenomics. Microbiol Mol Biol Rev. 2008;72(4):557–78. Table 578 Contents. doi:10.1128/MMBR.00009-08. PMC 2593568 Freely accessible. PMID 19052320

Kwon HH, Suh DH. Recent progress in the research about Propionibacterium acnes strain diversity and acne: pathogen or bystander? Int J Dermatol. 2016;55(11):1196–204. https://doi.org/10.1111/ijd.13282. Review.PMID: 27421121

Lane DJ, Pace B, Olsen GJ, Stahl DA, Sogin ML, Pace NR. Rapid determination of 16S ribosomal RNA sequences for phylogenetic analyses. Proc Natl Acad Sci. 1985;82(20):6955–9. Bibcode:1985PNAS...82.6955L. doi:10.1073/pnas.82.20.6955. PMC 391288 Freely accessible. PMID 2413450

Lau P, Cordey S, Brito F, Tirefort D, Petty TJ, Turin L, Guichebaron A, Docquier M, Zdobnov EM, Waldvogel-Abramowski S, Lecompte T, Kaiser L, Preynat-Seauve O. Metagenomics analysis of red blood cell and fresh-frozen plasma units. Transfusion. 2017;57(7):1787–800. https://doi.org/10.1111/trf.14148. Epub 2017 May 11.PMID: 28497550

Liu J, Yan R, Zhong Q, Ngo S, Bangayan NJ, Nguyen L, Lui T, Liu M, Erfe MC, Craft N, Tomida S, Li H. The diversity and host interactions of Propionibacterium acnes bacteriophages on human skin. ISME J. 2015;9(9):2078–93. https://doi.org/10.1038/ismej.2015.47. Epub 2015 Apr 7. Erratum in: ISME J. 2015 Sep; 9(9):2116.PMID: 25848871

Ma Y, Madupu R, Karaoz U, Nossa CW, Yang L, Yooseph S, Yachimski PS, Brodie EL, Nelson KE, Pei Z. Human papillomavirus community in healthy persons, defined by metagenomics analysis of human microbiome project shotgun sequencing data sets. J Virol. 2014;88(9):4786–97. https://doi.org/10.1128/JVI.00093-14. Epub 2014 Feb 12.PMID: 24522917

Martín R, Miquel S, Langella P, Bermúdez-Humarán LG. The role of metagenomics in understanding the human microbiome in health and disease. Virulence. 2014;5(3):413–23. https://doi.org/10.4161/viru.27864. Epub 2014 Feb 11. Review.PMID: 24429972

Mathieu A, Delmont TO, Vogel TM, Robe P, Nalin R, Simonet P. Life on human surfaces: skin metagenomics. PLoS One. 2013;8(6):e65288. https://doi.org/10.1371/journal.pone.0065288. Print 2013.PMID: 23776466

Mende DR, Waller AS, Sunagawa S, Järvelin AI, Chan MM, Arumugam M, Raes J, Bork P. Assessment of metagenomic assembly using simulated next generation sequencing data. PLoS One. 2012;7(2):e31386. Bibcode:2012PLoSO...731386M. doi:10.1371/journal.pone.0031386. ISSN 1932-6203. PMC 3285633 Freely accessible. PMID 22384016

Mitra S, Rupek P, Richter DC, Urich T, Gilbert JA, Meyer F, Wilke A, Huson DH. Functional analysis of metagenomes and metatranscriptomes using SEED and KEGG. BMC Bioinformatics. 2011;12(Suppl 1):S21. https://doi.org/10.1186/1471-2105-12-S1-S21. ISSN 1471-2105. PMC 3044276 Freely accessible. PMID 21342551

Nicola S, Waldron L, Ballarini A, Narasimhan V, Jousson O, Huttenhower C. Metagenomic microbial community profiling using unique clade-specific marker genes. Nat Methods. 2012;9(8):811–4. https://doi.org/10.1038/nmeth. 2066. PMC 3443552 Freely accessible. PMID 22688413

Pace NR, Stahl DA, Lane DJ, Olsen GJ. Analyzing natural microbial populations by rRNA sequences. ASM News. 1985;51:4–12. Archived from the original on 4 April 2012

Poinar HN, Schwarz C, Qi J, Shapiro B, Macphee RD, Buigues B, Tikhonov A, Huson D, Tomsho LP, Auch A, Rampp M, Miller W, Schuster SC. Metagenomics to paleogenomics: large-scale sequencing of mammoth DNA. Science. 2006;311(5759):392–4. https://doi.org/10.1126/science.1123360. Bibcode:2006Sci...311..392P

Rasheed Z, Rangwala H, Barbará D. 16S rRNA metagenome clustering and diversity estimation using locality sensitive hashing. BMC Syst Biol. 2013; 7(Suppl 4):S11. https://doi.org/10.1186/1752-0509-7-S4-S11. Epub 2013 Oct 23.PMID: 24565031

Tiffany C. Scharschmidt, Karin List, Elizabeth A. Grice, Roman Szabo, NISC Comparative Sequencing Program, Gabriel Renaud, Chyi-Chia R. Lee, Tyra G. Wolfsberg, Thomas H. Bugge, Julia A. Segre. Author manuscript; available in PMC 2010 Oct 1. J Invest Dermatol. 2009 129(10): 2435–2442. doi: https://doi. org/10.1038/jid.2009.104. PMCID: PMC2791707.

Schuster SC. Next-generation sequencing transforms today's biology. Nat Methods. 2007;5(1):16–8. https://doi.org/10.1038/nmeth1156.

Soares RC, Camargo-Penna PH, de Moraes VC, De Vecchi R, Clavaud C, Breton L, Braz AS, Paulino LC. Dysbiotic bacterial and fungal communities not restricted to clinically affected skin sites in dandruff. Front Cell Infect Microbiol. 2016;6:157. eCollection 2016.PMID: 27909689

Song H, Yoo Y, Hwang J, Na YC, Kim HS. Faecalibacterium prausnitzii subspecies-level dysbiosis in the human gut microbiome underlying atopic dermatitis. J Allergy Clin Immunol. 2016;137(3):852–60. https://doi.org/10.1016/j.jaci.2015. 08.021. Epub 2015 Oct 1.PMID: 26431583

Tanaka A, Cho O, Saito C, Saito M, Tsuboi R, Sugita T. Comprehensive pyrosequencing analysis of the bacterial microbiota of the skin of patients with seborrheic dermatitis. Microbiol Immunol. 2016;60(8):521–6. https://doi. org/10.1111/1348-0421.12398.

Tett A, Pasolli E, Farina S, et al. Unexplored diversity and strain-level structure of the skin microbiome associated with psoriasis. NPJ Biofilms and Microbiomes. 2017;3:14. https://doi.org/10.1038/s41522-017-0022-5.

Tse H, Tsang AK, Tsoi HW, Leung AS, Ho CC, Lau SK, Woo PC, Yuen KY. Identification of a novel bat papillomavirus by metagenomics. PLoS One. 2012;7(8):e43986. https://doi.org/10.1371/journal.pone.0043986. Epub 2012 Aug 24.PMID: 22937142

Urich T, Lanzen A, Qi J, Huson DH, Schleper C, Schuster SC. Simultaneous assessment of soil microbial community structure and function through analysis of the meta-transcriptome. PLoS One. 2008;3:e2527. [PubMed: 18575584]

Virgin HW, Todd JA. Metagenomics and personalized medicine. Cell. 2011;147:44.

Wan TW, Higuchi W, Khokhlova OE, Hung WC, Iwao Y, Wakayama M, Inomata N, Takano T, Lin YT, Peryanova OV, Kojima KK, Salmina AB, Teng LJ, Yamamoto T. Genomic comparison between Staphylococcus aureus GN strains clinically isolated from a familial infection case: IS1272 transposition through a novel inverted repeat-replacing mechanism. PLoS One. 2017;12(11):e0187288. https://doi.org/10.1371/journal.pone.0187288. eCollection 2017.PMID: 29117225

Weidinger S, Illig T, Baurecht H, Irvine AD, Rodriguez E, Diaz-Lacava A, et al. Loss-of-function variations within the filaggrin gene predispose for atopic dermatitis with allergic sensitizations. J Allergy Clin Immunol. 2006;118:214–9. [PubMed: 16815158]

White GM. Recent findings in the epidemiologic evidence, classification, and subtypes of acne vulgaris. J Am Acad Dermatol. 1998;39(2 Pt 3):S34–S37

Wilantho A, Deekaew P, Srisuttiyakorn C, Tongsima S, Somboonna N. Diversity of bacterial communities on the facial skin of different age-group Thai males. Peer J. 2017;5:e4084. https://doi.org/10.7717/peerj.4084. eCollection 2017. PMID: 29177119

Wooley JC, Godzik A, Friedberg I. A primer on metagenomics. PLoS Comput Biol. 2010;6(2):e1000667. https://doi.org/10.1371/journal.pcbi.1000667. PMC 2829047 Freely accessible. PMID 20195499. Bourne, Philip E., ed

Wylie KM, Mihindukulasuriya KA, Zhou Y, Sodergren E, Storch GA, Weinstock GM. Metagenomic analysis of double-stranded DNA viruses in healthy adults. BMC Biol. 2014;12:71. https://doi.org/10.1186/s12915-014-0071-7. PMID: 25212266

Zanvit P, Konkel JE, Jiao X, Kasagi S, Zhang D, Wu R, Chia C, Ajami NJ, Smith DP, Petrosino JF, Abbatiello B, Nakatsukasa H, Chen Q, Belkaid Y, Chen ZJ, Chen

W. Antibiotics in neonatal life increase murine susceptibility to experimental psoriasis. Nat Commun. 2015;6:8424. https://doi.org/10.1038/ncomms9424. PMID: 26416167

Zinicola M, Higgins H, Lima S, Machado V, Guard C, Bicalho R. Shotgun metagenomic sequencing reveals functional genes and microbiome associated with bovine digital dermatitis. PLoS One. 2015;10(7):e0133674. https://doi.org/10.1371/journal.pone.0133674. eCollection 2015.PMID: 26193110

21

Anti-inflammatory and anti-aging effects of hydroxytyrosol on human dermal fibroblasts (HDFs)

Seeun Jeon[1*] and Mina Choi[2*] ⓘ

Abstract

Background: Hydroxytyrosol is discovered in a form of elenolic acid ester oleuropein in olive leaf and oil. The anti-carcinogenic, antioxidant, and anti-inflammatory effects of hydroxytyrosol have been reported in the food, medical, pharmaceutical, and life science fields. But it has not been studied on skin biology field. This study is demonstrated using UVA-induced cellular aging model of human dermal fibroblast.

Methods: The cell survival rate was measured using the principle of water-soluble tetrazolium salt-1 assay, which is a measurement method for cell survival rate. The quantitative real-time PCR (qRT-PCR) was used to quantitatively analyze the gene expression changes in human dermal fibroblasts (HDFs) by hydroxytyrosol.
Senescence-associated β-galactosidase (SA-β-gal) assay was implemented to dye β-galactosidases (used as a cell aging biomarker) to measure HDF cell aging by UVA.

Results: Hydroxytyrosol decreased the SA-β-galactosidase activity in a dose-dependent manner in UVA-exposed HDFs. Also, the elevated expression of *MMP-1* and *MMP-3* by UVA were decreased by hydroxytyrosol in a dose-dependent manner. To examine the anti-inflammatory effect of hydroxytyrosol in UV exposed HDFs, the expression of inflammatory interleukins *IL-1β*, *IL-6*, and *IL-8* were analyzed. Quantitative RT-PCR showed that hydroxytyrosol decreased the expression of *IL-1β*, *IL-6*, and *IL-8* gene.

Conclusion: Through this research, we demonstrate that hydroxytyrosol has effects on anti-inflammatory and anti-aging in HDFs damaged by UVA. We suggest that hydroxytyrosol is fully worthy of using as a cosmetic material effective to anti-inflammatory and to delay cellular senescence on HDFs.

Keywords: Hydroxytyrosol, Fibroblasts, Anti-inflammatory, Cellular senescence, Anti-aging, Ultraviolet A

Background

Skin aging refers to a phenomenon where cells are unable to be regenerated or function properly as a result of cell loss or functional deterioration (Jones and Rando 2011; Kirkwood 2005). There are various biological, chemical, and physical causes of aging; skin aging as a result of continuous exposure to ultraviolet radiation is referred to as skin photoaging (Fisher et al. 1997; Wenk et al. 2001).

Exposure of the skin to a high level of ultraviolet rays causes direct cytotoxicity and subsequent apoptosis

(Netzel et al. 2002). When ultraviolet rays are irradiated onto incubated fibroblast in vitro or living tissues, matrix metallopeptidase (MMP) expression increases and collagen generation decreases; this ultimately damages connective tissues in the dermal skin layer (Brenneisen et al. 2002; Chung et al. 2002; Moon et al. 1992).

Continuous exposure to UVA, which affects a large number of living organisms, not only damages the DNA, but also affects cell survival and growth and induces protein denaturation, pigmentation, and creation of reactive oxygen species (Sinha and Haader 2002). Also, several research findings suggest that UVA and UVB damage DNA and generate reactive oxygen species, inducing apoptosis (Assefa et al. 2005), which directly or indirectly causes an inflammatory response (Bickers and

* Correspondence: jk35789@naver.com; cmn0424@naver.com
[1]Management Division, Swinner, 5F, 441, Teheran-ro, Gangnam-gu, Seoul 06158, Republic of Korea
[2]Liberal Arts Department, Jangan University, 1182, Samcheonbyeongma-ro, Bongdam-eup, Hwaseong-si, Gyeonggi-do, Republic of Korea

Athar 2006). If such response progresses in the skin for a long time, inflammatory factors are excessively secreted damaging normal tissues and cells, and thereby acting as causative factors for diseases such as cancer, high blood pressure, diabetes, and heart disease (Guzik et al. 2003; Patel et al. 2007). Recently, active researches are conducted on natural effective ingredients and traditional medical substances to treat intractable skin diseases and inhibit inflammatory skin diseases from progressing to their chronic stages. These researches are used as references for the production of cosmeceutical and health supplements (Kim et al. 2013a; Lee and Im 2011).

Olives have been extensively researched and utilized in many fields over the last few years, and besides having antioxidant effects, they also strengthen the immune system and boost the energy levels, and it has been reported that they are effective in treating respiratory diseases and skin wound infections and in relieving cold symptoms (Kitani et al. 2002). Olive leaves are considered as the best polyphenol complex with balanced super polyphenols such as hydroxytyrosol, tyrosol, caffeic acid, and oleuropein (Choi et al. 2008). It has been reported that DHPEA-EDA (hydroxytyrosol), also found in olive oil, is effective in protecting the red blood cells against oxidative damage, in comparison with other ingredients (Fatima et al. 2007). The researches on the inflammatory effects of hydroxytyrosol discuss its anti-cancer effects on colon and breast cancer (Sun et al. 2014; Warleta et al. 2011), its effects on osteoarthritis prevention and neuroprotection, and its inhibitive effects on oxidative stress and infection mediators (Facchini et al. 2014; Cabrerizo et al. 2013). Also, a skin-related study examined the photoprotective and anti-melanin effects of phenol compounds contained in olive leaf (*Olea europaea* L. var. Kalamata) extract on HaCaT cells (Ha et al. 2009). However, no research has been conducted on hydroxytyrosol as a cosmetic material. This study will examine the applicability of hydroxytyrosol, which contains a variety of bioactive substances, as a cosmetic ingredient, as a research on potential cosmetic ingredients for the further development of the cosmetic industry.

Materials and methods
Cell culture
The human dermal fibroblasts (HDFs) used in this study were purchased from Sigma-Aldrich Corporation (USA). To incubate HDF cells, Dulbecco's modified Eagle medium (DMEM; Hyclone, USA) containing 10% fetal bovine serum (FBS; Hyclone) and 1% penicillin/streptomycin (100 IU/mL penicillin, 100 µg/mL streptomycin; Invitrogen, USA) was used, and HDF cells were incubated in a cell incubator at 37 °C with 5% CO_2.

Sample treatment
When hydroxytyrosol (Sigma-Aldrich, USA) was used in a purified (> 90%) liquid state, it was dissolved in dimethyl sulfoxide (DMSO; Sigma-Aldrich) to achieve an appropriate concentration before use and was added to the medium for pre-processing for 6 h. A UVA lamp (UVP, USA) was used to irradiate UVA on cells, and the UVA wavelength was measured using a fiberoptic spectrometer system USB2000 (Ocean Optics, USA). The culture medium was removed from the cell culture tray, which was subsequently cleansed two times with phosphate-buffered saline (PBS, pH 7.4), and 1 mL PBS was added to the cleansed HDFs to prevent the cells from drying before UVA irradiation through the open lid of the cell culture dish. After irradiation, PBS was removed, a new medium was added, and the cells were incubated for 24 h and then used for the experiment.

Cell viability estimation
The cell survival rate was measured using the principle of water-soluble tetrazolium salt-1 (WST-1) assay, which is a measurement method for cell survival rate using formazan dye, generated by the reaction between mitochondrial dehydrogenase and water-soluble tetrazolium salts. After inoculation of HDFs (3×10^3 cells/well) on a 96-well plate and incubation for 24 h, hydroxytyrosol and UVA were treated in adequate concentrations and then cultured for 24 h. Further, 10 µL of the EZ-Cytox cell viability assay kit reagent (It's Bio, Korea) was added to the incubated cells, and 1 h later, the absorbance was measured using a microplate reader (Bio-Rad, USA). This experiment was repeated three times to calculate the mean and standard deviation of the cell survival rate.

RNA extraction and cDNA production
The incubated cells were dissolved in the Trizol reagent (Invitrogen, USA), and then 0.2 mL chloroform (Biopure, Canada) was added to react at room temperature. The supernatant fluid containing mRNA and infranatant fluid containing protein were separated by centrifugation for 20 min at 4 °C at 12000 rpm. Then, 0.5 mL isopropanol was added to the supernatant fluid, which was subsequently left to stand at room temperature for 10 min. Afterward, RNA was precipitated through centrifugation at 4 °C at 12,000 rpm, and it was cleansed with 75% ethanol and subsequently dried at room temperature with ethanol removed. RNase-free water was used to dissolve the dry mRNA that was used for the experiment. Nanodrop (Maestrogen, USA) was used to purify the extracted RNA, and only the RNA that exceeded the purity level, namely, a 260/280 nm ratio of 1.8, was used for the experiment. In order to produce cDNA from the extracted RNA, 1 µg RNA and 0.5 ng oligo dT18 were manufactured to total 10 µL in a PCR tube and then processed for

10 min at 70 °C to induce RNA denaturalization. M-MLV reverse transcriptase (Enzynomics, Korea) was used to synthesize cDNA through 1-h reaction at 37 °C.

Quantitative real-time PCR

The quantitative real-time PCR (qRT-PCR) was used to quantitatively analyze the gene expression changes in HDFs by hydroxytyrosol. A reaction solution was produced in qRT-PCR by mixing 0.2 μM primers, 50 mM KCl, 20 mM Tris/HCl pH 8.4, 0.8 mM dNTP, 0.5 U Extaq DNA polymerase, 3 mM MgCl, and 1X SYBR green (Invitrogen) in a PCR tube. PCR was carried out using LineGene K (BioER, China). The effectiveness of PCR was verified with a melting curve, and each gene expression was standardized with β-actin's expression for comparative analysis (Table 1).

Measurement of cellular aging

Senescence-associated β-galactosidase (SA-β-gal) assay was implemented to dye β-galactosidases (used as a cell aging biomarker) to measure HDF cell aging by UVA. SA-β-ga-lactosidase assay was incubated for 24 h after HDF (2×10^5 cells/well) incubation for 24 h with the senescence detection kit (Bio vision, USA). Afterward, hydroxytyrosol was treated in the concentrations of 5 and 10 μM and incubated for 24 h after 8 J/cm² UVA irradiation. The medium was removed from the incubated HDF, which was subsequently cleansed with 1 mL PBS and then added with 0.5 mL fixing solution, and then left at room temperature for 15 min to be immobilized. 0.5 mL mixed staining solution (staining solution 470 μL, staining supplement 5 μL, 20 mg/mL X-gal in dimethylformamide 25 μL) was added to the immobilized HDF to dye the cells through 24-h incubation at 37 °C. Afterward, the dyed cells were cleansed with PBS and measured with an optical microscope (Olympus, Japan) to analyze the ratio of aged cells.

Statistical process

Each independent experiment was repeated three times, and the results were shown in mean ± standard deviations.

Table 1 Lists of primers used in this study

Gene	Forward primer	Reverse primer
β-actin	GGATTCCTATGT GGGCGACGA	CGCTCGGTGAGG ATCTTCATG
MMP1	GGGCTTAGATCA TTCCTCAGTGCC	CAGGGTGACAC CAGTGACTGCAC
MMP3	GAGAGCAGAAG ACCGAAAGGA	CACAACACCAC GTTATCGGG
IL-1β	GATCCATTCTCC AGCTGCA	CAACCAAGTATT CTCCATG
IL-6	TAACAGTTCCTG CATGGGCGGC	AGGACAGGCAC AAACACGCACC
IL-8	CTCTCTTGGCAG CCTTCC	CTCAATCACTCT CAGTTCTTTG

The findings were verified through unpaired student's t tests and analyzed to be statistically significant when the p value was 0.05 or below.

Results
Cell viability analysis

Hydroxytyrosol was used to treat human dermal fibroblasts (HDFs) in the concentrations of 5, 10, 20, and 30 μM to determine the compound's cytotoxicity. As a result, the cell survival rate was 118% at 5 μM, 106% at 10 μM, 97% at 20 μM, and 100% at 30 μM. Therefore, it was concluded that hydroxytyrosol in a concentration of 30 μM or below is not cytotoxic. Therefore, the maximum concentration used for the experiment was 10 μM (Fig. 1).

The effect of hydroxytyrosol on anti-aging

In aged cells, oxygen free radicals increase, and protein and fat chromosomes are damaged by oxidative stress (Davalos et al. 2010a). Lysosome in normal cells shows β-galactosidase activity at pH 4.0, while that in aged cells shows the same activity at pH 6.0 (Wagner et al. 2001; Lee et al. 2006). Therefore, SA-β-galactosidase assay was used to measure the ratio of aged cells by calculating the numbers of all cells and dyed cells.

As a result, when HDFs were treated neither by hydroxytyrosol nor UVA, the β-galactosidase activity was 1, which rapidly increased to 7 when treated by UVA. Nevertheless, the activity decreased to 4 when treated by UVA after pre-processing of 5 μM hydroxytyrosol for 24 h and to 2.6 when treated by UVA after pre-processing of 10 μM, depending on the hydroxytyrosol concentration (Fig. 2).

The effects of hydroxytyrosol on MMP-1 and MMP-3 expressions

MMPs damage structural proteins at the dermis, which contains collagen and elastin, to induce wrinkles (Fagot et al. 2002). When the skin is irradiated by ultraviolet rays, MMP expression increases, leading to skin aging (Oh 2006).

This study examines the effects of hydroxytyrosol on the skin tissues in the dermis through MMP-1 and MMP-3 gene expression changes. MMP-1 expression that has been increased by 3.18 times by UVA consequently decreased by 1.59 and 1.14 times with 5 and 10 μM hydroxytyrosol, respectively, depending on concentration (Fig. 3a). MMP-3 expression is increased by 5.16 times by UVA and consequently decreased to 3.35 and 1.46 times with 5 and 10 μM of hydroxytyrosol, respectively, depending on the concentration (Fig. 3b).

The effects of hydroxytyrosol on IL-1β expression

The majority of skin-related diseases are accompanied by inflammation. Chronic inflammation not only aggravates

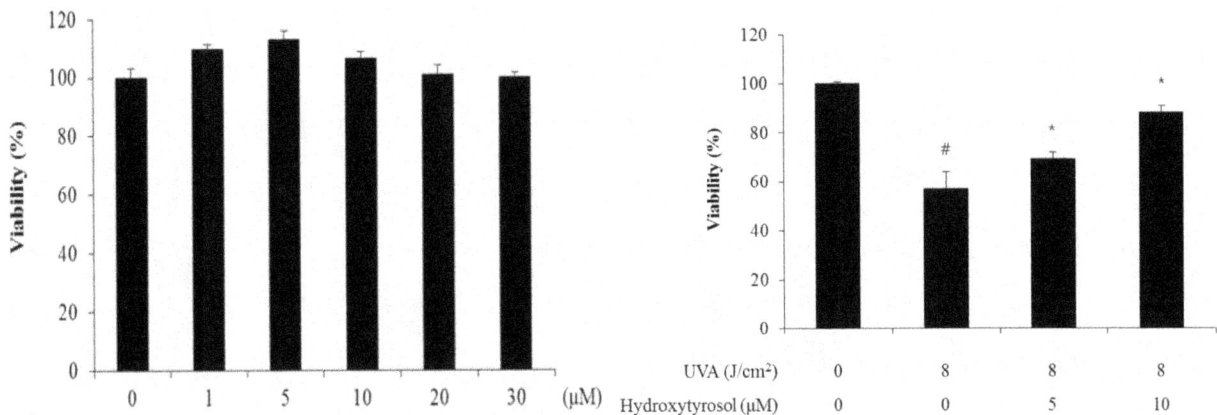

Fig. 1 Cytotoxicity of hydroxytyrosol on HDF. HDF (3×10^3 cells) were plated into a 96-well plate, cultured for 24 h, and pre-treated with hydroxytyrosol of various concentrations. After culturing it for 24 h, the cellular toxicity was measured by WST-1 analysis. The graph showed the averages of three experiments with error bars representing standard deviation (*$p < 0.05$)

but also accelerates aging (Abu et al. 2009; Shon et al. 2013; Lee et al. 2014). IL-1β is a pro-inflammatory cytokine that intervenes in a variety of inflammatory responses and stimulates the hypothalamic-pituitary-adrenal axis (HPA axis) to play an important role in tumor promotion and progression (Maes 2008).

This study examined how much hydroxytyrosol recovered *IL-1β* mRNA that had been increased by UVA. *IL-1β* mRNA in HDFs increased to 2.92 by treatment with UVA of 8 J/cm^2. This can be regarded as an increased inflammation by UVA. When hydroxytyrosol was added in concentrations of 5 and 10 μM to the group treated by UVA of 8 J/cm^2, *IL-1β* mRNA decreased to 2.13 and 1.54, respectively (Fig. 4a).

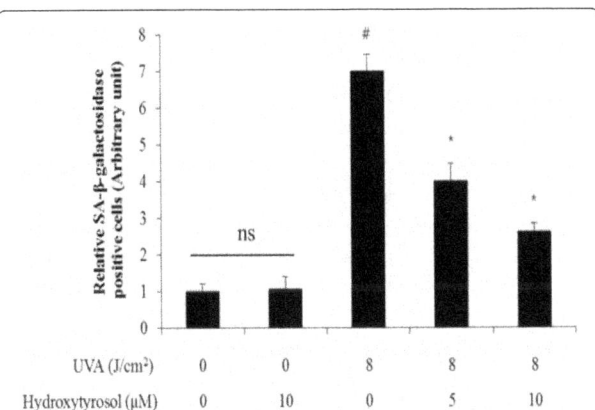

Fig. 2 Cell aging-inhibiting effects of hydroxytyrosol in UVA-irradiated HDF. HDF was cultured for 24 h and pre-treated with hydroxytyrosol of different concentrations for 6 h. Afterward, the cells were irradiated with UVA for 24 h. The SA-β-gal analytical method was used to measure aging. The staining solution was added to fixed cells for staining. The number of stained cells was counted to determine the aged cell ratio. The graph showed the averages of three experiments with error bars representing standard deviation (*$p < 0.05$)

The effects of hydroxytyrosol on *IL-6* expression

IL-6 is known as a cytokine formed from various cells, and it intervenes in cancer induction through various mechanisms, such as cellular multiplication, cell apoptosis inhibition, and promotion of the conversion from normal cells to cancer stem cells (Berner et al. 1998; Gasche et al. 2011; Hodge et al. 2005; Kim et al. 2013b).

This study examined how much hydroxytyrosol recovered *IL-6* mRNA that had been increased by UVA. *IL-6* mRNA in HDFs increased to 6.3 by treatment with UVA of 8 J/cm^2. This can be regarded as an increased inflammation by UVA. When hydroxytyrosol was added in concentrations of 5 and 10 μM to the group treated by UVA of 8 J/cm^2, *IL-6* mRNA decreased to 4.09 and 1.96, respectively (Fig. 4b).

The effects of hydroxytyrosol on *IL-8* expression

IL-8 is an inflammation-inducing chemokine that first reaches the area of tissue damage or microbial infection. It amplifies inflammation by mobilizing neutrophils and basophils to the inflamed part (Bachert et al. 1999).

This study examined how much hydroxytyrosol recovered *IL-8* mRNA that had been increased by UVA. *IL-8* mRNA in HDFs increased to 3.84 by treatment with UVA of 8 J/cm^2. This can be regarded as an increased inflammation by UVA. When hydroxytyrosol was added in concentrations of 5 and 10 μM to the group treated by UVA of 8 J/cm^2, *IL-8* mRNA decreased to 2.72 and 1.36, respectively (Fig. 4c).

Discussion

The inhibitive effects of hydroxytyrosol on human dermal fibroblasts aging by UVA

Cell aging generates mitochondria of various forms, reduces endoplasmic reticulum, and modifies Golgi apparatus (Dimri et al. 1995). Aged cells increase in size,

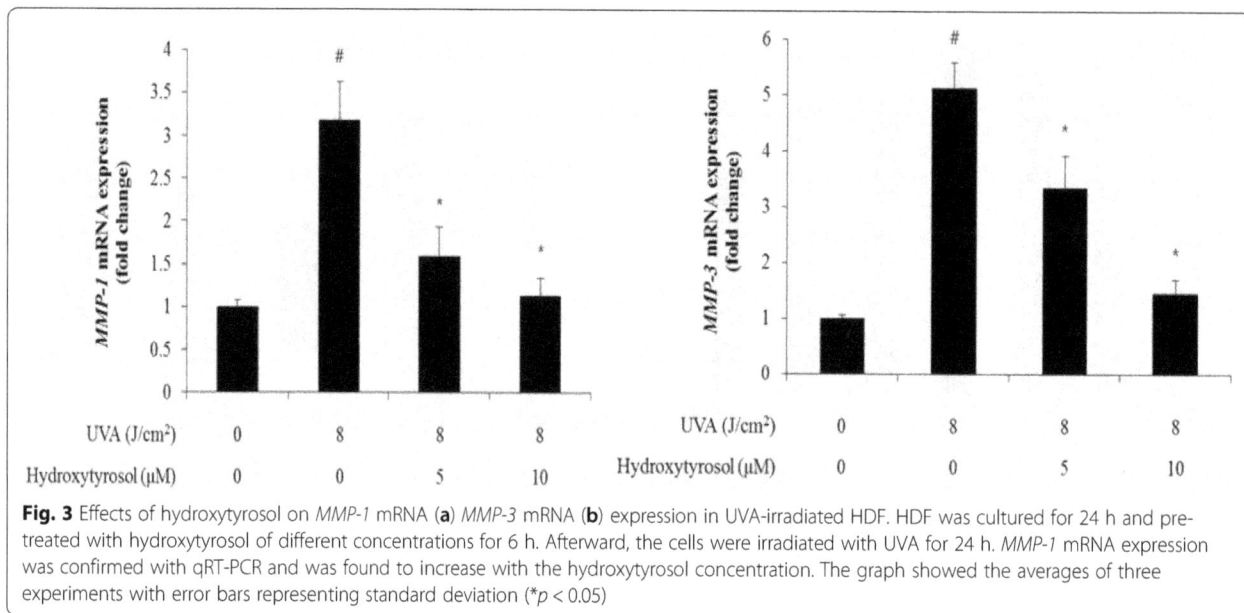

Fig. 3 Effects of hydroxytyrosol on *MMP-1* mRNA (**a**) *MMP-3* mRNA (**b**) expression in UVA-irradiated HDF. HDF was cultured for 24 h and pre-treated with hydroxytyrosol of different concentrations for 6 h. Afterward, the cells were irradiated with UVA for 24 h. *MMP-1* mRNA expression was confirmed with qRT-PCR and was found to increase with the hydroxytyrosol concentration. The graph showed the averages of three experiments with error bars representing standard deviation (*$p < 0.05$)

granule content, and SA-β-gal activities. In aged cells, the quantity of oxygen free radicals increases, and chromosome in protein and lipid is damaged by oxidative stress (Davalos et al. 2010b). Normal cells show β-galactosidase activity in pH 4.0 of the intracellular lysosome, while aged cells show β-galactosidase activity in pH 6.0 (Wagner et al. 2001; Lee et al. 2006). The aging effects of UVA on human dermal fibroblasts (HDFs) were examined using SA-β-galactosidase assay, an aging indicator. As a result, it was confirmed that β-galactosidase activity decreases depending on the increase in hydroxytyrosol concentration (Fig. 2). Therefore, these findings suggest that hydroxytyrosol cannot completely restore cell aging, but it reduces oxidative stress onto aged cells through to subsequently inhibit the progression of aging.

The effects of hydroxytyrosol on *MMP-1* and *MMP-3* expression in human dermal fibroblasts treated by UVA

MMPs damage structural proteins of the dermis, containing collagen and elastin, to increase wrinkles and intervene in aging (Fagot et al. 2002). In UV-irradiated skin, MMP expression increased, by which the constituents of skin tissues, including collagen, were intensely decomposed, ultimately leading to skin aging (Oh 2006). MMP-1 (interstitial or fibroblast collagenase) mainly decomposes collagen types 1, 2, and 3, which are the major constituents of atroma, while MMP-3 decomposes a broad array of extracellular matrix (ECM), as well as proteoglycan, laminin, fibronectin, gelatin, and collagen types 3 and 4 (Knauper et al. 1996). Therefore, *MMP* expression changes confirm the effect on the skin tissues

in the dermis to indicate the degree of skin aging. As a result of examining *MMP-1* and *MMP-3* mRNA expression changes that accelerate wrinkle formation, *MMP-1* and *MMP-3* mRNA expressions decreased by UVA depending on the concentration of hydroxytyrosol (Fig. 3). This is because collagen decomposition was accelerated by UVA that resulted in skin aging, and hydroxytyrosol reduced *MMP-1* and *MMP-3* mRNA expressions in a concentration-dependent manner to inhibit wrinkles in human dermal fibroblasts (HDFs) and protect skin from oxidative stress.

Anti-inflammatory effects of hydroxytyrosol on human dermal fibroblasts treated by UVA

IL-1β is known to intervene in various inflammatory responses, and it stimulates the hypothalamic-pituitary-adrenal axis (HPA axis) to play an important role in tumor promotion and progression through secretion of transposable elements and angiogenic factors (Maes 2008). *IL-6* is known as a cytokine produced by various cells including T lymphocytes, B lymphocytes, neuroepithelial cells, dendritic cells, macrophages, endothelial cells, and fibroblasts to play an important role in various inflammation diseases, including allergic rhinitis (Suzuki and Ikeda 2002). IL-8 is an inflammation-inducing chemokine that first reaches the area of tissue damage or microbial infection to mobilize neutrophils and basophils to the inflamed area and amplifies the inflammatory response (Bachert et al. 1999). This study examined the *IL-1β*, *IL-6*, and *IL-8* gene expression changes by treating the aged human dermal fibroblast by UV with hydroxytyrosol in different concentrations in order to

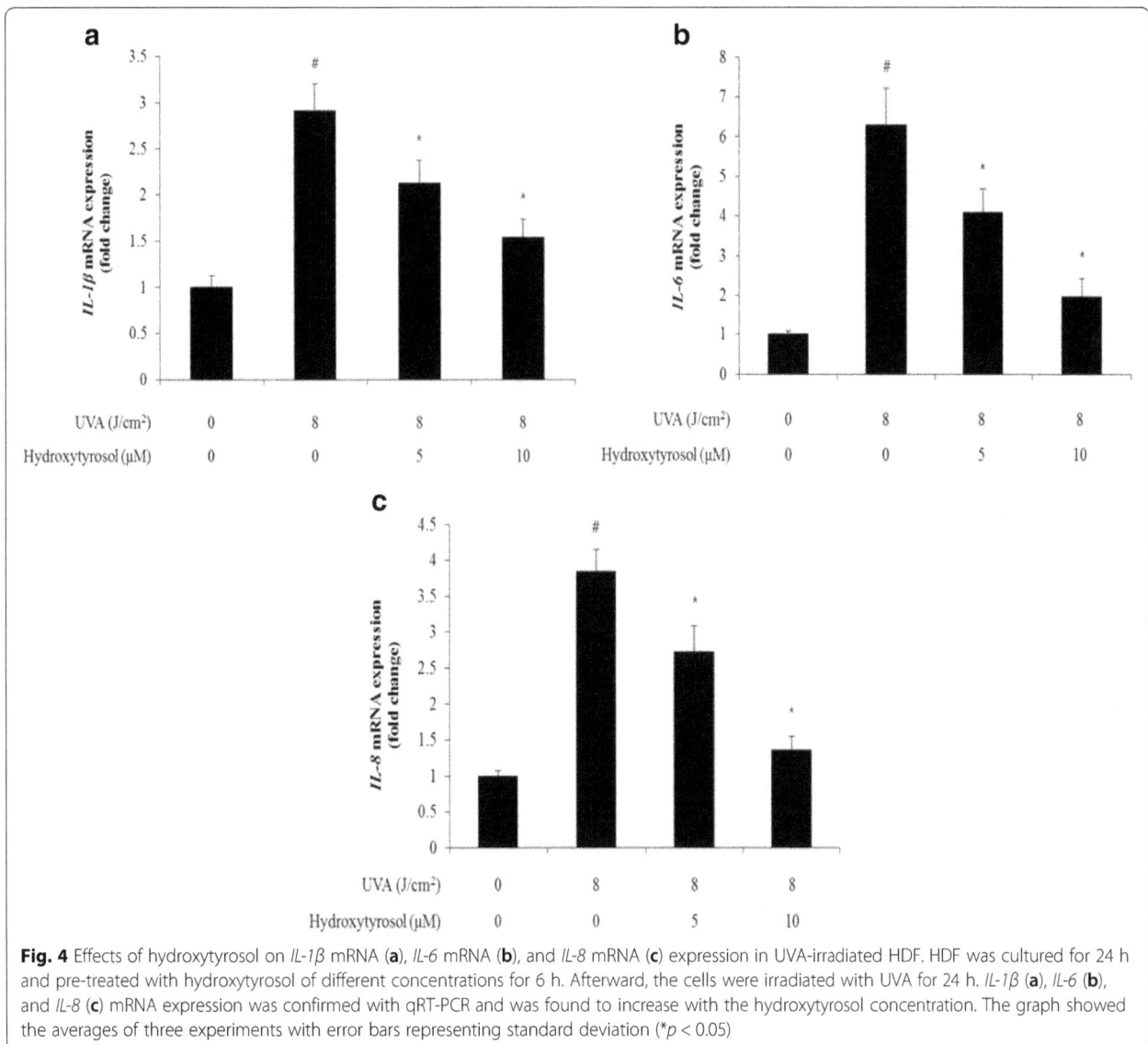

Fig. 4 Effects of hydroxytyrosol on *IL-1β* mRNA (**a**), *IL-6* mRNA (**b**), and *IL-8* mRNA (**c**) expression in UVA-irradiated HDF. HDF was cultured for 24 h and pre-treated with hydroxytyrosol of different concentrations for 6 h. Afterward, the cells were irradiated with UVA for 24 h. *IL-1β* (**a**), *IL-6* (**b**), and *IL-8* (**c**) mRNA expression was confirmed with qRT-PCR and was found to increase with the hydroxytyrosol concentration. The graph showed the averages of three experiments with error bars representing standard deviation (*$p < 0.05$)

identify the anti-inflammatory effects of hydroxytyrosol. The qRT-PCR technique was used to measure the changes, and it was concluded *IL-1β*, *IL-6*, and *IL-8* gene expressions decreased as the concentration of hydroxytyrosol increased (Fig. 4). These findings suggest the positive anti-inflammatory effects of hydroxytyrosol in human dermal fibroblasts (HDFs) damaged by UVA.

Conclusions

Hydroxytyrosol is found in olive fruit and oil as a major phenolic compound of olive oil. Due to its strong antioxidant effects, it has been studied in the fields of medicine, pharmaceuticals, and food (Poudyal et al. 2017; Lopez and Fonolla 2017; Visioli 2012). However, no study has been found on its effects on the skin. This study used a molecular biological mechanism to propose

the applicability of hydroxytyrosol as an anti-aging and anti-inflammatory ingredient.

First, senescence-associated β-galactosidase (SA β-Gal) activities were examined as an aging indicator. It was confirmed that when treated, hydroxytyrosol decreased its activity in a concentration-dependent manner and inhibited cell aging (Fig. 2). MMP expression changes affect the skin tissues in the dermis to indicate aging. Therefore, this study confirmed that increased *MMP-1* and *MMP-3* expressions by UVA (which accelerates wrinkle formations) decreased depending on the concentrations of hydroxytyrosol when treated (Fig. 3). The qRT-PCR technique was used to examine the effects on *IL-1β*, *IL-6*, and *IL-8* gene expressions as the pro-inflammatory cytokines that act as a catalyst of inflammatory responses. This study verified that as the concentration of hydroxytyrosol increased,

IL-1β, IL-6, and *IL-8* gene expressions decreased (Fig. 4). These findings show the anti-inflammatory effects of hydroxytyrosol in human dermal fibroblasts (HDFs) damaged by UVA.

Resultantly, this study confirmed the anti-aging and anti-inflammatory effects of hydroxytyrosol on the skin cells. Therefore, it will be applicable as an anti-aging and anti-inflammatory cosmeceutical ingredient for future clinical researches of products containing hydroxytyrosol.

Abbreviations

DMEM: Dulbecco's modified Eagle medium; DMSO: Dimethyl sulfoxide; FBS: Fetal bovine serum; HDFs: Human dermal fibroblasts; IL-1β: Interlukin-1 beta; IL-6: Interlukin-6; IL-8: Interlukin-8; MMP-1: Matrix metalloproteinase-1; MMP-3: Matrix metalloproteinase-3; PBS: Phosphate-buffered saline; qRT-PCR: Quantitative real-time polymerase chain reaction; SA-β-gal: Senescence-associated β-galactosidase; UV: Ultraviolet; WST: Water-soluble tetrazolium salts

Acknowledgements

Not applicable

Authors' contributions

MC did all of the research backgrounds such as experiments, data collection, and statistical analysis, and SJ wrote the draft manuscript. Both authors read and approved the final manuscript.

Competing interests

Both authors declare that they have no competing interests.

References

Abu SM, Noman NK, Ferdaus H, Imtiaz IEK, Jargalsaikhan D, Gantsetseg T, Shamima I, Yoshikazu N, Tomoaki Y, Takashi Y. Thalidomide inhibits lipopolysaccharide-induced tumor necrosis factor-a production via down-regulation of MyD88 expression. Innate Immunity. 2009;15:33–41.

Assefa Z, Van Laethem A, Garmyn M, Agostinis P. Ultraviolet radiation-induced apoptosis in keratinocytes: on the role of cytosolic factors. Biochim Biophys Acta. 2005;1755:90–106.

Bachert C, van Kempen M, Van Cauwenberge P. Regulation of proinflammatory cytokines in seasonal allergic rhinitis. Int Arch Allergy Immunol. 1999;118:375–9.

Berner R, Niemeyer CM, Leititis JU. Plasma levels and gene expression of granulocyte colony-stimulating factor, tumor necrosis factor-α, interleukin (IL)-1β, IL-6, IL-8, and soluble intercellular adhesion molecule-1 in neonatal early onset sepsis. Pediatr Res. 1998;44:469–77.

Bickers DR, Athar M. Oxidative stress in the pathogenesis of skin disease. J Investig Dermatol. 2006;126:2565–75.

Brenneisen P, Sies H, Scharffetter-Kochanek K. Ultraviolet-B irradiation and matrix metalloproteinases: from induction via signaling to initial events. Ann N Y Acad Sci. 2002;973:31–43.

Cabrerizo S, De La Cruz JP, López-Villodres JA, Muñoz-Marín J, Guerrero A, Reyes JJ, Labajos MT, González-Correa JA. Role of the inhibition of oxidative stress and inflammatory mediators in the neuroprotective effects of hydroxytyrosol in rat brain slices subjected to hypoxia reoxygenation. J Nutr Biochem. 2013;24:2152–7.

Choi NY, Lee JH, Shin HS. Antioxidant activity and nitrite scavenging ability of olive leaf (Olea europaea L.) fractions. Korean J. Food Sci. Thechnology. 2008;40:257–64.

Chung JH, Seo JY, Lee MK, Eun HC, Lee JH, Kang S, Fisher GJ, Voorhees JJ. Ultraviolet modulation of human macrophage metalloelastase in human skin in vivo. J Investig Dermatol. 2002;119:507–12.

Davalos AR, Coppe JP, Campisi J, Desprez PY. Senescent cells as a source of inflammatory factors for tumor progression. Cancer Metastasis Rev. 2010a;29:273–83.

Davalos AR, Coppe JP, Campisi J, Desprez PY. Senescent cells as a source of inflammatory factors for tumor progression. Cancer Metastasis Rev. 2010b;29:273–83.

Dimri GP, Lee G, Basile M, Acosta G, Scott C, Roskelley EE, Medrano M, Linskens I, Rubelj I, Pereira-Smith O. A biomarker that identifies senescent human cells in culture and in aging skin in vivo. Proc Natl Acad Sci. 1995;92:9363–7.

Facchini A, Cetrullo S, D'Adamo S, Guidotti S, Minguzzi M, Facchini A, Borzì RM, Flamigni F. Hydroxytyrosol prevents increase of osteoarthritis markers in human chondrocytes treated with hydrogen peroxide or growth-related oncogene α. PLoS One. 2014;9:e109724.

Fagot D, Asselineau D, Bernerd F. Direct role of human dermal fibroblasts and indirect participation of epidermal keratinocytes in MMP-1 production after UV-B irradiation. Arch Dermatol Res. 2002;93:576–83.

Fatima PM, Rui C, Susana F, Pedro F, Michael H. Effects of enrichment of refined olive oil with phenolic compounds from olive leaves. J Agric Food Chem. 2007;55:4139–82.

Fisher GJ, Wang ZQ, Datta SC, Varani J, Kang S, Voorhees JJ. Pathophysiology of premature skin aging induced by ultraviolet light. N Engl J Med. 1997;337:1419–28.

Gasche JA, Hoffmann J, Boland CR, Goel A. Interleukin-6 promotes tumorigenesis by altering DNA methylation in oral cancer cells. Int J Cancer. 2011;129:1053–63.

Guzik TJ, Korbut R, Adamek-Guzik T. Nitric oxide and superoxide in inflammation and immune regulation. J Physiol Pharmacol. 2003;54:469–87.

Ha JY, Choi HK, Oh MJ, Choi HY, Park CS, Shin HS. Photo-protective and anti-melanogenic effect from phenolic compound of olive leaf (Olea europaea L. var. Kalamata) extracts on the immortalized human keratinocytes and B16F1 melanoma cells. Food Sci Biotechnol. 2009;18:1193–8.

Hodge DR, Hurt EM, Farrar WL. The role of IL-6 and STAT3 in inflammation and cancer. Eur J Cancer. 2005;41:2502–12.

Jones DL, Rando TA. Emerging models and paradigms for stem cell ageing. Nat Cell Biol. 2011;13:506–12.

Kim MK, Lee KK, Jang AR. A study on cosmetic physiological activities of Sasa borealis root extracts. Kor. J. Aesthret. Cosmetol. 2013a;11:845–54.

Kim SY, Kang JW, Song X. Role of the IL-6-JAK1-STAT3-Oct-4 pathway in the conversion of non-stem cancer cells into cancer stem-like cells. Cell Signal. 2013b;25:961–9.

Kirkwood TB. Understanding the odd science of aging. Cell. 2005;120:437–47.

Kitani K, Minami C, Yamamoto T, Kanai S, Ivy GO, Carrillo MC. Pharmacological interventions in aging and age-associated disorders: potentials ofropargylamines forhuman use. Ann N Y Acad. 2002;959:259–307.

Knauper V, Lopez C, Smith B, Knight G, Murphy G. Biochemical characterization of human collagenase-3. J Biol Chem. 1996;271:1544–50.

Lee GY, Im DY. Skin-related biological activities of the extract and its fractions from Puerariae Flos. Kor J Aesthret Cosmetol. 2011;9:19–30.

Lee HJ, Sim BY, Bak JW, Kim DH. Effect of Gami-sopungsan on inflammation and DNCB-induced dermatitis in NC/Nga in mice. Kor J Orient Physiol Pathol. 2014;28:146–53.

Lee J, Jung E, Lee J, Huh S, Hwang CH, Lee HY, Kim EJ, Cheon YM, Hyun CG, Kim YS, Park D. Emodin inhibits TNF alpha-induced MMP-1 expression through suppression of activator protein-1(AP-1). Life Sci. 2006;79:2480–5.

Lopez H, Fonolla J. Hydroxytyrosol supplementation increases vitamin C levels in vivo. A human volunteer trial. Redox Biol. 2017;11:384–9.

Maes M. The cytokine hypothesis of depression: inflammation, oxidative & nitrosative stress (IO&NS) and leaky gut as targets for adjunative treatment in depression. Neuro Endocrinol Lett. 2008;29:287–91.

Moon CK, Park KS, Kim SG, Won HS, Chung JH. Brazilin protects cultured rat hepatocytes from BrCCl₃-induced toxicity. Drug Chem Toxicol. 1992;15:81–91.

Netzel S, Mitola DJ, Yanada SS, Holmbeck K. Collagen dissolution by keratinocytes requires cell surface plasmitogen activation are matrix metalloproteinase activity. J Biol Chem. 2002;277:451–4.

Oh JH. Role of PTEN in UVB-induced MMP secretion in cultured human dermal fibroblasts. Korea Advanced Institute of Science and Technology Thesis (doctoral), 2006.

Patel TN, Shishehbor MH, Bhatt DL. A review of high-dose statin therapy: targeting cholesterol and inflammation in atherosclerosis. Eur Heart J. 2007;28:664–72.

Poudyal H, Lemonakis N, Efentakis P, Gikas E, Halabalaki M, Andreadou I, Skaltsounis L, Brown L. Hydroxytyrosol ameliorates metabolic, cardiovascular and liver changes in a rat model of diet-induced metabolic syndrome: pharmacological and metabolism-based investigation. Pharmacol Res. 2017; 117:32–45.

Shon MS, Song JH, Kim JS, Jang HD, Kim GN. Anti-oxidant activity of oil extracted from Korean Red Ginseng and its moisturizing function. Kor J Aesthet Cosmetol. 2013;11:489–94.

Sinha RP, Haader DP. UV-induced DNA damaged and repair: a review. Photochem Photobiol Sci. 2002;1:225–36.

Sun L, Luo C, Liu J. Hydroxytyrosol induces apoptosis in human colon cancer cells through ROS generation. Food Funct. 2014;5:1909–14.

Suzuki H, Ikeda K. Mode of action of long-term low-dose macrolide therapy for chronic sinusitis in the light of neutrophil recruitment. Curr Drug Targets Inflamm Allergy. 2002;1:117–26.

Visioli F. Olive oil phenolics: where do we stand? Where should we go? J Sci Food Agric. 2012;9:2017–9.

Wagner M, Hampel B, Bernhard D, Hala M, Zwerschke W, Jansen DP. Replication senescence of human endothetial cells in vitro involves G1 areest, polyploidization and senescence associated apoptosis. Exp Gerontol. 2001;36: 1327–47.

Warleta F, Quesada CS, Campos M, Allouche Y, Beltrán G, Gaforio JJ. Hydroxytyrosol protects against oxidative DNA damage in human breast cells. Nutrients. 2011;3:839–57.

Wenk J, Brenneisen P, Meewes C, Wlaschek M, Peters T, Blaudschun R, Ma W, Kuhr L, Schneider L, Scharffetter-Kochanek K. UV-induced oxidative stress and photoaging. Curr Probl Dermatol. 2001;29:83–94.

22

Efficacy of Skinfill plus filler in the management of facial aging: a multicenter, post-marketing clinical study

Antonella Savoia[1], Nicoletta Onori[2] and Alfonso Baldi[3]* iD

Abstract

Background: Injectable dermal fillers are commonly used by physicians in the treatment of the signs of aging. The most commonly used dermal filler is hyaluronic acid. Skinfill plus (SFP) belongs to the family of monophasic monodensified fillers. In this post-marketing clinical study, we have evaluated the efficacy of SFP for the treatment of facial aging.

Methods: The study enrolled 109 patients in three different centers that were treated with various SFP fillers to treat facial aging. Analyses of the cosmetic effects were performed by using the Wrinkle Severity Rating Scale (WSRS) and the Global Aesthetic Improvement Scale (GAIS).

Results: Statistical analysis showed a significant effect on facial aging for all the SFP fillers used at all time-points studied. Moreover, a significant correlation was found, by analyzing the grade of facial aging, calculated by using the WSRS or the lifestyle of the patients (smokers or non-smokers) in relation to the cosmetic effects of the treatment.

Conclusions: The study confirms the good performance and safety of SFP for a range of facial indications in routine clinical practice.

Keywords: Dermal filler, Facial aging, Hyaluronic acid

Background

In recent years, injectable dermal fillers have challenged the use of more invasive esthetic surgical procedures, emerging into the armamentarium of products used by physicians in the treatment of the signs of aging (Brandt & Cazzaniga, 2008; Carruthers et al., 2009; Palm, 2014). The most commonly used dermal filler is hyaluronic acid (HA) (Lorenc et al., 2013). More than 1.6 million HA filler procedures were performed in 2014 in the USA, making it the second most commonly used non-surgical esthetic procedure after botulinum toxin. HA is a glucosaminoglycan biopolymer composed of strands of repeating chains of D-glucuronic acid and N-acetyl-D-glucosamine (Lee et al., 2015). It is a normal component of the extracellular matrix in humans as well as many other species. HA is commonly found in the muscle, synovial fluid, skin, and vitreous body of the eye, in the human body (Cheon et al., 2016). HA is extremely hydrophilic and can bind many times its own weight in water. These properties make it a lubricant and an important structural component of tissues. Moreover, HA, being highly biocompatible, displays a low incidence of antigenic adverse events (Lee et al., 2015). Nevertheless, in its natural state, HA shows reduced biomechanical properties as dermal fillers, because of its poor viscoelasticity and short half-life when injected into normal skin (Schante et al., 2011).

The first HA dermal fillers available on the market were biphasic fillers, made up by crosslinked particles suspended in a non-crosslinked HA matrix acting as a lubricant (Tran et al., 2014; Flynn et al., 2011). These products (e.g., Restylane®, Q-Med AB, Uppsala, Sweden, a wholly owned subsidiary of Galderma, Fort Worth, TX, USA; HA concentration 20 mg/mL) were manufactured with non-animal-stabilized hyaluronic acid (NASHA®) technology (Verpaele & Strand, 2006).

A large selection of HA dermal fillers have since been designed. In particular, monophasic monodensified fillers

* Correspondence: alfonsobaldi@tiscali.it
[3]Department of Environmental, Biological and Pharmaceutical Sciences and Technologies, Università degli Studi della Campania "L. Vanvitelli", Via Vivaldi, 43, 81100 Caserta, Italy
Full list of author information is available at the end of the article

do not undergo "sizing," a common phenomenon that happens when using biphasic gels and that disrupts the gel (Bogdan Allemann & Baumann, 2008). Indeed, they encompass a single phase of HA with a single density (Tran et al., 2014). Diverse families of monophasic monodensified fillers exist depending on the manufacturing technology; such is the case for Skinfill plus (SFP), which is the object of this article. In contrast to other monodensified fillers, SFP after crosslinkage is subjected to a micronization process. This process is carried out by injecting under pressure the material in a closed circuit in which it operates as a fluid (compressed air, superheated steam, inert gases) at a very high speed. The material particles, intimately mixed with the fluid, are dragged in the cycle. The continuous variations in speed and direction, due to the shape of the circuit, cause countless collisions among the particles themselves, which are thus subjected to repeated breaking actions. This process is called Coesix® and gives the extreme maneuverability and fluidity equivalent to the fillers which have the same concentration of HA and crosslinking agent. The final result is a gel with viscosity that is lower than that of other fillers used for the same indication. These properties provide a more homogeneous intradermal distribution of the material (Reinmüller, 2008). The SFP range of products offers different densities of HA (concentration ranging from 15 to 25 mg/mL) to suit different purposes regarding soft-tissue augmentation and rejuvenation. The objective of this paper is to describe the clinical evidence regarding the performance, tolerability, and safety of the SFP dermal fillers for soft-tissue augmentation and rejuvenation.

Methods
Skinfill

Skinfill plus (Promoitalia Group, Italy) is a pyrogen-free, colorless, transparent, viscoelastic, cohesive, and monophasic gel obtained by bacterial bio-fermentation and generated through crosslink of hyaluronate diluted in a solution buffered with phosphate (Schante et al., 2011). Skinfill plus is subjected to a physical process called micronization or micro-grinding, by crushing to very minute dimensions in the order of micrometers. The product is sterile and it is contained in two syringes of 1 mL each equipped with a needle of 30 or 27 G. Three variants (Silver, Gold, Diamond), which vary depending on the viscosity of the product, have been used in this protocol. In detail, (a) Silver is indicated for the correction of periocular wrinkles and it has to be injected in the superficial derma, (b) Gold is injected in the middle derma, and (c) Diamond is equipped with greater density and, therefore, indicated for the re-harmonization of facial contours, for the increase of soft tissues, and for the treatment of the folds of the nose genus furrow.

Patients

The study was conducted in accordance with the ethical standards of Good Clinical Practice, and the applicable sections of the national medical device law. All patients provided written informed consent before enrollment in the study. All the HA fillers of the SFP range were CE marked and were used as per labeling, that is, defects related to aging such as wrinkles, loss of volume, and treatment of wrinkles around the lips.

The inclusion criteria of the study were represented by a severe-moderate photo-aging. Moreover, they had to be free of diseases that could interfere in cutaneous aging evaluation and none of the patients had undergone other medical-aesthetical treatments (botulinic toxin, laser for skin resurfacing, intradermic RF) for the entire duration of the follow-up.

Criteria of exclusion from the study were as follows: previously received permanent implants; any facial surgery or invasive procedures such as laser therapy, chemical peeling, dermabrasion, and botulinum toxin injection, or treatment with dermal fillers in the same anatomical regions within the previous 12 months before enrollment; dermatological problem such as cutaneous lesions and hypertrophic scars; systemic diseases such as diabetes mellitus and connective tissue diseases or immune system disorders; a positive history for allergies to HA or cosmetic fillers; pregnant or lactating patients; patients taking any medication that in the investigator's judgment would prohibit inclusion in the study.

A total of 109 patients, predominantly women, aged 32 to 66 years, seeking esthetic treatment in the face were recruited from the investigators' patient pool. In detail, 21 patients have been treated with SFP Silver, 44 patients with SFP Gold, and 44 patients with SFP Diamond. The procedures, as well as the evaluations, were performed in three different centers by three different doctors.

Clinical evaluation

The clinical results have been based on two reference scales. The Wrinkle Severity Rating Scale (WSRS) scale which evaluates the condition of the wrinkle and, therefore, the degree of aging. This scale has been useful for grouping patients and for the follow-up at 6 and 9 months. The Global Aesthetic Improvement Scale (GAIS) supplies an instrument useful for the interpretation of the cosmetic result immediately after the first session, during the touch-up, at 3, 6, and 9 months. The WSRS and the GAIS are in turn supported by a photographic evaluation at 0, 3, 6, and 9 months. Finally, treated patients have filled a self-evaluation test to define the level of satisfaction.

Treatment procedure

The area to be treated was first cooled down with the application of ice for 10 min; then, local anesthesia was carried out with lidocaine topic at 2% an hour before the beginning of the filler procedure. Prior to treatment at the first visit (V1), patients' baseline characteristics were documented, and a severity assessment of the area to be treated was performed using the appropriate WSRSs. During this visit, the patients were treated in one or more areas of the face with the SFP HA filler(s) selected by the investigator according to their usual practice and patients' needs. The volume to be injected (up to a total of 2 mL) and the injection techniques were at the investigator's discretion. At a follow-up visit 14 days post-injection (V2), further assessments were performed, including optional touch-up injections, if required, in which case the same product as the one injected at V1 was used. The V2 follow-up visit coincided with the routine patient follow-up performed in clinical practice, typically scheduled for ~ 2 weeks after the initial treatment. Successively, the patients were re-checked at three (V3) and 9 months (V4) after the first treatment, to complete the follow-up.

All evaluations at a given site were carried out by the same investigator. Performance was assessed at rest using the GAIS at V1 (immediately post-injection) and at V2. In case of a touch-up injection at V2, the evaluation was performed prior to injection(s). For bilateral treatment, each side was scored separately. During the period of follow-up, also the eventual adverse reactions have been evaluated. Adverse reactions were defined as signs and symptoms linked to the injection of stabilized hyaluronic acid and in particular the following: reactions of hypersensitivity, inflammation, pain, hematomas in the injection site, and itching sensation. The incidence of reactions in the injection site has been evaluated after the first treatment session and during the 9 months of follow-up. The most common reactions observed during the follow-up have been the following: dyschromia, pustular rash, papules, and nodules.

Statistical analysis

Descriptive analysis was made using median values and 95% confidence interval (CI). The differences in the WSRSs and in the GAIS scores in the different time-points of each group were performed using Wilcoxon's test for nonparametric dependent continuous variables. Spearman Rho correlation tests were performed to define correlation between different parameters. SPSS software (version 17.00, SPSS, Chicago, USA) was used for statistical analysis. A p (two tailed) value of less than 0.05 was considered to indicate statistical significance.

Results

The treatment with the different fillers has caused minimum discomfort, without any post-treatment pain. All patients have returned to their daily accomplishments immediately after the treatment. In a small number of patients (10% of patients), hematomas have occurred and areas of hyperemia associated with itchiness or pain in case of pressure after the injection disappeared in a few days, following the application of anti-edemigen creams. Tables 1, 2, and 3 illustrate all the results obtained in this study using the WSRS and the GAIS described in the "Methods" section. The use of Skinfill plus Silver was limited to the correction of perioral and periocular wrinkles. It has determined an excellent therapeutic success in patients already at 15 days after the treatment with a statistically significant difference in the GAIS scores ($p = 0.0001$). In panels e and f of Fig. 1, an exemplificative case is shown. In the group of patients treated with Skinfill plus Gold, the injection was performed in the middle derma and resulted in an optimal cosmetic for the correction of facial wrinkles. The results were statistically significant starting from 15 days after the treatment ($p = 0.0001$). In panel c and d of Fig. 1, an exemplificative case is shown. The Skinfill plus Diamond is equipped with greater density and, therefore, was indicated for the re-harmonization of facial contours, for the increase of soft tissues and consequentially of the lips, and for the treatment of the folds of nose genus furrow. Its use has given good results with appreciable cosmetic effects, that were statistically significant already 15 days after the treatment ($p = 0.0001$). In panel a and b of Fig. 1, an exemplificative case is shown. To note, for all the filler used, the cosmetic effects were still visible and significantly different from time 0 to 9 months after the treatment ($p = 0.0001$). Interestingly, we performed also statistical analysis to define the correlation between the cosmetic effects still visible 9 months after the treatment and

Table 1 Wrinkle Severity Rating Scale (WSRS)

Score	Description	Number of patients at 15 days
5	Extreme	0 for Silver
		0 for Diamond
		0 for Gold
4	Severe	0 for Silver
		0 for Diamond
		0 for Gold
3	Moderate	1 for Silver
		4 for Gold
		6 for Diamond
2	Light	9 for Silver
		15 for Gold
		17 for Diamond
1	Absent	11 for Silver
		25 for Gold
		21 for Diamond

Table 2 Global Aesthetic Improvement Scale (GAIS); a total number of 109 patients were enrolled in the study

Score	Degree	Description	Number of patients at 15 days
1	Outstanding improvement	Excellent cosmetic result for the implant of the filler	11 for Silver
			21 for Diamond
			24 for Gold
2	Very improved	Marked improvement, but not completely excellent. A touch-up would improve the results.	9 for Silver
			17 for Diamond
			18 for Gold
3	Improved condition	An improvement compared to the initial condition but a touch-up is recommended.	1 for Silver
			6 for Diamond
			2 for Gold
4	Unaltered condition	The condition seems to be the same as the initial one.	0 for Silver
			0 for Diamond
			0 for Gold
5	Worsened condition	The appearance has worsened compared to the initial condition.	0 for Silver
			0 for Gold
			0 for Diamond

two different parameters: the grade of aging of the skin, as determined by the WSRS and the lifestyle of the patients (smokers or non-smokers). Indeed, we found a statistically significant inverse correlation, by using the Spearman correlation test for both parameters ($p = 0.023$ and $p = 0.024$). Finally, the self-evaluation test filled by the patients 9 months after the treatment confirmed the long-lasting good cosmetic effect of these procedures: 90% of the patients were within levels 1 and 2 of the scale (see Table 3)

Discussion

The performance of the filler is influenced by several rheological parameters such as the concentration of HA, the molecular weight, the crosslinking, and the elasticity and viscosity. The degree of crosslinking of a filler is instead related to its ability to retain water, and, then, to determine a post-treatment edema. It should also be considered that the physical-chemical properties (crosslinking, HA concentration, viscosity, etc.) also affect the stability and thus the longevity of the treatment, and, therefore, they involve medical assessments that take into account the specific patient and the specific problem to be treated. The Skinfill plus range ensures a variability of these parameters in order to select the most suitable characteristics for the treatment that will be run

Table 3 Self-evaluation test performed at the end of the treatment

Score 1 (Patient very satisfied)	56 patients
Score 2 (Patient satisfied)	44 patients
Score 3 (Patient not completely satisfied)	9 patients
Score 4 (Patient not satisfied)	0 patients

with a right balance between the physical and chemical characteristics of hyaluronic acid during the injection in order to minimize the occurrence of adverse events associated with it (Ginat & Schatz, 2012; Carruthers et al., 2010).

Regarding the concentration of the filler, the literature documents various concentrations, generally in the range of 1.5–3% (Brandt & Cazzaniga, 2008; Carruthers et al., 2009; Palm, 2014). The different concentrations are used to adapt the filler to the specific intended use and to the anatomical area. Indeed, the filler used in this study, has been formulated in three different concentrations to ensure a variable approach to different clinical conditions, as described in the "Methods" section. In fact, the different areas of the face vary in their underlying structures, requiring different product characteristics, injection volumes, and injection techniques.

This study enrolled 109 subjects who were predominantly women aged 32 to 66 years with severe-moderate photo-aging. The objectives of the study were to assess the safety and efficacy of Skinfill plus fillers in achieving significant correction in facial signs of aging and to assess whether these positive results obtained would persist over the 9-month duration of the study. This project was a multicenter, observational study in a clinical setting using three different crosslinked HA fillers of the Skinfill plus range. The choice of filler or their combination was based on the parameters defined in the "Methods" section. The study confirms the good performance and safety of SFP for a range of facial indications in routine clinical practice. The majority of patients showed an improvement on GAIS immediately after injection and after 9 months of observation posttreatment, when compared with the baseline. The percentage of responders was high for all facial

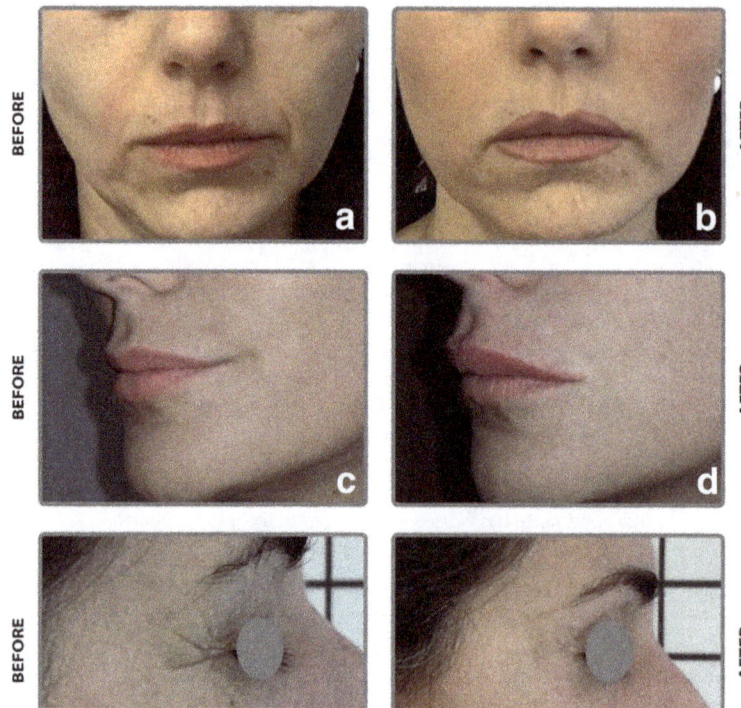

Fig. 1 Some examples of the results obtained with various Skinfill fillers on different body areas. **a** Patient at presentation with evident folds of nose genus furrow. **b** The same patients at 15 days of treatment with Skinfill Diamond. **c** Patient at presentation with wrinkles around lips. **d** The same patient at 6 months after treatment with SFP Gold. **e** Patient at presentation with periocular wrinkles. **f** The same patient at 9 months after treatment with Skinfill Silver

areas but was greatest for the lip area, followed by naso-labial folds.

Overall, patient satisfaction is a key parameter when evaluating the performance of dermal fillers, since esthetic interventions are optional and the patients play a decisive role in treatment choice. Our results, showing high patient satisfaction, corroborate the findings of several publications that show good patient outcomes, immediate results, and high satisfaction when using HA fillers for treatment of lines and wrinkles (Ginat & Schatz, 2012; Carruthers et al., 2010) and for volume restoration (Muhn et al., 2012). Volumes of < 8 mL were sufficient for optimal esthetic outcomes and this can be explained by the fact that SFP has optimal rheological properties and a homogeneous pattern of tissue integration after intra- or subdermal implantation (Goh et al., 2014; Tran et al., 2014).

The data collected during this study also support the good safety profile of the SFP HA fillers. The minor adverse events reported, such as redness, swelling, and bruising, are to be expected with any type of dermal filler injection and are usually temporary. The most common post-injection adverse event was edema of the lips. This could occur depending on the product used, the injector's experience, the vessel supply in the treated area, the injection technique, and/ or the speed of injection. The literature shows that crosslinked hyaluronic acid fillers are

considered safe and well tolerated, especially in cases where the HA is of bacterial origin (non-animal), and then characterized by a high biocompatibility (Savoia et al., 2011; Savoia et al., 2013).

Commonly observed adverse events are temporary, mild, and mainly related to the injection itself (burning, redness, itching, swelling, edema) (Brandt & Cazzaniga, 2008; Carruthers et al., 2009; Palm, 2014). Despite the high safety profile of hyaluronic acid, the literature documents rare isolated cases of more serious adverse events and/or delays such as granulomas of the skin at a distance up to 2 years after the first injection, which is not found in the follow-up of patients treated with SFP (Ginat & Schatz, 2012; Carruthers et al., 2010; Muhn et al., 2012).

Conclusions

In this context, the positive results and the good safety profile of the SFP HA fillers demonstrate the suitability of the fillers tested for comprehensive facial treatments in a normal clinical setting. Limitations of this study were the small number of patients in some of the treatment groups and the relatively short follow-up time. Moreover, it must be underlined the fact that GAIS and WSRS are commonly accepted scales to assess clinical efficacy of dermal fillers; nevertheless, they are essentially based on the subjective evaluation of the investigators and, consequently, can display significant bias. Considering also the fact that this was a single intervention cohort study, the results obtained, even if promising, must be confirmed and completed by further studies involving several cohorts of patients with a longer follow-up in order to better define the real efficacy of SFP for facial rejuvenation.

Abbreviations
GAIS: Global Aesthetic Improvement Scale; HA: Hyaluronic acid; SFP: Skinfill plus; WSRS: Wrinkle Severity Rating Scale

Acknowledgements
None

Funding
This research was partially supported by Promoitalia Group S.p.A.

Authors' contributions
AS performed some of the treatments and collected the data from the other centers; NO recovered the data and performed statistical analyses; AS together with AB conceived the work, analyzed the data, and wrote the paper. All authors read and approved the final manuscript.

Competing interests
AS and AB are scientific advisors of Promoitalia Group S.p.A.

Author details
[1]Buon Consiglio Hospital, Naples, Italy. [2]San Giovanni Addolorata Hospital, Rome, Italy. [3]Department of Environmental, Biological and Pharmaceutical Sciences and Technologies, Università degli Studi della Campania "L. Vanvitelli", Via Vivaldi, 43, 81100 Caserta, Italy.

References
Bogdan Allemann I, Baumann L. Hyaluronic acid gel (Juvederm) preparations in the treatment of facial wrinkles and folds. Clin Interv Aging. 2008;3:629–34.
Brandt FS, Cazzaniga A. Hyaluronic acid gel fillers in the management of facial aging. Clin Interv Aging. 2008;3:153–9.
Carruthers J, Cohen SR, Joseph JH, Narins RS, Rubin M. The science and art of dermal fillers for soft-tissue augmentation. J Drugs Dermatol. 2009;8:335–50.
Carruthers A, Carruthers J, Monheit GD, Davis PG, Tardie G. Multicenter, randomized, parallel- group study of the safety and effectiveness of onabotulinumtoxinA and hyaluronic acid dermal fillers (24-mg/ml smooth, cohesive gel) alone and in combination for lower facial rejuvenation. Dermatol Surg. 2010;36:2121–34.

Cheon C, Kim Y, Son S, Lee DY, Kim J, Kwon M, Kim Y, Kim S. Viscoelasticity of hyaluronic acid dermal fillers prepared by crosslinked HA microspheres. Polym. Korea. 2016;40:600–6.
Flynn TC, Sarazin D, Bezzola A, Terrani C, Micheels P. Comparative histology of intradermal implantation of mono and biphasic hyaluronic acid fillers. Dermatol Surg. 2011;37:637–43.
Ginat DT, Schatz CJ. Imaging Features of Midface Injectable Fillers and Associated Complications. AJNR Am J Neuroradiol PubMed PMID: 22837310 (2012)
Goh AS, Kohn JC, Rootman DB, Lin JL, Goldberg RA. Hyaluronic acid gel distribution pattern in periocular area with high-resolution ultrasound imaging. Aesthet Surg J. 2014;34:510–5.
Lee DY, Cheon C, Son S, Kim Y, Kim J, Jang J, Kim S. Influence of molecular weight on swelling and elastic behavior of hyaluronic acid dermal fillers. Polym Korea. 2015;39:976–80.
Lorenc ZP, Fagien S, Flynn TC, Waldorf HA. Review of key Belotero Balance safety and efficacy trials. Plast Reconstr Surg. 2013;132:33S–40S.
Muhn C, Rosen N, Solish N, et al. The evolving role of hyaluronic acid fillers for facial volume restoration and contouring: a Canadian overview. Clin Cosmet Investig Dermatol. 2012;5:147–58.
Palm MD. Filler frontier: what's new and heading West to the US market. Semin Cutan Med Surg. 2014;33:157–63.
Reinmüller J. Hyaluronsäure in der ästhetischen Medizin - Historie, Entwicklung, heutige Bedeutung [Hyaluronic acid in aesthetics - History, development, and today's importance]. J Dtsch Dermatol Ges. 2008;6:S4–9.
Savoia A, Vannini F, Baldi A. Radiofrequency waves with filling and peeling substances: An innovative minimally invasive technique for facial rejuvenation. Dermatol Ther (Heidelb). 2011;1:2–10.
Savoia A, Landi S, Baldi A. A new minimally invasive mesotherapy technique for facial rejuvenation. Dermatol Ther (Heidelb). 2013;3:83–93.
Schante CE, Zuber G, Herlin C, Vandamme TF. Chemical modifications of hyaluronic acid for the synthesis of derivatives for a broad range of biomedical applications. Carbohydr Polym. 2011;85:469–89.
Tran C, Carraux P, Micheels P, Kaya G, Salomon D. In vivo bio-integration of three hyaluronic acid fillers in human skin: a histological study. Dermatology. 2014; 228:47–54.
Verpaele A, Strand A. Restylane SubQ, a non-animal stabilized hyaluronic acid gel for soft tissue augmentation of the mid- and lower face. Aesthet Surg J. 2006;26:S10–7.

23

Verification of air brush effectiveness using cosmeceutical ingredients

Hyun Jung Kim, Min Sook Jung*⑩, Jeong Min Shin and Yu Kyung Hur

Abstract

Background: The development of the beauty industry has been accelerated by the combination of the basic desire of humans to look beautiful and the trend of the age in which the down-aging phenomenon is caused by an aging society. Previously, therapy, which has been provided by experts, has now expanded and changed its category into everyday home care. Thus, skin care devices became common and widespread. Also, public attention has been focused on functional cosmetics such as whitening and wrinkling improvements of a home care product. However, the results of validation of the effectiveness of functional components and the use of skin care devices are rare.

Methods: Middle-aged women were asked to apply 3 mL of ampule containing niacinamide 2% and adenosine 0. 04% to the face twice a day, once in the morning and the other in the evening, for 4 weeks. The control group (C) was asked to apply using hands while the experimental group (E) was asked to apply using airbrush.

Results: The moisture content of the entire face has increased in all clusters, resulting from a combination of the moisture content of the niacinamide and the increase in the collagen content of the adenosine. L* was increased in all groups, but only E showed significant results. a* was increased in C and showed a significant decrease in E only. b* decreased in group C and increased in group E. The overall size of the wrinkles, the depth of the wrinkles, and the width of the wrinkles showed significant improvements in all groups, with higher rates of improvement in E.

Conclusions: This study produced verification results on whitening effects of niacinamide, wrinkling improvement of adenosine, and the usefulness of air brushes. Previously, dermal absorption studies on soluble ingredients of cosmetics were limited to iontophoresis, while various methods of study design on the dispensing and physical effects of fine particles were expected. It also recommends a research design approach that is practical for home care, rather than approach using a professional program on the usefulness of skin care device.

Trial registration: Korea National Institute for Bioethics Policy, P01-201711-13-002, registered 16 November 2017, http://public.irb.or.kr/.

Keywords: Airbrush, Niacinamide, Adenosine, Skin care device, Cosmeceutical ingredient

Background

Entering the 2000s, the general public identified looks as a new differentiating factor, unlike conventional factors such as race, gender, religion, and ideology. Along with this, the term *lookism* emerged, which refers to appearance-oriented views, through a column published in The New York Times in 2000 (Safire 2000). The criteria for the ideal "modern look" have been standardized and disseminated via mass media and are now used as important tools that enable individuals to be recognized (Kim et al. 2005; Kim 2006; Lee and Kim 2015).

Moreover, South Korean society is rapidly aging. In 2020, the country's elderly population will account for over 14% of the total population. Therefore, modern Koreans who look to a centenarian era still intend to convey an image of high economic activity, regardless of their actual ages. Accordingly, this desire can drive an individual to attempt to look younger than his or her chronological age. This is referred to as the *down-aging phenomenon* (Jo and Hwang 2013).

* Correspondence: yunhai0540@naver.com
Dasan Skin Clinical Research Center, Dasan C & Tech, 42, Eonju-ro 81-gil, Gangnam-gu, Seoul 06223, Republic of Korea

Down-aging has accelerated the growth of the beauty industry in conjunction with an increasing demand for physical beauty. In the past, plastic surgeons were the primary providers of a range of services, from skin care and therapies to surgical treatments. Today, these treatments have penetrated the daily home care market. Skin care devices that are popularized and widely distributed throughout the general public include exfoliating devices, vibrating cleansers, galvanic devices, and light-emitting diode (LED) masks.

In addition, there is a new emphasis on functionality in the beauty industry as exemplified by generalization of products with whitening and anti-wrinkle functions, even including cosmetics such as air cushions. In 2001, functional cosmetics were established as an official category of cosmetics through enactment of regulations thus securing a legal status (Kim et al. 2014). Along with continuous legal amendments, as of May 2017, cosmetic functionalities, which were previously limited to whitening, anti-wrinkle, and sunscreen products, were broadened to encompass cosmetics for dyeing, bleaching, hair loss prevention, acne, atopy, and stretch mark care.

While the present study used niacinamide and adenosine, which are anti-wrinkle functional substances, few domestic studies have verified the effectiveness of these ingredients outside of the whitening function. Moreover, despite the launch of a variety of new skin care devices, little research has been done on their effectiveness.

Therefore, the present study aimed to analyze the effects of functional ingredients, niacinamide and adenosine, on skin physiology using an air brush skin care device, thereby examining the overall usefulness of air brushes for skin care.

Methods

This study was approved by the Institutional Review Board of the Korea National Institute for Bioethics Policy following a comprehensive review of study-related procedures (P01-201711-13-002).

Subjects

This study involved middle-aged women in their 30s–50s, who showed symptoms of hyperpigmentation (e.g., stains, freckles) and wrinkles around the eyes. They were divided into an experimental group (group E; $n = 10$) and a control group (group C; $n = 10$). The subjects were selected based on the guidelines for evaluating the effectiveness of functional cosmetics suggested by the Ministry of Food and Drug Safety (MFDS) and the results of a study conducted by Lee et al. (2013).

Exclusion criteria were as follows: (1) those who showed abnormal symptoms such as acute and chronic physical diseases involving the face, including facial skin diseases; (2) those with at least a 1-month history of facial application of a skin care product containing steroids; (3) those with medical histories of contact or photoallergic dermatitis caused by a topical ointment; and (4) those with sensitive or hypersensitive skin. In addition, the subjects were randomly divided into different clinical groups so as to minimize any variations in the experimental results.

The study was conducted between November 20, 2017, and February 5, 2018. The subjects were provided with a 3-mL test agent and instructed to apply it to their skin twice a day, once in the morning and once in the evening, over a 28-day period. They were instructed to wash their faces, smooth out their skin with a toner, and then apply the agent on their face. Group C subjects applied the test agent using their hands, whereas group E subjects applied the test agent using an air brush and left it to be absorbed without using their hands. All subjects were monitored by the researchers and were instructed to record the daily applications in a self-care chart that was later submitted to ensure compliance with test procedures. In addition, we requested they avoid other skin care or treatment modalities over the research period, including the use of cosmetics that could change their facial skin conditions. Subjects were also instructed to make no changes to their typical daily living routines. The subjects were completely informed that they should not use cosmetics that contained whitening or anti-wrinkle functional ingredients that could change their facial skin conditions during the research period, and they consented to do so. Moreover, based on a study conducted by Han et al. (2015), the subjects were allowed to use sunblock when going outside and wear light makeup and maintain their usual skin care cosmetics or makeup habits. However, they were instructed to not make any changes in their daily living patterns, such as exercise, because changes in living patterns could affect their skin conditions.

Regarding the measurement of facial skin conditions, a study conducted by Kim (2007) reported that at least 30 min of skin stabilization is necessary to measure all selected variables for the skin surface: temperature, color luminosity, transepidermal water loss, and oil. The study also reported that consistent measurement values could be obtained through skin stabilization regardless of environmental effects. Accordingly, skin stabilization was induced to all subjects in the present study for 30 min after facial wash, and all subjects underwent skin measurement. Nonetheless, to minimize any environmental effect, the skin measurement was performed indoors at temperatures between 20 and 24 °C and relative humidity levels between 40 and 60% based on a study conducted by Kim and Gang (2017).

All subjects underwent skin measurement before and after the experiment. All skin measures took place 30 min after facial washing to encourage skin stabilization. Additionally, group E subjects were trained by the researcher in the operation of the air brush at their first visit. The spraying method was based on the principle of lymphatic massage.

Research materials

The test agent administered to groups C and E is described in Table 1 and consisted of 2.00% niacinamide and 0.04% adenosine. Niacinamide is recognized as a whitening ingredient and adenosine as an anti-wrinkle ingredient by the MFDS. The test agent was considered safe for daily use. Niacinamide, which is used as a whitening functional ingredient, was purchased from company B as a 100% powder form, whereas adenosine, which is used as an anti-wrinkle functional ingredient, was purchased from company A in an undiluted form. According to the Globally Harmonized System of Classification and Labelling of Chemicals, these purchased ingredients were confirmed as identical with "niacinamide" and "adenosine" listed in the International Nomenclature of Cosmetic Ingredients. In addition, 2.00% niacinamide and 0.04% adenosine were applied to formulate the test agent in consideration of the subjects' stability pursuant to the notifications of the MFDS. The test agent was manufactured as 6 ml ampules and was provided to the subjects to ensure easier use, which is to apply one ampule each day. The main goal of the experiment was to have the subjects use accurate volumes of the test agent.

Research tools

The air brush (M66, Dasan C & Tech., Korea) used for this study consisted of a spray gun, air compressor, air hose, and adapter. It is shown in Fig. 1.

Spray gun

After putting liquid into the container and pulling the lever, a needle is pulled. This creates a space in the nozzle, and the liquid is mixed with the air that is injected by the compressor. This mixture of liquid and air is propelled from the device. With the spray gun used in this study, the stronger the lever is pulled, the greater is the volume of air exposure. Consequently, more liquid is sprayed. The spray gun's nozzle size is 0.35 mm.

Air compressor

This component delivers compressed air to the spray gun. The pressure of the air that is injected by the air compressor is approximately 0.7 kgf/cm^2.

Air hose

The air hose transmits the air from the air compressor to the spray gun, connecting the air compressor outlet with the spray gun inlet.

Adapter

Input: AC 100–240 V, 50–60 Hz, 1.5 A.
  Output: DC 13 V, 1.5 A.

  The air brush is rechargeable, with a charging time of approximately 2 h. It can be used for approximately 60 min after a single charge. The amount of battery life is indicated with LED lights.

Skin measurement tools

In this study, the SKIN-O-MAT (CORNEOMETER, SEBUMETER, SKIN-pH-METER, Cosmomed, Germany) was used to measure skin moisture levels, and the DSM II ColorMeter (DSM II ColorMeter reflectance test unit, Cortex Technology, Denmark) was used to measure skin color and luminosity. In addition, Antera 3D (Antera 3D CS, Miravex Limited, Ireland) imaged the deepest wrinkles in the lower orbit of the eye and measured wrinkle length, depth, and width.

Data analysis methods

SPSS 24.0 for Windows (IBM, New York, USA) was used to analyze all data. An independent t test was performed to test homogeneity between the two groups before the experiment, and a paired t test was used to analyze any changes before and after the experiment. In addition, a paired t test was conducted to identify the subjects' satisfaction with the condition of their skin before and after the experiment.

Table 1 Cosmetic ingredients applied to the group

Variable	Base		Active		Total unit (%)
	Ingredient	Quantity (%)	Ingredient	Quantity (%)	
C/E group	Water	87.36	Niacinamide	2.00	100
	Glycerin	3.00	Adenosine	0.04	
	Butylene glycol	5.00			
	PEG-60 hydrogenated castor oil	0.50			
	Isopropyl myristate	0.10			
	1,2-Hexanediol	2.00			

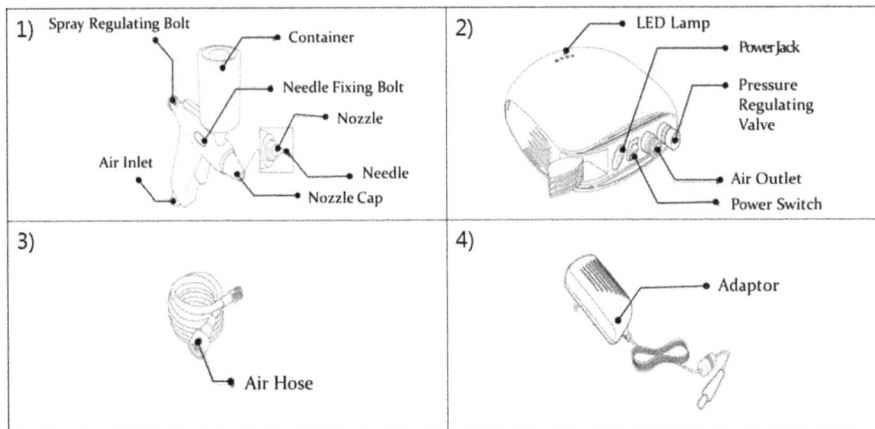

Fig. 1 (1) Air spray—put the liquid in the container and pull the lever to spray the liquid; the amount of injection can be adjusted according to the strength of pulling the lever. (2) Air compressor—the air compressor compresses a certain amount of air and delivers it to the spray gun. (3) Air hose—the air from the air compressor is supplied with the spray gun. (4) Adapter—its function is to charge the air compressor

Results

1. Verification of homogeneity between the groups
   Subjects' baseline facial skin conditions are presented in Table 2. Because these results did not show statistically significance differences between the two groups, pre-treatment group homogeneity was confirmed ($p > .05$).
2. Changes in skin moisture level in each group
   Skin moisture level changes for groups C and E are shown in Table 3. On the forehead surface, group C showed a significant increase of 4.76(M) in mean moisture content, from 59.60(M) to 64.37(M) post-treatment ($p < .05$). Group E showed an increase of 4.67(M) in mean moisture content, from 61.00(M)

to 65.68(M) post-treatment. On the chin surface, group C showed a mean moisture increase of 1.88(M), from 62.57(M) to 64.45(M), and group E showed an increase of 2.15(M), from 63.47(M) to 65.62(M). For the right cheek, the mean moisture increase for group C was 2.66(M), from 67.60(M) to 70.27(M) post-treatment, and that for group E was 4.44(M), from 64.85(M) to 69.29(M). For the left cheek, group C showed an increase of 5.05(M), from 64.81(M) to 69.86(M), and group E showed an increase of 4.16(M), from 65.80(M) to 69.97(M).
3. Changes in skin color luminosity in each group
   Changes in skin color luminosity for groups C and E are presented in Figs. 2 and 3. Group C showed an increase of brightness in the region of the upper-

Table 2 Verification of homogeneity between C and E groups

Variable			C (n = 10) M ± SD	E (n = 10) M ± SD	t	p
Moisture	Forehead		59.60 ± 8.12	61.00 ± 6.38	− .429	.673
	Jew		62.57 ± 6.15	63.47 ± 8.57	− .268	.792
	Rt. Cheek		67.60 ± 5.82	64.85 ± 7.18	.941	.359
	Lt. Cheek		64.81 ± 10.51	65.80 ± 8.97	− .226	.824
Skin Color Value	Rt. Lid Cheek	L*	35.77 ± 5.00	36.64 ± 3.60	− .446	.661
		a*	18.20 ± 1.77	18.89 ± 2.82	− .652	.523
		b*	16.05 ± 2.96	17.10 ± 3.11	− .778	.447
	Lt. Lid Cheek	L*	36.86 ± 3.47	35.81 ± 3.37	.690	.499
		a*	18.53 ± 1.40	19.90 ± 2.09	− 1.722	.102
		b*	16.29 ± 1.76	15.66 ± 3.38	.519	.610
Wrinkle	Overall size		12.98 ± 5.08	13.21 ± 4.98	−.102	.920
	Depth		0.049 ± 0.013	0.055 ± 0.018	−.802	.433
	Width		1.13 ± 0.18	0.97 ± 0.28	1.461	.161

Abbreviations: *C* control group, *E* experimental group, *M* mean, *SD* standard deviation

Table 3 Comparison of facial moisture (index: AU)

Variable	Group	Measurement (M ± SD)		t_1-t_2	t (p)	
		Before	After			
Forehead	C ($n = 10$)	59.60 ± 8.12	64.37 ± 5.83	− 4.76 ± 6.60	− 2.284	(.048*)
	E ($n = 10$)	61.00 ± 6.38	65.68 ± 5.96	− 4.67 ± 8.01	− 1.846	(.098)
Jew	C ($n = 10$)	62.57 ± 6.15	64.45 ± 4.56	− 1.88 ± 7.31	− .813	(.437)
	E ($n = 10$)	63.47 ± 8.57	65.62 ± 5.27	− 2.15 ± 7.10	− .959	(.363)
Rt. Cheek	C ($n = 10$)	67.60 ± 5.82	70.27 ± 4.86	− 2.66 ± 5.06	− 1.663	(.131)
	E ($n = 10$)	64.85 ± 7.18	69.29 ± 4.78	− 4.44 ± 6.54	− 2.147	(.060)
Lt. Cheek	C ($n = 10$)	64.81 ± 10.51	69.86 ± 5.20	− 5.05 ± 10.39	− 1.537	(.159)
	E ($n = 10$)	65.80 ± 8.97	69.97 ± 5.04	− 4.16 ± 8.01	− 1.645	(.134)

*$p < .05$
Abbreviations were the same as Table 2.

right cheekbone of 11.0%, from 35.77(M) to 39.71(M) post-treatment, and group E exhibited a statistically significant increase of 6.6%, from 36.64(M) to 39.06(M) ($p < .05$). In terms of red color intensity in the same region, group C showed an increase of 0.2%, from 18.20(M) to 18.23(M) post-treatment, and group E showed a statistically significant decrease of 16.3%, from 18.89(M) to 15.80(M) ($p < .05$). In terms of yellow color intensity in the same region, group C showed a decline of 4.4%, from 16.05(M) to 15.34(M) post-treatment, whereas group E exhibited an increase of 5.9%, from 17.10(M) to 18.11(M). In terms of the level of brightness in the upper-left cheekbone, group C showed an increase of 4.2%, from 36.86(M) to 38.42(M) post-treatment, and group E exhibited a statistically significant increase of 8.3%, from 35.81(M) to 38.81(M) ($p < .05$). In terms of red

color intensity in the same region, group C showed an increase of 2.9%, from 18.53(M) to 19.06(M) post-treatment, and group E exhibited a statistically significant increase of 18.0%, from 19.90(M) to 16.30(M) ($p < .001$). Meanwhile, group C showed a decrease of 8.1%, from 16.29(M) to 14.96(M) post-treatment, and group E showed a statistically significant increase of 15.9%, from 15.66(M) to 18.16(M) ($p < .05$) in yellow color intensity in the same region.

4. Changes in main wrinkles in each group
The changes in wrinkles around the left eye for groups C and E are shown in Table 4 and Fig. 4. In group C, the size of the main wrinkles significantly decreased by 16.6%, from 12.98(M) to 10.83(M) post-treatment ($p < .01$). In group E, there was a statistically significant decrease of 20.9%, from 13.21(M) to 10.45(M) ($p < .01$). In group C, the

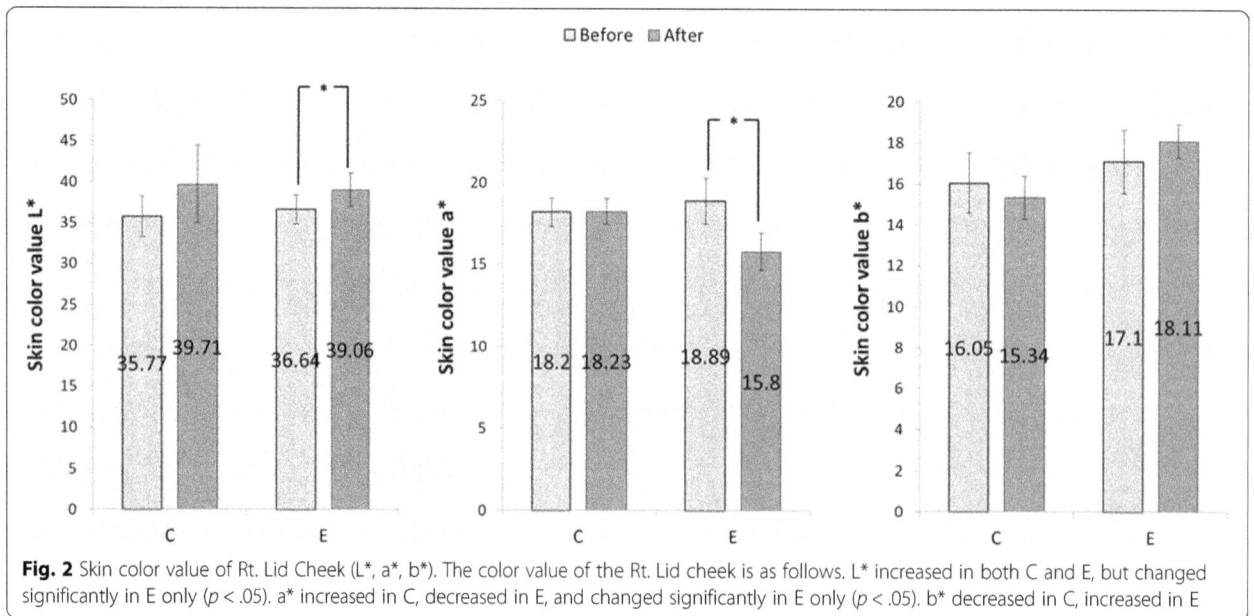

Fig. 2 Skin color value of Rt. Lid Cheek (L*, a*, b*). The color value of the Rt. Lid cheek is as follows. L* increased in both C and E, but changed significantly in E only ($p < .05$). a* increased in C, decreased in E, and changed significantly in E only ($p < .05$). b* decreased in C, increased in E

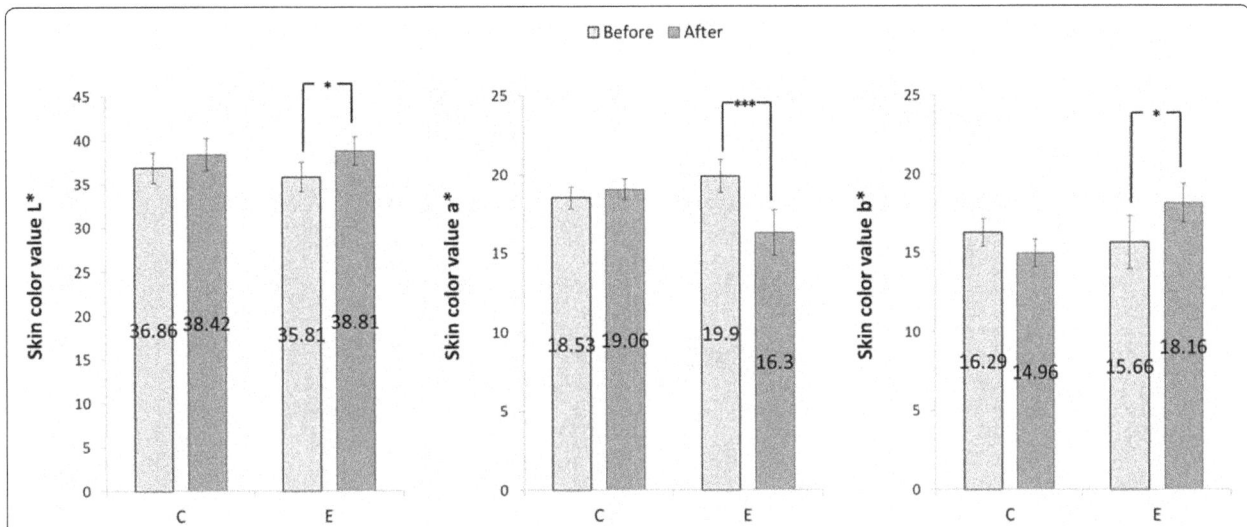

Fig. 3 Skin color value of Lt. Lid Cheek (L*, a*, b*). The color value of the Lt. Lid cheek is as follows. L* increased in both C and E, but changed significantly in E only ($p < .05$). a* increased in C, decreased in E, but changed significantly in E only ($p < .001$). b* decreased in C, increased in E, and changed significantly in E only ($p < .05$)

depth of the main wrinkles significantly decreased by 10.2%, from 0.049(M) to 0.043(M) post-treatment ($p < .05$). In group E, the depth significantly decreased by 12.7%, from 0.055(M) to 0.047(M) ($p < .05$). In group C, the width of the main wrinkles significantly decreased by 8.0%, from 1.13(M) to 1.04(M) post-treatment ($p < .01$). In group E, the width significantly decreased by 9.3%, from 0.97(M) to 0.88(M) ($p < .01$). Consequently, both groups showed statistically significant improvements in the overall size, depth, and width of the main wrinkles. However, group E achieved relatively more improvement in all variables compared to group C, which may point to the effectiveness of the air brush.

5. Changes in subjective satisfaction with skin conditions in each group

The reliability of the satisfaction evaluation tool used in this study is presented in Table 5. And

subjective satisfaction ratings are presented in Table 6. The selected items were scored based on a 5-point scale as follows: 1 point for "very unsatisfied," 2 points for "unsatisfied," 3 points for "average," 4 points for "satisfied," and 5 points for "very satisfied." A higher score corresponds to a higher level of satisfaction. In addition, the same items were administered to each subject pre- and post-treatment to treatment-related changes in perceived satisfaction.

In the items related to skin dryness and tightness, group C registered a statistically significant increase of 1.60(M) in satisfaction, from 2.20(M) to 3.80(M) post-treatment ($p < .01$). Group E also showed significant increase by 1.90(M), from 2.21(M) to 4.00(M) ($p < .01$). On items related to the formation of dead skin cells, group C showed a statistically significant increase of 1.40(M) in satisfaction, from 2.80(M) to 4.20(M) ($p < .01$) post-treatment. Group E also exhibited a statistically significant

Table 4 Comparison of facial wrinkle

Variable	Group	Measurement (M ± SD) Before	After	t_1-t_2	t (p)	
Overall size (AU)	C (n = 10)	12.98 ± 5.08	10.83 ± 5.19	2.15 ± 1.36	4.984	(.001**)
	E (n = 10)	13.21 ± 4.98	10.45 ± 4.03	2.76 ± 2.51	3.478	(.007**)
Depth (mm)	C (n = 10)	0.049 ± 0.013	0.043 ± 0.016	0.005 ± 0.006	3.023	(.014*)
	E (n = 10)	0.055 ± 0.018	0.047 ± 0.014	0.007 ± 0.009	2.475	(.035*)
Width (mm)	C (n = 10)	1.13 ± 0.18	1.04 ± 0.21	0.09 ± 0.07	4.150	(.002**)
	E (n = 10)	0.97 ± 0.28	0.88 ± 0.25	0.09 ± 0.06	5.010	(.001**)

*$p < .05$, **$p < .01$
Abbreviations were the same as Table 2

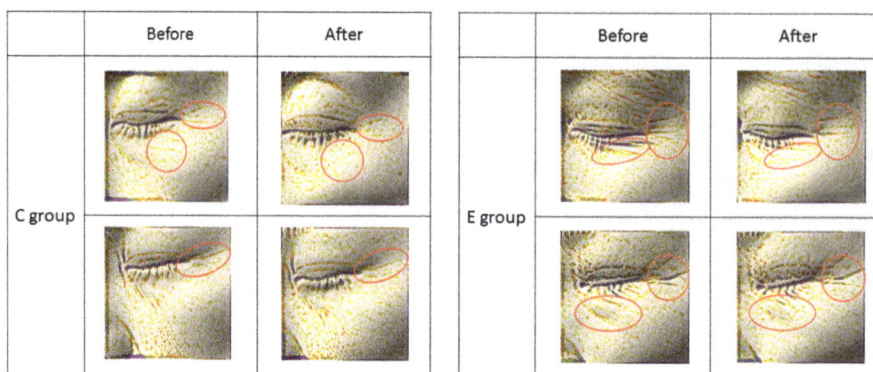

Fig. 4 Comparison of main wrinkles of the Lt. Eye. Main wrinkles of Lt. Eye have been indicated. Overall size, depth, and width of wrinkles decreased significantly in both C and E; however, it decreased more in E than in C

increase of 1.70(M), from 2.50(M) to 4.20(M) post-treatment ($p < .01$). In the items related to skin roughness, group C achieved a statistically significant improvement of 1.70(M) in satisfaction, from 2.70(M) to 4.40(M) post-treatment ($p < .01$). Group E also registered a statistically significant increase of 1.40(M) in satisfaction, from 2.90(M) to 4.30(M) ($p < .01$). In all items related to skin moisture, all subjects were "unsatisfied" with a mean score of fewer than 3 points pre-treatment, but all stated they were "satisfied" post-treatment, with a mean score of 4.15 points. In addition, these changes were statistically significant for all items. Given that the subjects were middle-aged women in their 30s–50s, this study showed significant improvements in overall satisfaction with skin moisture, even though the research was done in the late autumn and winter between November and February.

In the items related to skin pigmentation such as stains, freckles, and blemishes, group C showed a statistically significant increase of 2.50(M) in satisfaction, from 1.50(M) to 4.00(M) post-treatment ($p < .001$). Group E also showed a statistically significant increase of 2.30(M) in satisfaction, from 1.60(M) to 3.90(M) ($p < .001$). In the items related to the evenness of skin tone, group C showed a significant increase of 2.30(M) in satisfaction, from 1.90(M) to 4.20(M) post-treatment ($p < .001$). Group E also exhibited a statistically significant increase of 1.80(M) in satisfaction, from 2.20(M) to 4.00(M) ($p < .01$). In the items related to

skin whitening, all subjects were "unsatisfied" with a mean score of 1.80(M) pre-treatment, but they were "satisfied" with a mean score of 4.0(M) post-treatment. These changes were statistically significant for all items under the category. Overall, subjects showed higher levels of satisfaction with their level of skin whitening than with their ratings of skin moisture. As presented in Figs. 2 and 3, these results appear to verify the effectiveness of niacinamide as a whitening agent.

In the items related to skin redness, group C showed a statistically significant increase of 0.70(M) in satisfaction, from 3.30(M) to 4.00(M) post-treatment ($p < .005$). Group E also exhibited a statistically significant increase of 1.00(M) in satisfaction, from 3.10(M) to 4.10(M) ($p < .01$). Unlike the earlier results describing overall satisfaction with hyperpigmentation, group E showed higher overall satisfaction with hyperpigmentation compared to group C. This finding might relate to observations of reduced skin redness following air brushing. Skin redness most clearly contrasts the two groups when verifying air brush effectiveness.

In the items related to pores, group C showed a statistically significant increase of 1.70(M) in satisfaction, from 2.20(M) to 3.90(M) post-treatment ($p < .01$). Group E also exhibited a statistically significant increase of 1.50(M), from 2.40(M) to 3.90(M) ($p < .01$). In the items related to skin elasticity, group C showed a statistically significant increase of 1.90(M) in satisfaction, from 1.70(M) to 3.60(M) post-treatment ($p < .001$). Group E also showed a statistically significant increase of 2.10(M) in satisfaction, from 1.90(M) to 4.00(M) ($p < .001$). In the items related to wrinkles, group C showed a statistically significant increase of 1.90(M) in satisfaction, from 1.70(M) to 3.60(M) post-treatment ($p < .001$). Group E also exhibited a statistically significant increase of 2.00(M) in satisfaction, from 1.80(M) to 3.80(M) ($p < .001$). As shown in Table 4, these results appear to verify the effectiveness of adenosine as an anti-wrinkle agent.

Table 5 Reliability of the measurement tool

Category		The number of question	Alpha
Satisfaction of skin condition	Hydration	3	.940
	Pigmentation	3	
	Elasticity	3	
	Skin sensitization	1	

Table 6 Satisfaction after use

Variable	Group	Measurement (M ± SD)		t_1-t_2	t (p)	
		Before	After			
Dehydrated	C (n = 10)	2.20 ± 0.78	3.80 ± 1.03	− 1.60 ± 1.42	− 3.539	(.006**)
	E (n = 10)	2.21 ± 0.56	4.00 ± 0.81	− 1.90 ± 1.19	− 5.019	(.001**)
Flaking skin	C (n = 10)	2.80 ± 0.42	4.20 ± 0.78	− 1.40 ± 0.96	− 4.583	(.001**)
	E (n = 10)	2.50 ± 0.70	4.20 ± 0.78	− 1.70 ± 1.33	− 4.019	(.003**)
Rough skin	C (n = 10)	2.70 ± 0.82	4.40 ± 0.69	− 1.70 ± 1.15	− 4.636	(.001**)
	E (n = 10)	2.90 ± 1.10	4.30 ± 0.67	− 1.40 ± 1.17	− 3.772	(.004**)
Hyper-pigmentation	C (n = 10)	1.50 ± 0.52	4.00 ± 0.94	− 2.50 ± 0.97	− 8.135	(.000***)
	E (n = 10)	1.60 ± 0.69	3.90 ± 0.99	− 2.30 ± 1.33	− 5.438	(.000***)
Even skin tone	C (n = 10)	1.90 ± 0.31	4.20 ± 0.91	− 2.30 ± 0.94	− 7.667	(.000***)
	E (n = 10)	2.20 ± 0.63	4.00 ± 0.94	− 1.80 ± 1.22	− 4.630	(.001**)
Blush	C (n = 10)	3.30 ± 1.25	4.00 ± 0.81	− 0.70 ± 0.94	− 2.333	(.045*)
	E (n = 10)	3.10 ± 0.87	4.10 ± 0.56	− 1.00 ± 0.94	− 3.354	(.008**)
Pore condition	C (n = 10)	2.20 ± 0.78	3.90 ± 0.73	− 1.70 ± 1.05	− 5.075	(.001**)
	E (n = 10)	2.40 ± 0.69	3.90 ± 0.56	− 1.50 ± 0.97	− 4.881	(.001**)
Skin elasticity	C (n = 10)	1.70 ± 0.82	3.60 ± 1.07	− 1.90 ± 1.10	− 5.460	(.000***)
	E (n = 10)	1.90 ± 0.73	4.00 ± 1.05	− 2.10 ± 0.73	− 9.000	(.000***)
Wrinkle	C (n = 10)	1.70 ± 0.94	3.60 ± 1.07	− 1.90 ± 0.73	− 8.143	(.000***)
	E (n = 10)	1.80 ± 0.63	3.80 ± 0.91	− 2.00 ± 0.94	− 6.708	(.000***)
Skin sensitization	C (n = 10)	3.50 ± 1.08	3.70 ± 0.94	− 0.20 ± 1.03	− .612	(.555)
	E (n = 10)	3.70 ± 0.82	4.20 ± 0.91	− 0.50 ± 1.26	− 1.246	(.244)

$*p < .05$, $**p < .01$, $***p < .001$
Abbreviations were the same as Table 2

In the items related to skin sensitivity and allergies, group C showed a statistically significant increase of 0.20(M) in satisfaction, from 3.50(M) to 3.70(M) post-treatment. Group E also exhibited a statistically significant increase of 0.50(M) in satisfaction, from 3.70(M) to 4.20(M). There were no statistically significant post-treatment changes relating to skin sensitivity and allergies.

The items related to pigmentation such as stains, freckles, and blemishes, the items related to skin elasticity, and the items related to wrinkles showed the lowest levels of satisfaction prior to the application; interestingly, these items showed the overall greatest changes in satisfaction post-treatment. Certainly, there could be minor differences in the level of skin condition improvement between measures, using skin analysis devices and the subjects' subjective evaluations. However, as the degree to which individuals were satisfied with their skin is essentially based on naked-eye observations, these observations are inherently subjective. For this reason, certain differences between the subjects' own evaluations and objective data could be further validated. Nevertheless, the present study proved the functional utility of niacinamide and adenosine, based on both objective and subjective measures. These findings speak to this study's significance.

Discussion

Kim (2004) described the usefulness of niacinamide as a moisturizing agent. A study by Draelos et al. (2005) reported that a 4-week application of a moisturizer containing 2% niacinamide to the forearms of subjects in the experimental group resulted in a statistically significant increase in the mean moisture level of the skin compared to the control group ($p < .01$). A study by Draelos (2008) reported that a 24-day application of a topical ointment containing 2% niacinamide to the forearms of the subjects in the experimental group led to a statistically significant decrease in transepidermal water loss compared to the control group ($p < .002$). Adenosine, the second ingredient in the test agent, may have increased the dermal distribution of collagen, which could be attributed to adenosine's ability to increase collagen synthesis and inhibit collagen disintegration (Ha et al. 1998; Sohn et al. 2007). Thus, adenosine can increase skin moisture because of the moisture-friendly characteristics of collagen. In the present study, the observed increases in skin moisture may have resulted from the complex interactions of niacinamide and adenosine contained in the test agent.

Niacinamide is a functional whitening ingredient that inhibits the production of melanin by suppressing tyrosinase secretion (Go et al. 2013). A study by Hakozaki et al. (2002), which was conducted in an in vitro co-culture experiment, indicated that niacinamide effectively inhibited the transfer of melanosome by up to 68%. Based on this finding, our finding of increased brightness on both the left and right sides was attributed to the functional whitening effects of niacinamide.

Park et al. (2010) administered vitamin C to subjects twice a week over a 6-week period. Here, the experimental group underwent ion electrophoresis coupled with a micro-spray device, whereas the control group received only ion electrophoresis. The authors measured levels of pigmentation in both groups using the RSA (Robo Skin Analyzer CS50, Inforward, Japan). After receiving their respective treatments 12 times, the experimental group showed a statistically significant decrease of 4.38 ± 3.85 ($M \pm SD$) in the number of small-particle pigments ($p < .05$), but the control group exhibited an increase of 5.63 ± 8.90 ($p = .117$). In terms of the number of large-particle pigments, the experimental group exhibited a statistically significant decrease of 10.75 ± 7.44 ($p < .01$) and the control group showed an increase of 5.50 ± 10.53 ($p = .183$). These results suggest that using small particles that are sprayed increases the absorption of water-soluble cosmetic substances. In the present study, only group E showed a statistically significant change in the level of brightness, thereby suggesting that the air brush was effective.

Skin redness is caused by hemoglobin in the blood vessels underneath; close distribution of capillaries to the epidermis provides the face with a red tone (Yoo and Lee 2010). In this study, group C showed increased skin redness ($+ 16.3\%$) on both the left and right sides, whereas group E showed statistically significant decreases ($- 18.0\%$) in skin redness on the left and right sides. This result probably occurred because of reductions in skin surface temperature due to the air brush stimulation of the capillaries, which in turn produced reduced redness. In addition, as described earlier, increased distribution of collagens in the skin due to adenosine may have increased the physical distance between the capillaries and the skin surface.

Blueish tones in the lower orbit of the eye can be caused by complex factors such as structural problems arising from fat thickness imbalances, blood vessels or lower tissue layers visualized through thin skin tissues, and pigmentation (Shin et al. 2011). In the present study, group C showed decreases in skin yellowing on both the left and right sides, while group E exhibited increased yellowing on both sides. In other words, the blue color intensity may have increased in group C but decreased in group E. This can be explained in line with the observed decreases in skin redness due to collagen distribution and capillary contraction.

Park and Lee (2015) implemented a skin care program using a water-jet, and the program was administered two times in an interval of 2 days. Then, the changes in the wrinkles were measured based on the number of pixels by employing a shadow detection method. As a result, fine wrinkles around the orbicularis oris muscle showed a statistically significant reduction of 5.14 ± 2.90 pixels ($p < .001$). In this study, Park and Lee (2015) used a water-jet in conjunction with a skin care program in the subjects and measured the changes 20 min after the final treatment. This differs from the current study method where air brushes were used in the home setting. However, in both studies, statistically significant wrinkle improvements were achieved over the entire face.

Conclusions

This study attempted to verify the physiological activities of niacinamide as a functional whitening agent and adenosine as an anti-wrinkle agent, as well as the effectiveness of the air brush as a skin care device.

The study's findings showed increases in moisture content among all subjects. This may have been because the moisturizing effects of niacinamide were coupled with adenosine-induced increases in skin collagen content. This caused collagens, which are typically moisture-friendly, to further increase the moisture content of the skin. Both groups showed increased skin brightness post-treatment. These changes may have occurred because niacinamide acts as a functional whitening agent, which suppresses the production of melanin and the transfer of melanisome. However, statistically significant increases in the skin brightness were found only in group E. Consequently, these changes may actually reflect the effect of spraying fine particles using an air brush. In terms of the red color intensity, group C showed an increase, while group E showed a significant decrease. The increased distribution of collagens due to adenosine application may have increased the physical distance between the capillaries and the skin surface. In addition, temperature decrease on the skin surface caused by the air brush may have effectively constricted the capillaries. This result seems to agree with our observation that group C showed an increase in blue intensity, whereas group E showed a decrease in blue intensity. Both groups achieved statistically significant improvements in the overall size, depth, and width of the main wrinkles. This may reaffirm the beneficial effects of adenosine. However, the relatively greater improvements observed in group E compared to group C appeared to verify the usefulness of the air brush as a skin care device. When we evaluated patient satisfaction, items related to pigmentation and skin elasticity showed the greatest changes. This result was meaningful and, once again, appeared to validate the use of niacinamide and adenosine for improving perceived skin satisfaction.

The present study also verified the usefulness of niacinamide and adenosine as they relate to skin physiology, and the effectiveness of the air brush as a skin care device. Existing studies on skin care devices are limited in that they were mostly conducted within expert-run programs. Therefore, future studies may be required to verify the effects of skin care devices within the home environment. In addition, while studies on the dermal absorption of water-soluble substances have thus far been confined to the application of ionospheresis, some previous studies have suggested the potential for enhanced dermal absorption of water-soluble substances through physical actions (Park et al. 2010).

The dermis only absorbs approximately 0.1–0.5% of the total volume of water-soluble substances. These substances are quickly absorbed via sebaceous glands and then activated (Yoo and Lee 2010). Additional studies are needed on the dermal absorption of water-soluble substances. In particular, studies using air brushes in order to induce physical changes through air pressure-driven spray of fine particles are needed.

Abbreviations

LED: Light-emitting diode; MFDS: Ministry of Food and Drug Safety

Funding

This study was performed through a joint research contract between Dasan C & Tech and Aphrozone in 2017 and was funded by Aphrozone.

Authors' contributions

HJK designed the study and wrote the manuscript. MSJ reviewed the study and edited the manuscript. JMS and YKH performed the research background such as the experiments and data collection. All authors read and approved the final manuscript.

Competing interests

The authors declare that they have no competing interests.

References

Draelos ZD. Clinical situations conducive to proactive skin health and anti-aging improvement. J Investig Dermatol Symp Proc. 2008;13:25–7. http://www.riss.kr/link?id=O48885692 Accessed 2008

Draelos ZD, Ertel K, Berge C. Niacinamide-containing facial moisturizer improves skin barrier and benefits subjects with rosacea. Cutis. 2005;76:135–41. http://www.riss.kr/link?id=O43267714 Accessed 2005

Go HJ, Kim NS, Kim EH, Um MS, Oh JS. New cosmetology. Seoul: Gadam books; 2013. p. 110–1. http://www.riss.kr/link?id=M13762516 Accessed 2013

Ha YH, Yu SU, Kim DS, Lim SJ, Choi YW. Hydrolysis, skin permeation and in vivo whitening effect of kojic acid monostearate as an antimelanogenic agent. 1998;42:39–45. http://www.riss.kr/link?id=A100402513 Accessed 1998

Hakozaki T, Minwalla L, Zhuang J, Chhoa M, Matsubara A, Miyamoto K, et al. The effect of niacinamide on reducing cutaneous pigmentation and suppression of melanosome transfer. Br J Dermatol. 2002;14:20–31. http://www.riss.kr/link?id=O32050979 Accessed 2002

Han SM, Hong IP, Woo SO, Cheon SN, Han CS. The effect of cosmetic included purified bee venom on the improvement of skin wrinkle. 2015;21:288–292. http://www.riss.kr/link?id=A100486555 Accessed 2015.

Jo SY, Hwang SM. A study of effects of gap between actual age and self-perceived age in middle-age women on their appearance management behavior and self-esteem. Kor J Aesthet Cosmetol. 2013;11:1137–46. http://www.riss.kr/link?id=A99908555 Accessed 2013.12

Kim EH. A study on professional unmarried men's clothing purchase·appearance management behavior and self-respect. Seoul, Korea: Unpublished master's thesis, Kyunghee University; 2006. p. 1–2. http://www.riss.kr/link?id=T10697500 Accessed 2006.08

Kim JE. Stabilization of facial skin physiological parameters after exposure to summer and winter climatic condition. Theses for Master's Degree at Korea University, 2007:43–44. http://www.riss.kr/link?id=T11086500 Accessed 2007.08.

Kim JH, Park OL, Lee DC. The study on the consumer's clothing satisfaction and fashion consciousness according to shopping orientation of male consumers. J Korean Data Anal Soc. 2005;7:533–48. http://www.riss.kr/link?id=A101600342 Accessed Apr 2005

Kim KS, Gang SM. The skin safety and effects of the fermented broth of Lactobacillus rhamnosus for improving the neck skin. J Korean Acad Nurs. 2017;23:101–14. http://www.riss.kr/link?id=A103064107 Accessed 2017

Kim KY, Bea YK, Lee EJ, Kim SM, Kim EA, Ahn SL. Essence cosmetology. Paju-si: Jigu Publishing Co; 2014. p. 161. http://www.riss.kr/link?id=M13421745 Accessed 2014

Kim YM. Medical skin care2. Seoul: Imsong Books; 2004. p. 246–7. http://www.riss.kr/link?id=M9369963 Accessed 2004

Lee JH, Moon JS, Choi TB. Effect of the cosmetics containing schizandra chinesis extracts on the skin of the middle aged women. J Korea Soc Cosmetol. 2013; 19:634–41. http://www.riss.kr/link?id=T13244819 Accessed 2013.8

Lee KJ, Kim HJ. Correlation of body image, self-esteem, and appearance management behavior. Kor J Aaesthet Cosmetol. 2015;13:203–11. http://www.riss.kr/link?id=A100537798 Accessed 2015

Park JY, Kang SM, Lee OK. Effect of fine particles injection by vitamin C on the skin change. Kor J Aesthet Cosmetol. 2010;8:253–62. http://www.riss.kr/link?id=A82373498 Accessed 2010

Park KS, Lee HH. Development of a water sprayer for skin care and its effects on moisture and wrinkle improvements. Kor J Aesthet Cosmetol. 2015;13:603–13. http://www.earticle.net/article.aspx?sn=257397 Accessed 2015

Safire W. On language; lookism. In: The New York Times Magazine; 2000. https://www.nytimes.com/2000/08/27/magazine/the-way-we-live-now-8-27-00-on-language-lookism.html Accessed 27 Aug 2000.

Shin JI, Kwon IO, Kim CY. Strategy for the treatment of infraorbital dark circles. 2011;17:91–98. http://www.riss.kr/link?id=A104566924 Accessed 2011.

Sohn ED, Hwang JS, Chang IS. R & D trend of functional anti-wrinkle cosmetics. News Inf Chem Eng. 2007;25:133–8. http://www.riss.kr/link?id=A75313705 Accessed 2007

Yoo EA, Lee HA. Rediscovery of cosmetics, vol. 41. Seoul: Sungshin Women's University Press; 2010. p. 59–61. http://www.riss.kr/link?id=M12183745 Accessed 2010

24

Exploring vitiligo susceptibility and management

Razia Rahman and Yasha Hasija[*]

Abstract

Background: Vitiligo is a common dermatological disorder of chronic depigmentation which is phenotypically characterized by white macules on the skin caused as a result of the systematic destruction of functional melanocytes. This review provides an overview of vitiligo, its etiopathogenesis and disease management, and also discusses the scope of network-interaction studies and polypharmacological studies in understanding vitiligo disease module.

Methods: A narrative review of the relevant published literatures known to the authors that comprehensively discussed about vitiligo and its implications was conducted.

Results: Emerging evidence underlines the existing connection between deregulated miRNA function and vitiligo pathogenesis. It has also been linked with autoimmunity for the cause of melanocyte death in susceptible individuals. Alteration of genetic factors involved in immune responses and melanogenesis along with environmental factors are central to disease manifestation. Screening methods as such are not available for vitiligo, and the diagnosis is based on the assessment of the absence of melanocytes from the lesions in the affected area. With the occurrence of vitiligo at any age, most people typically develop it at a young age. Depending on the disease course and duration, clinical management primarily involves disease stabilization either by repigmentation or depigmentation of the skin.

Conclusions: Several questions remain unsolved which indeed makes vitiligo an excellent model for studying autoimmune and degenerative processes. An understanding of the underlying degenerative mechanisms and unraveling the biological mediators of melanocyte loss will open up avenues for testing novel therapeutic approaches in vitiligo management. Such studies can revolutionize our apprehension of the molecular interconnections that underpin vitiligo pathogenesis.

Keywords: Vitiligo, Autoimmunity, Genetics, Disease management

Background

Evolutionary studies indicated that skin pigmentation was the result of adaptive responses to the environment (UV radiation) after the loss of hair coat in humans. Pigmentation provides photoprotection and participates in skin barrier function and antimicrobial defenses of the skin, hence, is essential for maintaining body homeostasis (Jablonski and Chaplin 2010). Dermatological disorders have a significant psychosocial impact on the quality of patients' lives since their symptoms are visible. Although dermatological conditions are not life-threatening, it is the product of this morbidity multiplied by the high prevalence of skin disease which results in a large burden of the disease in absolute terms. Vitiligo is one such dermatological disorder that is inflicted upon almost all age groups irrespective of gender and skin type. Vitiligo is a complex acquired depigmentation disorder characterized by white non-scaly patches with distinct sharp margins distributed unilaterally in the skin. It results in the episodically selective disappearance of functional melanocytes which leads to pigment dilution in the affected areas (Le Poole et al. 1993; Ezzedine et al. 2012a, b). Vitiligo is usually asymptomatic and can appear anywhere on the skin commonly affecting the areas of the face and hands, and the genitals (Ezzedine et al. 2012a, b). It might also lead to whitening of hair although the skin and hair are affected to different degrees depending on the disease course which is unpredictable in most cases with phases of stabilized depigmentation eventually with the duration of the disease (Picardo et al. 2015).

* Correspondence: yashahasija06@gmail.com
Department of Biotechnology, Delhi Technological University, Shahbad Daulatpur, Main Bawana Road, Delhi 110042, India

The onset of vitiligo and its subsequent progression is thought to be impelled by several inherited genes and can develop at any age irrespective of the type of skin, gender, race, or geographical location. Additional stochastic or environmental factors are also likely to further influence the pathogenesis of vitiligo (Spritz 2013). It affects the life of patients both biologically and psychologically due to its unsightly appearance inflicting significant psychological stress and exerting a pernicious influence on the quality of life in patients concerning self-esteem and social interactions. The development of new lesions resulting in enlarged macules is classified as an active form of the disease that warrants more aggressive therapy (Taieb 2012). Friction has also been indicated to trigger vitiligo development in areas such as the neck, elbows, and ankles, a phenomenon known as the Koebner phenomenon (Gauthier et al. 2003). It has been proposed that in some vitiligo cases, Koebner phenomenon could be used to predict and analyze the clinical profile and disease course (van Geel et al. 2012). Various genetic, experimental, and clinical studies have unraveled significant pathways in vitiligo pathogenesis that have helped in identifying targets for the development of efficient treatment approaches for disease management.

Epidemiology and prevalence

Vitiligo is the most common depigmentation disorder with an overall estimated worldwide prevalence of 0.5 to 2% (Krüger and Schallreuter 2012) but a higher prevalence rate up to 8.8% has been reported in India (Sehgal and Srivastava 2007). It has also been reported to occur at an early age in the women population. The largest epidemiological study of the prevalence of vitiligo was carried out on 47,033 inhabitants on the island of Bornholm in Denmark in 1977, where vitiligo was found to affect 0.4% of the population (Howitz et al. 1977). Similar results were obtained in French West Indies, predominantly in the black population (Boisseau-Garsaud et al. 2000). Reports from China, Mexico, and Japan also indicate high incidences of vitiligo with an overall prevalence rate of 0.6% (Sehgal and Srivastava 2007; Wang et al. 2013).

The vitiligo prevalence rates of 0.06 to 2.3% in the general population and 0 to 2.2% in children have been reported in earlier studies (Nicolaidou et al. 2012). Findings also indicate an increased rate of prevalence with respect to age (Alikhan et al. 2011) (Table 1), increasing from 0.5% in children of less than 1 year of age to 1% in children of 1–5 years of age and further expanding to 2.1% in 5–12 year olds. The onset of vitiligo before the age of 12 years is reported to range from 0–2.6% (Halder 1997; Nicolaidou et al. 2012). In almost half of the patients, vitiligo develops before the age of 20 years with nearly about 70 to 80% developing it before 30 years of age. Segmental vitiligo also tends to occur at a younger age with 87% of cases reported in patients before 30 years of age and 41.3% cases before 10 years of age

Table 1 Increased prevalence rate of vitiligo with respect to age

Prevalence rates	Percentage
General population	0.06–2.3%
Children	0–2.2%
Of less than 1 year	0.5%
1–5 years of age	1%
5–12 year olds	2.1%
Before the age of 12 years	0–2.6%
Onset of disease	Percentage
Before 20 years of age	50%
Before 30 years of age	70–80%

(Ezzedine et al. 2012a, b). Discrepancies between prevalence and incidence data leads to variability in epidemiological data which is attributable to the diverse populations and its genetics, differences in disease classification, cultural and social differences, lack of screening or diagnostic tests, social and cultural stigma attached to the disease, and inconsistent reporting by patients. Despite the same prevalence ratio of 1:1 in males and females, the ratio of treatment requests is 1:2. This signifies that females seek treatments more frequently, which apparently might be due to the ramifications of greater social burden (Alikhan et al. 2011).

Classification of vitiligo

Figure 1 shows the major classifications of vitiligo, namely, non-segmental or generalized vitiligo, segmental vitiligo, and mixed vitiligo according to international consensus (Ezzedine et al. 2012a, b). The onset of mixed vitiligo is the same as segmental vitiligo which eventually develops into non-segmental vitiligo, thus, the name mixed vitiligo.

In non-segmental (generalized) vitiligo, which is the most common form of vitiligo, the depigmented patches develop on both sides of the body and usually progresses slowly (Picardo et al. 2015). While in segmental vitiligo, the patches are limited to only one side of the body, particularly in the face and trunk area, and do not usually cross the midline of the body. It initially progresses rapidly which spontaneously stabilizes after a period of 6 months (Ezzedine et al. 2012a, b). In segmental vitiligo, typical distribution patterns on the face and trunk have been described, which aid in differential diagnosis (Kim et al. 2011; Geel et al. 2014). Mixed vitiligo, on the other hand, has been described as a rare combination of both segmental vitiligo and non-segmental vitiligo. The onset of mixed vitiligo is the same as segmental vitiligo which eventually develops into non-segmental vitiligo, thus the name mixed vitiligo (Ezzedine et al. 2011). The markedly different distribution patterns aid in recognition of the type of vitiligo as the evolution and the kind of treatment are different for the different subtypes of vitiligo.

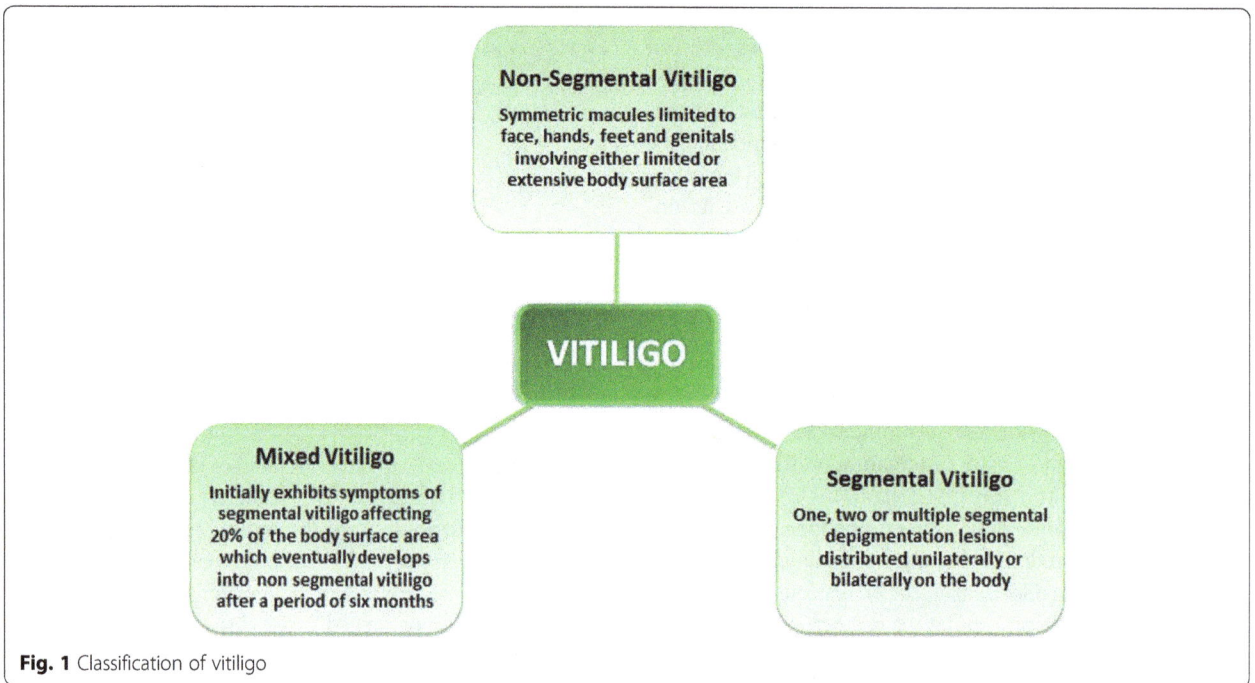

Fig. 1 Classification of vitiligo

Etiopathogenesis of vitiligo

Stress responses in the skin eliciting an autoimmune response in genetically susceptible individuals are thought to be instigated by a trigger event that eventually targets the melanocytes predisposing individuals to develop vitiligo. Though recent studies have started to reveal the etiopathogenesis of vitiligo, the mechanisms leading to vitiligo are yet a debatable topic. However, several hypotheses have been presented signifying its association with the development of vitiligo (Fig. 2). Among the different theories developed, namely, autoimmunity, oxidative stress, melanocyte growth and defective melanocyte adhesion, viral infections, and neural mechanisms, the autoimmune theory is currently considered and accepted

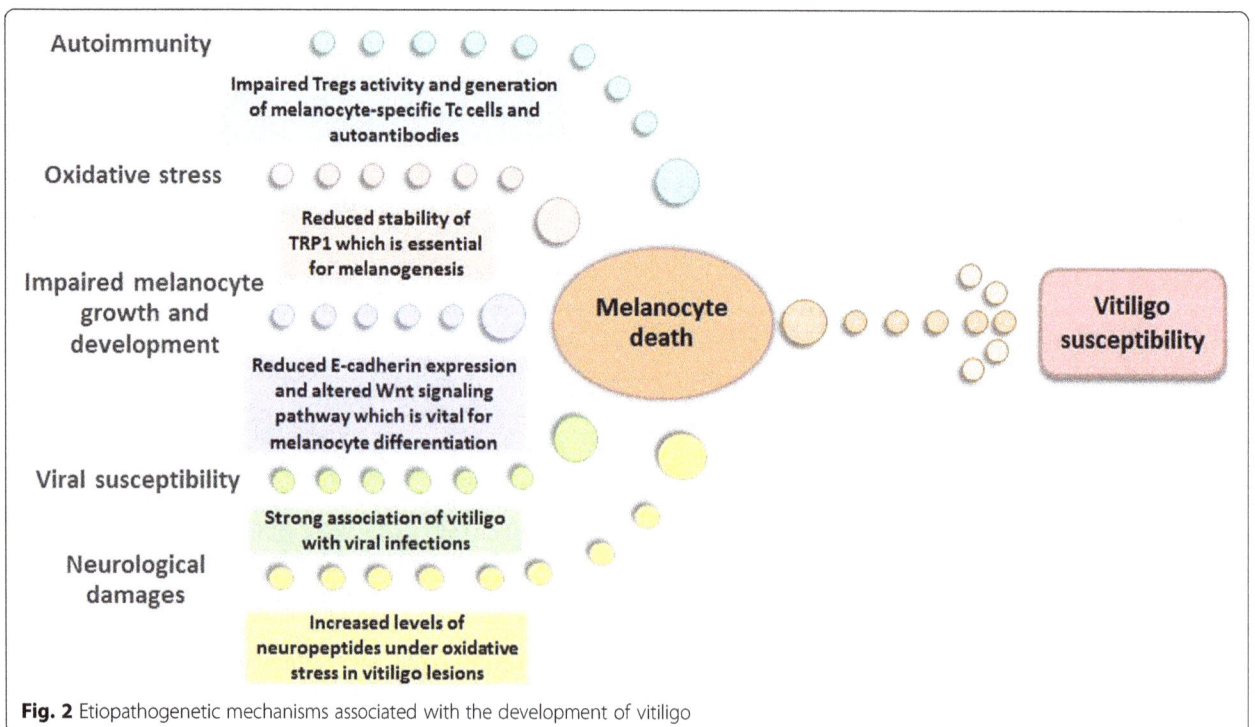

Fig. 2 Etiopathogenetic mechanisms associated with the development of vitiligo

as the leading theory globally, which has been substantiated by several reports on the frequent association of vitiligo with autoimmune diseases (Rezaei et al. 2007; Le Poole and Luiten, 2008; Kasumagic-Halilovic et al. 2013; Strassner and Harris 2016). Also, the association of vitiligo with halo naevus, which is characterized by depigmented halo-like area circumscribing a mole encompassing dense immune cell infiltrate, further supports the importance of immune mechanisms in vitiligo development (Spritz 2010).

Autoimmune theory

The loss of self-tolerance in the pathogenesis of vitiligo is unclear and not yet well understood. High levels of circulating melanocyte autoantibodies recognized by T cells specifically against tyrosinase (TRP-1 and TRP-2) have been found in many vitiligo patients with their role being linked to the destruction of keratinocytes and melanocytes (Jimbow et al. 2001; Kemp et al. 2011). Autoimmunity in vitiligo has been suggested to develop owing to the failure of inherent mechanisms which are intended to control melanocyte proliferation (Le Poole and Luiten 2008). Other antigenic proteins related to disease activity, namely, glycoprotein 100 (gp100) and melanoma antigen recognized by T cells 1 (MART-1) have also been detected in the blood and tissues of vitiligo patients (Lang et al. 2001). Several studies have shown the accumulation of T helper (TH) and T cytotoxic (TC) cells suggesting the formation of a silent micro-inflammatory process that kills melanocytes in the junction of the dermal and epidermal area of vitiligo lesion implying cell-mediated immune response activity (Oyarbide-Valencia et al. 2006). Certain major histocompatibility complex (MHC) alleles have been suggested to be associated with vitiligo as a vital link between the disease etiology and the aberrant self-antigen presentation to the T cells. Moreover, human leukocyte antigen (HLA)-A2 restricted, melanocyte-specific CD8+ T lymphocytes identified to kill melanocytes in the perilesional skin, has been detected in vitiligo patients (Van Den Boorn et al. 2009; Spritz 2010). Also, the fundamental role of regulatory T cells (Tregs) in the pathogenesis of vitiligo has been implicated in several reports with a reduction in their number in the peripheral blood of vitiligo patients along with their dysfunctional activity (Ben Ahmed et al. 2012; Lili et al. 2012). Also considered as a Th1-related disease, a significant increase in the concentration of the cytokines, namely, TNF-α, IFNG, IL-10, IL1B, and IL-17 has also been reported to be associated with the onset as well as persistence of vitiligo in patients (Taher et al. 2009; Levandowski et al. 2013). Therefore, vitiligo serves as an eminent disease model to understand the initiation and progression of organ-specific autoimmune diseases.

Oxidative stress theory

Oxidative stress, which is the result of an increase in the levels of reactive oxygen species (ROS) and subsequent reduction of antioxidant enzymes, compromises the function of cellular proteins and membrane lipids, thus impairing the activity of the antioxidant system in both lesional and non-lesional skin (Maresca et al. 1997). This imbalanced status of the antioxidant system in vitiligo has been indicated to cause increased sensitivity of melanocytes to oxidative stress leading to cellular death. Excess levels of ROS have been reported in active vitiligo skin suggesting oxidative stress as the plausible cause of vitiligo pathogenesis (Jimbow et al. 2001). Superoxide dismutase, an antioxidant enzyme, has been reported to be altered in vitiligo skin indicating that ROS generation causes an alteration in the expression of the antioxidant system affecting melanocyte function (Sravani et al. 2009). Oxidative stress-driven reduction of TRP1 expression triggers the production of intermediates of toxic melanin leading to subsequent immune-mediated melanocyte destruction (Dell'anna and Picardo 2006). Experimental data revealed a close association between oxidative stress and immune responses that promote intrinsic damage. Histological analysis shows the expression of NLR family pyrin domain containing 1 (NLRP1), IL-1, and catalase (CAT) in developing lesions (Marie et al. 2014). Several polymorphisms have been reported in the CAT gene, which impairs the enzyme function of X-box binding protein 1 (XBP1) which is primarily involved in mitigating stress-induced inflammation (Wood et al. 2008). These factors are involved in stress responses which ultimately triggers innate immune responses.

Deficient melanocyte adhesion and melanocyte growth theory

Evidence of the decreased adhesive property of melanocytes in vitiligo has been reported in earlier studies (Gauthier et al. 2003). Reduced expression levels of E-cadherin have been observed in melanocytes prior to depigmentation development in vitiligo skin. During oxidative or mechanical stress, an altered E-cadherin expression incites the loss of adhesion in epidermal melanocytes due to the increased levels of anti-adhesion molecule, tenascin (Le Poole et al. 1997; Wagner et al. 2015). Loss of melanocytes from the epidermal layer due to deficient adhesion of melanocytes could be an early phenomenon in vitiligo. Also, alteration in the factors influencing successful differentiation and proliferation of melanocytes due to oxidative stress, such as altered Wnt signaling, may also render susceptibility to vitiligo.

Viral theory

Several studies have depicted a strong association between vitiligo and hepatitis C virus (HCV) and hepatitis B virus (HBV) infections in vitiligo patients (Akbayir et al. 2004;

Akcan et al. 2006). Also, the association of cytomegalo-virus (CMV) infection with vitiligo was also suggested to provoke the deterioration of skin conditions in vitiligo (Toker et al. 2007). Furthermore, the suspicious association of herpes virus and the human immunodeficiency virus (HIV) infection with vitiligo has also been reported (Niamba et al. 2007).

Neuronal mechanisms theory

Clinical observations addressing the correlation of local neurological damage to skin depigmentation (whitening) suggest that neuronal mechanisms do have a role to play in vitiligo pathogenesis. Current evidence of the detection of neuropeptides in vitiligo lesions supports the neural hypothesis which might be the effect of inflammation rather than a triggering factor. An increased level of neuropeptides such as neuropeptide Y (NPY) has been observed in the marginal areas of vitiligo lesions triggered under the conditions of oxidative stress that is thought as a reason for the induction of vitiligo (Lazarova et al. 2000).

Diagnosis and screening

The diagnosis of vitiligo does not require confirmatory laboratory tests in the majority of cases irrespective of its clinical subtype. The absence of melanocytes from lesions can be assessed by in vivo confocal microscopy (non-invasive) or a skin biopsy with the use of specific markers. There are no screening methods available for vitiligo (Ezzedine et al. 2012a, b). The clinical screening of associated disorders on the diagnosis of vitiligo is currently a debatable topic. However, female patients and those with longer disease duration and involving greater body surface area are more likely to have autoimmune thyroid disease. Therefore, proper thyroid function and the presence of anti-thyroglobulin and anti-thyroid peroxidase antibodies need to be checked regularly in vitiligo patients (Gey et al. 2013).

Therapeutic options and management of vitiligo

The management of vitiligo becomes challenging considering its complex etiopathogenesis. There is no definite cure available for vitiligo. Therefore, the current optimal management options according to the recent consensus guidelines involves a personalized approach with the therapeutic choice influenced by several factors such as disease course and its impact, skin type, age, gender, age, affected area and its extent, and social and cultural life influences (Taieb 2012). Also, general measures of avoiding factors of mechanical stress, Koebner phenomenon and UV-exposure might be helpful in limiting depigmentation conditions (van Geel et al. 2012). Figure 3 shows a flowchart depicting the clinical management of vitiligo depending on the disease course and treatment outcomes.

Topical corticosteroids, immunomodulators, and antioxidants

Topical corticosteroids being the first-line of treatment option manage disease progression by initiating anti-inflammatory responses with trivial outcomes. Although repigmentation is observed in the face and neck, the trunk area and the extremities show limited repigmentation. Oral corticosteroid involving moderate dosage of corticosteroids (mini-pulse therapy) is used to arrest disease progression in active disease conditions where the repigmentation outcomes are rare (Njoo et al. 1998). However, the associated side effects oral corticosteroids limit its long-term use.

Topical immunomodulators such as tacrolimus and pimecrolimus attenuate the production of proinflammatory cytokines by inhibiting T cell activity, thereby enhancing melanocyte migration and pigmentation in vitiligo patients (Ormerod 2005). Similar to corticosteroids, the results mostly show repigmentation in the face with moderate effects at other sites of the body.

Although, according to the current consensus guidelines, the use of topical antioxidants is not recommended, however, they are frequently prescribed in relatively limited trials (Leone and Paro 2015). The use of oral antioxidants in combination therapy is sometimes considered in patients undergoing phototherapy.

Phototherapy

Narrow-band UVB (NB-UVB) phototherapy is an effective treatment choice that has long been recognized to induce repigmentation. The majority of the patients are observed to develop the signs of repigmentation with phototherapy. Topical treatments are also advised after completed phototherapy sessions to prevent recurrence of depigmentation (Sitek et al. 2007).

Photochemotherapy is also an option, but the recurrent side effects often accompany carcinogenic risk along with limited successful outcomes which restrict its use over NB-UVB where such risks are less evident (Bhatnagar et al. 2007).

Surgery

Pigment cell transplantation techniques such as cellular and tissue graft transplantation may offer a valuable alternative treatment option. The necessity of the disease stability, which is the primary criteria linked to successful outcomes, limits this treatment option to selective patients only (van Geel et al. 2010). It is effective in both stable non-segmental and segmental vitiligo patients. Regardless of the technique used, the stability of the lesions is a major criterion related to the outcome of the procedure.

Combination therapy

The complexity of the disease makes it necessary to use a combination of different treatments to address both

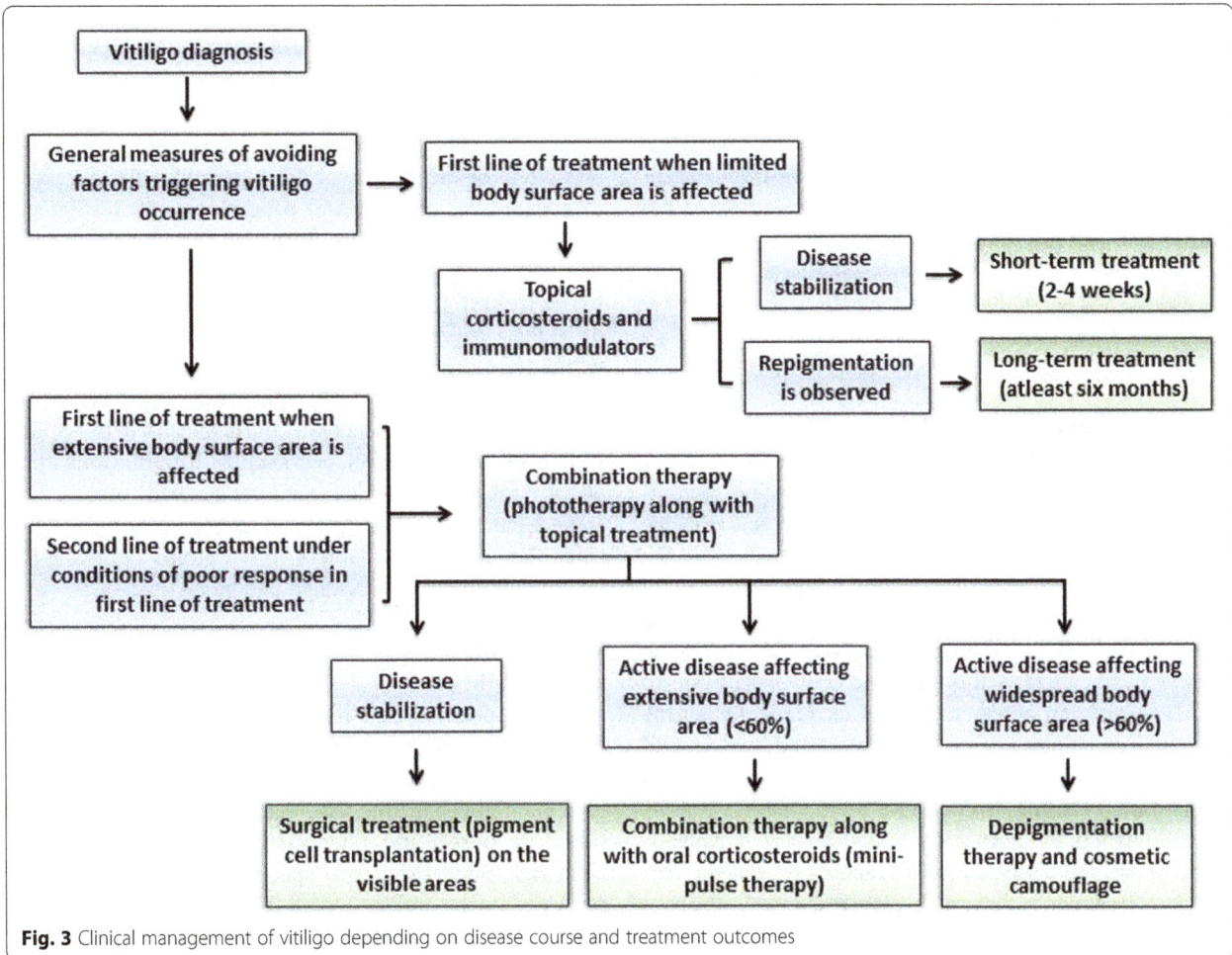

Fig. 3 Clinical management of vitiligo depending on disease course and treatment outcomes

inflammatory responses on melanocyte differentiation and proliferation. Currently, NB-UVB is prescribed along with topical corticosteroids and immunomodulators, instead of its use as a monotherapy. Such combination therapies have been shown to accelerate the repigmentation rates (Nordal et al. 2011). However, the risk of skin cancer due to the combined use of immunosuppressants is a topic of both concern and debate.

Depigmentation and cosmetic camouflage

In conditions of extensive vitiligo where most parts of the body are affected by depigmentation, depigmenting the remaining pigmented areas is considered as a better option instead of repigmentation treatments. Bleaching creams, laser therapy, and cryotherapy are some of the options for depigmentation therapy (AlGhamdi and Kumar 2011). Regardless of this treatment method, repigmentation on the treated depigmented areas might occur and as such a permanent cure cannot be assured.

Camouflaging the depigmented areas with cosmetic products could aid to reduce the daily impact of the disease on social life (Hossain et al. 2016). However,

specialized advice is required to be taken before going for such alternatives of cosmetic exposure to vitiligo skin.

Association with other diseases

Due to the polygenic nature of vitiligo, it is frequently associated with several autoimmune or autoinflammatory diseases, namely, thyroid disorders (Kasumagic-Halilovic et al. 2011), psoriasis, atopic dermatitis (Ezzedine et al. 2012a, b), diabetes mellitus, pernicious anemia, and Addison's disease (Rezaei et al. 2007). Antibodies directed against melanocytes and other organ-specific tissues have been found in vitiligo patients. Recent observations strongly point to vitiligo as an autoimmune disease sharing genes with other autoimmune disorders (Zhang and Xiang 2014). Recent studies reported the expression of markers on vitiligo melanocytes that have been detected in cells from neurodegenerative diseases, such as Alzheimer's (Bellei et al. 2013). Therefore, vitiligo might represent a degenerative disease model as well. Although the definite link between vitiligo and melanoma has not been fully elucidated yet, it has been reported that they both share an inverse relationship meaning that vitiligo-affected people are relatively protected having a much lower risk of developing melanoma' and vice-versa (Spritz 2010). Melanoma patients experiencing successful treatment responses were observed to consequently develop vitiligo. Both melanoma and vitiligo share CD8+ T cell antigens, and the allelic variants associated with vitiligo were found to confer protection from melanoma directly (Paradisi et al. 2014). This observation has contributed significantly to the development of improved therapeutic interventions to regulate melanoma in patients and depicts the similarity in the generation of immune responses and the target of similar antigens in both vitiligo and melanoma.

Impact on the quality of life

The implications of disease progression influence the potential psychiatric comorbidity associated with vitiligo. Skin integrity is considered relevant in many cultural and religious contexts, and any modification in the color or aspect of the skin influences the physical functioning and psychological state of the affected ones. Vitiligo has a major impact on the quality of patients' life relating to social and cultural stigma that eventually affects self-esteem and self-concept due to negative evaluation by others. Several factors including the patients' age at the onset of disease, the extent and distribution of the depigmented patches in the body, and stigmatization causing psychological trauma have a considerably influences the impact that vitiligo has on its patients. Furthermore, the discrepancies prevailing between the efficiency of treatment strategy, therapy response evaluation, and expectations of the patient and overall clinical management further add to the consternation of both the patients and their families (Kruger and Schallreuter 2013). Stigmatization has been shown to be the most influential factor in patient well-being and perceived quality of life, even more than disease duration and treatment inefficiency. In most cases, patients have reported discomfort owing to the uncontrolled progression of the disease rather than noting the development of new lesions in visible areas (Teovska Mitrevska et al. 2012). This suggests that the impaired quality of life is linked to the activity of the disease at a greater extent rather than to the involvement of exposed areas well indicating that the presence of visible lesions did not much affect the global pattern.

The onset of vitiligo in adolescence can have a long-lasting impact on a child's self-esteem directly affecting their psychological state causing interaction anxiousness and depression and thus pose as a risk factor for impaired quality of life in such children. Vitiligo has been found to cause more embarrassment and self-consciousness as children with vitiligo grow older with almost 95% of the teenagers within the age group of 15 to 17 years to be tribulated by their condition as compared to children (50%) of age group between 6 to 14 years (Parsad et al. 2013).

Stress and anxiety caused by vitiligo being a precipitating factor for considerable psychosocial stress can be mitigated by self-help cognitive behavioral therapy (Shah et al. 2014). Treatment according to disease severity might not alone address a patient's suffering adequately. Increased awareness of the quality of life impairments is necessary to address the physical and psychological state that encompasses several factors from the patient's perspective and will help to assure that vitiligo patients are not under-treated and under-appreciated. More than a third of vitiligo patients experience symptoms of depression without necessarily fulfilling the criteria for clinical depression (Parsad et al. 2013). New vitiligo-specific impact scales that better reflects the burden caused by vitiligo have been recently developed such as VitQoL (Lilly et al. 2013), Vitiligo Life Quality (Senol et al. 2013), and Vitiligo Impact Patient Scale (Gupta et al. 2014; Salzes et al. 2016) since the high rate of depressive symptoms signifying the psychological impact in vitiligo patients is evident.

Role of miRNAs and genetic variants on vitiligo susceptibility

Vitiligo appears to be a multifaceted disorder underlying both genetic and non-genetic factors in a complex interactive manner. A comprehensive understanding of the molecular mechanisms that determine disease susceptibility, its onset, and phenotypic expression remains a challenge since the entire spectrum of this disorder is not yet clearly understood. Recent advances in genetic studies have led to the considerable progress in defining the genetic epidemiology and pathogenesis of vitiligo, and its relationships to other autoimmune diseases offering a real insight into its biological framework (Spritz 2013). These studies have improved our knowledge on vitiligo pathogenesis and have opened up new avenues for novel targeted therapies for lack of melanocyte regeneration in vitiligo leading to effective treatment approach as well as disease prevention.

miRNA signatures

MicroRNAs are conserved, small, endogenous non-coding RNA molecules that regulate post-transcriptional gene expression and promote translational repression leading to the cleavage and degradation of mRNA. Recent studies have shown that miRNAs play prime roles in various cellular, regulatory, and signaling processes maintaining physiological homeostasis. They are also essential for cellular morphogenesis, and any disruption in its architecture leads to disease development and progression. Serum miRNA expression profiles have been observed in vitiligo patients (Shi et al. 2013). Moreover, deregulated miRNA metabolism has been reported to be indicative of inflammatory skin conditions and linked to vitiligo pathogenesis (Mansuri et al. 2016). At present, characterization of interpretative miRNA expression and function in human melanocytes has elucidated them to be promising biomarkers for disease prognosis.

The collective role of miRNAs in oxidative stress and autoimmunity results in melanocyte destruction and leads to further progression of the disease. The expression levels of miR-1, miR-135a, and miR-9 targeting sirtuin 1 (SIRT1) which regulates stress response and inflammation have been found to increase in response to oxidative stress (Saunders et al. 2010), while heme oxygenase 1 (HO1) mRNA targeted by miR-183 is a stress-responsive antioxidant and anti-inflammatory factor (Chang et al. 2011). Increased expression of these miRNAs has been found in vitiligo patients suggesting their potential role in the destruction of melanocyte and formation of inflammatory micro-environment in the skin lesions caused as a result of oxidative stress. Increased levels of miR-133b expression have been observed in the lesional skin of vitiligo patients that suggests its role in the pathogenesis of vitiligo (Mansuri et al. 2014). let-7c targets the 3′ UTR of IL10 and regulates its expression which is a pleiotropic cytokine possessing both anti-inflammatory and immunosuppressive properties (Jiang et al. 2012). A decrease in the level of IL10 expression has been noted in skin biopsies, peripheral blood mononuclear cells, and sera obtained from vitiligo patients well indicating towards its contribution to disease development (Ratsep et al. 2008). An increased expression of miR-99b, miR-125b, miR-155, and miR-199a-3p has also been reported in vitiligo-affected skin which is related to the inhibition of expression of melanogenesis-associated genes which demonstrates that the expression of these miRNAs are dysregulated in the skin of patients with vitiligo and suggests its contribution to vitiligo pathogenesis (Sahmatova et al. 2016). Another miRNA, miR-30b targets platelet-derived growth factor receptor β (PDGFRB) mRNA and represses its ability to regulate cell proliferation in melanocytes resulting in melanocyte death in vitiligo patients (Shi et al. 2013). A significant increase in miR-183, miR-30a-3p, and miR-487a expression have also been shown in the lesional skin of vitiligo patients suggesting the importance of miR-183, miR-30a-3p, and miR-487a expression in rendering vitiligo susceptibility (Ruksha et al. 2017). Apart from the upregulated expression of miRNAs being responsible for vitiligo disease pathogenesis, individual miRNAs have been found to be significantly downregulated in the lesional skin as compared to controls. A downregulated miR-145 can restrict melanocyte proliferation and cause melanocyte death by inducing apoptosis via caspase-3 and caspase-7 activation, thereby playing a prime role in disease initiation (Sahmatova et al. 2016). The expressions of miR-211, miR-141, miR-136, miR-296, and miR-328 have been found to be specifically downregulated in vitiligo skin exhibiting their potential role in the development and progression of the disease (Mansuri et al. 2016).

Genetic susceptibility

In the recent years, several genome-wide association and linkage studies have been conducted in vitiligo which is a polygenic disorder with a complex mechanism of pathogenesis. Although multiple studies have demonstrated the genetic background of vitiligo development, however, the genetic risk is not absolute. Strong evidence for genetic factors in the pathogenesis of generalized vitiligo from various gene expression and association studies identified candidate genes. These candidate genes were found to be involved in encoding components of biological networks that primarily regulate the elements of the immune system and their targeted destruction of melanocytes mediating vitiligo susceptibility (Spritz 2012). Accordingly, several potent disease-contributing loci has been identified to be associated with vitiligo. Between 15 and 20% of patients have one or more familial first-degree relatives with vitiligo indicating the sporadic nature of occurrence of non-segmental vitiligo. Moreover, a 23% concordance of the disease has been noted in monozygotic twins (Spritz 2013). This signifies the penetrance of the genetic predisposition to vitiligo and heritability of vitiligo-associated genes (Alikhan et al. 2011). Identifying vitiligo susceptibility genes and characterizing the stress responses against trigger events that delineate autoimmune components causing disease progression would impel towards significant progress in understanding vitiligo etiology. Various studies have identified that the majority of the susceptible gene variants inculpates modulation of the immune system along with genes linked with melanocytes proliferation and migration (Zhang and Xiang 2014). It is the modulation and alteration exerted by specific genetic variations and their interactions that predispose inflammatory responses targeting melanocyte death owing to the onset of vitiligo.

Genetic studies have identified a majority of the genes that are associated with vitiligo to be a subset of immune regulatory genes concerning immuno-modulatory functions. However, a small number of genes have been identified to be linked to functions involving the regulation of melanocytes growth and proliferation, thus supporting immune regulatory mechanisms as the process that manifest vitiligo. The functional role of the many identified susceptibility loci in the pathogenesis of vitiligo is not known yet which remarkably overlaps with the genes that influence other autoimmune disorders underlining our incomplete knowledge of the disease mechanism (Shen et al. 2016). Genetic mutations that have the potential to modulate both the innate and adaptive immune responses increase the risk for vitiligo susceptibility. Table 2 lists the genetic variants that have been reported to be associated with vitiligo susceptibility. Mutations in several genes in the HLA class I and II regions encoding MHC have been discovered to be associated with vitiligo (Spritz 2012; Shen et al. 2016). MHCs are responsible for the processing and presentation

Table 2 Vitiligo susceptible genetic variants

Gene	Locus	Protein	Role
BACH2	6q15	BTB domain and CNC homolog 2	B cell regulator
BTNL2	6p21.32	Butyrophilin-like 2	T cell regulator
CASP7	10q25.3	Caspase 7	Apoptosis
CAT	11p13	Catalase	Oxidative stress regulator
CCR6	6q27	C-C motif chemokine receptor 6	B cell, T cell and dendritic cell regulator
CD44	11p13	CD44 antigen	T cell regulator
CD80	3q13.33	T-lymphocyte activation antigen CD80	T cell priming by B cells, T cells and dendritic cells
CLNK	4p16.1	Cytokine-dependent hematopoietic cell linker	Positive regulator of mast cells
C1QTNF6	22q12.3	Complement C1q tumor necrosis factor-related protein 6	Immune response-induced apoptosis
CTLA4	2q33.2	Cytotoxic T-lymphocyte protein 4	T cell inhibition
CXCR5	11q23.3	C-X-C motif chemokine receptor 5	B cell activity
FGFR1OP	6q27	Fibroblast growth factor receptor 1 oncogene partner	Cell growth and proliferation
FOXP3	Xp11.23	Forkhead box protein P1	T cell activity and development
GSTP1	11q13.2	Glutathione S-transferase Pi 1	Oxidative stress regulator
GZMB	14q12	Granzyme B	Cytotoxic T lymphocyte-mediated death
HLA-A, HLA-B and HLA-C	6p22.1	Human leukocyte antigen A, B and C	Peptide antigen presentation
HLA-DQB1 and HLA-DRB1	6p21.32	Human leukocyte antigen DQB1 and DRB1	Peptide antigen presentation
IFIH1	2q24.2	Interferon-induced helicase C domain containing protein 1	Innate immune activity
IFNAR1	21q22.11	Interferon alpha and beta receptor subunit 1	T cell signaling
IKZF4	12q13.2	Zinc finger protein Eos	T cell regulator
IL2RA	10p15.1	Interleukin-2 receptor subunit alpha	Interleukin 2-dependent T cell activation
LTA	6p21.33	Lymphotoxin alpha	Immune response-induced apoptosis
MC1R	16q24.3	Melanocortin 1 receptor	Melanogenesis regulator
MTHFR	1p36.22	Methylenetetrahydrofolate reductase	Oxidative stress regulator
NLRP1	17p13.2	NLR family pyrin domain containing 1	Innate immune Activity
OCA2	15q12-13-1	P protein	Melanosomal transporter
PMEL	12q13.2	Premelanosome protein	Melanosomes regulator
PTPN22	1p13.2	Tyrosine-protein phosphatase non-receptor type 22	T cell signaling
RERE	1p36.23	Arginine-glutamic acid dipeptide repeats protein	Lymphoid co-repressor
SH2B3	12q24.12	SH2B adaptor protein 3	T cell signaling
SLA	8q24.22	Src-like adaptor	T cell signaling
SOD2 and SOD3	6q25.3, 4p15.2	Superoxide dismutase 2 and 3	Oxidative stress regulator
TICAM1	19p13.3	Toll-like receptor adaptor molecule 1	Innate immune activity
TLR2 and TLR4	4q31.3, 9q33.1	Toll-like receptor 2 and 4	Innate immune activity
TNF	6p21.33	Tumor necrosis factor	Cell proliferation, differentiation and apoptosis
TYR	11q14.3	Tyrosinase	Melanogenesis regulator
UBASH3A	21q22.3	Ubiquitin associated and SH3 domain containing A	T cell signaling
ZMIM1	10q22.3	Zinc finger MIZ-type containing 1	Transcriptional co-activator

of antigens and are associated with autoimmune diseases in the incidence of derailed recognition of self-antigens. Failure of the immune system to recognize self-antigens leads to the development of autoreactive T cells that eventually restrict the formation of an efficient regulatory T cell (Treg) population (Simmonds and Gough 2007). Also, genetic variants of CTLA4 that are involved in T cell inhibition have been implicated to have a role in vitiligo pathogenesis (Birlea et al. 2009). Genome-wide association studies (GWAS) have found alteration in the genes that encode for factors involved in B cell regulation (BACH2), T cell development and priming (CD44, CD80), T cell receptor signaling (SLA, PTPN22, UBASH3A, CLNK, IFNAR1), and T cell activation (IKZF4, IL2RA, BTNL2, FOXP3) to be associated with vitiligo. Altered expression of the genes that regulate the innate immune response (IFIH1, NLRP1, TICAM1, TLR) and chemokine or cytokine receptors (CXCR5, CCR6, SH2B3) have also been found to be associated with vitiligo (Jin et al. 2012; Karaca et al. 2013; Shen et al. 2016).

Polymorphisms in non-immune-related genes have also been identified as risk factors. The melanocyte-specific genes (TYR, PMEL, MC1R, OCA2) encode for proteins or enzymes that participate in melanin production, and the ZMIZI gene is involved in the regulation of melanocyte development and survival (Sun et al. 2014). Genetic variants of these genes may serve as T cell antigens (autoantigens) which facilitates the initiation of an anti-melanocyte immune response contributing to cellular stress and melanocyte damage resulting in the development of vitiligo (Jin et al. 2010; Spritz 2013). Variation in the genes FGFR1OP, RERE, and CASP7 which have a central role in apoptosis along with GZMB, C1QTNF6, LTA, and TNF which are involved in immune response-induced apoptosis has also been linked with vitiligo (Lee and Bae 2015; Shen et al. 2016). Recently, an elevated plasma level of homocysteine has been described in patients with vitiligo which is associated with the polymorphic expression of MTHFR. MTHFR regulates homocysteine levels in the plasma, and an increased expression renders higher susceptibility to oxidative stress thereby contributing to the damage of melanocytes in vitiligo patients (Chen et al. 2014). Additionally, the genes GSTP1, SOD, and CAT are all broadly expressed in defense against oxidative stress wherein altered expression of these genes impairs their defense mechanisms contributing to ROS-induced melanocyte death in vitiligo patients (Wood et al. 2008; Liu et al. 2009; Laddha et al. 2013).

Scope of network-interaction studies and polypharmacological studies in understanding vitiligo disease module

Network science and analysis involve systemic cataloging of molecular interactions that offer unforeseen perspective prospects to understand and analyze the internal cellular organization and the interconnections between disease-related genes and functional proteins. Network-based studies facilitate in elucidating the extensive complex cellular networks presenting an ideal framework of their cellular organization. Protein-protein interaction networks composed of multiple nodes connected by edges accommodate better estimation of network statistics contributing to a comprehensive assistance in discerning the cellular organizing principles and molecular mechanisms that dictate the manifestation of a disease cycle (Barabasi and Oltvai 2004). This is particularly propitious when interpreting polygenic disorders having intricate patterns. Protein-protein interactions are of prime importance for various cellular and regulatory processes. Genetic variation alters or damages protein structure inciting disruption in protein-protein interactions constituting the pretext of disease development. These interaction networks usually consist of a few essential nodes (called hubs) that show maximum interaction to a large number of neighboring nodes. According to the phenomena of the centrality-lethality rule, the identification of such hub proteins and their inhibition may be lethal for the network. The magnitude of the change in structure caused by the removal of a node in a network determines the relative importance of the node in the network. Removal of such structurally critical nodes (hubs) in a network is widely believed to reflect the significance of the network architecture to better ascertain the network functionality (He and Zhang 2006). These hubs in a protein-protein interaction network may represent potential drug candidates. Since drug discovery and development is a complicated and expensive process, polypharmacology has emerged as the next paradigm of drug discovery. The transformation in the philosophy of current drug designing from one drug-one target to multiple targets of a single drug incorporates polypharmacological analysis that intends to discover the unknown targets for the existing drugs (Yildirim et al. 2007). Polypharmacology-based integrated systems biology approaches along with computational modeling, pharmacological, and clinical studies are productive for identification of novel molecular determinants essential in drug discovery and development. It also aids in unraveling the understanding of the significant impact of a new drug on complex human diseases (Rahman et al. 2018). A drug showing connections with multiple nodes (targets) in a network implies its high efficacious potential to control or inhibit the function of the particular target that is detrimental for regulatory pathways (Boran and Iyengar 2010). The identification of such hub proteins in vitiligo disease network together with polypharmacological studies will serve as an effective practical approach towards improved therapeutic interventions for better vitiligo management.

Conclusions

Cellular and molecular genetics studies have improved our knowledge on disease pathogenesis opening possibilities for new targeted therapies. An understanding of the mechanisms leading to melanocyte degeneration and autoimmunity and how melanocytes interact with their surroundings may help to unravel the rationale for the lack of melanocyte regeneration in vitiligo. Also, profiling the biological mediators of disease mechanisms might identify new therapeutic targets that may arrest disease progression and promote cell regeneration thereby stimulating repigmentation in the affected areas. Improved therapeutic and diagnostic modalities would substantially increase the compliance and satisfaction of patients. Also, the association of vitiligo with other diseases indicates that the knowledge of vitiligo pathogenesis could be of importance other than the skin as well.

Abbreviations

CMV: Cytomegalovirus; GWAS: Genome-wide association studies; HBV: Hepatitis B virus; HIV: Human immunodeficiency virus; HLA: Human leukocyte antigen; HO1: Heme oxygenase 1; MART-1: Melanoma antigen recognized by T cells 1; MHC: Major histocompatibility complex; NB-UVB: Narrow-band UVB; NLRP1: NLR family pyrin domain containing 1; NPY: Neuropeptide Y; PDGFRB: Platelet-derived growth factor receptor β; ROS: Reactive oxygen species; SIRT1: Sirtuin 1; TRP: Tyrosinase; UTR: Untranslated region; XBP1: X-box binding protein

Acknowledgements

Not applicable.

Funding

This work was supported by the Department of Biotechnology, Government of India [No.BT/PR5402/BID/7/508/2012].

Authors' contributions

YH conceived and designed the study. RR and YH prepared the manuscript. Both the authors read and approved the final manuscript.

Competing interests

The authors declare that they have no competing interests.

References

Akbayir N, Gokdemir G, Mansur T, Sokmen M, Gündüz S, Alkim C, Barutcuoglu B, Erdem L. Is there any relationship between hepatitis C virus and vitiligo? J Clin Gastroenterol. 2004;38:815–7.

Akcan Y, Kavak A, Sertbas Y, Olut AI, Korkut E, Bicik Z, Kisacik B. The low seropositivity of hepatitis B virus in vitiligo patients. J Eur Acad Dermatol Venereol. 2006;20(1):110–1.

AlGhamdi KM, Kumar A. Depigmentation therapies for normal skin in vitiligo universalis. J Eur Acad Dermatol Venereol. 2011;25(7):749–57.

Alikhan A, Felsten LM, Daly M, Petronic-Rosic V. Vitiligo: a comprehensive overview Part, I Introduction, epidemiology, quality of life, diagnosis, differential diagnosis, associations, histopathology, etiology, and work-up. J Am Acad Dermatol. 2011;65:473–91.

Barabasi AL, Oltvai ZN. Network biology: understanding the cell's functional organization. Nat Rev Genet. 2004;5(2):101–13.

Bellei B, Pitisci A, Ottaviani M, Ludovici M, Cota C, Luzi F, Dell'Anna ML, Picardo M. Vitiligo: a possible model of degenerative diseases. PLoS One. 2013;8(3):e59782.

Ben Ahmed M, Zaraa I, Rekik R, Elbeldi-Ferchiou A, Kourda N, Belhadj Hmida N, Abdeladhim M, Karoui O, Ben Osman A, Mokni M, Louzir H. Functional defects of peripheral regulatory T lymphocytes in patients with progressive vitiligo. Pigment Cell Melanoma Res. 2012;25(1):99–109.

Bhatnagar A, Kanwar AJ, Parsad D, De D. Comparison of systemic PUVA and NB-UVB in the treatment of vitiligo: an open prospective study. J Eur Acad Dermatol Venereol. 2007;21(5):638–42.

Birlea SA, LaBerge GS, Procopciuc LM, Fain PR, Spritz RA. CTLA4 and generalized vitiligo: two genetic association studies and a meta-analysis of published data. Pigment Cell Melanoma Res. 2009;22(2):230–4.

Boisseau-Garsaud AM, Garsaud P, Cales-Quist D, Helenon R, Queneherve C, Claire RC. Epidemiology of vitiligo in the French West Indies (Isle of Martinique). Int J Dermatol. 2000;39(1):18–20.

Boran AD, Iyengar R. Systems approaches to polypharmacology and drug discovery. Curr Opin Drug Discov Devel. 2010;13(3):297.

Chang CL, Au LC, Huang SW, Fai Kwok C, Ho LT, Juan CC. Insulin up-regulates heme oxygenase-1 expression in 3T3-L1 adipocytes via PI3-kinase- and PKC-dependent pathways and heme oxygenase-1-associated microRNA downregulation. Endocrinology. 2011;152:384–93.

Chen JX, Shi Q, Wang XW, Guo S, Dai W, Li K, Song P, Wei C, Wang G, Li CY, Gao TW. Genetic polymorphisms in the methylenetetrahydrofolate reductase gene (MTHFR) and risk of vitiligo in Han Chinese populations: a genotype-phenotype correlation study. Br J Dermatol. 2014;170(5):1092–9.

Dell'Anna ML, Picardo M. A review and a new hypothesis for non-immunological pathogenetic mechanisms in vitiligo. Pigment Cell Melanoma Res. 2006;19(5):406–11.

Ezzedine K, Diallo A, Leaute-Labreze C, Seneschal J, Boniface K, Cario-Andre M, Prey S, Ballanger F, Boralevi F, Jouary T, Mossalayi D. Pre-vs. post-pubertal onset of vitiligo: multivariate analysis indicates atopic diathesis association in pre-pubertal onset vitiligo. Br J Dermatol. 2012a;167(3):490–5.

Ezzedine K, Gauthier Y, Leaute-Labreze C, Marquez S, Bouchtnei S, Jouary T, Taieb A. Segmental vitiligo associated with generalized vitiligo (mixed vitiligo): a retrospective case series of 19 patients. J Am Acad Dermatol. 2011;65(5):965–71.

Ezzedine K, Lim HW, Suzuki T, Katayama I, Hamzavi I, Lan CC, Goh BK, Anbar T, Silva de Castro C, Lee AY, Parsad D. Revised classification/nomenclature of vitiligo and related issues: the vitiligo global issues consensus conference. Pigment Cell Melanoma Res. 2012b;25(3)

Gauthier Y, Cario-Andre M, Lepreux S, Pain C, Taieb A. Melanocyte detachment after skin friction in non lesional skin of patients with generalized vitiligo. Br J Dermatol. 2003;148(1):95–101.

Geel N, Bosma S, Boone B, Speeckaert R. Classification of segmental vitiligo on the trunk. Br J Dermatol. 2014;170(2):322–7.

Gey A, Diallo A, Seneschal J, Leaute-Labreze C, Boralevi F, Jouary T, Taieb A, Ezzedine K. Autoimmune thyroid disease in vitiligo: multivariate analysis indicates intricate pathomechanisms. Br J Dermatol. 2013;168(4):756–61.

Gupta V, Sreenivas V, Mehta M, Khaitan BK, Ramam M. Measurement properties of the Vitiligo impact Scale-22 (VIS-22), a vitiligo-specific quality-of-life instrument. Br J Dermatol. 2014;171(5):1084–90.

Halder RM. Childhood vitiligo. Clin Dermatol. 1997;15:899–906.

He X, Zhang J. Why do hubs tend to be essential in protein networks? PLoS Genet. 2006;2(6):e88.

Hossain C, Porto DA, Hamzavi I, Lim HW. Camouflaging agents for vitiligo patients. J Drugs Dermatol. 2016;15(4):384–7.

Howitz J, Brodthagen H, Schwartz M, Thomsen K. Prevalence of vitiligo: epidemiological survey on the Isle of Bornholm, Denmark. Arch Dermatol. 1977;113(1):47–52.

Jablonski NG, Chaplin G. Human skin pigmentation as an adaptation to UV radiation. Proc Natl Acad Sci USA. 2010;107(Supplement 2):8962–8.

Jiang L, Cheng Z, Qiu S, Que Z, Bao W, Jiang C, Zou F, Liu P, Liu J. Altered let-7 expression in myasthenia gravis and let-7c mediated regulation of IL-10 by directly targeting IL-10 in Jurkat cells. Int Immunopharmacol. 2012;14:217–23.

Jimbow K, Chen H, Park JS, Thomas PD. Increased sensitivity of melanocytes to oxidative stress and abnormal expression of tyrosinase-related protein in vitiligo. Br J Dermatol. 2001;144(1):55–65.

Jin Y, Birlea SA, Fain PR, Ferrara TM, Ben S, Riccardi SL, Cole JB, Gowan K, Holland PJ, Bennett DC, Luiten RM. Genome-wide association analyses identify 13 new susceptibility loci for generalized vitiligo. Nat Genet. 2012;44(6):676.

Jin Y, Birlea SA, Fain PR, Gowan K, Riccardi SL, Holland PJ, Mailloux CM, Sufit AJ, Hutton SM, Amadi-Myers A, Bennett DC. Variant of TYR and autoimmunity susceptibility loci in generalized vitiligo. N Engl J Med. 2010;362:1686–97.

Karaca N, Ozturk G, Gerceker BT, Turkmen M, Berdeli A. TLR2 and TLR4 gene polymorphisms in Turkish vitiligo patients. J Eur Acad Dermatol Venereol. 2013;27(1):e85–90.

Kasumagic-Halilovic E, Ovcina-Kurtovic N, Jukic T, Karamehic J, Begovic B, Samardzic S. Vitiligo and autoimmunity. Med Arch. 2013;67(2):91.

Kasumagic-Halilovic E, Prohic A, Begovic B, Ovcina-Kurtovic N. Association between vitiligo and thyroid autoimmunity. J Thyroid Res. 2011;3:938257.

Kemp EH, Emhemad S, Akhtar S, Watson PF, Gawkrodger DJ, Weetman AP. Autoantibodies against tyrosine hydroxylase in patients with non-segmental (generalised) vitiligo. Exp Dermatol. 2011;20:35–40.

Kim DY, Oh SH, Hann SK. Classification of segmental vitiligo on the face: clues for prognosis. Br J Dermatol. 2011;164(5):1004–9.

Krüger C, Schallreuter KU. A review of the worldwide prevalence of vitiligo in children/adolescents and adults. Int J Dermatol. 2012;51(10):1206–12.

Kruger C, Schallreuter KU. Cumulative life course impairment in vitiligo. Curr Probl Dermatol. 2013;44:102–17.

Laddha NC, Dwivedi M, Gani AR, Shajil EM, Begum R. Involvement of superoxide dismutase isoenzymes and their genetic variants in progression of and higher susceptibility to vitiligo. Free Radic Biol Med. 2013;65:1110–25.

Lang KS, Muhm A, Moris A, Stevanovic S, Rammensee HG, Caroli CC, Wernet D, Schittek B, Knauss-Scherwitz E, Garbe C. HLA-A2 restricted, melanocyte-specific CD8+ T lymphocytes detected in vitiligo patients are related to disease activity and are predominantly directed against MelanA/MART1. J Invest Dermatol. 2001;116(6):891–7.

Lazarova R, Hristakieva E, Lazarov N, Shani J. Vitiligo-related neuropeptides in nerve fibers of the skin. Arch Physiol Biochem. 2000;108(3):262–7.

Le Poole IC, Das PK, van den Wijngaard RM, Bos JD, Westerhof W. Review of the etiopathomechanism of vitiligo: a convergence theory. Exp Dermatol. 1993;(4):145–53.

Le Poole IC, Luiten RM. Autoimmune etiology of generalized vitiligo. Curr Dir Autoimmun. 2008;10:227–43.

Le Poole IC, van den Wijngaard RM, Westerhof W, Das PK. Tenascin is overexpressed in vitiligo lesional skin and inhibits melanocyte adhesion. Br J Dermatol. 1997;137(2):171–8.

Lee YH, Bae SC. Associations between TNF-α polymorphisms and susceptibility to rheumatoid arthritis and vitiligo: a meta-analysis. Genet Mol Res. 2015;14(2):5548–9.

Leone G, Paro VA. Effect of an antioxydant cream versus placebo in patients with vitiligo in association with excimer laser: a pilot randomized, investigator-blinded, and half-side comparison trial. G Ital Dermatol Venereol. 2015;150(4):461–6.

Levandowski CB, Mailloux CM, Ferrara TM, Gowan K, Ben S, Jin Y, McFann KK, Holland PJ, Fain PR, Dinarello CA, Spritz RA. NLRP1 haplotypes associated with vitiligo and autoimmunity increase interleukin-1β processing via the NLRP1 inflammasome. Proc Natl Acad Sci U S A. 2013;110(8):2952–6.

Lili Y, Yi W, Ji Y, Yue S, Weimin S, Ming L. Global activation of CD8+ cytotoxic T lymphocytes correlates with an impairment in regulatory T cells in patients with generalized vitiligo. PLoS One. 2012;7:e37513.

Lilly E, Lu PD, Borovicka JH, Victorson D, Kwasny MJ, West DP, Kundu RV. Development and validation of a vitiligo-specific quality-of-life instrument (VitiQoL). J Am Acad Dermatol. 2013;69(1):e11–8.

Liu L, Li C, Gao J, et al. Genetic polymorphisms of glutathione S-transferase and risk of vitiligo in the Chinese population. J Invest Dermatol. 2009;129(11):2646–52.

Mansuri MS, Singh M, Begum R. miRNA signatures and transcriptional regulation of their target genes in vitiligo. J Dermatol Sci. 2016;84(1):50–8.

Mansuri MS, Singh M, Dwivedi M, Laddha NC, Marfatia YS, Begum R. MicroRNA profiling reveals differentially expressed microRNA signatures from the skin of patients with nonsegmental vitiligo. Br J Dermatol. 2014;171:1263–7.

Maresca V, Roccella M, Roccella F, Camera E, Del Porto G, Passi S, Grammatico P, Picardo M. Increased sensitivity to peroxidative agents as a possible pathogenic factor of melanocyte damage in vitiligo. J Invest Dermatol. 1997;109(3):310–3.

Marie J, Kovacs D, Pain C, Jouary T, Cota C, Vergier B, Picardo M, Taieb A, Ezzedine K, Cario-Andre M. Inflammasome activation and vitiligo/nonsegmental vitiligo progression. Br J Dermatol. 2014;170(4):816–23.

Niamba P, Traore A, Taieb A. Vitiligo in a black patient associated with HIV infection and repigmentation under antiretroviral therapy. Ann Dermatol Venereol. 2007;134:272.

Nicolaidou E, Antoniou C, Miniati A, Lagogianni E, Matekovits A, Stratigos A, Katsambas A. Childhood- and later-onset vitiligo have diverse epidemiologic and clinical characteristics. J Am Acad Dermatol. 2012;66:954–8.

Njoo MD, Spuls PI, Bos JT, Westerhof W, Bossuyt PM. Nonsurgical repigmentation therapies in vitiligo: meta-analysis of the literature. Arch Dermatol. 1998;134(12):1532–40.

Nordal EJ, Guleng GE, Rönnevig JR. Treatment of vitiligo with narrowband-UVB (TL01) combined with tacrolimus ointment (0.1%) vs. placebo ointment, a randomized right/left double-blind comparative study. J Eur Acad Dermatol Venereol. 2011;25(12):1440–3.

Ormerod AD. Topical tacrolimus and pimecrolimus and the risk of cancer: how much cause for concern? Br J Dermatol. 2005;153(4):701–5.

Oyarbide-Valencia K, van den Boorn JG, Denman CJ, Li M, Carlson JM, Hernandez C, Nishimura MI, Das PK, Luiten RM, Le Poole IC. Therapeutic implications of autoimmune vitiligo T cells. Autoimmun Rev. 2006;5(7):486–92.

Paradisi A, Tabolli S, Didona B, Sobrino L, Russo N, Abeni D. Markedly reduced incidence of melanoma and nonmelanoma skin cancer in a nonconcurrent cohort of 10,040 patients with vitiligo. J Am Acad Dermatol. 2014;71(6):1110–6.

Parsad D, Dogra S, Kanwar AJ. Quality of life in patients with vitiligo. Health Qual Life Outcomes. 2013;1:58.

Picardo M, Dell'Anna ML, Ezzedine K, Hamzavi I, Harris JE, Parsad D, Taieb A. Vitiligo. Nat Rev Dis Primers. 2015;1:15011.

Rahman R, Sharma I, Gahlot LK, Hasija Y. DermaGene and VitmiRS: a comprehensive systems analysis of genetic dermatological disorders. Biomed Dermatol. 2018;2(1):18.

Ratsep R, Kingo K, Karelson M, Reimann E, Raud K, Silm H, Vasar E, Koks S. Gene expression study of IL10 family genes in vitiligo skin biopsies, peripheral blood mononuclear cells and sera. Br J Dermatol. 2008;159:1275–81.

Rezaei N, Gavalas NG, Weetman AP, Kemp EH. Autoimmunity as an aetiological factor in vitiligo. J Eur Acad Dermatol Venereol. 2007;21(7):865–76.

Ruksha TG, Komina AV, Palkina NV. MicroRNA in skin diseases. Eur J Dermatol. 2017;27(4):343–52.

Sahmatova L, Tankov S, Prans E, Aab A, Hermann H, Reemann P, Pihlap M, Karelson M, Abram K, Kisand K, Kingo K. MicroRNA-155 is dysregulated in the skin of patients with vitiligo and inhibits melanogenesis-associated genes in melanocytes and keratinocytes. Acta Derm Venereol. 2016;96(6):742–8.

Salzes C, Abadie S, Seneschal J, Whitton M, Meurant JM, Jouary T, Ballanger F, Boralevi F, Taieb A, Taieb C, Ezzedine K. The Vitiligo Impact Patient Scale (VIPs): development and validation of a vitiligo burden assessment tool. J Investig Dermatol. 2016;136(1):52–8.

Saunders LR, Sharma AD, Tawney J, Nakagawa M, Okita K, Yamanaka S, Willenbring H, Verdin E. miRNAs regulate SIRT1 expression during mouse embryonic stem cell differentiation and in adult mouse tissues. Aging (Albany NY). 2010;2:415–31.

Sehgal VN, Srivastava G. Vitiligo: compendium of clinico-epidemiological features. Indian J Dermatol Venereol Leprol. 2007;73(3):149.

Senol A, Yucelten AD, Ay P. Development of a quality of life scale for vitiligo. Dermatology. 2013;226(2):185–90.

Shah R, Hunt J, Webb TL, Thompson AR. Starting to develop self-help for social anxiety associated with vitiligo: using clinical significance to measure the potential effectiveness of enhanced psychological self-help. Br J Derm. 2014;171:332–7.

Shen C, Gao J, Sheng Y, Dou J, Zhou F, Zheng X, Ko R, Tang X, Zhu C, Yin X, Sun L. Genetic susceptibility to vitiligo: GWAS approaches for identifying vitiligo susceptibility genes and loci. Front Genet. 2016;7:3.

Shi YL, Weiland M, Li J, Hamzavi I, Henderson M, Huggins RH, Mahmoud BH, Agbai O, Mi X, Dong Z, Lim HW. MicroRNA expression profiling identifies potential serum biomarkers for non-segmental vitiligo. Pigment Cell Melanoma Res. 2013;26(3):418–21.

Simmonds MJ, Gough SC. The HLA region and autoimmune disease: associations and mechanisms of action. Curr Genomics. 2007;8(7):453–65.

Sitek JC, Loeb M, Ronnevig JR. Narrowband UVB therapy for vitiligo: does the repigmentation last? J Eur Acad Dermatol Venereol. 2007;21(7):891–6.

Spritz RA. The genetics of generalized vitiligo: autoimmune pathways and an inverse relationship with malignant melanoma. Genom Med. 2010;2(10):78.

Spritz RA. Six decades of vitiligo genetics: genome-wide studies provide insights into autoimmune pathogenesis. J Invest Dermatol. 2012;132(2):268–73.

Spritz RA. Modern vitiligo genetics sheds new light on an ancient disease. J Dermatol. 2013;40(5):310–8.

Sravani PV, Babu NK, Gopal KV, Rao GR, Rao AR, Moorthy B, Rao TR. Determination of oxidative stress in vitiligo by measuring superoxide dismutase and catalase levels in vitiliginous and non-vitiliginous skin. Indian J Dermatol Venereol Leprol. 2009;75(3):268.

Strassner JP, Harris JE. Understanding mechanisms of autoimmunity through translational research in vitiligo. Curr Opin Immunol. 2016;43:81–8.

Sun Y, Zuo X, Zheng X, Zhou F, Liang B, Liu H, Chang R, Gao J, Sheng Y, Cui H, Wang W. A comprehensive association analysis confirms ZMIZ1 to be a susceptibility gene for vitiligo in Chinese population. J Med Genet. 2014; 51(5):345–53.

Taher ZA, Lauzon G, Maguiness S, Dytoc MT. Analysis of interleukin-10 levels in lesions of vitiligo following treatment with topical tacrolimus. Br J Dermatol. 2009;161(3):654–9.

Taieb A. Vitiligo as an inflammatory skin disorder: a therapeutic perspective. Pigment Cell Melanoma Res. 2012;25(1):9–13.

Teovska Mitrevska N, Eleftheriadou V, Guarneri F. Quality of life in vitiligo patients. Dermatol Ther. 2012;25(Suppl. 1):S28–31.

Toker SC, Sarycaoglu H, Karadogan SK, Mistik R, Baskan EB, Tunaly S. Is there any relation between vitiligo and cytomegalovirus? J Eur Acad Dermatol Venereol. 2007;21:141–2.

Van Den Boorn JG, Konijnenberg D, Dellemijn TA, Van Der Veen JW, Bos JD, Melief CJ, Vyth-Dreese FA, Luiten RM. Autoimmune destruction of skin melanocytes by perilesional T cells from vitiligo patients. J Invest Dermatol. 2009;129(9):2220–32.

van Geel N, Speeckaert R, De Wolf J, Bracke S, Chevolet I, Brochez L, Lambert J. Clinical significance of Koebner phenomenon in vitiligo. Br J Dermatol. 2012; 167(5):1017–24.

van Geel N, Wallaeys E, Goh BK, De Mil MA, Lambert J. Long-term results of noncultured epidermal cellular grafting in vitiligo, halo naevi, piebaldism and naevus depigmentosus. Br J Dermatol. 2010;163(6):1186–93.

Wagner RY, Luciani F, Cario-Andre M, Rubod A, Petit V, Benzekri L, Ezzedine K, Lepreux S, Steingrimsson E, Taieb A, Gauthier Y. Altered E-cadherin levels and distribution in melanocytes precede clinical manifestations of vitiligo. J Investig Dermatol. 2015;135(7):1810–9.

Wang X, Du J, Wang T, Zhou C, Shen Y, Ding X, Tian S, Liu Y, Peng G, Xue S, Zhou J, Wang R, Meng X, Pei G, Bai Y, Liu Q, Li H, Zhang J. Prevalence and clinical profile of vitiligo in China: a community-based study in six cities. Acta Derm Venereol. 2013;93(1):62–5.

Wood JM, Gibbons NC, Chavan B, Schallreuter KU. Computer simulation of heterogeneous single nucleotide polymorphisms in the catalase gene indicates structural changes in the enzyme active site, NADPH-binding and tetramerization domains: a genetic predisposition for an altered catalase in patients with vitiligo? Exp Dermatol. 2008;17(4):366–71.

Yildirim MA, Goh KI, Cusick ME, Barabasi AL, Vidal M. Drug-target network. Nat Biotechnol. 2007;25(10):1119–26.

Zhang Z, Xiang LF. Genetic susceptibility to vitiligo: recent progress from genome-wide association studies. Dermatol Sin. 2014;32(4):225–32.

25

Inhibitory effect of naringenin on LPS-induced skin senescence by SIRT1 regulation in HDFs

Kye Hwa Lim[1] and Gyu Ri Kim[2*]

Abstract

Background: This study aims to investigate the ability of naringenin to regulate the expression of nuclear factor-κB, the upper gene of lipopolysaccharide-induced SIRT1; regulate signal transduction in the extracellular matrix, which plays an important role in the dermis; and alter the matrix metalloproteinase 1 and matrix metalloproteinase 3 gene expression, therefore having suppressing effect on skin cell senescence and deoxyribonucleic acid protection and cell protection effects and confirm naringenin's potential as an important cosmetic ingredient.

Methods: The efficacy of naringenin was assessed through reactive oxygen species assay, water-soluble tetrazolium salt assay, nuclear factor-κB luciferase assay, enzyme-linked immunosorbent assay, nicotinamide adenine dinucleotide phosphate oxidase activity assay, and quantitative real-time polymerase chain reaction.

Results: Sirt1, which regulates naringenin upstream of the nuclear factor-κB pathway, inhibits nuclear factor-κB activity and decreases matrix metalloproteinase expression level and SIRT1 gene dose-dependently. The results confirmed naringenin had an anti-aging effect on lipopolysaccharide-induced skin senescence. Various age-related biomarkers were used to analyze the inhibitory effect naringenin had on cell senescence progress and oxidative activity. Further experiments also showed naringenin also acted on NADPH oxidase, which produces superoxide (O2-), resulting in inhibiting NADPH oxidase activity. Experimental results reported that naringenin regulated the activity of SIRT1, which is the cause of modern skin cell aging, and in turn had a regenerative effect on reactive oxygen species-induced skin cellular senescence which affects skin elasticity and wrinkles.

Conclusions: This study confirmed that naringenin inhibits cellular senescence and regenerates human dermal fibroblasts damaged by lipopolysaccharide, and suggests that naringenin will be a cosmetic ingredient that has cell regenerative effects and anti-aging effects.

Keywords: Naringenin, Lipopolysaccharide, SIRT1, Human dermal fibroblasts, Nuclear factor-κB, Cellular aging, Skin cell regeneration, Antioxidation

Background

More than 300 theories have been proposed to explain the basic mechanisms for the progression of aging (Medvedev 1990). Among the three major theories, the first theory of reactive oxygen is a key mechanism of innate immunity (Harman 2006). The theory of free radicals was first introduced by Dr. Gerschman in 1954, but was developed by Dr. Denham Harman. In the free radical theory, it is

known that reactive oxygen species (ROS), which are generated abnormally, can induce DNA damage and oxidation of proteins, nucleic acids, and lipids (Nakayama et al. 2016). Secondly, in the programmed cellular senescence theory (Aubert and Lansdorp 2008), the major mechanisms involved in the senescence process, which include the insulin/IGF-1 signaling pathway and the mTOR pathway as well as the AMP kinase (AMPK), and Sirtuin protein were found to be aging factors. Thirdly, according to the inflammation theory, immune responses decrease with aging, contributing to the increased

* Correspondence: grkim@eulji.ac.kr
[2]Department of Beauty and Cosmetic Science, Eulji University, 553, Sanseong-daero, Sujeong-gu, Seongnam-si, Gyeonggi-do 13135, Republic of Korea
Full list of author information is available at the end of the article

incidence of different chronic diseases with an inflammatory component (Coppe et al. 2010).

With increased levels of the pro-inflammatory cytokines, interleukin (IL)-1β, IL-6, and IL-8 are the senescence-associated secretory phenotype (SASP). While these theories aid the overall understanding of aging, the mechanism for skin disease and aging is difficult to define (Fagiolo et al. 1993).

Cells that are involved in skin wrinkles are fibroblasts, granulocytes, macrophages, and mast cells that are present in the dermis, which is a visible characteristic of skin aging that is of most importance to modern women. Decreased synthesis of collagen types I and III due to incomplete mechanical stimulation of the tissue forming the skin tissue and matrix metalloproteinase (MMP) activity forms skin sagging and deep wrinkles (Sardy 2009). Phenomenons caused by aging include changes in cell contact, insecure DNA replication at the end of chromosome, reduction of DNA repair ability, histone methylation modification, stem cell exhaustion, loss of quality of proteostasis ability of protein, mitochondrial dysfunction, nutritional control disorder, and increased senile senescence. As a typical phenomenon, cell senescence and telomere portions become shorter, and aging cells change the tissue microenvironment associated with matrix metalloproteinases, a kind of secretory phenotypes (Tchkonia et al. 2013), and induced matrix metalloproteinases, and in turn matrix metalloproteinases inhibit the synthesis of a generation of collagen in the body and thus represent an important feature of skin aging (Wondrak et al. 2003; Kimura et al. 2014).

Recent studies have shown that SIRT1 (silent mating type information regulation 2 homolog, Sirtuin 1), a SIR2 mutein that acts to enhance the viability of mammalian cells belonging to the longevity gene that regulates the activity of NF-κB, is a nicotinamide adenine dinucleotide (NAD +) which is a class III deacetylase that is involved in a number of biological processes including DNA repair, energy metabolism, tumor suppression, and mitochondrial stabilization (Michan and Sinclair 2007). SIRT1-associated SIR2 is a type of sirtuin, a deacetylase that is dependent on nicotinamide adenine dinucleotide (NAD +), and these genes have been shown to have an effect on life prolongation in yeast and Drosophila (Cohen et al. 2004). Recent studies have also shown that SIRT1 plays a positive role in stress, metabolism, apoptosis, and premature aging. Environmental stresses such as smoking and air pollution are reported to reduce the production of SIRT1 in lungs, causing lung diseases (Rajendrasozhan et al. 2008). In addition, activation of NF-κB and activation of JNK, ERK, p38, and MAP kinase through SIRT1 expression inhibition lead to increased production of ROS. SIRT1 is mainly found in the nucleus and is known to deacetylate various proteins including p53, FOXO, NK-κB, Ku70, and histone (Haigis and Guarente 2006; Kimura et al. 2014).

SIRT1 plays an important role in cell survival by acting on cell cycle molecules and deacetylation of apoptosis regulatory proteins (Noh et al. 2013). As a factor controlling the development and differentiation of neurons, it has been recently reported to effectively inhibit neuronal dysfunction and nerve cell death in neurodegenerative diseases such as Alzheimer's disease and Parkinson's disease (Finkel and Holbrook 2000).

SIRT1 inhibits the secretion of inflammatory cytokines TNF-α and IL-6 and increases the secretion of anti-inflammatory cytokine IL-10 (Lu et al. 2008) and has anti-inflammatory effects by downregulating the expression of various inflammatory cytokines in endothelial cells and macrophages (Michishita 2005; Stein and Matter 2011). As the expression level of SIRT1 decreases, the expression level of MMPs increases. Furthermore, by inhibiting the expression of MMP1, SIRT1 promotes the synthesis of extracellular matrix (Razaq et al. 2010).

SIRT1 and NF-κB system regulation, one of the most important causes of various common skin problems in modern people, represents an ancient signaling pathway that regulates metabolism and metabolism. This reaction inhibits the inflammatory cells of mammals through opposite regulation mechanisms (Salminen 2008; Kauppinena et al. 2013). Prevention of skin aging, anti-pollution, and inflammation treatments are primarily aimed at the cosmetic and medical industries; however, they are still insufficient (Rajendrasozhan et al. 2008).

Recently, reported anti-aging molecules have been developed to minimize intrinsic or extrinsic aging factors and to produce intracellular signaling molecules involved in collagen synthesis and its degradation (Rajendrasozhan et al. 2008; Mukherjee et al. 2011; Hwang et al. 2014). These antioxidants include antioxidants of natural raw materials through in vitro experiments, such as Ligularia fischeri, Rubus coreanus Miquel, Korean pine nut shells, lotus leaf, and bolus terminated chitosan, which is a seawood.

Through in vivo or human application tests, citrus, Oenanthe javanica, dandelion, soybean, Saururus chinensis, and Peucedanum japonicum Thunberg were proven as natural raw material antioxidants (Na et al. 2016).

Naringenin (4′,5,7-trihydroxy flavanone), a yellow crystalline powder, is hydrolyzed from a form of rutinoside of flavanone to an aglycone form. When the convert is complete, absorption is promoted and present at a higher concentration in plasma, bile, urine, etc., thus exhibiting anti-inflammatory effects in RAW 264.7 cell lines and anti-cancer effects in cancer cells (Fuhr and Kummert 1995; Tripoli et al. 2007).

Naringenin has a polyphenol structure capable of eliminating active oxygen groups and active oxygen generated by hydrogen/electron transfer in the 4-hydroxyl group of group B, and shows anti-inflammatory activity and antioxidant activity (Vafeiadou et al. 2009).

This study focused on the lack of research on naringenin's effects on skin, especially its potent as a cosmetic ingredient and its intracellular mechanism of action, and carried out experiments to investigate how naringenin regulates the activity of SIRT1, which in turn controls the activity of nuclear factor-κB, a major cause of modern skin aging, and has inhibitory effects on the reactive oxygen species production.

Methods

Cell culture

In this study, human dermal fibroblasts (HDFs) were purchased from Lonza Switzerland and cultured in Dulbecco's modified Eagle medium (DMEM; Hyclone, USA) supplemented with 10% fetal bovine serum (FBS; Hyclone), 1% penicillin/streptomycin (100 IU/mL penicillin, 100 μg/mL streptomycin; Invitrogen, USA) and cultured at 37 °C and 5% CO_2.

Sample treatment

Naringenin (Sigma-Aldrich, USA) was used to dissolve the purified powder (> 99%) in a suitable concentration in dimethyl sulfoxide (DMSO; Sigma-Aldrich). Lipopolysaccharide (LPS), a cell-stimulating agent, was purchased from Sigma-Aldrich. For the experiment, the solution was dissolved in dimethyl sulfoxide (DMSO; Sigma-Aldrich) at a proper concentration. HDFs (1×10^6 cells/well) were incubated in a 60-mm cell culture dish for 24 h. An appropriate concentration of naringenin was added to the culture medium. Lipopolysaccharide was co-treated at a constant concentration for 24 h and analyzed 3 h later. The significance of PCR was validated using a melting curve. The gene expressions were compared for analysis by normalizing the β-actin expression.

Cell viability estimation

WST-1 Cell Proliferation Assay System used a chromogenic material, formazan, which is formed from tetrazolium salts (WST-1) by intracellular mitochondrial dehydrogenase, to quantify cell proliferation and cell viability. Human dermal fibroblasts were inoculated into metabolically active 96-well plates, at a concentration of 3×10^3 cells/well, and cultured for 24 h. HDFs were simultaneously treated with various samples such as naringenin and LPS and cultured for 24 h. Ten microliters of EZ-Cytox cell viability assay kit reagent (ItsBio, Korea) was added to the cultured cells and incubated for 1 h. The absorbance was measured at 490 nm using a microplate reader (Bio-Rad, USA). The mean and standard deviation of cell viability were calculated after repeating the procedure three times.

qRT-PCR analysis

Changes of gene expression caused by naringenin in the cells were quantitatively confirmed. qRT-PCR was performed by mixing 0.2 μM primers, 50 mM KCl, 20 mM Tris/HCl pH 8.4, 0.8 mM dNTP, 0.5 U Extaq DNA polymerase, 3 mM MgCl 2, and 1X SYBR green (Invitrogen). PCR was validated by melting curve. The melting curve confirmed the validity of PCR. Expression of each gene was standardized and compared. The primers used in this experiment are shown in Table 1.

ROS assay

To investigate the effect of naringenin on the removal of reactive oxygen species, ROS scavenging assay was performed. Human dermal fibroblasts were seeded in a 60-mm culture dish at 2×10^5 cells/well and cultured for 24 h. Cells were treated appropriately, cultured for an additional 24 h, added 10 μM of dichlorofluorescein diacetate (DCF-DA), and then cultured for 30 min. After cells were harvested and analyzed for changes in ROS using a flow cytometer (BD Biosciences, USA). N-Acetyl-L-cysteine (NAC; Calbiochem, USA) serving as a ROS scavenger was also measured in the same manner.

Nuclear factor-κB luciferase assay ·

To investigate the effect of naringenin on the nuclear factor-κB transcriptional activity, the nuclear factor-κB promoter luciferase assay was used. In this experiment, the nuclear factor-κB reporter NIH-3T3 stable cell line (Panomics, USA) containing the reporter gene with the nuclear factor-κB promoter consensus sequence was used in the promoter region. Nuclear factor-κB reporter NIH-3T3 stable cells were inoculated in a 60-mm culture dish at a concentration of 2×10^5 cells, cultured for 24 h, treated with appropriate conditions, and cultured for additional 24 h. The cultured cells were harvested; passive lysis buffer (Promega, USA) was added, put in ice for 10 min, dissolved, then centrifuged at 12,000 rpm at 4 °C for 30 min to recover the supernatant. A sample containing the same amount of protein was added to a black 96-well plate (80 μg each), followed by luciferin (Promega, USA). The luminescence of luciferin was measured using a luminometer (Veritas, USA).

Table 1 Lists of primers

Gene	Forward primer	Reverse primer
β-actin	GGATTCCTATGTGGGCGACGA	CGCTCGGTGAGGATCTTCATG
SIRT1	GCAGGTTGCGGGAATCCAA	GGCAAGATGCTGTTGCAAA
MMP1	TCTGACGTTGATCCCAGAGAGCAG	CAGGGTGACACCAGTGACTGCAC
MMP3	ATTCCATGGAGCCAGGCTTTC	CATTTGGGTCAAACTCCAACTGTG
HO-1	GCCTGCTAGCCTGGTTCAAG	AGCGGTGTCTGGGATGAACTA

Enzyme-linked immunosorbent assay (ELISA)

MMPs (Merck, USA; sandwich) and PGE2 (Cayman chemical, USA; competitive) were evaluated using an enzyme-linked immunosorbent assay (ELISA) kit according to the instruction manual for the HDF culture medium. Prostaglandin E2, MMPs, and monoclonal antibody were immobilized on plastic cell culture dish wells. One hundred microliters of each culture medium was dispensed (at room temperature for 2 h). After washing five times each with a single washing buffer, 100 μL horseradish peroxidase (HRP)-conjugated anti-MMP1 antibody was added for 1 h at room temperature, and 100 μL of tetramethylbenzidine (TMB) was added and incubated for 30 min in a dark room. The absorbance was measured at 405–420 nm (PGE2) and 450 nm (MMPs).

Nicotinamide adenine dinucleotide phosphate oxidase assay

Naringenin has an antioxidative effect on the oxidase activity of reduced NADP, NADPH, which directly influences superoxide anion (O2-) production, which in turn plays the most fundamental role in ROS production. To study the antioxidative effect of naringenin on NADPH oxidase activity, using HDFs, 100 μL of homogenates was added to each well and 900 μL of 50 mM phosphate buffer (1 mM EGTA, 150 mM sucrose, 5 mM lucigenin, 100 mM NADPH, pH 7.0) was added which was examined through lucigenin chemiluminescence assay.

Statistical process

All experiments were performed independently three times, and the results were expressed as mean ± standard deviation. Student's t test was used to analyze all findings, with a p value of 0.05, 0.01, or 0.001 below considered as statistically significant (*$p < 0.05$, **$p < 0.01$, ***$p < 0.001$).

Results

Cytotoxicity of naringenin and lipopolysaccharide

Lipopolysaccharide acts as an endotoxin in cells, activating signals such as MAPK, NF-κB, and IRF-3 and promoting excessive secretion of inflammatory cytokines (Lu et al. 2008). Lipopolysaccharide induced nuclear factor-κB activity through IκB phosphorylation and its degradation. In this study, WST-1 assay was performed to determine the cytotoxicity of naringenin in human dermal fibroblasts. Human dermal fibroblasts were treated with untreated control group and naringenin-treated group at 1-, 2-, 5-, and 10-μM dose levels, each respectively, for 24 h.

Cell viability of untreated control group was set as 100%, and up to 1-μM dose level, the survival rate was shown to be 100% or more. When naringenin was treated at 1-, 2-, 5-, and 10-μM dose levels, the cell viability levels of 101%, 107%, 117%, and 110% did not decrease, confirming almost no toxicity (Fig. 1a). To confirm the changes in the survival rate of cells, HDFs was treated with LPS at 1-, 2-, 3-, 4-, and 5-μg dose levels, respectively, and the survival rate was 94% at 1 μg/mL (Fig. 1b).

Protective effect of naringenin on LPS-induced cell senescence in HDFs

Changes in Sirt1 expression

SIRT1 inhibits NF-κB, a protein complex that promotes inflammatory responses. Furthermore, by inhibiting the MMP1 production, SIRT1 promotes the synthesis of extracellular matrix (Wang et al. 2012).

qRT-PCR was performed to study the SIRT1 expression. Compared to the control group, SIRT1 expression was decreased to 0.56 level at 1-μg dose of LPS. However, when naringenin treatment was applied, SIRT1 gene expression increased back in a dose-dependent manner, resulting in 0.64 level at 5 μM and 0.86 level at 10 μM (Fig. 2a).

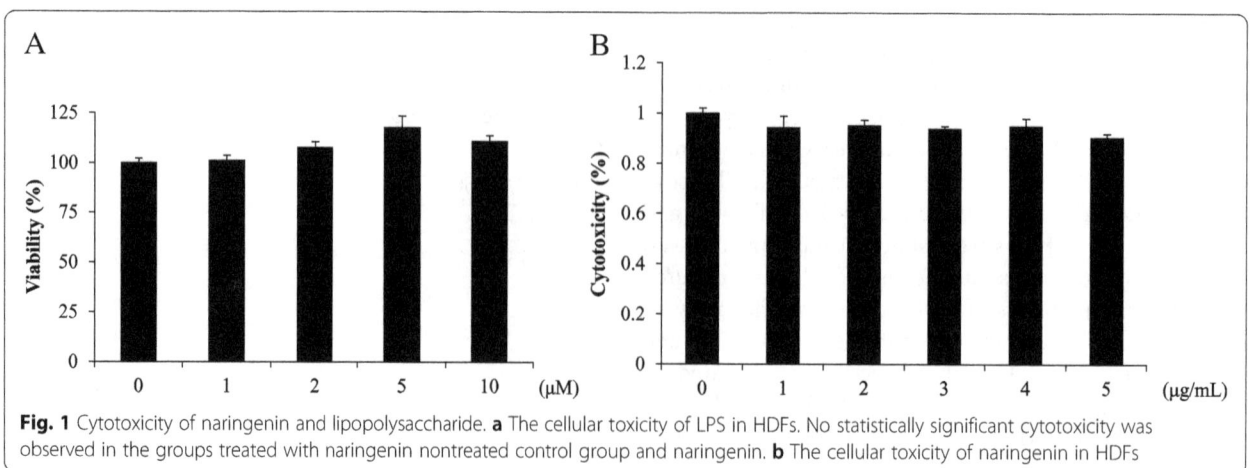

Fig. 1 Cytotoxicity of naringenin and lipopolysaccharide. **a** The cellular toxicity of LPS in HDFs. No statistically significant cytotoxicity was observed in the groups treated with naringenin nontreated control group and naringenin. **b** The cellular toxicity of naringenin in HDFs

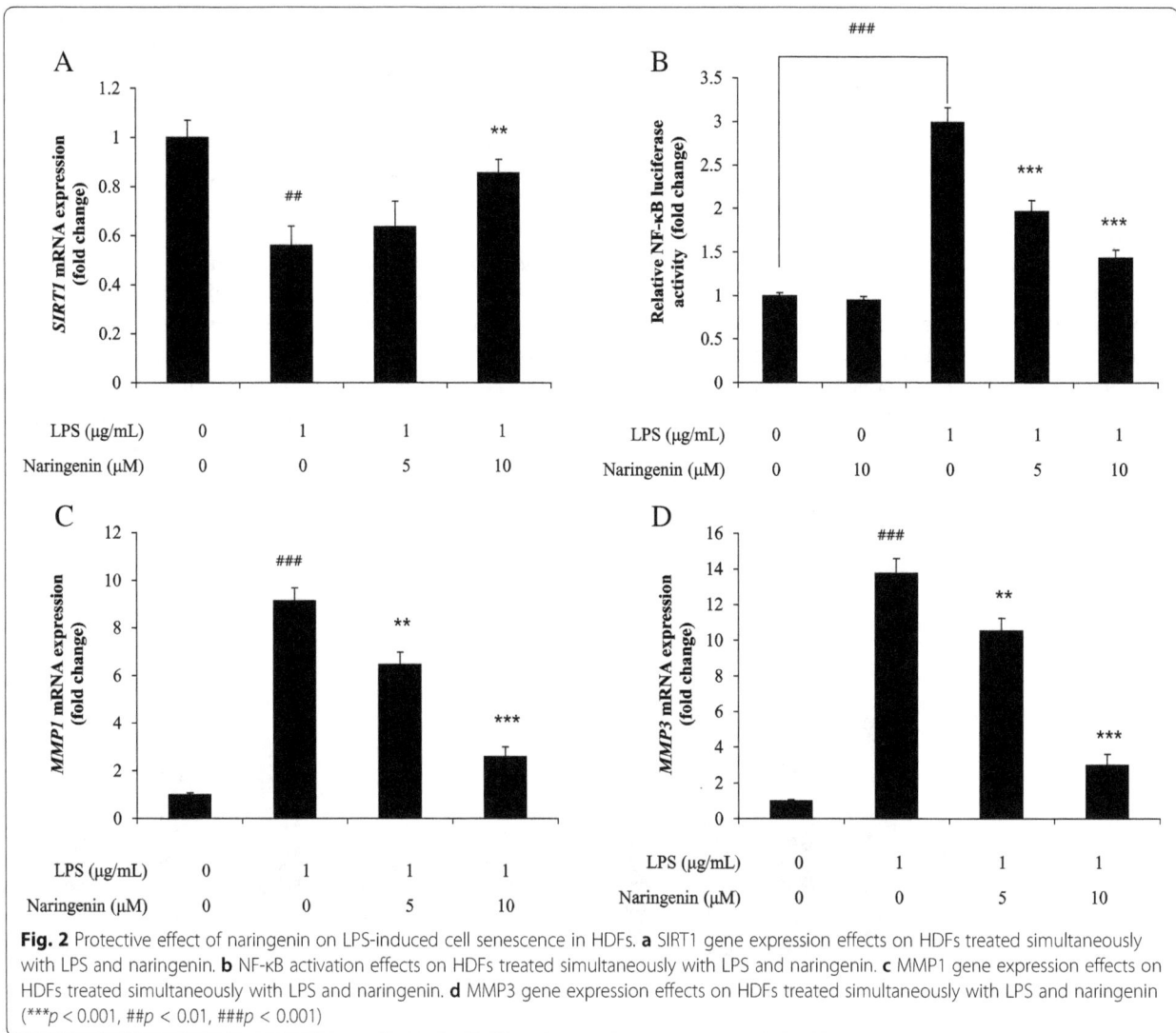

Fig. 2 Protective effect of naringenin on LPS-induced cell senescence in HDFs. **a** SIRT1 gene expression effects on HDFs treated simultaneously with LPS and naringenin. **b** NF-κB activation effects on HDFs treated simultaneously with LPS and naringenin. **c** MMP1 gene expression effects on HDFs treated simultaneously with LPS and naringenin. **d** MMP3 gene expression effects on HDFs treated simultaneously with LPS and naringenin (***$p < 0.001$, ##$p < 0.01$, ###$p < 0.001$)

Changes in nuclear factor-κB expression

In NF-κB signaling pathway, NF-κB is activated by LPS through phosphorylation and is then translocated to the nucleus, promoting the transcription of inflammatory cytokines and mediators, initiating various diseases (Lvashkiv 2011; Schett et al. 2013).

When LPS was treated with NF-κB luciferase assay, cell expression level increased to 3.0. When naringenin was treated with 5- and 10-μM dose levels, cell expression level each decreased to 2 and 1.4. Therefore, cell interval level was dose-dependently reduced by naringenin (Fig. 2b).

Changes in MMP1 and MMP3 expression

ELISA was performed to determine the effect of naringenin on the dermis by assaying the antigen or antibody using antigen-antibody reaction after binding the enzyme to the antibody, in order to investigate the effect of naringenin on the dermal structure of the skin through the changes of MMPs, an anti-aging index, and to examine the changes in gene expression of MMP1 and MMP3, which break down type I collagen of dermis related to skin wrinkles.

When HDFs were not treated with naringenin and LPS, the level of MMP1 gene expression was 1.0, and when treated by LPS, the level increased to 9.1. However, the level of MMP1 gene expression was decreased by naringenin in a dose-dependent manner to 6.4 at 5 μM treatment and 2.5 at 10 μM treatment (Fig. 2c). In addition, when HDFs were not treated with naringenin and LPS, MMP3 gene expression level was 1.0 and when treated with LPS, MMP3 gene expression level increased to 14. However, MMP3 expression decreased in a dose-dependent manner with naringenin, with MMP3 gene expression level decreasing from 11 to 3 when pretreatment of 5 μM and 10 μM were each applied (Fig. 2d). Therefore, naringenin was shown to inhibit MMP1 and MMP3 gene expression in the dermis.

Protective effect of naringenin on oxidative stress by LPS in HDFs

Expression changes in ROS production

ROS activates NF-κB, a transcriptional factor of inflammatory response through LPS stimulation, and in turn activates pro-inflammatory factors such as cytokines, NO, PGE2, iNOS, COX2, IL-1β, MCP-1, MIP-1, IL-16, IL-18, and M-CSF, which contributes to the development of chronic diseases (Levi et al. 1998; Knott et al. 2000; Rivest 2003).

To investigate the effect of naringenin on the total intracellular amount of ROS in LPS-treated HDFs, fluorescent probe DCF-DA was performed. When naringenin and NAC treatment were not present, LPS treatment increased the total amount of ROS level to 2.1. At 5 μM dose, naringenin decreased the level to 1.7 and further decreased the level to 1.2 at 10 μM. When the control group NAC was treated with 10 mM, the total amount of ROS level decreased to 1.0.

The results showed that at a low concentration of 10 μM, naringenin reduced ROS in a dose-dependent manner compared to the 10 mM of NAC applied on the positive control group, showing inhibiting effects on normal skin cell function impairment which resulted in excellent antioxidant activity (Fig. 3a).

Changes in NADPH oxidase expression

NADPH oxidase exists in vascular smooth muscle cells and endothelial cells and is also a major source of peroxidation that causes vascular disease and atherosclerosis. NADPH oxidase is a multiple enzyme complex consisting of large gp91phox known as Nox2, a small protein p22phox, and three cytosolic components p40phox, p47phox, p67phox, and Rac (Zalba et al. 2005). Cellular stimulation directly produces superoxide (O2-) and is produced by the activity of NADPH oxidase.

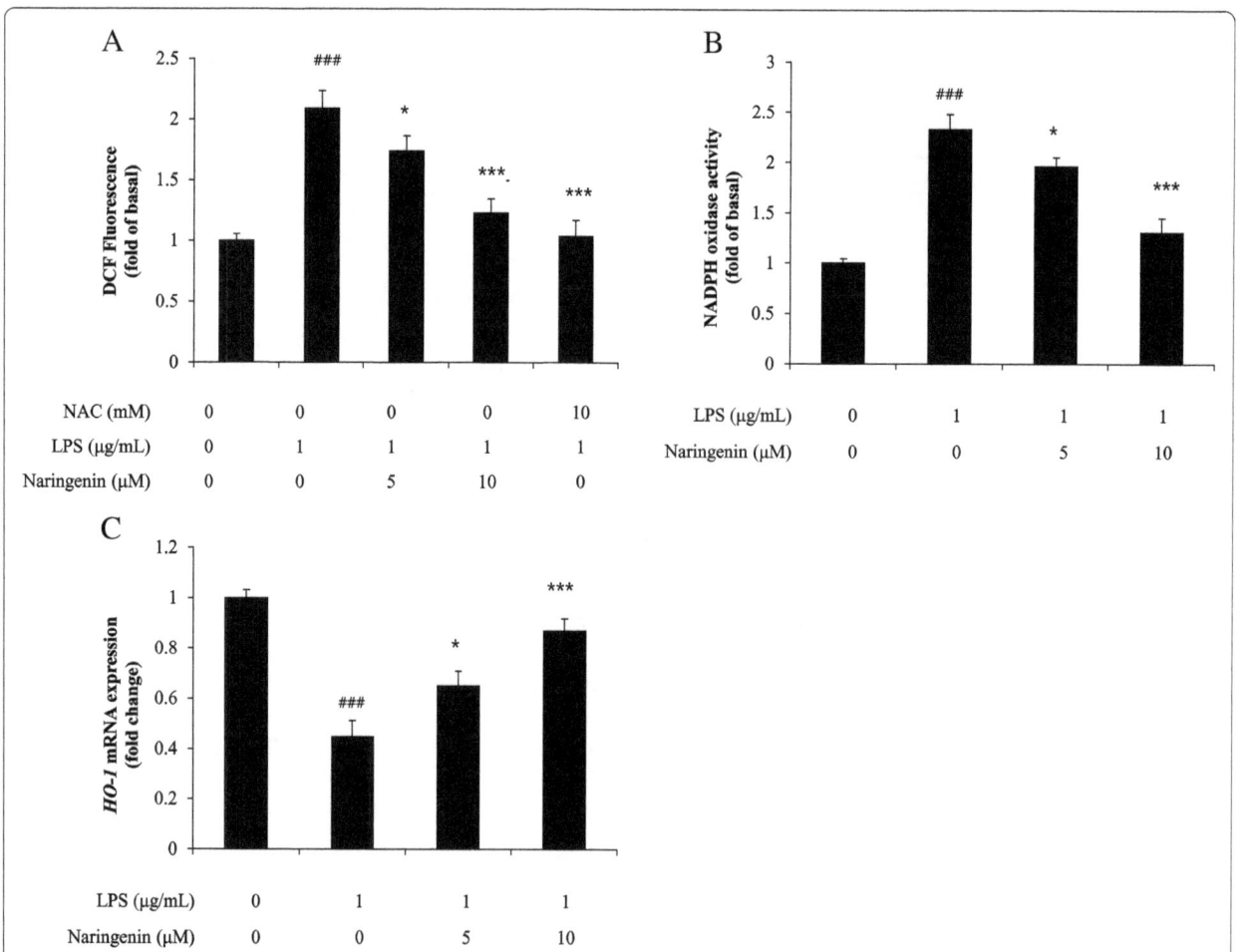

Fig. 3 Protective effect of naringenin on oxidative stress by LPS in HDFs. **a** Intracellular ROS scavenging activity on HDFs. **b** The effect of NADPH oxidase activity on HDFs treated simultaneously with LPS and naringenin. **c** HO-1 gene expression effects on HDFs treated simultaneously with LPS and naringenin. HDF human dermal fibroblast, LPS lipopolysaccharide, DCF dichlorodihydrofluorescein diacetate, NADPH nicotinamide adenine dinucleotide phosphate, HO-1 heme oxygenase-1. (*$p < 0.05$, ***$p < 0.001$, ###$p < 0.001$)

When LPS was treated with naringenin, cell interval level increased to 2.3. When naringenin was treated with 5 and 10 µM concentrations, the cell interval levels decreased to 2.0 and 1.3. Therefore, naringenin was shown to have dose-dependent reducing effect (Fig. 3b).

Changes in HO-1 expression

Heme oxygenase-1 (HO-1), one of the representative protective enzymes in the human body, shows protective effects through strong anti-apoptosis and antioxidant action during hepatic ischemia and reperfusion (40, 41).

To study the effect naringenin has on the dermal structure, the changes in HO-1 expression was analyzed through qRT-PCR assay. When LPS was treated with naringenin, the cell interval level increased to 0.4. When naringenin was treated at 5 and 10 µM concentrations, the level increased to 0.7 and 0.9. Therefore, it was confirmed that naringenin increased HO-1 expression again in a dose-dependent manner (Fig. 3c).

Discussion

Inhibitory effect of naringenin on aging HDFs in SIRT1

Aging cells release several factors called SASPs, which have deleterious effects on surrounding cells as well as tissues. Molecular activation of the inflammation-inducing gene by the redox signal pathway ultimately leads to inflamed tissues and organs, or aging (Cheng et al. 2011; Hall et al. 2003). We found that an increase in NF-κB activation and expression of inflammatory molecules, in addition to an increase in oxidative stress, causes exogenous aging and photoaging. We also found that endogenous aging occurs due to a combination of various internal factors over time and is mainly represented by cellular senescence. The main cause of cellular senescence is oxidative stress, which stops cell division and growth by blocking the cell cycle. MMP1, which is widely distributed in human tissues, is secreted by fibroblasts and mainly degrades type II collagen, a major component of cartilage matrix, as well as types VII and VI collagen (Roberts et al. 2006; Donmez 2012). In addition, when MMP1 cleaves the middle portion of collagen fibers, MMP3 and MMP9 subdivide and cleave the collagen further. HDFs regulate collagen metabolism through interaction of MMP1, tissue inhibitor of metalloproteinase 1 (TIMP1), type I collagen, transforming growth factor beta 1 (TGF-β1), and various cytokines. SIRT1, a major anti-senescence agent that inhibits the activity of these MMPs, is activated through nuclear histones, transcription factors, and protein deacetylation of cell-signaling mediators, which causes cell signaling, anti-aging, gene expression of cell protection, and neuronal differentiation (Wang et al. 2012; Correia et al. 2017). Recently, SIRT1 activation has been reported to suppress endoplasmic reticulum stress in renal tubular cells. In addition, resveratrol, polyphenol, and

SIRT1 activators mimic the anti-aging effects of calorie restriction in lower organisms, mitigate insulin resistance, and increase mitochondrial content in rats with a high-fat diet, resulting in their prolonged survival. SIRT1 also inhibits NF-κB, a protein complex that promotes inflammatory responses. Furthermore, by inhibiting MMP1 expression, SIRT1 promotes ECM synthesis (Wang et al. 2012). The degree of skin wrinkles and thickened skin formed by ROS controls MMP activity, which is highly correlated with aging features such as skin sagging and may lead to tumors due to their imbalance. It has been reported that ROS inhibits the transcriptional activity of Smad by inhibiting TGF-β, a growth-promoting factor, and so inhibits the expression of downstream collagen genes (Quan et al. 2010; Otterbein et al. 2003).

Using quantitative real-time polymerase chain reaction (qRT-PCR) assay and enzyme-linked immunosorbent assay (ELISA), we examined how naringenin affects the expression of the NF-κB upstream gene, *SIRT1*, and the downstream genes, *MMP1* and *MMP3*. The results showed that naringenin increases the expression of *SIRT1* and decreases the expression of *MMP1* and *MMP3* in a dose-dependent manner.

In conclusion, naringenin regulates the expression of *NF-κB*; regulates signal transduction in the ECM, which has important functions in the dermis; and alters *SIRT1*, *MMP1*, and *MMP3* expression. Therefore, naringenin has a suppressing effect on skin cell senescence, DNA protection, and cell protection, indicating that it can be an important cosmetic ingredient.

Inhibition of oxidation by naringenin through inhibition of ROS activity

NADPH oxidase directly influences the production of the superoxide anion (O^{2-}), which plays the most fundamental role in ROS production, and the inducible form of nitric oxide synthase (iNOS), which is related to the immune response in NOS and produces NO, which is important for immune cell signaling. $ONOO^-$, a potent oxidant that forms naturally in cells by the reaction of NO and O^{2-}, induces apoptosis and inflammation.

O^{2-} is an oxygen molecule produced in cells. It is then converted to H_2O_2 through a spontaneous reaction or enzymatic catalysis. In addition, when a transition metal (Fe, Cu) is present, Fenton's reaction reduces O^{2-} to H_2O_2 which are eliminated by the antioxidative enzymes superoxide dismutase (SOD) and catalase. However, the body lacks controlling enzymes for OH^-, which is harmful and is known to the human body (Chen and Ames 1994). Heme oxygenase-1 (HO-1) removes cause stains, wrinkles, and freckles through oxidation of inflammatory, toxic-free heme (Fe^{2+}), treats damaged cells, and protects the body from oxidative stress by increasing bilirubin, a bile pigment that removes ROS. HO-1 is also a cell-protecting enzyme that produces biliverdin and iron and is a potent antioxidant that protects the body against various oxidative stress-related diseases. HO-1 can also inhibit endoplasmic reticulum stress (Hu et al. 2015).

In conclusion, naringenin inhibits NADPH oxidase activity, which produces O^{2-}, removes ROS, and increases *HO-1* gene expression. The results of this study suggested that naringenin inhibits the damaging and aging effects of toxic substances that cause aging and skin inflammation.

Conclusions

Naringenin is a flavanone known to have physiological antioxidant and active oxygen-scavenging properties. It has a polyphenol structure capable of eliminating active oxygen groups and active oxygen generated by hydrogen/electron transfer in the 4-hydroxyl group of group B and has anti-inflammatory effects and antioxidant properties (Lee et al. 2016; Hee et al. 2018). SIRT1 inhibits NF-κB, a protein complex that promotes inflammatory responses and is correlated with common skin diseases caused by harmful particulate matter (PM) and environmental pollutants. Furthermore, by inhibiting the expression of MMP1, SIRT1 promotes ECM synthesis.

This study analyzed the anti-aging and antioxidative effects of naringenin by observing changes in the expression of the longevity gene *SIRT1* and the downstream genes *MMP1* and *MMP3* in the cell senescence model of LPS-induced HDFs. The results showed that naringenin increases *SIRT1* expression and decreases *NF-κB*, *MMP1*, and *MMP3* expression in a dose-dependent manner. Additional experiments confirmed the ability of NADPH oxidase to inhibit O^{2-} activity, remove ROS, and increase *HO-1* gene expression.

In conclusion, this in vitro research confirmed that naringenin not only increases SIRT1 activity but, by blocking the NF-κB pathway, also inhibits the gene expression of inflammatory factors (which are major components of SASPs) and substances that produce ROS. Naringenin can be used as an effective cosmetic ingredient to prevent age-induced skin elasticity reduction and wrinkled skin, troublesome skin diseases, and premature skin aging caused by harmful environmental pollutants, PM, etc.

Acknowledgements
Not applicable.

Funding
Not applicable.

Authors' contributions
KHL and GRK did all of the research background such as experiments, data collecting, and statistical analysis as well as drafting the manuscript. Both authors read and approved the final manuscript.

Competing interests
The authors declare that they have no competing interests.

Author details
[1]Department of Beauty Care, Sangji Youngseo College, 84, Sangjidae-gil, Wonju-si, Gangwon-do 26339, Republic of Korea. [2]Department of Beauty and Cosmetic Science, Eulji University, 553, Sanseong-daero, Sujeong-gu, Seongnam-si, Gyeonggi-do 13135, Republic of Korea.

References
Aubert G, Lansdorp PM. Telomeres and aging. Physiol Rev. 2008;88:557–79.
Chen Q, Ames BN. Senescence-like growth arrest induced by hydrogen peroxide in human diploid fibroblast F65 cells. Proc Natl Acad Sci. 1994;91:4130–4.
Cheng J, Phong B, Wilson DC, Hirsch R, Kane LP. Akt fine-tunes NF-kappaB-dependent gene expression during T cell activation. J Biol Chem. 2011;286:36076–85.
Cohen HY, Miller C, Bitterman KJ, Wall NR, Hekking B, Kessler B, Howitz KT, Gorospe M, de Cabo R, Sinclair DA. Calorie restriction promotes mammalian cell survival by inducing the SIRT1 deacetylase. Science. 2004;305:390–2.
Coppe JP, Desprez PY, Krtolica A, Campisi J. The senescence-associated secretory phenotype: the dark side of tumor suppression. Annu Rev Pathol. 2010;5:99–118.
Correia M, Perestrelo T, Rodrigues AS, Ribeiro MF, Pereira SL, Sousa MI, Ramalho-Santos J. Sirtuins in metabolism, stemness and differentiation. Biochim Biophys Acta. 2017;1861:3444–55.
Donmez G. The neurobiology of sirtuins and their role in neurodegeneration. Trends Pharmacol Sci. 2012;33:494–501.
Fagiolo U, Cossarizza A, Scala E. Increased cytokine production in mononuclear cells of healthy elderly people. Eur J Immunol. 1993;23:2375–8.
Finkel T, Holbrook NJ. Oxidants, oxidative stress and the biology of ageing. Nature. 2000;408:239–47.
Fuhr U, Kummert AL. The fate of naringin in humans: a key to grapefruit juice-drug interactions? Clin Pharmacol Ther. 1995;58:365–73.
Haigis MC, Guarente LP. Mammalian sirtuins-emerging roles in physiology, aging and calorie restriction. Genes Dev. 2006;0:2913–21.
Hall MC, Young DA, Waters JG, Rowan AD, Chantry A, Edwards DR. The comparative role of activator protein 1 and Smad factors in the regulation of Timp-1 and MMP-1 gene expression by transforming growth factor-beta 1. J Biol Chem. 2003;278:10304–13.
Harman D. Free radical theory of aging: an update: increasing the functional life span. Ann N Y Acad Sci. 2006;1067:10–21.
Hee JY, Kim GR, Ahn JJ, An IS, Kim YS. Inhibition of apoptosis and anti-inflammatory effects of embelin. Asian J Beauty Cosmetol. 2018;16:103–12.
Hu Y, Duan M, Liang S, Wang Y, Feng Y. Senkyunolide I protects rat brain against focal cerebral ischemia-reperfusion injury by up-regulating p-Erk1/2, Nrf2/HO-1 and inhibiting caspase 3. Brain Res. 2015;1605:39–48.
Hwang E, Park SY, Lee HJ, Lee TY, Sun ZW, Yi TH. Gallic acid regulates skin photoaging in UVB-exposed fibroblast and hairless mice. Phytother Res. 2014;28:1778–88.
Kauppinena A, Suuronen T, Ojalab J, Kaarniranta K, Salminen A. Antagonistic crosstalk between NF-κB and SIRT1 in the regulation of inflammation and metabolic disorders. Cell Signal. 2013;25(10):1939–48.
Kimura Y, Sumiyoshi M, Kobayashi T. Whey peptides prevent chronic ultraviolet B radiation-induced skin aging in melanin-possessing male hairless mice. J Nutr. 2014;144:27–32.
Knott C, Shern G, Wilkin GP. Inflammatory regulators in Parkinson's disease: iNOS, lipocortin-1, and cyclooxygenase-1 and -2. Mol Cell Neurosci. 2000;16:724–39.
Lee SJ, Han HS, An IS, Ahn KJ. Effects of amentoflavone on anti-inflammation and cytoprotection. Asian J Beauty Cosmetol. 2016;14:201–11.
Levi G, Minghetti L, Aloisi F. Regulation of prostanoid synthesis in microglial cells and effects of prostaglandin E2 on microglial functions. Biochimie. 1998;80:899–904.
Lu YC, Yeh WC, Ohashi PS. LPS/TLR4 signal transduction pathway. Cytokine. 2008;42:145–51.
Lvashkiv LB. Inflammatory signaling in macrophages: transitions from acute to tolerant and alternative activation states. Eur J Immunol. 2011;41:2477–81.

Medvedev ZA. An attempt at a rational classification of theories of aging. Biol Rev. 1990;65:375–98.

Michan S, Sinclair D. Sirtuins in mammals: insights into their biological function. Biochem J. 2007;404:1–13.

Michishita E. Evolutionarily conserved and nonconserved cellular localizations and functions of human SIRT proteins. Mol Biol Cell. 2005;16(10):4623–35.

Mukherjee T, Kim WS, Mandal L, Banerjee U. Interaction between Notch and Hif-alpha in development and survival of Drosophila blood cells. Science. 2011; 332:1210–3.

Na EJ, Jang HH, Kim GR. Review of recent studies and research analysis for anti-oxidant and anti-aging materials. Asian J Beauty Cosmetol. 2016;14(4):481–91.

Nakayama H, Nishida K, Otsu K. Macromolecular degradation systems and cardiovascular aging. Circ Res. 2016;118:1577–92.

Noh SJ, Kang MJ, Kim KM. Acetylation status of P53 and the expression of DBC1, SIRT1, and androgen receptor are associated with survival in clear cell renal cell carcinoma patients. Pathology. 2013;45:574–80.

Otterbein LE, Soares MP, Yamashita K, Bach FH. Heme oxygenase-1: unleashing the protective properties of heme. Trends Immunol. 2003;24(8):449–55.

Quan T, Shao Y, He T, Voorhees JJ, Fisher GJ. Reduced expression of connective tissue growth factor (CTGF/CCN2) mediates collagen loss in chronologically aged human skin. J Invest Dermatol. 2010;130:415–24.

Rajendrasozhan S, Yang SR, Kinnula VL, Rahman I. SIRT1, an antiinflammatory and antiaging protein, is decreased in lungs of patients with chronic obstructive pulmonary disease. Am J Respir Crit Care Med. 2008;177(8):861–70.

Razaq S, Wilkins RJ, Urban JP. The effect of extracellular pH on matrix turn over by cells of the bovine nucleus pulposus. Eur Spine J. 2010;12:341–9.

Rivest S. Molecular insights on the cerebral innate immune system. Brain Behav Immun. 2003;17:13–9.

Roberts S, Evans H, Trivedi J, Menage J. Histology and pathology of the human intervertebral disc. J Bone Joint Surg Am. 2006;88:10–4.

Salminen A. Interaction of aging-associated signaling cascades: inhibition of NF-kappaB signaling by longevity factors FoxOs and SIRT1. Cell Mol Life Sci. 2008;65(7–8):1049–58.

Sardy M. Role of matrix metalloproteinases in skin ageing. Connect Tissue Res. 2009;50:132–8.

Schett G, Elewaut D, McInnes IB, Dayer J, Neurath MF. How cytokine networks fuel inflammation: toward a cytokine-based disease taxonomy. Nat Med. 2013;19:822–4.

Stein S, Matter CM. Protective roles of SIRT1 in atherosclerosis. Cell Cycle. 2011;10:640–7.

Tchkonia T, Zhu Y, van Deursen J, Campisi J, Kirkland JL. Cellular senescence and the senescent secretory phenotype: therapeutic opportunities. J Clin Invest. 2013;123:966–72.

Tripoli E, Guardia ML, Giammanco S, Majo DD, Giammanco M. Citrus flavonoids: molecular structure, biological activity and nutritional properties. Food Chem. 2007;104:466–79.

Vafeiadou K, Vauzour D, Lee HY, Rodriguez-Mateos A, Williams RJ, Spencer JPE. The citrus flavanone naringenin inhibits inflammatory signalling in glial cells and protects against neuroinflammatory injury. Arch Biochem Biophys. 2009; 484(1):100–9.

Wang DW, Hu ZM, J Hao. SIRT1 inhibits apoptosis of degenerative human disc nucleus pulposus cells through activation of Akt pathway. AGE. 2013;35: 1741–53.

Wondrak GT, Roberts MJ, Cervantes-Laurean D, Jacobson MK, Jacobson EL. Proteins of the extracellular matrix are sensitizers of photo-oxidative stress in human skin cells. J Invest Dermatol. 2003;121:578–86.

Zalba G, SanJosé G, Moreno MU, Fortuño A, Díez J. NADPH oxidase mediated oxidative stress: genetic studies of the p22(phox) gene in hypertension. Antioxid Redox Signal. 2005;7(9–10):1327–36.

26

A new piece of an old puzzle: lack of association between C-Rel (rs13031237-rs842647) single nucleotide polymorphisms and non-segmental vitiligo

Eman Salah[1]* ⓘ and Alshymaa A. Ahmed[2]

Abstract

Background: The exact pathogenesis of vitiligo is still unclear; however, studies mostly support autoimmune mechanisms including altered T-regulatory cells and FOXP3. C-Rel is a NF-κB family member affecting the normal development of FOXP3⁺ regulatory T cells.

Methods: The aim was to examine the association between 2 C-Rel gene polymorphisms (rs13031237 and rs842647) and non-segmental vitiligo patients. Genomic DNA was isolated from blood samples of 100 patients plus 100 controls for genotyping using restriction fragment length polymorphism and DNA sequencing analyses. Statistical analysis was performed using SPSS program version 21 (IBM Corp., Chicago, IL, USA).

Results: The genotype frequencies did not differ significantly from non-segmental vitiligo patients to controls for both alleles.

Conclusions: C-Rel (rs13031237 and rs842647) polymorphisms are not associated with increased risk for non-segmental vitiligo. We recommend testing additional mutations in vitiligo patients from different populations to unravel Rel aspects among different autoimmune disorders.

Keywords: Melanocytes, Depigmentation, Autoimmune, T-regulatory cells, FOXP3

Background

Rel is a transcription factor encoded by C-Rel gene that is located on chromosome 2p16.1. It belongs to nuclear factor kappa-light-chain-enhancer of activated B cell (NF-κB) family, and its signaling pathway plays a critical role in several autoimmune disorders (Chen et al. 2016). C-Rel is expressed utmost only in mature hemopoietic cells but is not necessary for normal hematopoiesis and lymphopoiesis according to C-Rel knockout mice studies. However, C-Rel stays a prerequisite for various specific functions in mature T and B cells (Gilmore and Gerondakis 2011) such as antigen presentation and

CD40 signaling cascade (Chen et al. 2016). Furthermore, C-Rel is present at smaller levels in normal endothelial and epithelial cells including the skin. In the skin, loss of NF-κB activity is known to initiate a strong inflammatory response (Gilmore and Gerondakis 2011). Subsequently, C-Rel has been linked as a susceptibility locus to some autoimmune diseases including systemic lupus erythematosus (Zhou et al. 2012), rheumatoid arthritis (Gregersen et al. 2009; Eyre et al. 2010; Ali et al. 2013), Behcet's disease (Chen et al. 2016), psoriasis (Ali et al. 2013), and celiac disease (Gilmore and Gerondakis 2011; Varadé et al. 2011).

Vitiligo is a de-pigmenting skin disorder resulting in selective destruction of melanocytes. The exact pathogenesis of vitiligo is not clear; however, autoimmunity has been strongly implicated (Dwivedi et al. 2015). The first observation suggesting the involvement of defective T-regulatory cells (Tregs) in vitiligo originated after

* Correspondence: esmohamed@zu.edu.eg; connexin1980@yahoo.com
[1]Dermatology, Venereology & Andrology department, Faculty of Medicine, Zagazig University, Zagazig, Egypt
Full list of author information is available at the end of the article

experiments on murine melanomas. In those studies, reduction of Tregs count triggered the generation of cytotoxic T cells against melanoma cells. This ended in the successful destruction of melanoma, however unexpectedly triggered vitiliginous lesions (Zhang et al. 2007). Additionally, histopathological examination of lesional skin in vitiligo has shown increased CD8+ cytotoxic T lymphocytes and decreased CD4+ CD25+ FOXP3+ Tregs. This may explain the lost tolerance toward melanocytes with anti-melanocyte reactivity in non-segmental vitiligo (Jahan et al. 2013).

Among different markers expressed by Tregs, FOXP3 is by far the most distinctive (de Boer et al. 2007). As a transcription factor, FOXP3 has a critical role in Tregs differentiation and function. Surprisingly, Ruan et al. 2009 have found that the development of FOXP3+ Tregs requires C-Rel through a complex called the "C-Rel enhanceosome." Additionally, an association between increased susceptibility to non-segmental vitiligo and FOXP3 promoter (rs3761548) polymorphism was found in an Indian population (Jahan et al. 2013).

Herein, we sought to investigate two putative C-Rel single nucleotide polymorphisms (SNPs) (rs13031237 and rs842647) in peripheral blood of non-segmental vitiligo patients as a possible susceptibility risk candidate in comparison to healthy controls. The choice of these SNPs is based on the consideration of previously reported genetic associations with other autoimmune diseases (Chen et al. 2016; Gilmore and Gerondakis 2011; Zhou et al. 2012; Gregersen et al. 2009; Eyre et al. 2010; Varadé et al. 2011; Ali et al. 2013), and rs13031237 and rs842647 are the most frequently reported SNPs. The SNP rs13031237 is a G→T transition located in the fourth intron of *REL* gene (chromosomic location 61136129). The SNP rs842647 is an A→G transition located in the second intron of *REL* gene on chromosome 2 (chromosomic location 61119471).

Methods

Ethical approvals

The Institutional Review Board (IRB) and ethical committee at Zagazig University Hospitals approved this work. Before enrollment, all subjects provided a well-informed and written consent.

Subjects

This study includes a 100 of clinically diagnosed non-segmental vitiligo patients recruited from the outpatient clinic at the Dermatology, Venereology and Andrology Department of our Hospital. All patients underwent complete history taking including age, sex, disease onset, family history of vitiligo, associated disorders, disease severity using vitiligo area scoring index (VASI), and stability or activity. Stable vitiligo was considered in lack of

new lesions, a progression of existing lesions, depigmentation after successful re-pigmentation and of Koebner phenomenon during the last 6 months. All included patients were not receiving any therapy for vitiligo for at least 6 months before analysis. The control group involved one 100 healthy age and sex-matched volunteers. Initially, we tested 30 patients and 30 controls for C-Rel mutations (unpublished work) by PCR, then we extended the subjects count and confirmed the first provisional findings by DNA sequencing as follows.

C-Rel gene polymorphism genotyping by PCR-RFLP

Two milliliters of anticoagulated whole-blood samples using EDTA were withdrawn from every subject. C-Rel gene single nucleotide polymorphisms (SNPs) (rs13031237 & rs842647) were genotyped as follows: (1) Genomic DNA extraction was obtained using (QIAamp Blood Kit; Qiagen GmbH, Hilden, Germany) spin column technique, following the manufacturer's guidelines. (2) Amplification of the gene targets by PCR was carried out according to Persico et al. 2006 with modification. The primers for *rs13031237* were 5'-GAGTTGTTATGAGAGTAAAAGG CTGC-3' and 5'-AAGTACACAAGTTCTGCCTAGGGT AA-3'. While those for *rs842647* were 5'-TGCTTG TCTCTGATTCTCTGGGTC-3' and 5'-CTGGGCGACA AGTGTGAAA CTC-3'. PCR was carried out in 25 μl reaction mixture containing 12.5 μL of MyTaq, Red Master Mix (bioline, UK), 10 pmol of each primer, 100 ng of genomic DNA, and nuclease-free water up to 25 μl. PCR began first with denaturation at 95 °C for 5 min, then 35 cycles of denaturation at 95 °C for 30 s, annealing at 62 or 63 °C for rs13031237 and rs842647, respectively, for 40 s, and 72 °C for 30 s, followed by the last extension step at 72 °C for 3 min. PCR yields were checked out on 2.0% agarose gel electrophoresis as bands at 268 bp and 193 bp for rs13031237 and rs842647 respectively. (3) Restriction of RFLP products using enzyme Csp6I (Thermo Fisher Scientific Inc., Ontario, Canada) for rs13031237 in 37 °C and HpyCH4 III for rs842647 (Thermo Fisher Scientific Inc.,Ontario, Canada) in 65 °C was according to the manufacturer's guidelines. (4) PCR-RFLP product interpretation. Products were visualized on 2.0% agarose gel stained with ethidium bromide on an ultraviolet transilluminator. The candidate mutations in this study came at the cut point of the used restriction enzymes, so the wild alleles will be digested while the mutated ones will not. Homozygous wild genotypes will appear as two bands which are shorter than the original amplification band. While homozygous mutated genotypes will appear as one band at the site of the amplified one. A heterozygous case will appear as three bands, i.e., for rs13031237, they will be at 79 and 189 bp while for rs842647, they will be at 58 and 135 bp. While homozygous mutated genotypes will appear as one band at the site of the amplified one. A heterozygous case will appear as three bands.

REL gene polymorphism genotyping by DNA sequencing

Ambiguous samples were genotyped and 10% of samples were double-checked using direct Sanger sequencing as follows: (1) TopTaq Master Mix Kit (250) (Qiagen GmbH, Hilden, Germany) in 50 uL reaction volume with the previously mentioned protocol was used for PCR amplification. (2) Amplified PCR products underwent the first purification using QIAquik PCR Purification Kit (50) (Qiagen GmbH, Hilden, Germany) using the manufacturer's guidelines. (3) Cycle sequencing performed using Bigdye Terminator V3.1 cycle sequencing kit (Thermo Fisher Scientific Inc., Ontario, Canada) followed by the second purification of the products using BigDye X Terminator Purification Kit (Thermo Fisher Scientific Inc., Ontario, Canada), according to the manufacturer's guidelines. (4) The Applied Biosystems 3500 Genetic Analyzer (Thermo Fisher Scientific Inc., Ontario, Canada) was used for sequencing of the purified products. (5) Nucleotide Blast online program (https://blast.ncbi.nlm.nih.gov) was used for data analysis and interpretation of results.

Statistical analysis

SPSS program version 21 (IBM Corp., Chicago, IL, USA) was used for statistical analysis. Hardy-Weinberg equilibrium was conducted on the control group by using the chi-square test. Frequencies of each genotype, as well as allele, were expressed as numeral and percentage. Differences in C-Rel allele frequencies were analyzed using the chi-square test and the two-tailed Fisher's exact test for the results ≤ 5. The odds ratios (ORs), as well as the 95% confidence intervals, were calculated. $P \leq 0.05$ was considered as an indicator for statistically significant differences.

Results

This work included 70 females and 30 males with non-segmental vitiligo as well as a 100 of healthy volunteers as controls. Patients' ages ranged from 9 to 55 years old with a mean of 29.0 years, and VASI scores ranged from 20 to 70. Table 1 describes the clinical characteristics of the studied patients. Genotypes and allele distribution of the two tested SNPs among patients and controls were summarized in Table 2 and Fig. 1. There was no significant association between these mutations and disease occurrence. Independent sample t test was used to compare the mean age of onset of positive versus negative patients for each SNP to clarify whether these mutations affect the age of onset of vitiligo or not. For rs13031237, the mean age of onset of positive patients (GT and TT genotypes) was 30 years old while for the negative cases (GG genotype), it was 21.5 years old ($p = 0.06$); for

Table 1 Clinical characteristics of non-segmental vitiligo patients

Character	n (total = 100)	%
Females	70	70
Males	30	30
Family history for vitiligo	30	30
Associated other disorders		
Diabetes mellitus type-1	15	15
Hypothyroidism	5	5
Stable vitiligo	40	40
Active vitiligo	60	60

rs842647, the mean ages were 27 and 24.1 years old for AG and GG, and AA, respectively, ($p = 0.7$). Also, there was no significant association between the studied mutations and disease activity. It is worth mentioning that 20 patients have an associated disease (diabetes mellitus-type1 or hypothyroidism) and are positive for rs13031237 (GT genotype).

Discussion

In the present study, we have tested the possible link between C-Rel SNPs and non-segmental vitiligo. We decided to analyze the most commonly reported C-Rel mutations to be associated with other autoimmune disorders. Two specific mutations (namely, rs13031237 and rs842647) were more frequently associated with immune-mediated diseases (Chen et al. 2016) such as celiac disease (Trynka et al. 2009), rheumatoid arthritis (Gregersen et al. 2009; Eyre et al. 2010; Varadé et al. 2011), SLE (Zhou et al. 2012), psoriasis (Ali et al. 2013), and Behcet's disease (Chen et al. 2016). In spite the fact that "rs13031237" is the most commonly studied C-Rel SNP in autoimmune diseases, it was also interesting to study rs842647 in vitiligo, as its GG genotype and G

Table 2 Frequencies of alleles and genotypes of REL polymorphisms in non-segmental vitiligo patients and controls

SNP	Genotype/allele	Cases $n = 100$	Controls $n = 100$	P value	OR (95% CI)
rs13031237	GG	53	46	0.3	1.3(0.75–2.3)
	GT	40	46	0.4	0.8(0.44–1.4)
	TT	7	8	0.8	0.9(0.3–2.4)
	G	93	92	0.5	1.1(0.7–1.9)
	T	47	54	0.5	0.8(0.5–1.4)
rs842647	AA	75	69	0.3	1.3(0.7–2.5)
	AG	20	30	0.1	0.6(0.3–1.1)
	GG	5	1	0.1	5.2(0.6–45)
	A	95	99	0.6	1.1(0.7–2.2)
	G	25	31	0.6	0.8(0.5–1.5)

SNP single nucleotide polymorphism, *OR* odds ratio, *CI* confidence interval

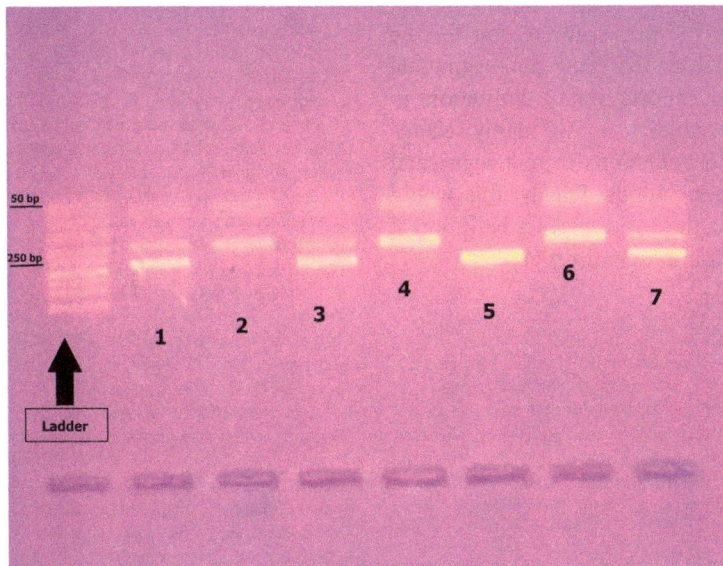

Fig. 1 Agarose gel electrophoresis for restriction fragments of C-Rel gene (rs 13031237). (Chen et al. 2016; Zhou et al. 2012; Ali et al. 2013) heterozygous (GT genotype), (Gilmore and Gerondakis 2011; Gregersen et al. 2009; Varadé et al. 2011) homozygous wild (GG genotype), (Eyre et al. 2010) homozygous mutated (TT genotype)

allele was associated with a more risk for cutaneous lesions in patients with Behcet's disease. This finding may indicate that rs842647 polymorphism can affect the occurrence of autoimmune disease as well as the tendency to show skin manifestations (Chen et al. 2016).

In the present work, we could not detect a significant association between the two tested C-Rel SNPs and non-segmental vitiligo in the study population. Perhaps other different and less common Rel mutations are linked to non-segmental vitiligo which necessitates further studies. Another possible explanation would be a different and distinct unknown autoimmune cascade that is involved in vitiligo and not in other autoimmune disorders. Also, previous conflicting results about the role of Rel in mouse and human models have been reported for both diabetes mellitus and bronchial asthma (Fullard et al. 2012). Herein, it is worth mentioning that 20 of our patients who have an associated diabetes mellitus-type1 or hypothyroidism are positive for rs13031237 (GT genotype) which have been linked previously to SLE (Zhou et al. 2012), rheumatoid arthritis (Gregersen et al. 2009; Eyre et al. 2010; Varadé et al. 2011), psoriasis (Ali et al. 2013), and celiac disease (Trynka et al. 2009). We believe that it would be more interesting if we can test such cases for presence or absence of autoantibodies, e.g., anti-islet cell antibodies and anti-thyroid antibodies. Furthermore, we could not find previous studies about Rel and hypothyroidism which would be a good research point for interested colleagues.

Vitiligo is an old puzzle and different hypotheses have been suggested to explain its pathogenesis (Iannella et al.

2016). Recently, the role of Tregs has been linked to vitiligo pathogenesis. Several studies revealed either reduction of Tregs count in peripheral blood and/or functional abnormalities in vitiligo patients. These deviations may increase the count and activity of cytotoxic T cells leading to loss of melanocytes (Dwivedi et al. 2015). The "enhanceosome" model described by Ruan et al. 2009 perfectly explains the link between C-Rel and the development of FOXP3+ Tregs. They proposed that antigen-presenting cells can bind to TCR and CD28 in the presence of TGF-β. This binding leads to the activation of IKKb, which phosphorylates IkBα resulting in C-Rel and p65-free release. Then "C-Rel-p65" dimer migrates to the nucleus and attaches to a FOXP3 promoter. Finally, this prompts the creation of Tregs-specific multifactorial transcriptional complex or the "enhanceosome" to switch on/or off Tregs differentiation (Ruan et al. 2009). Furthermore, Grigoriadis et al. 2011 reports the requirement of C-Rel for conversion of FOXP3– Tregs precursors into FOXP3+ Tregs through IL-2 and IL-15. In vitiligo, cumulative observations indicated an impaired FOXP3 expression that might disturb Tregs norms (Dwivedi et al. 2015).

However, the lack of association between the two tested C-Rel SNPs in our study population could also be a similar finding to some previous studies who failed to replicate the association of C-Rel with SLE (Zhou et al. 2012; Varadé et al. 2011; Cen et al. 2013) in contrast to several other studies. To add more complexity, C-Rel may show diverse patterns among different autoimmune disorders and even within the same immune-mediated disorder in different populations.

Conclusions

To our knowledge, this is the first study to test for the potential link between C-Rel SNP and non-segmental vitiligo. Lack of previous reports was a limitation to compare our data to other studies. So, we highly recommend testing further C-Rel mutations in non-segmental vitiligo and in different populations. Finally, this would provide an explanation for the controverting behavior of C-Rel among different autoimmune disorders.

Abbreviations

DNA: Deoxyribonucleic acid; EDTA: Ethylenediaminetetraacetic Acid; FOXP3: Forkhead box P3; IkBα: Nuclear factor of kappa light polypeptide gene enhancer in B-cells inhibitor alpha; IKKb: Inhibitor of nuclear factor kappa-B kinase; IL: Interleukin; IRB: Institutional review board; NF-κB: Nuclear factor kappa-light-chain-enhancer of activated B cells; PCR-RFLP: Polymerase chain reaction-restriction fragment length polymorphism; SLE: Systemic lupus erythematosus; SNP: Single nucleotide polymorphism; Tregs: T-regulatory cells; VASI: Vitiligo area scoring index

Acknowledgements

All molecular techniques performed at Zagazig University Hospitals, Clinical Pathology Department, Immunology, and Research Unit Laboratory.

Funding

This research did not receive any specific grant from funding agencies in the public, commercial, or not-for-profit sectors.

Authors' contributions

Both authors read and approved the final manuscript. ES was responsible for the research idea, the patients' enrollment, and writing the major part of the manuscript. AA was responsible for the Lab section for the gene study and statistical analysis and shared in writing as well as revising the manuscript.

Competing interests

The authors declare that they have no competing interests.

Author details

[1]Dermatology, Venereology & Andrology department, Faculty of Medicine, Zagazig University, Zagazig, Egypt. [2]Clinical Pathology department, Faculty of Medicine, Zagazig University, Zagazig, Egypt.

References

Ali FR, Barton A, Smith RL, et al. An investigation of rheumatoid arthritis loci in patients with early onset psoriasis validates association of the REL gene. Br J Dermatol. 2013;168(4):864–6.

Cen H, Zhou M, Leng RX, et al. Genetic interaction between genes involved in NF-κB signaling pathway in systemic lupus erythematosus. Mol Immunol. 2013;56(4):643–8.

Chen F, Xu L, Zhao T, et al. Genetic variation in the REL gene increases risk of Behcet's disease in a Chinese Han population but that of PRKCQ does not. PLoS One. 2016;11(1):e0147350.

de Boer OJ, van der Loos CM, Teeling P, et al. Immunohistochemical analysis of regulatory T cell markers FOXP3 and GITR on CD41CD251 T cells in normal skin and inflammatory dermatoses. J Histochem Cytochem. 2007;55:891–8.

Dwivedi M, Kemp EH, Laddha NC, et al. Regulatory T cells in vitiligo: implications for pathogenesis and therapeutics. Autoimmun Rev. 2015;14:49–56.

Eyre S, Hinks A, Flynn E et al 2010. Confirmation of association of the REL locus with rheumatoid arthritis susceptibility in the UK population. Ann Rheum Dis 2010;69(8):1572–1573.

Fullard N, Wilson CL, Oakley F. Roles of c Rel signalling in inflammation and disease. Int J Biochem Cell Biol. 2012;44(6):851–60.

Gilmore TD, Gerondakis S. The c-Rel transcription factor in development and disease genes cancer. 2011;2(7):695–711.

Gregersen PK, Amos CI, Lee AT, et al. 2009. REL, encoding a member of the NF-kappaB family of transcription factors, is a newly defined risk locus for rheumatoid arthritis. Nat Genet. 2009;41(7):820–3.

Grigoriadis G, Vasanthakumar A, Banerjee A, et al. c-Rel controls multiple discrete steps in the thymic development of Foxp3 (+) CD4 regulatory T cells. PLoS One. 2011;6(10):e26851.

Iannella G, Greco A, Didona D, et al. Vitiligo: pathogenesis, clinical variants and treatment approaches. Autoimmun Rev. 2016;15(4):335–43.

Jahan P, Cheruvu R, Tippisetty S, et al. Association of FOXP3 (rs3761548) promoter polymorphism with nondermatomal vitiligo: a study from India. J Am Acad Dermatol. 2013;69(2):262–6.

Persico M, Capasso M, Persico E, et al. Interleukin-10-1082 GG polymorphism influences the occurrence and the clinical characteristics of hepatitis C virus infection. J Hepatol. 2006;45(6):779–85.

Ruan Q, Kameswaran V, Tone Y, et al. Development of Foxp3 (+) regulatory t cells is driven by the c-Rel enhanceosome. Immunity. 2009;31(6):932–40.

Trynka G, Zhernakova A, Romanos J, et al. Coeliac disease associated risk variants in TNFAIP3 and REL implicate altered NF kappaB signaling. Gut. 2009;58(8):1078–83.

Varadé J, Palomino-Morales R, Ortego-Centeno N, et al. Analysis of the REL polymorphism rs13031237 in autoimmune diseases. Ann Rheum Dis. 2011;70(4):711–2.

Zhang P, Côté AL, de Vries VC, et al. Induction of postsurgical tumor immunity and T-cell memory by a poorly immunogenic tumor. Cancer Res. 2007;1:6468–76.

Zhou XJ, Lu XL, Nath SK, et al. Gene-gene interaction of BLK, TNFSF4, TRAF1, TNFAIP3, and REL in systemic lupus erythematosus. Arthritis Rheum. 2012;64(1):222–31.

27

Protective effect of protocatechuic acid against inflammatory stress induced in human dermal fibroblasts

Ji Hye Son[1,2], Soo-Yeon Kim[3], Hyun Hee Jang[4], Sung Nae Lee[5] and Kyu Joong Ahn[6*]

Abstract

Background: Protocatechuic acid (PCA) is an anthocyanin metabolite with a high antioxidant property. It is also known for having anticancer and anti-inflammatory capacities with diverse medicinal activities. As one of the active ingredients in plant sources, PCA has been studied and has revealed various mechanisms, but effects on cosmetology are not sufficient. This paper suggests the effects of PCA on cosmeceutical via antioxidant and senescence-inhibiting activities.

Methods: Prior to demonstrating PCA efficacy, we performed cell viability of PCA of 0–100 μM with or without lipopolysaccharide (LPS) using water-soluble tetrazolium salt (WST-1). Then, to evaluate the antioxidant capacity, especially excessive generated reactive oxygen species (ROS), researchers carried out ROS scavenging activity of PCA through 2′,7′-dichlorodihydrofluorescein diacetate (DCFH-DA) fluorescence intensity. Cellular senescence was assessed by senescence-associated β-galactosidase (SA-β-gal)-positive value, and extracellular matrix (ECM)-associated gene expression, collagen type I, alpha 1 chain (COL1A1), and matrix metalloproteinase-1 (MMP1) were estimated through quantitative real-time polymerase chain reaction (qRT-PCR).

Results: PCA has not shown cellular toxicity under 100 μM, with or without LPS. The results demonstrated that PCA exerted an antioxidant effect on LPS-treated human dermal fibroblasts (HDFs), via ROS scavenging activity. Furthermore, PCA has shown the senescence attenuating efficacy in HDFs through reducing senescent cells and regulating COL1A1 and MMP1 gene expression.

Conclusion: This work suggests the potential benefits of PCA against LPS-induced excessive ROS generation and cellular senescence, for the first time.

Keywords: Protocatechuic acid, Human dermal fibroblast, Lipopolysaccharide, Antioxidant, Senescence

Background

Polyphenols, the most focused dietary antioxidant for decades, have been reported to have not only antioxidant capacity but also biological efficacy. Phenolic acids, one of a major class of polyphenols, are naturally occurring in the plant kingdom including diverse edible plants (Tsao, 2010; Manach et al., 2004; Piazzon et al., 2012). PCA is a widely distributed phenolic compound common in human dietary plants and fruits, including plums, grapes, nuts (almonds), onion (*Allium cepa* L.), grain brown rice (*Oryza sativa* L.),

and olives (*Oleaeuropaea*). PCA has been researched about its biological and pharmacological properties including particular disease models. According to previous studies, PCA has anti-inflammatory, antioxidant, and free radical scavenging properties in both in vitro and in vivo reports (Khan et al., 2015; Kakkar & Bais, 2014; Semaming et al., 2015). Aside from its antioxidant property, it is important and necessary to examine whether PCA has other potential benefits such as anti-aging effects.

Fibroblasts are the most omnipresent cells in the human dermis and are important in maintaining and structuring organs via remodeling extracellular matrix (ECM) components (Tracy et al., 2016; Eleftheriadis et al., 2011; Darby & Hewitson, 2007; Kisseleva &

* Correspondence: kjahn@kuh.ac.kr
[6]Department of Dermatology, Konkuk University School of Medicine, 120 Neungdong-ro, Gwangjin-gu, Seoul 05029, Republic of Korea
Full list of author information is available at the end of the article

Brenner, 2008). The cells, fibroblasts, are also known to generate diverse cytokines to interfere with the immune system under certain conditions (Jordana et al., 1994). The endotoxin, LPS, is the major component of the outer membrane of gram-positive bacteria. It also covers about 90% of the cell surface and then serves as a physical barrier (Rosenfeld & Shai, 2006; Hancock & Diamond, 2000; Nikaido, 1989; Papo & Shai, 2005). In biological properties, it has been reported that LPS recruits immune cells to human dermal fibroblasts (HDFs) via inducing the progression of inflammatory processes through secretion of soluble mediators (Gasparrini et al., 2017; Tardif et al., 2004; Wheater et al., 2012). Moreover, the ECM is also capable of influencing cell migration, senescence, and gene expression of the fibroblasts (Tracy et al., 2016; Majno et al., 1971). Focusing on the above results, this study aims to investigate LPS-induced ROS scavenging capacity and suppressing activity of PCA in cellular senescence phenomena. This study is the first to verify the protective effect of PCA on LPS-induced damages in HDF cells.

Methods
Cell culture
The HDFs derived from human skin cells were obtained from the Lonza Group (Basel, Switzerland) and were maintained in DMEM supplemented with 10% heat-inactivated FBS, 100 units/mL penicillin, and 100 µg/ml streptomycin in a humidified atmosphere of 5% CO_2 at 37 °C. For subculture, the medium was eliminated and cells were rinsed with PBS twice. Then, cells detached using trypsin-EDTA were cultured with fresh complete growth medium in a ratio of 1:5 every 72 h. Protocatechuic acid was diluted with the culture medium before treatment, and final concentrations were adjusted using DMSO.

Cell cytotoxicity
The cytotoxicity was determined using an WST-1 assay kit following the manufacturer's protocol. Briefly, the cells were seeded in the culture plate, incubated for 24 h, and then treated with diverse concentrations of protocatechuic acid (25, 50, 75, and 100 µM) for 24 h with or without 1 µg/mL of LPS. Then, 10 µL of EZ-Cytox cell viability assay kit reagent (ItsBio, Korea) was added to the cultured cells and the cells were incubated for 1 h. The absorbance was measured at 490 nm using a microplate reader (Bio-Rad, Hercules, CA, USA). The mean and standard deviation of cell viability was calculated after repeating the procedure three times.

DCFH-DA scavenging assay
The intracellular ROS generation was measured using the fluorescence dye DCFH-DA, which produces a detectable fluorescence when the non-fluorescent DCFH reacts with ROS in cells. The treated cells were incubated with 25 µM DCFH-DA at 37 °C for 1 h and then the fluorescence intensity was measured using a BD fluorescence-activated cell sorting calibur (FACSCalibur, flow cytometer, BD Biosciences, San Jose, CA, USA), at excitation and emission wavelengths of 485 and 535 nm, respectively.

SA-β-gal activity
SA-β-gal staining was carried out according to the manufacturer's instructions, and senescence cell staining was detected 24 h after treatment. Briefly, the cells were rinsed twice with PBS, fixed with 0.5 ml fixative solution (4% formaldehyde and 0.5% glutaraldehyde in PBS, pH 7.2) for 20 min, rinsed again with PBS, and then were incubated with the staining solution for 24 h at 37 °C. Then, the staining solution was removed, and 70% glycerol was added to each well before the stained cells were examined for senescence using a microscope (Olympus Microscope System IX51, Olympus, Japan).

RNA isolation and qRT-PCR
The total RNA of each sample was isolated using the TRIzol reagent following the manufacturer's protocol. After the purified RNA had been validated using a spectrophotometer (MaestroNano, Maestrogen, NV, USA), 1 µg of the total RNA was used for cDNA synthesis using a miScript II RT kit. The mRNA expression was quantitatively assessed using Evagreen dye with the Line-Gene K software (BioER, Hangzhou, China), according to the manufacturer's protocol. The primers for the qRT-PCR are *β-actin* (Forward: GGATTCCT ATGTGGGCGACGA, Reverse: CGCTCGGTGAGG ATCTTCATG), *COL1A1* (Forward: AGGGCCAAGACG AAGACATC, Reverse: AGATCACGTCATCGCACAA CA) and *MMP1* (Forward: TCTGACGTTGATCCCAGA GAGCAG, Reverse: CAGGGTGACACCAGTGACTGC AC). And the experiment was performed in triplicate.

Statistics
All the results are presented as the mean percentage ± standard deviation (SD) of three independent experiments. p values < 0.05, 0.01, and 0.001 were considered statistically significant and were determined using Student's t test.

Results
Cytotoxicity of LPS and PCA in HDF cells
We observed cytotoxicity of LPS and PCA on HDF cells using WST-1 assay. Researchers treated PCA (0–100 µM) on HDF cells for 24 h with or without LPS (1 µg/mL). As shown in Fig. 1, indicated concentrations of PCA and LPS have no significant cytotoxicity. Based on these results, we

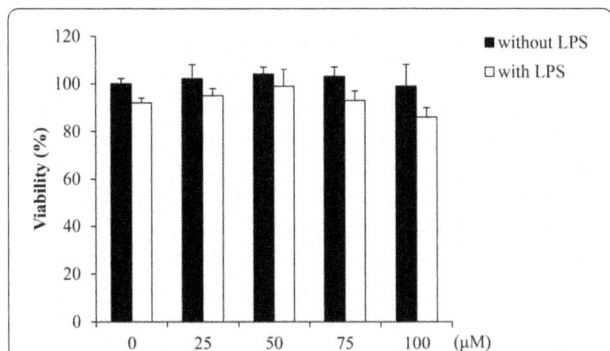

Fig. 1 Cytotoxicity of PCA with or without LPS in HDF cells. Cell viability in HDF cells were measured by WST-1 assay with different concentrations of PCA (0–100 μM) and LPS (1 μg/mL) for 24 h. Black bar represents the cell viability of indicated concentrations of PCA without LPS treatment. White bar represents the cell viability of PCA co-treated with LPS. Data are expressed as mean ± standard deviation

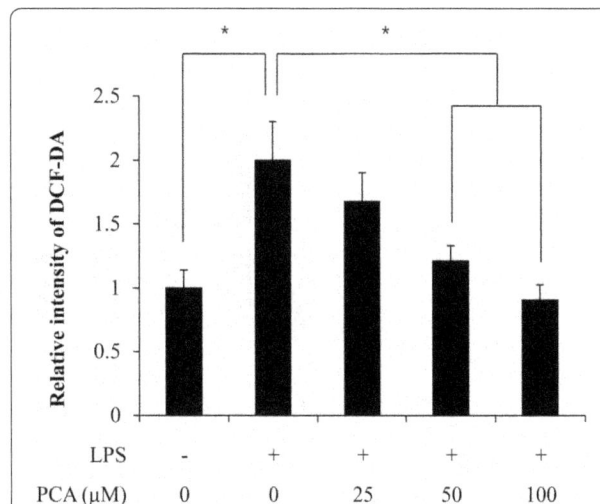

Fig. 2 Excessive ROS scavenging effect of PCA in HDF cells. Effect of PCA on excessive-generated intracellular ROS scavenging capacity was determined by DCF-DA fluorescent intensity. HDF cells had been treated with LPS (1 μg/mL) and PCA for 24 h and then were reacted with DCFH-DA (25 μM). Data are expressed as mean ± standard deviation of triplicate experiments ($*p < 0.05$)

examined further experiments, antioxidant effect by measuring ROS scavenging capacity and antisenescence efficacy via senescent cell counting, and ECM-modulating gene expression analysis, at various concentrations of PCA.

Intracellular excessive ROS scavenging effect of PCA in HDF cells

Estimating intracellular ROS concentrations could explain the quantitative oxidative stress induced by a stimulus. LPS, an endotoxin released from gram-negative bacteria, has been reported to induce intracellular ROS production and acute injuries (Kim et al., 2012). Thus, this study demonstrated whether PCA reduces intracellular ROS induced by LPS in HDF cells via DCFH-DA assay. As a result, 1 μg/mL LPS-treated HDFs for 24 h showed increased DCF fluorescent intensity while cells treated with diverse PCA with LPS indicated significantly reduced DCF intensity (Fig. 2). A significant reduction in the DCF fluorescent intensity compared to the LPS treatment was 50 and 100 μM of PCA-treated cells ($*p < 0.05$).

Attenuation effects of PCA on cellular senescence and ECM-modulating gene expression in HDF cells

Next, researchers carried out the efficacy of PCA on LPS-induced cellular senescence. As shown in Fig. 3a, the LPS-treated cells prominently expressed cellular senescence 3.8-fold (30.7 ± 4.1) more than the non-treated control cells (8.0 ± 1.9). The increased senescent proportion by LPS was significantly reduced in a dose-dependent manner of PCA. The cellular senescence of HDFs was diminished to 16.3 ± 1.1 and 11.9 ± 2.0 at 50 and 100 μM of PCA, respectively. In accordance with cellular senescence estimation, mRNA expression of COL1A1 and MMP1 were measured using qRT-PCR. In this study, LPS-treated cells indicated downregulated COL1A1 expression whereas PCA co-treated cells presented significantly

induced expression (Fig. 3b). Interestingly, cells treated with LPS showed increasing MMP1 mRNA expression while the PCA co-treated cells reduced expression in a dose-dependent manner of PCA (Fig. 3c).

Discussion

PCA, one of phenolic acid, is widely distributed in edible plants and fruits and has been reported to have biological activities such as antioxidant, antibacterial, anticancer, antiviral, and anti-inflammatory. In this study, the data showed novel potential of PCA focused on skin cellular mechanisms. In indicated concentrations (0–100 μM), PCA had no cytotoxicity in HDF cells with or without LPS (1 μg/mL). According to previous studies, LPS has been reported to contribute to inflammatory response including ROS generation. For this reason, it is important to investigate how dermal fibroblasts regulate LPS-induced stress and research cellular senescence. PCA treatment had efficacious consequences on preventing LPS-induced cellular senescence and ECM-related gene expression, especially COL1A1 and MMP1 mRNA. Collagen, the most abundant protein in the animal kingdom, is identified with 28 types; even collagen I comprises approximately 90% of the total collagen in the skin (Tracy et al., 2016; Eyre, 1980). And MMPs, which remodel ECM through degradation, are upregulated to diminution of collagen matrices via downregulation of type I collagen in the normal healing process (Tracy et al., 2016). It is also reported in inflammatory process that MMPs induce degradation of ECM for making easier

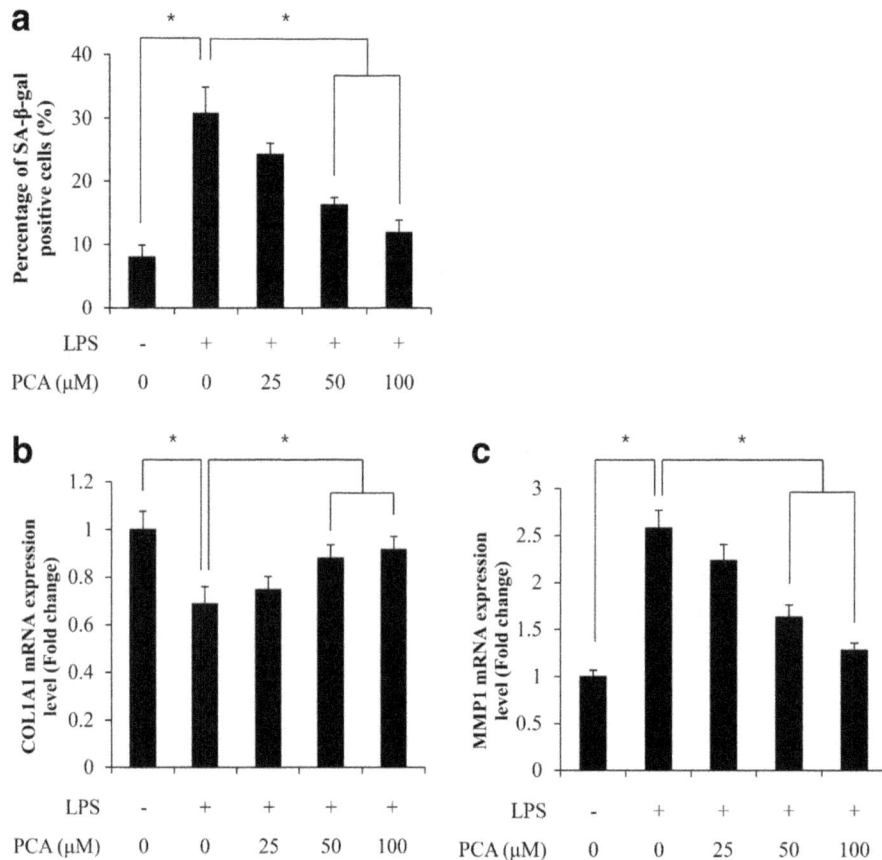

Fig. 3 Senescence-attenuating effect of PCA in HDF cells. **a** Effect of PCA on cellular senescence was determined by SA-β-gal assay. HDF cells had been co-treated with LPS (1 μg/mL) and the indicated concentration of PCA for 24 h, then SA-β-gal assay was conducted to determine cellular senescence. **b** *COL1A1* and **c** *MMP1* mRNA expression were determined by qRT-PCR, and β-actin expression was used for normalization. HDF cells were treated with LPS (1 μg/mL) and the indicated concentration of PCA for 24 h. Data are expressed as mean ± standard deviation (*$p < 0.05$)

invasion and damages (Eleftheriadis et al., 2011). In detail, 50 and 100 μM of PCA showed a significant result that reduced senescent cell portion and ECM collapse promoting enzymes and *MMP1* gene expression. Also, *COL1A1*, gene of type I collagen which is the most abundant structural protein of ECM expression, was increased in 50 and 100 μM of PCA-treated fibroblast cells. In this study, 25 μM of PCA is not sufficient for suppressing LPS-induced stress, while 50 and 100 μM of PCA reveal significant efficacy on the aims of this study.

Conclusion

Intracellular ROS are elaborately modulated by diverse antioxidant mechanisms under normal circumstances. But the excessive generation of ROS via intrinsic or extrinsic stimuli could lead to imbalance of cellular homeostasis which eventually causes damages or functional disorder in organisms. Skin, the outermost organ which protects the body from dehydration and physical or chemical irritations, has been regarded to be a representative and tangible object for

figuring out aging phenomena. Focused on this point, researchers investigated how PCA protects HDF cells from LPS-induced stress through estimation of ROS scavenging capacity, senescent cell, and senescence-associated gene expression analysis. As shown in this study, PCA adduces efficacy on excessive-generated ROS scavenging and attenuating dermal fibroblast senescence. This is not enough to fully suggest cellular mechanisms of PCA on the skin but, after further studies about detailed cellular or clinical efficacy trials, could reveal the potential of PCA against varied occasions including LPS-induced symptoms.

Abbreviations

COL1A1: Collagen type I alpha 1 chain; DCFH-DA: 2′,7′-Dichlorodihydrofluorescein diacetate; ECM: Extracellular matrix; HDFs: Human dermal fibroblasts; LPS: Lipopolysaccharide; *MMP1*: Matrix metalloproteinase-1; PCA: Protocatechuic acid; qRT-PCR: Quantitative real-time polymerase chain reaction; ROS: Reactive oxygen species; SA-β-gal: Senescence-associated β-galactosidase; WST-1: Water-soluble tetrazolium salt

Acknowledgements

This work was supported by a grant from the Korean Health Technology R&D Project (Grant No. HN13C0075), Ministry of Health & Welfare, Republic of Korea.

Funding
Not applicable.

Authors' contributions
JHS and KJA conducted the study and drafted the manuscript. All authors analyzed data and reviewed literatures. JHS and KJA wrote the manuscript. All authors read and approved the final manuscript.

Competing interests
The authors declare that they have no competing interests.

Author details
[1]Department of Bioengineering, Graduate School of Konkuk University, Seoul 05029, Republic of Korea. [2]Lemon Beauty Academy, Busan 47837, Republic of Korea. [3]Department of Beauty Art, Doowon Technical University, Paju-si, Gyeonggi-do 10838, Republic of Korea. [4]School of Cosmetology, Kyungbok University, Namyangju-si, Gyeonggi-do, Republic of Korea. [5]Department of Cosmetology, Kyungin Women's University, Incheon 21041, Republic of Korea. [6]Department of Dermatology, Konkuk University School of Medicine, 120 Neungdong-ro, Gwangjin-gu, Seoul 05029, Republic of Korea.

References
Darby IA, Hewitson TD. Fibroblast differentiation in wound healing and fibrosis. Int Rev Cytol. 2007;257:143–79.

Eleftheriadis T, Liakopoulos V, Lawson B, Antoniadi G, Stefanidis I, Galaktidou G. Lipopolysaccharide and hypoxia significantly alters interleukin-8 and macrophage chemoattractant protein-1 production by human fibroblasts but not fibrosis related factors. Hippokratia. 2011;15:238–43.

Eyre DR. Collagen: molecular diversity in the body's protein scaffold. Science. 1980;207:1315–22.

Gasparrini M, Forbes-Hernandez TY, Giampieri F, Afrin S, Mezzetti B, Quiles JL, et al. Protective effect of strawberry extract against inflammatory stress induced in human dermal fibroblasts. Molecules. 2017; https://doi.org/10.3390/molecules22010164.

Hancock RE, Diamond G. The role of cationic antimicrobial peptides in innate host defences. Trends Microbiol. 2000;8:402–10.

Jordana M, Särnstrand B, Sime PJ, Ramis I. Immune-inflammatory functions of fibroblasts. Eur Respir J. 1994;7:2212–22.

Kakkar S, Bais S. A review on protocatechuic acid and its pharmacological potential. ISRN Pharmacol. 2014; https://doi.org/10.1155/2014/952943.

Khan AK, Rashid R, Fatima N, Mahmood S, Mir S, Khan S, Jabeen N, Murtaza G. Pharmacological activities of protocatechuic acid. Acta Pol Pharm. 2015;72:643–50.

Kim CO, Huh AJ, Han SH, Kim JM. Analysis of cellular senescence induced by lipopolysaccharide in pulmonary alveolar epithelial cells. Arch Gerontol Geriatr. 2012;54:e35–41.

Kisseleva T, Brenner DA. Fibrogenesis of parenchymal organs. Proc Am Thorac Soc. 2008;5:338–42.

Majno G, Gabbiani G, Hirschel BJ, Ryan GB, Statkov PR. Contraction of granulation tissue in vitro: similarity to smooth muscle. Science. 1971;173:548–50.

Manach C, Scalbert A, Morand C, Rémésy C, Jiménez L. Polyphenols: food sources and bioavailability. Am J Clin Nutr. 2004;79:727–47.

Nikaido H. Outer membrane barrier as a mechanism of antimicrobial resistance. Antimicrob Agents Chemother. 1989;33:1831–6.

Papo N, Shai Y. A molecular mechanism for lipopolysaccharide protection of gram-negative bacteria from antimicrobial peptides. J Biol Chem. 2005;280:10378–87.

Piazzon A, Vrhovsek U, Masuero D, Mattivi F, Mandoj F, Nardini M. Antioxidant activity of phenolic acids and their metabolites: synthesis and antioxidant properties of the sulfate derivatives of ferulic and caffeic acids and of the acyl glucuronide of ferulic acid. J Agric Food Chem. 2012;60:12312–23.

Rosenfeld Y, Shai Y. Lipopolysaccharide (Endotoxin)-host defense antibacterial peptides interactions: role in bacterial resistance and prevention of sepsis. Biochim Biophys Acta. 2006;1758:1513–22.

Semaming Y, Pannengpetch P, Chattipakorn SC, Chattipakorn N. Pharmacological properties of protocatechuic acid and its potential roles as complementary medicine. Evid Based Complement Alternat Med. 2015; https://doi.org/10.1155/2015/593902.

Tardif F, Ross G, Rouabhia M. Gingival and dermal fibroblasts produce interleukin-1 beta converting enzyme and interleukin-1 beta but not interleukin-18 even after stimulation with lipopolysaccharide. J Cell Physiol. 2004;198:125–32.

Tracy LE, Minasian RA, Caterson EJ. Extracellular matrix and dermal fibroblast function in the healing wound. Adv Wound Care (New Rochelle). 2016;5:119–36. https://www.ncbi.nlm.nih.gov/pubmed/26989578

Tsao R. Chemistry and biochemistry of dietary polyphenols. Nutrients. 2010;2:1231–46.

Wheater MA, Falvo J, Ruiz F, Byars M. Chlorhexidine, ethanol, lipopolysaccharide and nicotine do not enhance the cytotoxicity of a calcium hydroxide pulp capping material. Int Endod J. 2012;45:989–95.

28

Comparison of efficacy of commercially available vs. freshly prepared salicylic acid peel in treatment of acne

Dhwani Rathod[1], Purna Pandya[1*], Ishan Pandya[2], Gaurav Shah[3], Rima Shah[4] and Bela Padhiyar[1]

Abstract

Background: Chemical peeling is increasingly used in dermatology nowadays. Salicylic acid peels have been widely used in Asian patients since long ago, but very few published literature is there focusing on the efficacy and safety of it in Asian population. This study was planned to compare the efficacy of salicylic acid (SA) peel either commercially available or freshly prepared in treatment of acne.

Methods: A prospective, randomized, open-label, parallel-group study was carried out in patients with acne. A total of 126 patients were randomized to receive 30% salicylic acid peel either commercially available (group A, $n = 60$) or freshly prepared (group B, $n = 63$). Assessment of acne lesions was done at baseline and at 2, 4, 6, 8, 10, and 12 weeks. Objective assessment was carried out using total acne score and subjective assessment using visual analog scale and were compared.

Results: Mean age of patients was 22.4 ± 3.1 years with female predominance. After six sessions with commercially available SA peel, reduction in average number of comedones was 88.45% ($P = 0.002$), in inflammatory papules 89.16% ($P = 0.01$), in pustules 31.47% ($P = 0.06$), and in nodules/cyst 50% ($P = 0.5$). After six sessions with freshly prepared SA peel, reduction in average number of comedones was 89% ($P = 0.0001$), in inflammatory papules 90.36% ($P = 0.0001$), in pustules 28.3% % ($P = 0.05$), and in nodules 96% ($P = 0.05$). Significant reduction of both non-inflammatory and inflammatory acne was seen in both groups ($P < 0.05$). Both of the agents led to a highly significant ($P < 0.001$) improvement in the total acne score; freshly prepared SA peel showed improvement significantly earlier at 6 weeks onwards. VAS score was significantly high for the freshly prepared SA group ($P = 0.05$).

Conclusion: This study has shown equivalence in therapeutic efficacy of both commercially available and freshly prepared SA peels both in terms of objective and subjective assessments in acne treatment with more patient satisfaction with freshly prepared peel.

Keywords: Acne, Salicylic acid peel, Commercially available vs. freshly prepared SA peel, Efficacy comparison, Total acne score

* Correspondence: dr.purnapandya2017@gmail.com
[1]Department of Dermatology, GMERS Medical College, Gandhinagar, Gujarat, India
Full list of author information is available at the end of the article

Background

Acne vulgaris is considered as one of the most prevalent skin disease requiring visits to dermatologists. It typically starts in the adolescent age group and resolves naturally also (Dudhiya et al. 2015). Acne vulgaris is a disease of the pilosebaceous unit characterized by seborrhea, comedones, papules, pustules, nodules, and, in few cases, scarring (Layton 2010). Acne not only causes cosmetic problems but it causes social, psychological, and emotional distress as well as self-perception of poor health leading to deteriorating quality of life of patients (Al Robaee 2009). Current treatment modalities for acne mainly target multiple factors contributing to development of acne including topical and systemic retinoids, antimicrobials, and other adjuvant therapies like peeling (Kim and Armstrong 2011). While retinoids and antimicrobials remain the mainstay of conventional treatment of acne, novel adjunctive treatment like chemical peeling, laser, and photodynamic therapy are on rise as patients and clinicians seek to circumvent antibiotic resistance, reduce adverse effect, and employ new technologies in acne care (Ross 2005; Taub 2007).

Chemical peeling is the application of a chemical agent to the skin that causes controlled destruction of part/ whole epidermis with/without dermis leading to exfoliation and removal of superficial lesions followed by rejuvenation of new epidermal and dermal tissues (Khunger 2008). Various chemical peels are available like glycolic acid, salicylic acid, mandelic acid, and lactic acid. Salicylic acid (SA) is a member of a group of compounds known as hydroxy acids, which are widely used for a number of cosmetic indications because of their many important properties (Kornhauser et al. 2010). Salicylic acid has been used as a well-tolerated and safe peeling agent in all skin types in cosmetic dermatology by various researchers. Most of the available literature on chemical peels focuses on its role in skin rejuvenation and the correction of dyschromias. Salicylic acid peels have been widely used in Asian patients since long ago, but very few published literature is there focusing on the efficacy and safety of it in Asian population. Various formulations are available for salicylic acid peels in the market with huge price differences.

Therefore, the present study is planned to study the efficacy of freshly prepared salicylic acid vs. commercially available salicylic acid peel in treatment of acne vulgaris.

Methods

A randomized open-label study spread over 1 year was carried out in the dermatology department of a tertiary care teaching hospital in Western India. The study protocol was approved by the Human Research Ethics Committee of the institute prior to commencement of study. Permission from the hospital superintendent and head of the dermatology department was also obtained before conducting the study.

Participant selection

A total 126 patients attending the dermatology outpatient department and diagnosed with acne vulgaris were included in the study.

Inclusion criteria

Diagnosis of acne was mainly based on clinical examination by the qualified dermatologist. Patients of age 12 years and more for both genders with mild to moderate acne with facial lesions only were included in the study. Only those newly diagnosed and those who did not take any treatment for the last 15 days were included for the study.

Exclusion criteria

Pregnant and lactating mothers, patients with known history of hypersensitivity reaction to salicylates or aspirin, patients with history of herpes simplex, patients with drug-induced acne, and patients with history of keloid formation were excluded from the study. Patients not willing to participate in the study and not willing to give written informed consent were also excluded.

Study duration

These 126 patients were enrolled from March 2017 to August 2017. The first examination started in March 2017, and, considering follow-up visits, the last patient was enrolled in May 2017 so that the 12-week follow-up could be completed in August 2017.

Study procedure in detail

All the patients participating in the study were given a clear explanation about the purpose and nature of the study in the language they understood. Written informed consent was obtained before including them in the study. In the case of a minor, written informed consent from the parent/legal guardian was obtained in addition to assent from the adolescent. All outdoor patients, new as well as old, meeting the inclusion criteria attending the dermatology department were interviewed for the first time on the day of enrollment, and their case sheets were reviewed to gather necessary information—as on that day—to fill up case record forms. Detailed history and examination was carried out by the treating dermatologist. Details of the symptoms, duration, site, and type of lesions; any keloidal tendencies in the patient or in the family; and presence of viral infection, local tumors, and evolving dermatoses were noted. Counting of lesions was done in good natural light with the help of a hand lens. Acne grading was done using lesion count: grade 1 (total number of lesions $< 10/100 \ cm^2$), grade 2 (10–20/

100 cm^2), grade 3 (20–30/100 cm^2), and grade 4 (> 30/ 100 cm^2) (Tutakne and Chari 2003).

Evaluation of active acne was done using a method devised by Michaelsson and colleagues (Table 1) (Michaelsson et al. 1977). By multiplying the number of each type by its severity index and adding each sum, a total acne score was obtained. Assessment of acne lesions was done at baseline (0 weeks) and at each visit (2, 4, 6, 8, 10, and 12 weeks).

Randomization and group allocation

All patients were randomly assigned into groups A and B using random number table.

Group A: Patients with acne vulgaris treated with commercially available 30% salicylic acid peeling

Group B: Patients with acne vulgaris treated with freshly prepared 30% salicylic acid peeling (which was prepared by adding 3 g of salicylic acid powder into 10 ml of denatured spirit)

Intervention—SA peel

Six peeling sessions were conducted for each group at weeks 0, 2, 4, 6, 8, and 10. Patients were also called at the end of the 12th week for follow-up visit, but peeling was not applied on that session. At the first visit of enrollment, hypersensitivity testing was done in all patients. A hypersensitivity test with 10% SA peel both commercially available and freshly prepared was performed on a small 1-cm area in the right retro-auricular area. The patients were reviewed after 1 week, and if they tolerated the peel well, they were taken up for full-face peels. Patients were asked to first wash their face with water then asked to lie down in a 45° semi-reclining position with eyes closed. All patients were given a surgical cap to pull back their hair and cover the ears. Degreasing was done by scrubbing with cotton gauze soaked with spirit, followed by one soaked with cleansing lotion. Sensitive areas of the face like the lips and nasolabial folds were protected with a thin layer of petrolatum. Commercially or freshly prepared SA peel will be then applied over the face using a fan-shaped

sable brush in a predetermined clockwise manner starting over the forehead, right cheek, chin, left cheek, nose, upper lip, and lastly the infraorbital areas, taking 30 to 35 s to accomplish and using approximately 0.8 to 1 ml solution per session. With SA peeling, the patients experience a stinging sensation that usually lasted for 3 to 5 min. After the cessation of this stinging sensation, most patients developed a uniform white crystalline precipitate, "pseudofrost," in the peeled areas (indicating the deposition of salicylic acid after its hydroethanolic vehicle had volatilized) which was considered as the end point of peeling. In patients who did not develop the pseudofrost, the cessation of the stinging sensation was considered the end point. The total duration of the peeling sessions varied from 3 to 5 min with SA peeling. As soon as the end point was reached, the peel was neutralized by asking the patients to wash their faces with copious amounts of cool tap water. Patients were then asked to pat, and not rub, the face dry. The patients were asked to apply a sunscreen with a sun protection factor (SPF) of greater than 30 on their faces before leaving the dermatology department. Patients were allowed to go home with instructions to apply a non-comedogenic moisturizing cream if the facial skin felt too dry, to avoid or minimize sun exposure, and to apply sunscreen whenever exposed to the sun. They were cautioned not to apply any cream or face wash containing AHAs, salicylic acid, or retinoids. All the patients were followed up every 15 days till 3 months and improvement in acne was recorded.

Outcome measures

The treating physician made an objective assessment of the changes in active acne lesions, post-acne scarring, and hyperpigmentation at each visit. For the objective assessment, each type of lesion was counted in number like number of comedones, papules, pustules, and cyst, and standard deviation for the mean of each lesion count was also calculated. Reduction/change in the number of lesion count was noted, and time to achieve this reduction was also compared between the two groups. For post-acne scarring and hyperpigmentation, clinical examination in appropriate light was carried out by two different qualified dermatologists. The reduction in post-acne scarring and hyperpigmentation was evaluated clinically by both dermatologists consensually, and then time to achieve this reduction was also noted. In cases of conflict of opinion among two dermatologists, the clinical examination by the head of the dermatology department was carried out and results were recorded accordingly. The patient's subjective assessment was also made using a 100-cm visual analog scale. It was graded as excellent (> 80%), good (60–80%), average (30–60%), poor (< 30%), no change, and worse. Clinical photographs using standardized positioning were taken at baseline and at 4, 8, and 12 weeks.

Table 1 Evaluation of active acne*

Lesion	Severity	Index definition*
Comedone	0.5	Horny follicular plug and pinhead-sized follicular papules
Papule	1.0	Infiltrated papules 2–8 mm
Pustule	2.0	Pustules 42 mm with surrounding inflammation
Infiltrate	3.0	Nodules and infiltrates: 48 mm and coalescent papules where individual papules cannot be distinguished
Cyst	4.0	Lesions where infiltrate has broken down to form discharging cyst

*Michaelsson et al. (1977); Cosmetic Surgery National Data Bank (2003)

Table 2 Baseline characteristics of study patients with acne ($n = 123$)

Characteristic	No. of patients in commercially available SA peel group; $n = 60$(%)	No. of patients in freshly prepared SA peel group; $n = 63$(%)	Total $n = 123$(%)	Chi-square test (P value)
Age in years				
12–20	24	18	42 (34.15)	
21–30	30	38	68 (55.28)	0.05
31–40	6	7	13 (10.57)	
Mean age (mean ± SD)	23.47 ± 5.62	22.99 ± 6.35	–	0.62
Gender (M:F)	0.62:1	0.66:1	–	0.54
Skin type				
2	2	3	5 (4.07)	0.71
3	21	25	46 (37.40)	0.64
4	34	30	64 (52.03)	0.42
5	3	5	8 (6.50)	0.5
Common presentation				
Papules	60	63	123(100)	0.45
Pustules	12	16	28 (22.76)	0.68
Nodules	6	9	15 (12.20)	0.42
Comedones	56	54	110 (89.43)	0.53
Grading of acne				
Grade 1	23	27	50	0.08
Grade 2	32	30	62	0.06
Grade 3	5	4	9	0.68
Grade 4	0	2	2	0.53

Chi-square test; P value < 0.05 is considered significant
SD standard deviation, M:F male to female ratio

Statistical analysis

All data were analyzed with the help of Microsoft excel 2010. Data were represented as actual frequency, mean, percentage, and standard deviation as appropriate. Chi-square test was used for analysis and association of qualitative data. Unpaired t test was used for comparison between the groups, and paired t test was used for within-group comparisons. P values < 0.05 were considered significant.

Results

Out of the total 126 patients enrolled, 123 completed the study while the rest three patients were lost to follow-up. The mean age of the patients was 23.47 ± 5.62 and 22.99 ± 6.35 years in the commercially and freshly prepared SA groups, respectively. 55.28% of patients belong to 21–30 years of age with female preponderance. Baseline details of the study participants are shown in Table 2.

Onset of acne occurred between the ages of 14 and 16 in 52.7% of the patients. The interval between onset of acne and scarring was 2 to 4 years in 57.4% of patients.

Objective assessment

Objective evaluation of treatment outcomes done by the treating physician revealed the following. As shown in Table 3, there was reduction of both non-inflammatory and inflammatory acne with commercially available SA

Table 3 Objective evaluation of acne after peeling with commercially available SA peel

Morphology of lesions	Commercially available SA peel (day 0) (mean)	Commercially available SA peel (at 12 week) (mean)	Mean percentage of reduction	P value*
Comedones	6.27 + 2.4	1.24 + 0.79	88.45 + 0.15	0.002
Papules	7.11 + 4.35	1.58 + 0.6	89.16 + 0.15	0.01
Pustules	2.06 + 1.8	0.17 + 0.37	31.47 + 0.45	0.06
Nodules	1.04 + 0.23	0.04 + 0.2	50.0 + 0.22	0.5

*Paired t test; P < 0.05 was considered significant

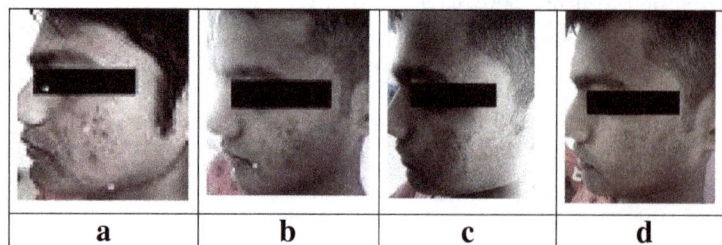

Fig. 1 Efficacy of commercially available salicylic acid peel **a** at baseline, **b** at 4 weeks, **c** at 8 weeks, and **d** at 12 weeks

peel. After six sessions, the reduction in average number of comedones was 88.45% ($P = 0.002$), reduction in inflammatory papules was 89.16% ($P = 0.01$), and reduction in pustules was 31.47% ($P = 0.06$) and nodules/cysts were reduced by 50% ($P = 0.5$). On clinical examination of the patient, it showed improvement in superficial scarring and skin texture. It also resolved post-acne hyperpigmentation to some extent (Fig. 1a–d).

Table 4 shows response of the patients with freshly prepared salicylic acid peel. Reduction of both non-inflammatory and inflammatory acne was observed. After six sessions, the reduction in average number of comedones was 89% ($P = 0.0001$), reduction in inflammatory papules was 90.36%, with $P = 0.0001$; pustules were reduced by 28.3% ($P = 0.05$) and nodules were reduced by 96% ($P = 0.05$). On clinical examination, it showed improvement in post-acne hyperpigmentation and overall appearance. It also resolved post-acne scarring to some extent (Fig. 2a–d).

Total acne score

Although both of the agents led to highly significant ($P < 0.001$) improvement in the total acne score, freshly prepared SA peel showed improvement significantly earlier at 6 weeks. The change in total acne score (week 0 to week 12) was 78.3% with commercially available peel and 80.1% with freshly prepared SA peel ($P > 0.05$) (Table 5).

Subjective assessment

The visual analog scale scores as assessed by the patient are shown in Table 5. Mean VAS scores were 84.3 and 90.1 in the commercially available and freshly prepared

SA peel groups, respectively, which were statistically significant ($P = 0.05$).

Acne lesions at baseline and after 4, 8, and 12 weeks for both the commercially available and freshly prepared SA peel groups are shown in Figs. 1 and 2 respectively.

Discussion

Acne is a one of the most common disease encountered in the dermatology department all over the world. Topical agents such as clindamycin, erythromycin, benzoyl peroxide, and retinoic acid have been mainstays in the treatment of acne vulgaris for the past two decades (Al Robaee 2009; Kim and Armstrong 2011; Ross 2005; Taub 2007), but new modalities like chemical peelings, laser, and other minimally invasive technologies are increasingly used nowadays. According to statistics from the American Society for Aesthetic Plastic Surgery, a total 495,415 chemical peels were performed in 2002 (Cosmetic Surgery National Data Bank 2003). The chemical peel is among the top 5 cosmetic procedures performed in the USA, and it has been increasingly used in developing countries like India. Several researchers have studied the role of salicylic acid as a superficial chemical peeling agent. There has been an increasing trend toward the use of more superficial chemical peels in the treatment of actinic damage and pigmentation. This study was aimed at comparative evaluation of efficacy of commercially available salicylic acid peel with freshly prepared salicylic acid peel in treatment of acne vulgaris in a tertiary care teaching hospital.

In this study, a maximum number of patients was from the age group of 21–30 years with female preponderance. The findings are well coinciding with the

Table 4 Objective evaluation of acne after peeling with freshly prepared SA peel

Morphology of lesions	Commercially available SA peel (day 0) (mean)	Commercially available SA peel (at 12 week) (mean)	Mean percentage of reduction	P value*
Comedones	6.18 ± 2.45	0.67 ± 0.70	89.00 ± 0.21	0.0001
Papules	7.29 ± 1.43	0.10 ± 0.74	90.36 ± 0.13	0.05
Pustules	5.91 ± 1.05	0.20 ± 0.34	28.3 ± 0.42	0.05
Nodules	1.04 ± 0.25	0.01 ± 0.00	96.0 ± 0.42	0.05

*Paired t test; $P < 0.05$ was considered significant

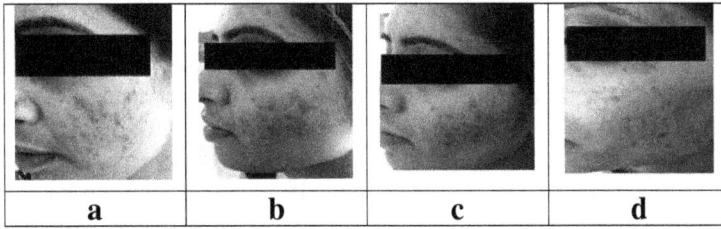

Fig. 2 Efficacy of freshly prepared salicylic acid peel **a** at baseline, **b** at 4 weeks, **c** at 8 weeks, and **d** at 12 weeks

studies by Atzori et al. (1999) and Sharma et al. (2016) and other available literature. This is because of hormonal changes at adolescent age which are more pronounced in the female gender. Moreover, females are more conscious about cosmetic appearance in India as compared to males, making more females visit the dermatology department.

SA peel has been established as an effective treatment modality in this study. Both commercially available and freshly prepared SA peels were effective in reducing the number of comedones and papules but less effective in treating nodules and pustules. However, a few studies have used salicylic acid for treatment of acne. Lee and Kim evaluated the use of 30% salicylic acid in treatment of acne in 35 Asian patients (Lee and Kim 2003). The salicylic acid was used fortnightly for 12 weeks. They found a significant decrease in mean total facial lesion count, non-inflammatory lesions, and mean acne grade reduction at the end of treatment. Grimes used two 20% and three 30% salicylic acid peels at fortnightly intervals in 25 dark-skinned patients with different dermatoses, out of whom 9 had acne vulgaris (Grimes 1999). Moderate (51–

75%) to significant (> 75%) clearing of acne was seen in 89% of patients. Non-inflammatory and inflammatory lesions were seen to clear faster than would ordinarily have occurred with traditional therapy.

Salicylic acid is a betahydroxy acid that has a phenolic ring in its chemical structure (Kim 2005). It is an excellent keratolytic agent by way of its ability to dissolve intercellular cement thereby reducing corneocyte adhesion (Lee and Kim 2003; Kessler et al. 2008). Due to its lipophilicity, it has better penetration into the pilosebaceous unit. This property of salicylic acid accounts for its strong comedolytic effect and its utility in the treatment of acne (Lee and Kim 2003; Kim 2005; Hashimoto et al. 2008; Kligman and Kligman 1997a; Ahn and Kim 2006; Lai and Mercurio 2009). The anti-inflammatory activity of SA makes it useful in rapidly decreasing facial erythema (Berger 1997).

Because both of the preparations of peeling agents are superficial peels, they serve only to resurface the upper layers of the epidermis. Through an indirect, as-yet-unknown mechanism, it stimulates the dermal fibroblasts to deposit more collagen, elastin, and glycosaminoglycans in the

Table 5 Comparison of outcomes in commercially vs. freshly prepared SA peels

	Commercially available SA peel		Freshly prepared SA peel			
	Objective: mean improvement in total acne score	Subjective: VAS	Objective: mean improvement in total acne score	Subjective: VAS	P value for total acne score*	P value for VAS**
At day 0	–	–	–	–	–	–
At 2 weeks	25.4	30	27.5	40	0.08	0.07
At 4 weeks	30.1	51	38.4	65	0.06	*0.05*
At 6 weeks	36.8	67.5	50	70.4	*0.04*	0.63
At 8 weeks	50.4	78.3	68	81.6	*0.05*	0.57
At 10 weeks	73.3	81	75.8	89.5	0.8	*0.05*
At 12 weeks	78.3	84.3	80.1	90.1	0.05	*0.05*
	$P < 0.05$[#]	$P < 0.05$[#]	$P < 0.05$[#]	$P < 0.05$[#]		

The italics $P < 0.05$ value was considered significant for the analysis

*Unpaired t test for comparison of the commercially available and freshly prepared SA peel groups

**Chi-square test for comparison of VAS between the commercially available and freshly prepared SA peel groups

[#]Within-group comparison; paired t test

papillary dermis. A more orderly and parallel arrangement of the fibers is also seen with use of SA peel (Kligman and Kligman 1997b). Thus, a gradual and slight decrease in the number of superficial scars and a decrease in the depth of deeper scars are observed. In addition, Ahn and Kim (2006) showed salicylic acid to have a whitening effect on the skin. This effect was seen in the present study too, with patients reporting diffuse lightening of their facial complexion.

On analyzing subjective assessment for peels, the mean visual analog scale scores were significantly higher for the freshly prepared SA peel group rather than the commercially available SA peel in this study. Acetyl salicylic acid is an easily available laboratory-grade ingredient and also one of the over-the-counter medications for pain and fever as "aspirin." This study has shown that if properly prepared considering the concentration of the peel, freshly prepared peels are equally efficacious as the commercially available chemical SA peel in terms of both subjective and objective outcome evaluation. Caution is required and skill has to be learned for preparing fresh SA peel like measuring the exact quantity of acetyl salicylic acid, its proper dilution in appropriate vehicle, and its use on the patients.

This study has established the equivalence in therapeutic efficacy of both commercially available and freshly prepared SA peels in treatment of acne vulgaris. To the best of our knowledge, this is the kind of first published study comparing freshly prepared peels and commercially available peels. Although homemade freshly prepared peels are routinely used as homemade remedies in India since long ago, its comparison with the commercially available preparations was less studied. The single center and the limited number of patients are among the few limitations of the study. Also, different types of formulations like gel base, cream, and solution may differ in some characteristics and may affect the outcome of peeling procedure when commercially available preparations are used which could not be studied here. Larger studies with multiple centers and longer follow-up duration are required in this area.

Conclusions

Chemical peeling is used increasingly for treatment of acne vulgaris either alone or in combination with traditional therapy like topical antimicrobial agents, benzyl peroxide,0 and retinoic acid. This study has shown that if properly prepared considering the concentration of the peel, freshly prepared peels are equally efficacious as the commercially available chemical SA peel in terms of both subjective and objective outcome evaluation. Total acne scores were reduced significantly and VAS showed significant more patients' satisfaction with the

freshly prepared peel. Chemical peeling with the freshly prepared SA peel can be an affordable treatment option performed in any dermatologist's office, if caution is required while preparing the peel. Postgraduate students and dermatologists can be trained in preparing and using freshly prepared SA peel which can serve as an effective treatment option.

Acknowledgements

The authors would like to thank Dr. Bipin Nayak, Hospital Superintendent, for allowing the research in the Department of Dermatology, Civil Hospital, Gandhinagar—a tertiary care teaching rural hospital in Western India.

Authors' contributions

PP has designed the idea and concept of the study, performed the salicylic acid peeling procedure, analyzed the data, and interpreted the results. DR has performed procedures on most patients and gathered the data of the patients. IP has performed the procedure of peeling on patients, collected the data, analyzed the data, and prepared the results. GS has helped in the statistical analysis of the data, results analysis, and writing of the manuscript. RS has helped in the study design, data analysis, and writing of the manuscript. BP has helped in the interpretation of the data and writing of the manuscript. All authors read and approved the final manuscript.

Competing interests

The authors declare that they have no competing interests.

Author details

[1]Department of Dermatology, GMERS Medical College, Gandhinagar, Gujarat, India. [2]Department of Dermatology, SBKS Medical Institute and Research Centre, Piparia, Waghodiya, Vadodara, Gujarat, India. [3]Department of Oral and Maxillofacial Surgery, NIIMS Dental College, Jaipur, Rajasthan, India. [4]Department of Pharmacology, GMERS Medical College, Gandhinagar, Gujarat, India.

References

Ahn HH, Kim IH. Whitening effect of salicylic acid peels in Asian patients. Dermatol Surg. 2006;32:372–5.

Al Robaee AA. Assessment of general health and quality of life in patients with acne using a validated generic questionnaire. Acta Dermatovenerol Alp Panonica Adriat. 2009;18(4):157–64.

Atzori L, Brundu MA, Orru A, Biggio P. Glycolic acid peeling in the treatment of acne. J Eur Acad Dermatol Venereol. 1999;12(2):119–22.

Berger R. Initial studies show salicylic acid promising as antiaging preparation. Cosmet Dermatol. 1997;10:31–2.

Cosmetic Surgery National Data Bank. 2002 Statistics. New York, NY: American Society for Aesthetic Plastic Surgery; 2003.

Dudhiya S, Shah RB, Agrawal P, Shah A, Date S. Efficacy and safety of clindamycin gel plus either benzoyl peroxide gel or adapalene gel in the treatment of acne: a randomized open-label study. Drugs Ther Perspect. 2015. https://doi.org/10.1007/s40267-015-0208-y.

Grimes PE. The safety and efficacy of salicylic acid chemical peels in darker racial-ethnic groups. Dermatol Surg. 1999;25:18–22.

Hashimoto Y, Suga Y, Mizuno Y, Hasegawa T, Matsuba S, Ikeda S, et al. Salicylic acid peels in polyethylene glycol vehicle for the treatment of comedogenic acne in Japanese patients. Dermatol Surg. 2008;34:276–9.

Kessler E, Flanagan K, Chia C, Rogers C, Glaser DA. Comparison of alpha and beta hydroxyl acid chemical peels in the treatment of mild to moderately severe facial acne vulgaris. Dermatol Surg. 2008;34:45–50.

Khunger N. Standard guidelines of care for chemical peels. Indian J Dermatol Venerol Leprol. 2008;74:S5–S12.

Kim IH. Salicylic acid peel (acne peel). Hong Kong J Dermatol Venereol. 2005;13:83–5.

Kim RH, Armstrong AW. Current state of acne treatment: highlighting lasers, photodynamic therapy, and chemical peels. Dermatol Online J. 2011;17(3):2.

Kligman D, Kligman AM. Salicylic acid as a peeling agent for the treatment of acne. Cosmetic Dermatol. 1997a;10:44–7.

Kligman D, Kligman AM. Salicylic acid as a peeling agent for the treatment of acne. Cosmet Dermatol. 1997b;10:44–7.

Kornhauser A, Coelho SG, Hearing VJ. Applications of hydroxy acids: classification, mechanisms, and photoactivity. Clin Cosmet Investig Dermatol. 2010;3:135–42.

Lai KW, Mercurio MG. Update on the treatment of acne vulgaris. J Clin Outcomes Manag. 2009;16:115–26.

Layton AM. Disorders of sebaceous glands. In: Burns T, Breathnach S, Cox N, Griffith C, editors. Rook's Textbook of Dermatology. 8th ed. Vol 2, vol. 42. Oxford: Blackwell publishers; 2010. p. 17.

Lee HS, Kim IH. Salicylic acid peels for the treatment of acne vulgaris in Asian patients. Dermatol Surg. 2003;29:1196–9.

Michaelsson G, Zuhlin L, Vahlquist A. Effects of oral zinc and vitamin A in acne. Arch Dermatol. 1977;113:31–6.

Ross EV. Optical treatments for acne. Dermatol Ther. 2005;18(3):253–66.

Sharma P, Shah A, Dhillon AS. Study of glycolic acid and salicylic acid peels as a sole therapy in treatment of acne vulgaris. Int J Med Res Rev. 2016;4(12): 2205–10 doi: 10.17511 /ijmrr. 2016.i12.21.

Taub AF. Procedural treatments for acne vulgaris. Dermatol Surg. 2007;33(9):1005–26.

Tutakne MA, Chari KVR. Acne, rosacea and perioral dermatitis. In: Valia RG, Valia AR, editors. IADVL textbook and atlas of dermatology. 2nd ed. Mumbai: Bhalani publishing House; 2003. p. 689–710.

29

DermaGene and VitmiRS: a comprehensive systems analysis of genetic dermatological disorders

Razia Rahman[†], Isha Sharma[†], Lokesh K. Gahlot and Yasha Hasija[*]

Abstract

Background: The interaction of genetic variants and their distribution in the genome is firmly believed to contribute to genetic dermatological disorders. For the convenience of clinicians and researchers to explore such genetic variants, we identified and validated the genetic association of human SNPs with dermatological disorders through manual curation and computational analysis.

Methods: Multiple online resources were investigated for creating a comprehensive list of dermatological disorders followed by identification and manual curation of data description of the SNP–disease relationship. The process for database creation involved extensive review of published literature and relevant articles that probed association of miRNAs and SNPs with vitiligo. Furthermore, computational analysis for deleterious SNPs and polypharmacological studies was performed with an effort to provide potential novel drug candidates for optimal therapeutic interventions.

Results: We established a dedicated database on dermatological disorders, DermaGene, which proffers a user-friendly interface to enable systematic querying and analysis of SNPs associated with dermatological disorders. Based on our disease network analysis, we further extended our present work to construct another comprehensive database, VitmiRS (Vitiligo associated miRNAs and SNPs), which furnishes detailed information on each miRNA and SNP association that renders susceptibility to vitiligo. Also, our systems analysis approach unraveled potential molecular determinants that may pose as novel drug candidates and can be targeted for efficient therapeutic approaches in vitiligo treatment.

Conclusions: Both the databases are freely accessible and will serve as a significant resource providing insights into previously undiscovered disease–gene and disease–SNP relationships. Our analysis unveiled significant findings that we believe may furnish a comprehensive understanding of the biological mechanisms that mediate vitiligo disease pathogenesis, thereby, driving the way towards better therapeutic interventions for disease management.

Keywords: miRNAs, SNPs, Dermatological disorders, Vitiligo

Background

The importance of systems and personalized medicine in the field of healthcare has grown vastly, especially in the last decade. Recent research has growingly demonstrated that many of the seemingly disparate diseases have a common molecular mechanism and strong association among them. This signifies the deeper interplay of genes, in contrast to one gene-one disease commonality well indicating towards the possibility of the related diseases to occur together in an individual (Yu et al. 2015). The exhibition of comorbidity association suggests that the occurrence of one disease will increase the likelihood of the other thereby contributing to compounded healthcare costs and multiplex clinical management. Also, a higher degree of interaction between many diseases indicates a greater prevalence and mortality rate associated with it. Due to the contribution of disease comorbidities as a burden on societies at large, it becomes

* Correspondence: yashahasija06@gmail.com
[†]Equal contributors
Department of Biotechnology, Delhi Technological University, Shahbad Daulatpur, Main Bawana Road, Delhi 110042, India

crucial for risk stratification and charting treatment course. One of the most powerful approaches in the present times, the Genome-Wide Association Studies (GWAS), serves as the primary pipeline for identifying disease variants and researching association of diseases and their phenotypes (Lewis et al. 2011). The complete sequen

The advent of SNP genotyping of dermatological disorders has revolutionized our understanding of the genetics of such disorders (Maruthappu et al. 2014). Relevant information from several published literature concerning the disease–SNP association in dermatological disorders are interspersed which impels the need for a repository that stores SNPs having prime roles in the initiation of dermatological disorders. Such a resource would be valuable for clinicians and researchers making it convenient for them to study the regulatory mechanisms of SNPs that underpin disease pathogenesis and translate their discoveries into clinical practice. We, therefore, aimed to fulfill this void concerning a dedicated genetic dermatological disorder database. DermaGene is the first attempt at providing information pertaining to human genetic dermatological disorders establishing itself as the primary pipeline for identifying disease variants and researching association of dermatological diseases and their phenotypes. The database as of now stores 114 unique diseases, as described by 244 different genes along with 871 associated SNPs and have been made freely accessible online. The present work not only provides information on experimentally validated dermatological disorders associated SNPs curated from a large scale of literature but also offers computationally predicted insights into previously undiscovered disease–gene and disease–SNP relationships.

Our disease association network analysis highlighted vitiligo to exhibit maximum interactions with different genes from our database. Vitiligo is a chronic, acquired depigmentation disorder of the skin resulting in an episodically progressive loss of functional melanocytes causing pigment dilution in the affected areas of the skin (Picardo et al. 2015). Affecting 0.5–1% of the world population (Boisseau-Garsaud et al. 2000; tHowitz et al. 1977) and with a prevalence rate of 0.5–2.5% in India (Handa and Kaur 1999), vitiligo can develop at any age irrespective of the type of skin, gender, race, or geographical location underlying both genetic and non-genetic factors in a complex interactive manner. We, therefore, investigated the role of specific miRNAs and SNPs reported to be associated with vitiligo in the human genome to identify their plausible effect on vitiligo susceptibility using computational platforms. The cataloging of susceptible miRNAs and SNPs is essential for narrowing down the plausible concomitant genetic determinants of vitiligo. Protein–protein interactions are virtually intrinsic for

every cellular and regulatory process, and a damaging alteration in such interactions have been deduced to cause and sometimes even accelerate human diseases. The regulation or impediment of a known detrimental protein–protein interaction delineates a principal target for drug discovery. Hence, a systems biology approach was implemented that unveiled significant interconnections and revealed intricate patterns of disease association. Such a network analysis is helpful in studying the gene expressions and analyzing a large set of disease-associated proteins (Barabasi and Oltvai 2004). Furthermore, we prioritized a few proteins in our protein–protein interaction network as pertinent hub proteins which may be targeted for treating vitiligo. We performed computational analysis for harmful SNPs and scrutinized drug–target and drug–similarity interactions with an effort to provide potential novel drug candidates for optimal therapeutic interventions. Subsequently, we manually curated all miRNAs and SNPs and established a vitiligo specific database, VitmiRS (Vitiligo associated miRNAs and SNPs), to provide a comprehensive, user-friendly interface to detailed information on each miRNA and SNP association that renders susceptibility to vitiligo supported with pertinent data. VitmiRS currently houses 41 miRNAs and 134 associated SNPs for 84 genes which have been made online allowing easy retrieval of data. Till date, no systematic efforts have been made for the compilation of such data in a single platform that is specifically designed for dermatological disorders thereby contributing to the uniqueness of both the databases. A comprehensive view of the databases is shown in Fig. 1. We hope they serve as a significant resource that would benefit the scientific community. The present polypharmacogenomic network integration approach in vitiligo disease module is novel to the best of our knowledge that attempts to furnish a comprehensive understanding of the biological mechanisms that mediate vitiligo disease pathogenesis and offering novel interventional drug targets for efficient therapeutic interventions for genetically susceptible individuals. The graphical representation of the workflow is shown in Fig. 2.

Methods
Construction of DermaGene: data sourcing, curation, and reassessment

We initiated by creating a comprehensive list of dermatological disorders by referring to various online and offline resource databases followed by identification and mining of data to make every entry in our database descriptive of the SNP–disease relationship. The three top databases that we referred to included UniProt, DisGeNET (Pinero et al. 2015), and OMIM.

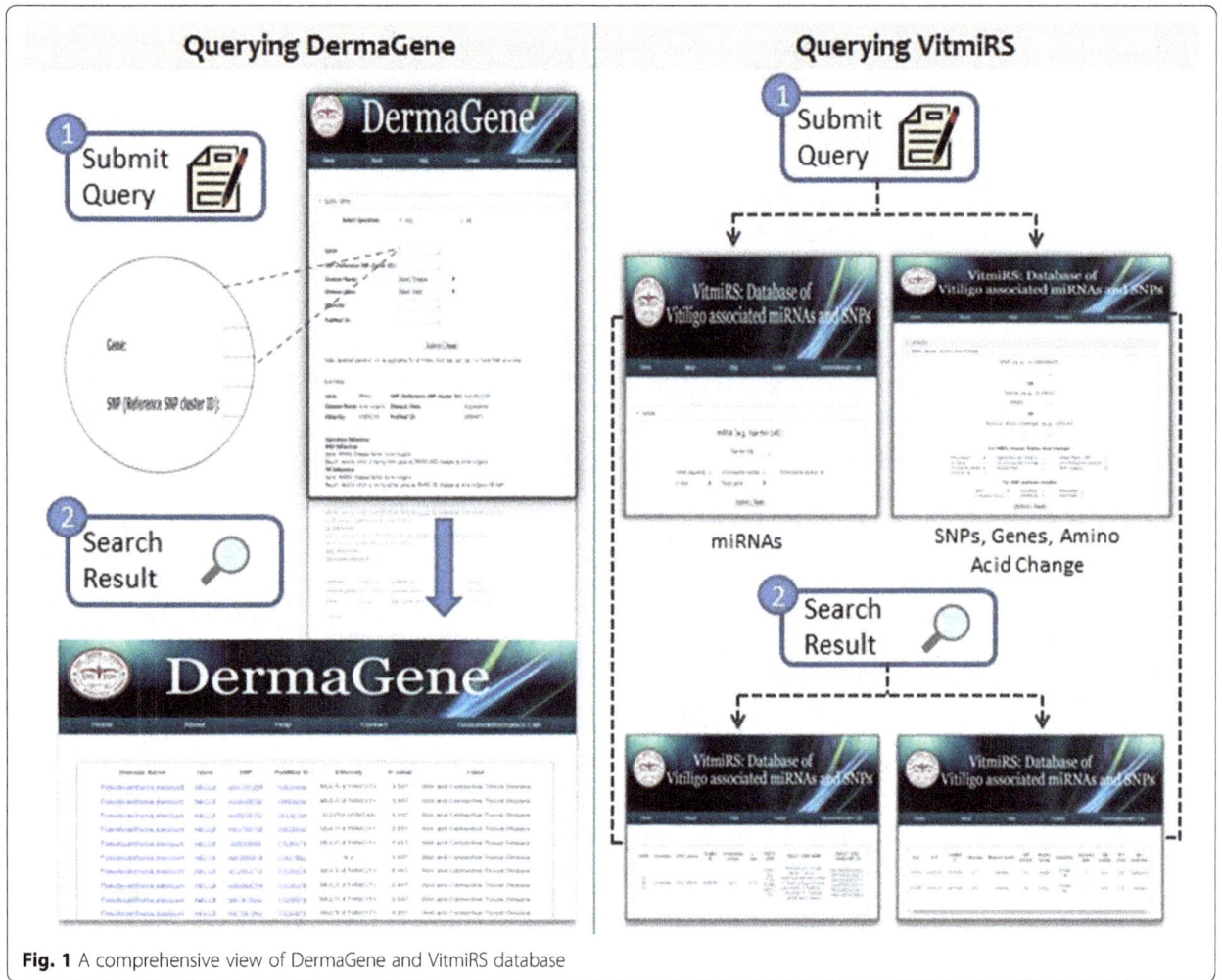

Fig. 1 A comprehensive view of DermaGene and VitmiRS database

Database creation was initiated by procuring the entire UniProt database, followed by converting the data obtained into the suitable and workable MS Excel format. A significant volume of data downloaded was delimited which required to be segregated into distinct columns, and we applied text to column—delimited to get a succinct view. This first stage download of database was subjected to filters from where we manually selected every possible dermatological disorder from the pool of 74,177 entries. This was achieved by referring to our previously generated comprehensive list of dermatological disorders. At this stage, we had the Gene name and rs ID indicating the SNP and the corresponding disease name. We thus reduced our database to 5000 entries, followed by removal of incomplete or duplicate entries thereby condensing it further to 2800 entries described by three attributes.

As the next step, we utilized disGeNET, to individually query every single gene (obtained from the UniProt database) to identify the p value and the PubMed ID. This was achieved by manually matching the results obtained with their corresponding rs IDs. Additionally, we populated the database with corresponding PubMed ID, p value, and disease class. Further, OMIM was put to use to support filling of gaps in the database. Extensive research helped us identify the missing values, which we were required to eliminate owing to insufficient data, thus reducing the database to 1116 entries.

Once we were finished with supplementing the database in its creation stage with requisite data, we proceeded to utilize PubMed as our primary source and to access all the research papers linked through their PubMed ID with our database. The work culminated into exhaustive reading of research papers to discern the ethnicities associated with the research conducted. Exhaustive study of research papers enabled us to determine ethnicities and to subsequently complete the database. Once the database was generated, the data was carefully re-assessed to ensure authenticity, through manual analysis of input data with the intention to establish the veracity of information as sourced from the specified databases. Besides, identification of alternative names for the specific diseases allowed for scope expansion of the database.

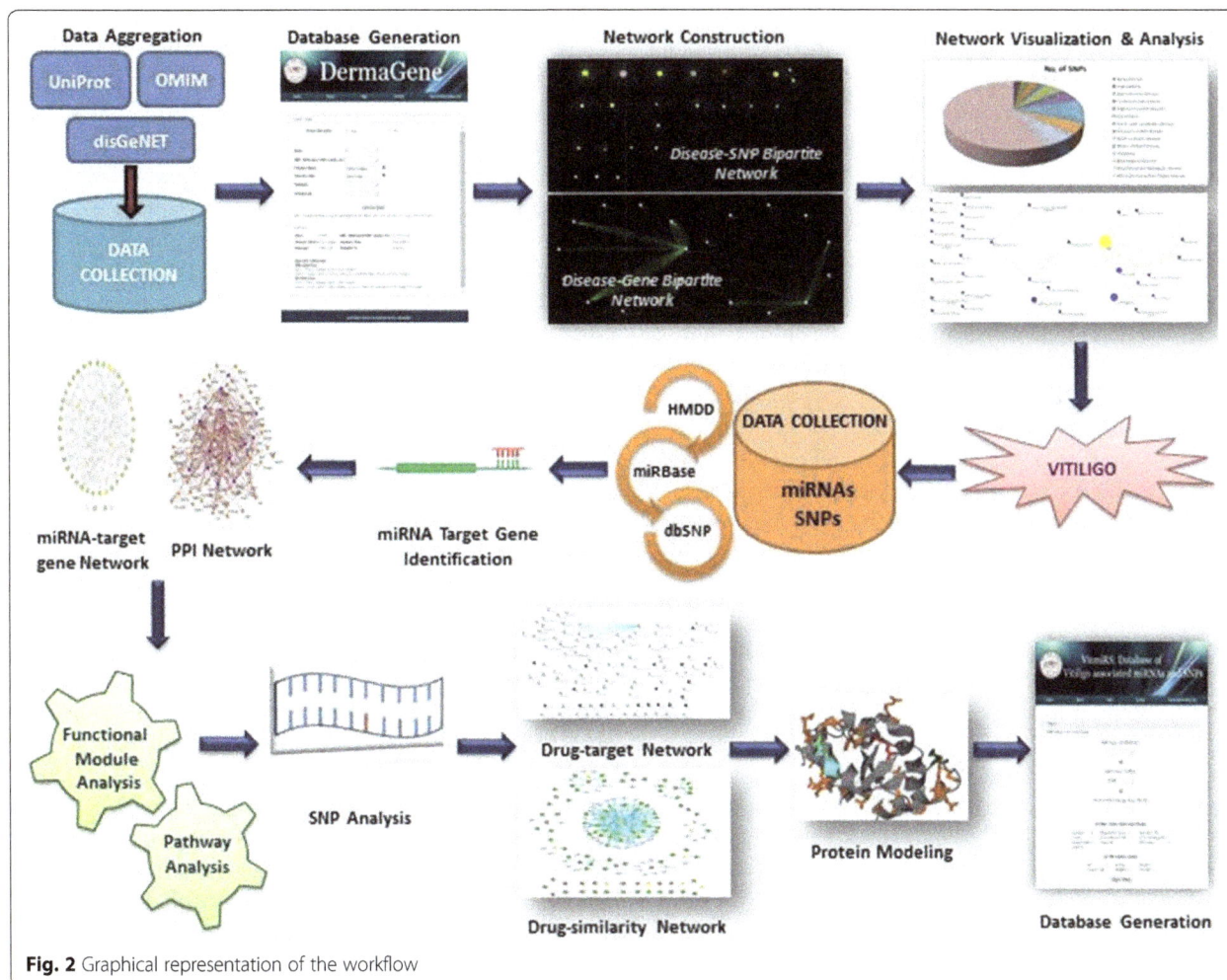

Fig. 2 Graphical representation of the workflow

Each entry in this database therefore describes the genes, the SNPs associated with diseases, the PubMed IDs of texts referred, and the frequency of disease occurrence along with the population ethnicity where it exists. Also, we have taken into consideration the ethnicity of the genotypic variation to identify disease susceptibility in specific populations, the p value for the occurrence of genetic dermatological disorders which enables recognition of how strongly a particular gene influences the mentioned diseases. We thus have included six fields, and the data obtained was subsequently used to chart patterns within multiple genes and diseases. The information sourced aims to provide in-depth knowledge on common dermatological disorders, subsequently provisioning us to analyze the risk of genetic variants on their contribution to disease susceptibility.

Disease classification and network analysis of DermaGene data

Network theory involves the analysis of complex systems and serves as a potent biological tool, thereby, facilitating a better understanding of gene interactions and their role in causing diseases. To perform disease association network analysis, we constructed disease–gene bipartite network (DGN) and disease–SNP bipartite network (DSN) using Cytoscape (Shannon et al. 2003) with each network comprising a pair of disjoint set of nodes. The two sets of nodes are chosen such that there is no intra-connection but capable of exhibiting inter-connection. The nodes communicate with each other via edges, where the edges are the representatives of the nature of the interaction between the pair of nodes. In DGN, all the genes present in our database formed one set of nodes and the other set of nodes were reflected by all the known dermatological disorders in DermaGene. An edge connected the two sets of nodes if a disease–gene association was found. Whereas in DSN, all the diseases in our database formed one set of nodes and the other set of nodes comprised of the associated SNPs. The diseases were linked only if they showed common genetic variants. We also illustrated the correlation between the diseases as a result of a shared gene between the two. The diseases were selected as nodes while the edge attributes represented the genes common between them.

Data collection for vitiligo disease module analysis

To analyze the role of miRNAs associated with vitiligo, the miRNA information was obtained from published literatures available in NCBI PubMed server (https://www.ncbi.nlm.nih.gov/pubmed/) and mined publicly available online databases, namely, HMDD v2.0 (the Human microRNA Disease Database) (Li et al. 2014), Entrez GENE database of NCBI, and miRBase (Griffiths-Jones 2006) for relevant entries. A total of 41 types of miRNAs were found to be associated with vitiligo.

On the other hand, we extracted the information of genes associated with vitiligo and its SNPs from the GENE database and dbSNP of NCBI. The build 141 of NCBI dbSNP database is the latest release containing nearly 44 million validated human SNPs (Sherry et al. 2001). A total of 186 genes were reported to be associated with the disease among which 134 polymorphisms for 84 genes were reported to be positively associated. UniProt IDs of the proteins were also noted.

Identification of miRNA target genes and construction of miRNA–target gene network

The miRNAs identified to be associated with vitiligo were used to find their respective target genes. TargetScanHuman 7.1 (Agarwal et al. 2015) was used to detect targets in the 3′UTR of the protein-coding transcripts by base-pairing rules where predictions with both broadly conserved and poorly conserved sites are provided. These target sites are the conserved sites that match or are complementary to the seed region of the miRNA that ultimately facilitates the binding of miRNA with the mRNA to functionally degrade the mRNA thereby resulting in gene silencing.

A structured network layout explaining network integrity is the core requirement to justify the interaction between miRNA and disease. A miRNA–target gene interaction network was therefore constructed and analyzed to understand the miRNA–target gene relationship and validate the miRNA–disease association. The miRNA–target gene bipartite network consists of two sets of nodes—one set represents the miRNAs, and the other set represents the target genes. Nodes from the two sets were connected if a particular miRNA is associated with a particular target gene. The datasheet prepared which included all the miRNAs associated with vitiligo along with their target genes was used to generate the network in Cytoscape (Shannon et al. 2003).

Construction of vitiligo-associated protein–protein interaction network

Interactions between genes whose expression profiles are correlated with disease pathogenesis may contribute to the progression of the disease (Srivastava et al. 2017). To identify such interactions, we constructed the protein–protein interaction network using STRING (The Search Tool for the Retrieval of Interacting Genes) (Von Mering et al. 2005). It is a comprehensive database capable of providing an overall view of all the known and predicted protein–protein interactions of physical and functional associations. The PPI network generated based on STRING online database was then visualized in Cytoscape whose common feature lies in combing biological interaction networks with relevant large databases into a unified framework.

Functional module and enrichment analysis

Considering the connectivity properties of a network, we resolved to identify the significant clusters or modules enriched in biological processes from the complex bipartite network to extract biologically meaningful interactions. The modular analysis can provide a better insight into the relationship of the interconnected proteins assuming that the highly connected nodes in a network could form a cluster. As we know, cellular processes and functions are modular; therefore, it is more feasible to predict the structural and functional behavior of a particular module than that of an individual gene. Such module analysis has played a significant role in the past in determining disease mechanisms (Mitra et al. 2013). We used Markov Clustering Algorithm (MCL) method among the other clustering algorithms as it is the most widely used unsupervised clustering algorithms for functional module analysis and assigns a fast and reliable scalable method for finding functionally enriched clusters in complex networks. The granularity parameter for MCL clustering was kept at 1.8.

To interpret the biological impetus of the clusters in the network, we further performed functional enrichment analysis of the clustered gene groups using DAVID (The Database for Annotation, Visualization and Integrated Discovery) 6.8 (Huang et al. 2009). Functional enrichment analysis uses statistical approaches to identify the clusters of genes or proteins that are highly expressed or enriched in a large set of genes or proteins which may have an association with disease (Huang et al. 2008). All the genes were mapped into DAVID with the default settings selected as *"Homo sapiens"* in both the species background as well as the current background for the analysis.

Pathway analysis

To analyze the pathways in which these genes are involved, we conducted a pathway analysis using KEGG (Kyoto Encyclopedia of Genes and Genomes) pathways in DAVID 6.8. KEGG Pathway database is the most comprehensive and widely used database of annotation information. The pathway classification with $p \leq 0.001$ and Benjamini–Hochberg FDR ≤ 0.01 was considered to have the most biological significance. Pathway analysis helps to interpret the data in the context of biological interactions and identify related proteins within a pathway.

A single protein may be involved in multiple pathways that are of importance to many biological processes. The biological cause of a disease can be explored by examining the changes in gene expression in a pathway. Also, the same pathway can be targeted for novel drug candidates (Wang et al. 2010). Deciphering the pathways which are explicitly targeted by the essential proteins may provide insight into their regulatory mechanisms. To better analyze the pathway analysis results, we constructed a protein pathway network to elucidate which pathways were eminently targeted by the proteins, specifically, the hub proteins. Such pathways, in turn, can be targeted for therapy and treatment approaches.

SNP analysis

The feasibility of the identification of the nsSNPs that vest susceptibility or resistance to human diseases has been improved with the use of in silico tools. To elucidate of the function of mutations in vitiligo-susceptible genes, we investigated the pathogenic effect of 134 SNPs which were reported to be associated with vitiligo. Among the 134 SNPs, the functional context of 36 nsSNPs was analyzed by employing various computational platforms. We used a combination of computational tools, namely, SIFT (Kumar et al. 2009), PolyPhen 2.0 (Adzhubei et al. 2010), PROVEAN (Choi et al. 2012), SNPs&GO (Magesh and Doss 2014), I-Mutant Suite 3.0 (Capriotti et al. 2008), and PANTHER Evolutionary Analysis of Coding SNP (Mi et al. 2005) to identify the nsSNPs that potentially affect the structure and function of proteins associated with vitiligo.

Additionally, MutPred 2 (Pejavar et al. 2017) was used to interpret the possible molecular cause of disease-inducing amino acid substitutions. Furthermore, NetSurfP (Petersen et al. 2009) was used to analyze the effect of such mutations in the stability of the protein by predicting the solvent accessibility of the substituted residue.

The information from different computational platforms was combined to prioritize the deleterious SNPs to increase the predictive power and accuracy of the results of the in silico techniques.

Construction of drug–target network and drug–similarity network

A single drug can target multiple proteins. To analyze this relationship between drug and protein targets (disease-gene products) and to understand how they intervene therapeutically in disease processes, we constructed a drug–target network (Yildirim et al. 2007). We extracted information about drugs with respect to our drug

candidates from DrugBank (Knox et al. 2011), which is a chemo-informatics resource that is updated and maintained with the Food and Drug Administration (FDA) information. We used known FDA drugs (both approved and approved-investigational) concerning to the protein targets to generate the drug–target bipartite network.

To identify which drugs act similarly on the same target, we constructed a drug–similarity network to analyze the interactions of drugs and its action on protein targets. DrugBank provides clinically relevant drug interactions, and the information of the interacting drugs and its interacting mechanism with respect to a particular drug was taken from DrugBank. Such a network can provide insights on drug–drug interaction for a potential drug candidate where an interacting drug can act synergistically or antagonistically with another drug altering the benefit or effectiveness of the drug on disease conditions. An interacting drug of a particular drug can also pose as a potential drug for the protein targeted by that drug.

Protein modeling of TLR2

Finding the 3D structure of proteins is helpful in predicting the impact of SNPs on the structural level and in showing the degrees of alteration. To elucidate the molecular dynamic behavior of the SNP in TLR2 protein, we performed preliminary protein modeling by G23D (Genomic variant to 3D protein data) (Solomon et al. 2016) which is a tool for the conversion of human genomic coordinates to protein structures. G23D allows the mapping of evolutionary related as well as identical protein of genomic variants in a 3D model structure assisting in the feasibility of structural insight. Along with the mutated sites, it also displays the wild-type residue and other functional sites on the modeled 3D protein structure to facilitate better interpretation of the variant.

We further carried out TLR2 protein–protein interaction analysis to analyze its interaction with other proteins which might be influenced by the mutation in TLR2 protein.

Construction of VitmiRS

The primary data in VitmiRS constitutes the collection of miRNAs and SNPs that have been reported to be associated with vitiligo. The process for database creation relied on extensive review of high-quality published journals, relevant articles published in PubMed, and multiple online resources discussing the association of miRNAs and SNPs with vitiligo for the identification and the subsequent extrication of relevant mentions of the fields that we explored. Information from multiple comprehensive and relevant databases, namely, dbSNP (Sherry et al. 2001), UniProt, HMDD v2.0 (Li et al., 2014), miR-Base (Griffiths-Jones 2006), and GENE database, was also taken into consideration. Every paper was read manually to eliminate the errors that may arise from machine-generated information. The information included was filtered at the thresholds of p value ≤ 0.05 and carefully re-assessed through manual analysis to ensure authenticity. A user-friendly web interface was developed for the ease of data retrieval. Apache was used as the application server and PHP as the programming language. The presentation layer of VitmiRS was created using XHTML and CSS, while for the backend database, MySQL was used.

Results
DermaGene

We curated a total of 244 unique genes in our database, with each gene exhibiting multiple SNPs and describing 114 diseases. A total of 871 unique SNPs exist that exhibits both pleiotropy and epistasis over dermatological disorders. The present DermaGene version relies on the review of over thousand literature sources to generate a comprehensive source comprising of 1116 tuples described through six attributes. It provides a user-friendly interface for easy retrieval of data to query detailed information on each SNP–disease association and hopes to facilitate analysis of the comorbidity associations asserted between human variation and observed disease conditions.

Disease classification and network analysis of DermaGene data
Disease classification

Analysis of DermaGene database revealed the existence of maximum SNPs accounting for dermatological disorders to lie on chromosome 17. The distribution of SNPs was also analyzed to observe their association with the different disease classes included in our database. We identified that the primary disease class which exists in our database is skin and connective tissue diseases (632). This indicates that the maximum number of SNPs, as in our database accounts for the skin and connective tissue class of diseases, followed by neoplasia (116) and nutritional and metabolic diseases (78). The results are summarized in Fig. 3. Our database reveals the possibility for disease comorbidity existence. We have identified few diseases that share the SNP with other diseases, indicating association among them and the subsequent combinatorial occurrence of the diseases. This shows that in the presence of co-morbid associations, the incidence of one of them in an individual may elevate the possibility of another disease to occur. An additional file (see Additional files 1 and 2) lists the 12 incidences of disease comorbidity arising from shared SNPs and 22 disease–gene associations, identified from DermaGene respectively which may be responsible for comorbid associations.

Disease–gene bipartite network (DGN)

Our analysis of DGN (Fig. 4a) identified vitiligo from our database to be under the influence of a maximum number of different genes since it exhibited maximum disease correlations, therefore, indicating a probable multi-factorial genetic inheritance. From our database, various genes are showed a higher degree of influence compared to other genes which are defined by the number of diseases it influences (Fig. 4b). The genes that exhibit maximum association include IL2RA, PTPN22, and FGFR2 and are shown in Fig. 5. We observed that the gene IL2RA causes three distinct diseases—alopecia areata, urticaria pigmentosa, and vitiligo. At the same time, another gene PTPN22 accounts for alopecia areata, systemic lupus erythematosus, and vitiligo (Fig. 5a). The third gene IKZ4 also contributes to alopecia and vitiligo, which confronts us with possible idea of a genetic association between these diseases. The relationship between alopecia and vitiligo has been validated through previously conducted research studies (Huang et al. 2013; Krishnaram et al. 2013). Similarly, the gene FGFR2 contributes to Apert syndrome, Crouzon syndrome, and Beare–Stevenson cutis gyrata syndrome (Fig. 5b), in spite of the absence of definite literature, indicating epistasis, if at all. This means a probable novel finding which can be useful for doctors and researchers alike.

Disease–SNP bipartite network (DSN)

From our DSN (Fig. 6), we inferred that most SNPs are associated with single diseases, although we also report the occurrence of few SNPs that exhibit pleiotropic effect since they are linked to multiple diseases. We identified the SNPs rs28931615, rs121912737, rs2476601, rs121913478, rs28931594, rs11540654, rs1042522, rs59856285, and rs60723330 from our DermaGene database to reveal a probable pleiotropy effect defined through association with multiple diseases. Published studies explicitly authenticate our findings for the already existing relationship between acanthosis nigricans and Crouzon syndrome (Mir et al. 2013); acrokeratosis verruciformis and Darier disease (Harman et al. 2016); systemic lupus erythematosus and vitiligo (Nath and Kelly 2001); alopecia and vitiligo (Krishnaram et al. 2013); alopecia and systemic lupus erythematosus (Werth et al. 1992); ichthyosis hystrix with deafness and keratitis–ichthyosis–deafness syndrome (Dalamon et al. 2016); associations of ectodermal dysplasia (ED) and incontinentia pigmenti (IP) caused by IBKG gene, as resulting from complete loss of function in case of IP and X-linked recessive inheritance as in the case of ED (Zonana et al. 2000); Costello syndrome and seborrheic keratosis caused by germline mutation of Ras/MAPK signaling pathway (Hafner and Groesser 2013); and keratoderma palmoplantar which is often accompanied by

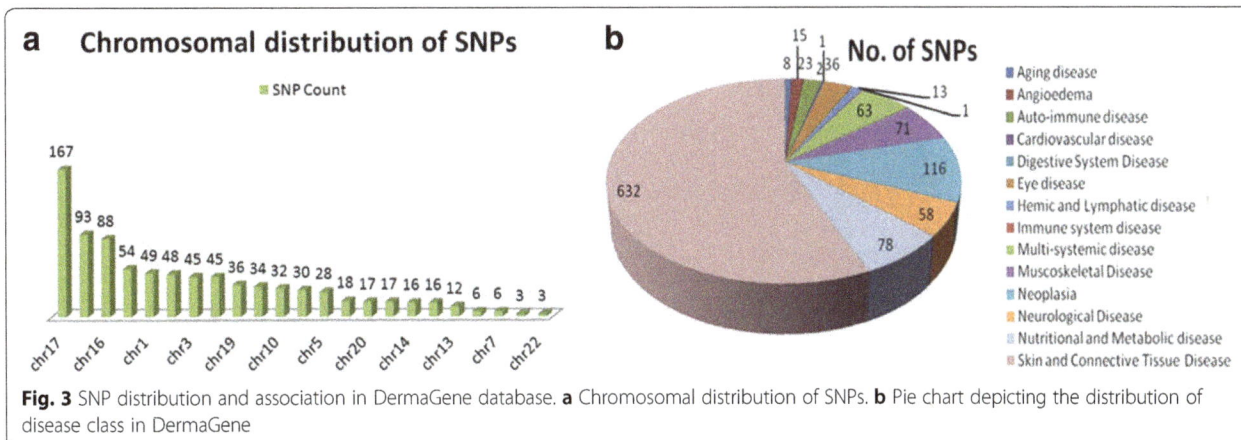

Fig. 3 SNP distribution and association in DermaGene database. **a** Chromosomal distribution of SNPs. **b** Pie chart depicting the distribution of disease class in DermaGene

pachyonychia congenita as described by Smith et al. (2000). There is thus a likelihood of epistatic effect and that the shared SNPs serve as an index of the biological relationship existing between them with subsequent co-manifestation of these diseases.

We also found that diseases xeroderma pigmentosum and keloid share two SNPs rs1042522 and rs11540654, which served as a revelation on the previously unidentified association between the two (Fig. 6a). Our database sheds light on the relationship between the diseases Beare–Stevenson cutis gyrata and Brooke–Spiegler syndrome as caused by the SNP rs121913478 which exhibits no prior known correlation (Fig. 6b).

We have identified various other genetic associations through network analysis as well, wherein we observe the role of a single gene in causing various dermatological disorders. Published evidence for a probable relationship between alopecia and Marie–Una syndrome can be inferred from a published study conducted on a seven generation British family, although the study is not directly indicative of the particular association as such (Marren et al. 1992). Xeroderma pigmentosum (XP) and Cockayne syndrome (CS), although

phenotypically different, share genetic similarities, since the gene ERCC5 is responsible for both the cases and this is probably because the several mutations accounting for UV sensitivity may also account for somatic and brain growth failure, thus resulting in neurological problems. Additionally, an existence of literature for LMNA gene contributing to both Hutchinson–Gilford progeria syndrome and congenital muscular dystrophy establish the authenticity of our findings from the DermaGene database (Barateau et al. 2017). Also, we find that Menkes syndrome is a more severe variant of cutis laxa, the latter being initiated during early middle childhood. Both the diseases arising from a mutation in ATP2A2 gene exhibit loose skin as a phenotypic contribution to the affected individual. Lastly, previous reports show clear progression of chilblain lupus erythematosus to systemic lupus erythematosus (SLE) (Bansal and Goel 2014), with around 20% individuals developing SLE (Hedrich et al. 2008).

We also identified the gene ABCC6 located at chromosome 16 on short arm (p) at position 13.11, to have the maximum SNPs as shown in Fig. 7. This gene contributes to pseudoxanthoma elasticum and hence

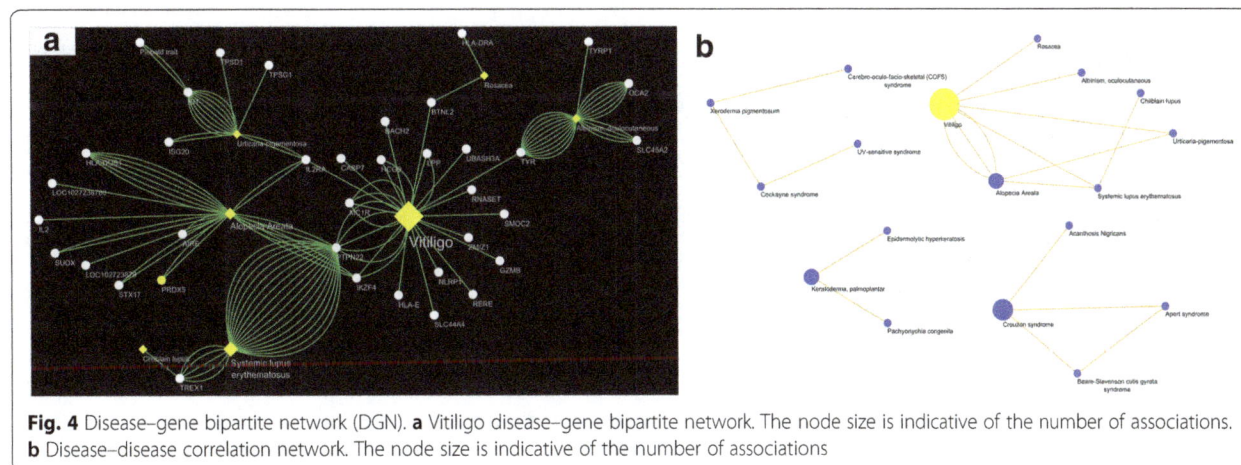

Fig. 4 Disease–gene bipartite network (DGN). **a** Vitiligo disease–gene bipartite network. The node size is indicative of the number of associations. **b** Disease–disease correlation network. The node size is indicative of the number of associations

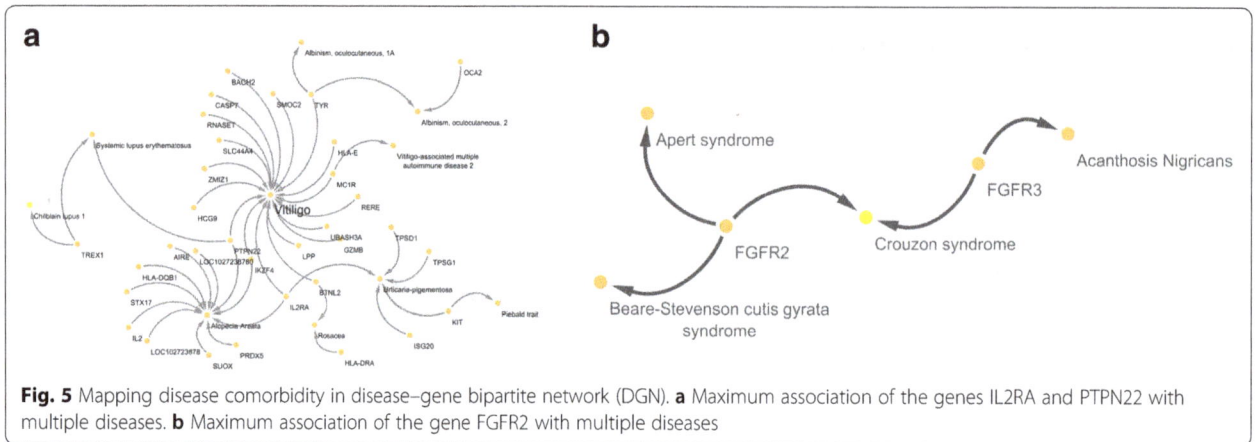

Fig. 5 Mapping disease comorbidity in disease–gene bipartite network (DGN). **a** Maximum association of the genes IL2RA and PTPN22 with multiple diseases. **b** Maximum association of the gene FGFR2 with multiple diseases

can play a key in disease prognosis. With a total of 91 SNPs within the gene, ABCC6 gene serves as a disease hotspot, with the existence of multiple SNPs contributing to the same disease. This reveals that ABCC6 gene is a relatively large gene, of size 74,766 bp to allow for a high number of SNPs.

Data collection for vitiligo analysis

We found 41 miRNAs to be associated with vitiligo with 34 upregulated and 7 downregulated in disease conditions. A total of 134 polymorphisms for 84 genes were found to be associated with vitiligo. Among the 134 SNPs, 36 are nsSNPs, 7 are coding synonymous SNPs, and 68 SNPs were found in the non-coding region.

Identification of miRNA target genes and construction of miRNA–target gene network

The respective target genes of the miRNAs were identified to explicate the biological targets of these miRNAs whereby they control gene expression and ultimately regulate the cellular and molecular responses during disease development and progression. The miRNA–target

gene bipartite network represented a total of 41 miRNAs and 98 unique target genes consisting of 139 nodes and 220 edges (Fig. 8). The target genes are considered to be connected in the network if they share a common miRNA. To identify the hub miRNAs and target genes associated with vitiligo, among the number of methods available for hub identification, we chose maximum clique centrality (MCC) along with two other topological parameters, namely, betweenness centrality and bottleneck (Chin et al. 2014), and normalized the data to identify the top hubs in the network. In our analysis, we found seven hub miRNAs (hsa-miR-99b, hsa-miR-577, hsa-miR-9, hsa-miR-155, hsa-miR-211, hsa-miR-10a, and hsa-miR-145).

Protein–protein interaction network

Protein–protein interaction network of vitiligo-associated proteins exhibited significant interconnections between the proteins. It comprised of 71 nodes and 322 edges (Fig. 9). The proteins are considered to be connected in the network if they interact with each

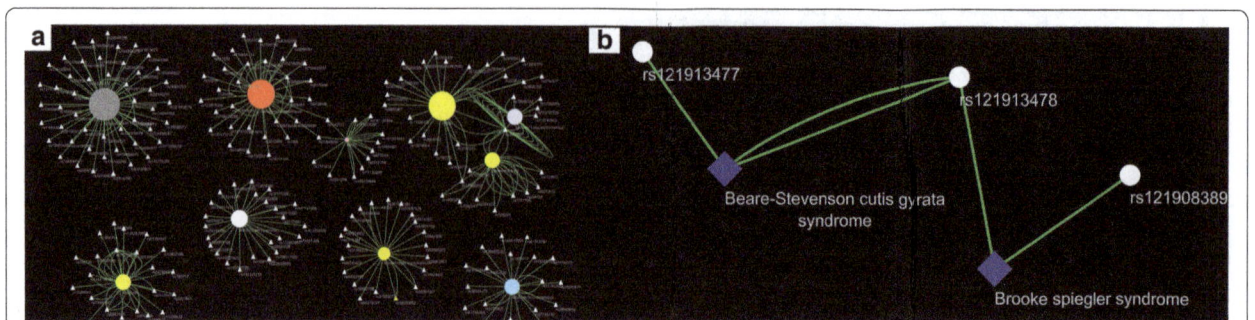

Fig. 6 Disease–SNP bipartite network (DSN). The triangular nodes represent the SNPs, and circular nodes indicate the disease. The size of circular nodes is proportional to the SNPs that the particular disease is associated with. **a** The diseases xeroderma pigmentosum and keloid share two SNPs rs1042522 and rs11540654. **b** Relationship between the diseases Beare-Stevenson cutis gyrata and Brooke–Spiegler syndrome as caused by the SNP rs121913478

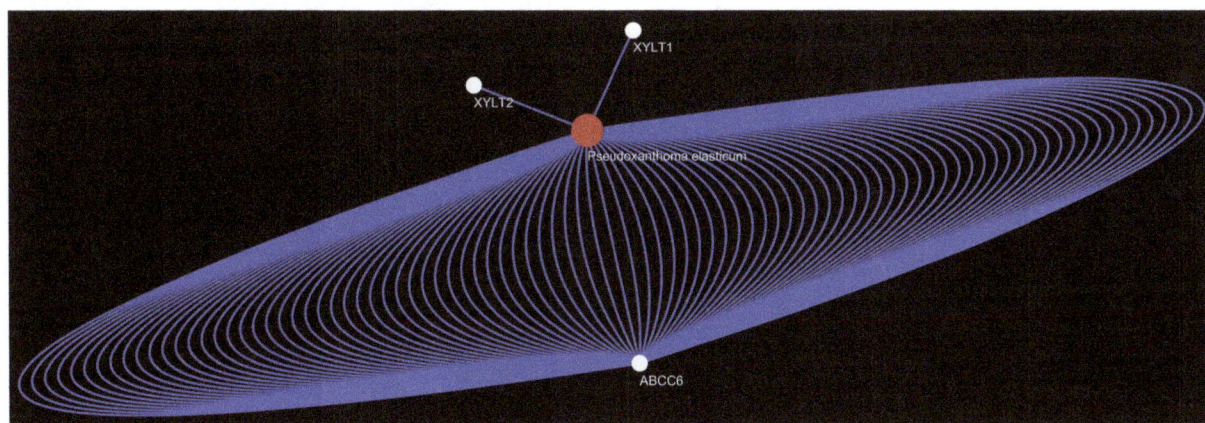

Fig. 7 Mapping ABCC6 gene to pseudoxanthoma elasticum. Multiple SNPs of ABCC6 gene are shown to be contributing to the same disease pseudoxanthoma elasticum

other. If each protein is not inclined to interact with another protein or specifically interacts with a single protein, then the bipartite network would be disconnected into many single nodes corresponding to specific or unique proteins with few or no edges between the nodes. Rather, the protein–protein interaction network generated displayed many interactions between the proteins. For prioritizing proteins as hubs, we chose MCC along with betweenness centrality and bottleneck as topological parameters (Chin et al. 2014) and normalized the data to identify the top 15 hubs in the network. These 15 essential (hub) proteins are IL10, IFNG, IL4, CD44, IL1B, CTLA4, GZMB, FOXP3, TNF, IL2RA, CAT, ESR1, TLR2, HLA-A, and GSTP1.

Functional module and enrichment analysis

The functional module analysis of vitiligo-associated proteins revealed four functional modules (Fig. 10). The average size of the clusters was 17.75, and they were ranked by their modularity score of 1. The majority of the proteins were found to form a single large cluster. This implies that these proteins have a biological similarity in their functions.

We performed functional enrichment analysis of the larger functional module consisting of 64 proteins using DAVID 6.8. Keeping the classification stringency at highest and considering the enrichment score value ≤ 1.3 to be significant, the given set of target genes was classified into nine functionally enriched clusters (see Additional file 3) that involved 15 genes from the given set of 64 genes. All the nine clusters were observed to be primarily associated with the immune system regulatory processes, such as MHC class I/II-like antigen recognition protein, conserved site of immunoglobulin/major histocompatibility complex, conserved site of interleukin-10, positive regulation of JAK-STAT cascade, apoptotic signaling, chemokines, and TNF.

Pathway analysis

According to the threshold of hypergeometric test $p \leq 0.001$ and Benjamini–Hochberg FDR ≤ 0.01, the mapped genes were found to be enriched in a total of 30 pathways, which involved a total of 40 genes from the given gene set. The most significant pathway was found to be the allograft rejection pathway with a p value of 5.70E–17 and FDR value of 1.51E–14 involving 13 genes. Among these 30 pathways, almost half of the pathways (15 pathways) were associated with immune system responses and related disorders, and autoimmunity, while 14 pathways were associated with infectious (viral, bacterial, and parasitic) disease pathways that have been reported to impair the proper regulation of the immune system.

In the protein–pathway network, a protein is connected to a pathway if the protein is known to be involved in that particular pathway. The network consisted of 71 nodes and 270 interactions representing 40 proteins and 30 pathways (Fig. 11).

Based on degree value, TNF showed maximum interaction in the network implying its participation in most of the pathways. Among the 30 pathways, TNF was found to be associated with 24 pathways. Similarly, IL1B, IFNG, IL10, and TLR2 were found to be involved in 19, 18, 15, and 14 pathways respectively. It was also observed that TLR2 was specifically associated with the infectious disease pathways that were responsible for deregulating the immune system processes as depicted in the results of KEGG pathway see analysis. An additional file (see Additional file 4) lists the pathways in which the hub proteins were found to be involved. Among the 15 hub proteins identified in the protein–protein interaction network, 11 were found in this network suggesting that these 11 essential proteins are involved in the filtered significant pathways.

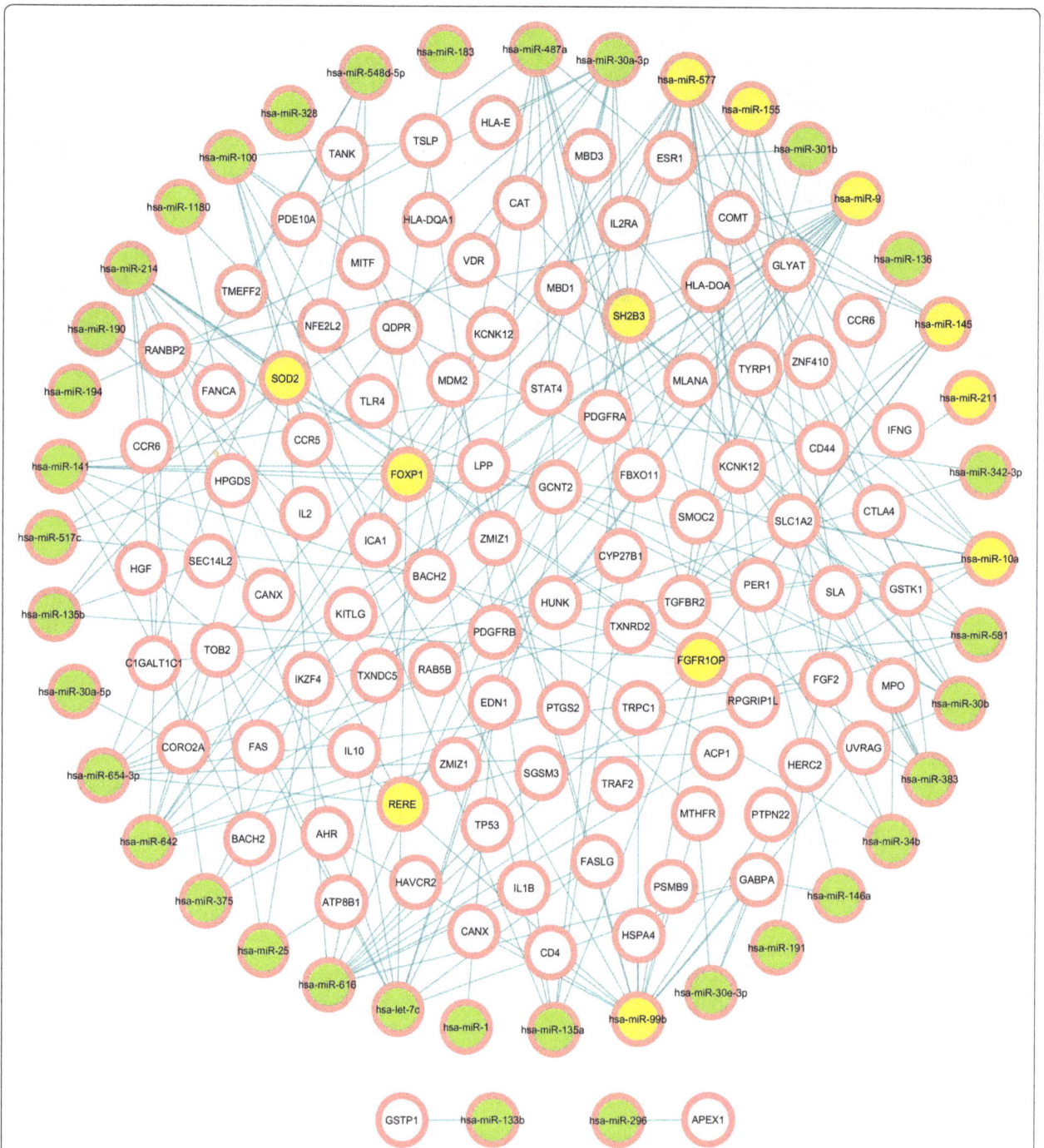

Fig. 8 miRNA–target gene interaction network. The green colored nodes represent the miRNAs, the white colored nodes represent the target genes, and yellow colored nodes represent the hub miRNAs along with the target genes of the highest degree in the network

SNP analysis

Among the 134 SNPs, 36 (26.9%) are nsSNPs and 7 (5.2%) are SNPs, while 68 (50.8%) SNPs were found in the non-coding region. SNPs in the non-coding region comprises of 44 (32.8%) SNPs in the intronic region, 19 (14.2%) in the near-gene region, and 5 (3.8%) in the mRNA UTR region. The rest 23 (17.1%)

among 134 SNPs are intergenic. The distribution of the SNPs is shown in Fig. 12a.

For our analysis, we selected the nsSNPs and UTR-region SNPs since UTRs are central for the post-transcriptional regulation of gene expression, and alterations in the functional UTR region can lead to severe pathology (Conne et al. 2000). The 36 nsSNPs

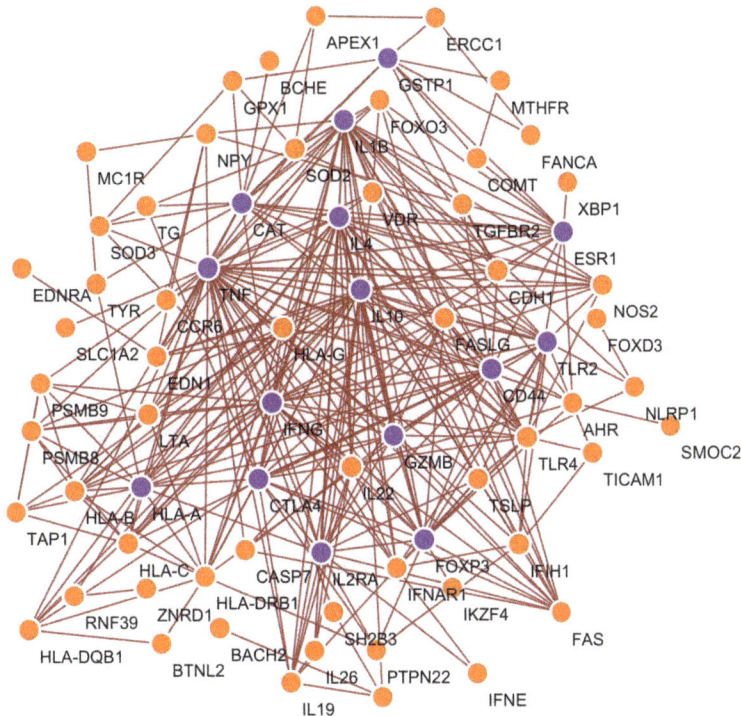

Fig. 9 Protein–protein interaction network. The purple nodes represent the hub proteins in the network

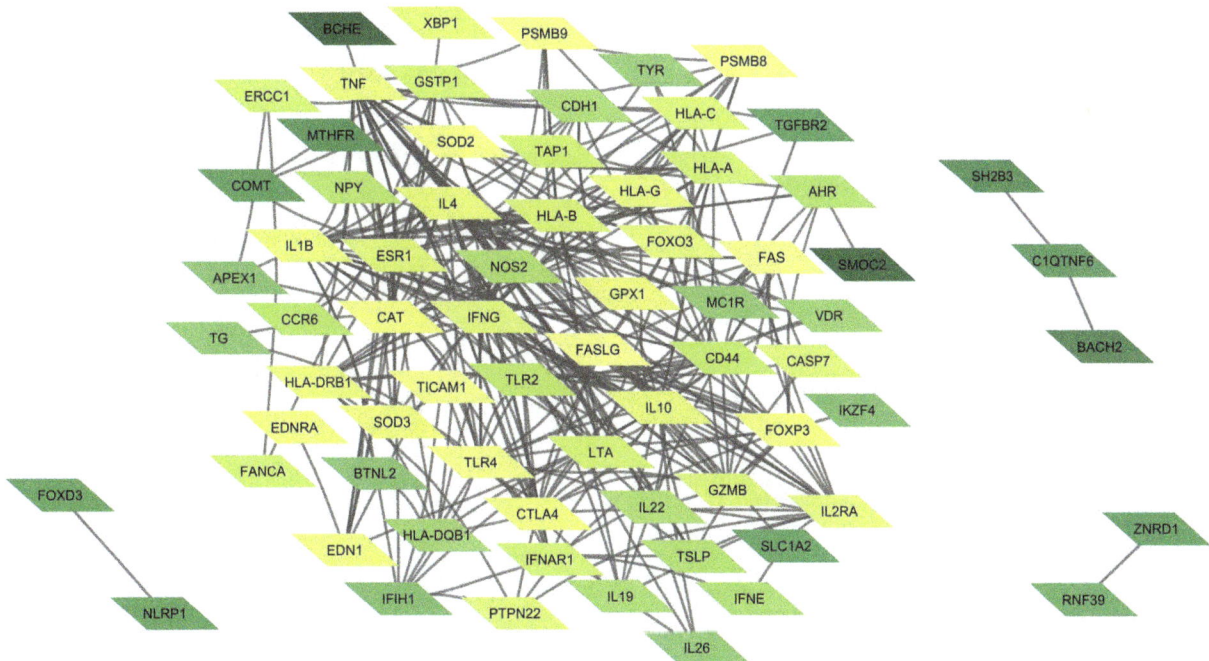

Fig. 10 Functional module (clusters) network. The shades of green color, from light to dark, represent the decrease in the number of interactions. The genes with the maximum number of interactions show lighter shades in the cluster

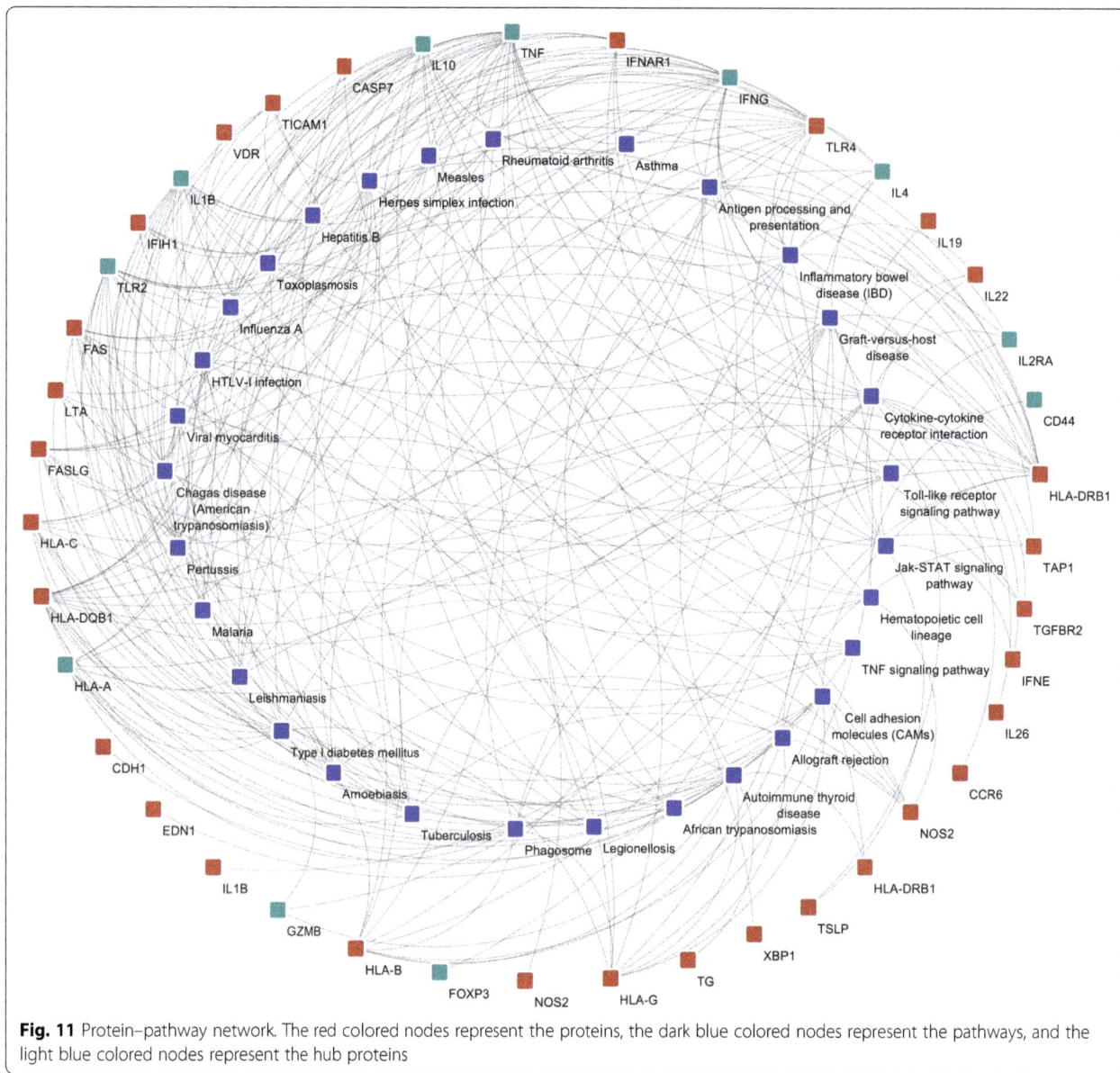

Fig. 11 Protein–pathway network. The red colored nodes represent the proteins, the dark blue colored nodes represent the pathways, and the light blue colored nodes represent the hub proteins

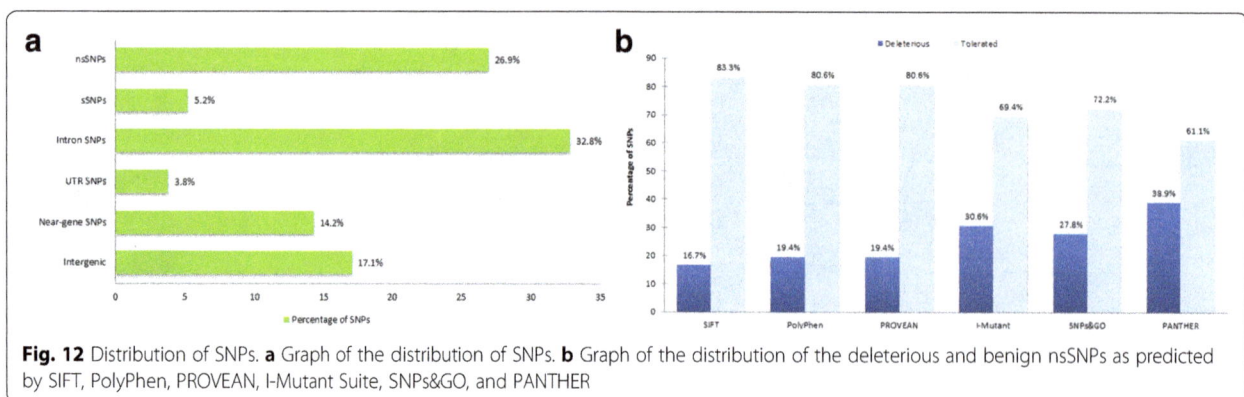

Fig. 12 Distribution of SNPs. **a** Graph of the distribution of SNPs. **b** Graph of the distribution of the deleterious and benign nsSNPs as predicted by SIFT, PolyPhen, PROVEAN, I-Mutant Suite, SNPs&GO, and PANTHER

were analyzed by using a combination of SIFT, PolyPhen, PROVEAN, SNPs&GO, I-Mutant Suite, and PANTHER Evolutionary Analysis of Coding SNP tools.

SIFT predicted six nsSNPs (16.7%) to be deleterious with a tolerance score cut off which is ≤ 0.05. Further analysis of the nsSNPs using PolyPhen predicted two nsSNPs to be "probably damaging" and five nsSNPs to be "possibly damaging" with a tolerance cut off score ≥ 0.5. Consequently, seven nsSNPs (19.4%) were characterized as damaging. Analysis using PROVEAN revealed a similar result as that of PolyPhen tool. Based on a tolerance cut off score value ≤ 0.05, it predicted seven nsSNPs (19.4%) to be damaging. Of these seven nsSNPs, one (rs5743708) was reported to be highly damaging with a tolerance score of 0.

To improve the prediction accuracy, we used I-Mutant Suite and SNPs&GO tools for further analysis. The output results in I-Mutant Suite predict the free energy change (DDG) and classifies it into any three of the mentioned classes, namely, largely unstable (DDG < – 0.5 kcal/mol), largely stable (DDG > 0.5 kcal/mol), or neutral (– 0.5 ≤ DDG ≤ 0.5 kcal/mol). The output result of a protein as largely unstable indicates the effect of a deleterious nsSNP. In our I-Mutant Suite results, we found that 11 nsSNPs (30.6%) exhibited a DDG value of less than – 0.5, which indicates that these are largely unstable resulting in disease-associated mutations. Whereas, SNPs&GO predicted 10 nsSNPs (27.8%) to be related to disease-associated mutations by using a tolerance cut off score ≥ 0.5.

A disease-causing mutation in the highly conserved regions of the genome may pose a high risk of that particular mutation to be damaging which is why we decided to carry out SNP conservation analysis. The probability of a mutation to cause a disease increases monotonically with the increase in the degree of site conservation (Vitkup et al. 2003). Conservation analysis by PANTHER Evolutionary Analysis of Coding SNP predicted 14 nsSNPs (38.9%) to be deleterious based on their preservation time. A longer preservation time implies a greater possibility of functional impact on a protein (Mi et al. 2005). Since different in silico tools have a diverse set of alignments and molecular characteristics, the results of the six tools were slightly different. Accordingly, we combined the results of SIFT, PolyPhen, PROVEAN, SNPs&GO, I-Mutant Suite, and PANTHER Evolutionary Analysis of Coding

SNP (see Additional file 5) to predict the deleterious nsSNPs common in all the analysis.

Figure 12b shows the distribution of deleterious and benign nsSNPs obtained using SIFT, PolyPhen, PROVEAN, I-Mutant Suite, SNPs&GO and PANTHER.

Of all of the predictions, 16.7%, 19.4%, 19.4%, 30.6%, 27.8%, and 38.9% deleterious nsSNPs were specifically found by SIFT, PolyPhen, PROVEAN, SNPs&GO, I-Mutant Suite and PANTHER respectively. Combining the results of all the six tools, three nsSNPs, namely, rs1801133 (MTHFR), rs5743708 (TLR2), and rs11575993 (SOD2), were predicted to be functionally significant. Tables 1 and 2 presents the deleterious nsSNPs obtained through the SIFT, PolyPhen, PROVEAN, I-Mutant Suite, SNPs&GO, and PANTHER analysis of the vitiligo-associated nsSNPs.

MutPred predicted the molecular cause of the nsSNPs to become deleterious in MTHFR (rs1801133), TLR2 (rs5743708), and SOD2 (rs11575993). Analysis of the results showed an interrelation of the SNPs to be damaging with respect to the solvent accessibility of the protein. The type of mutated residue and its position in the sequence affect the stability of the protein which due to mutation decreases with the decrease in solvent accessibility of a residue (Vitkup et al. 2003).

NetSurfP predicted the surface solvent accessibility of amino acids by using the protein FASTA sequence as a query. The solvent accessibility is predicted to be buried or exposed, based on the accessibility of the amino acid residues to the solvent. The reliability of relative surface accessibility is verified in the form of Z-score which highlights the surface prediction reliability. As given in Table 3, the class assignment does not change for the three nsSNPs. Although there were very minimal changes in the relative surface accessibility (RSA) values for the three nsSNPs, a considerable drift in the Z-score was not observed between the wild-type and mutant-type proteins. A decrease in RSA value has been observed in the mutant types of MTHFR and SOD2 while there was an increase in the RSA value of the TLR2 mutant type.

Drug–target network and drug–similarity network
Drug–target network

The bipartite network of drug–protein target interaction consisted of 109 nodes and 84 interactions (Fig. 13a). A drug and protein are considered to be connected to each

Table 1 nsSNPs found to be deleterious using SIFT, PolyPhen, and PROVEAN

SNP	Genes	SIFT score	SIFT prediction	PolyPhen score	PolyPhen prediction	PROVEAN score	PROVEAN prediction
rs1801133	MTHFR	0.043	Deleterious	0.998	Probably damaging	0.002	Damaging
rs5743708	TLR2	0.016	Deleterious	1	Possibly damaging	0	Damaging
rs11575993	SOD2	0.014	Deleterious	1	Possibly damaging	0.001	Damaging

Table 2 nsSNPs found to be deleterious using I-Mutant Suite, SNPs&GO, and PANTHER

SNP	Genes	I-Mutant score	I-Mutant prediction	SNPs&GO score	SNPs&GO prediction	PANTHER prediction
rs1801133	MTHFR	− 0.78	Disease-related mutation	0.88	Disease-associated variation	Probably damaging
rs5743708	TLR2	− 2.78	Disease-related mutation	0.7	Disease-associated variation	Possibly damaging
rs11575993	SOD2	− 1.4	Disease-related mutation	0.66	Disease-associated variation	Probably damaging

other if the protein is a known target of the drug, giving rise to a drug–target network.

In our analysis, we found that the most of the drugs targeting a particular protein did not show any interaction with other protein targets in the network except for the two drugs, etanercept and carfilzomib. Etanercept targets both TNF and LTA while carfilzomib targets PSMB8 as well as PSMB9. Also, we found that out of the 15 hub proteins, only 9 protein targets were found to be present in this network. This illustrates the other 6 hub proteins (IL10, IL4, GZMB, FOXP3, TLR2, AND HLA-A) as potential drug candidates for which drug information is currently not available. Also, we found that 4 hub proteins, namely, CD44, CD152, CAT, and GSTP1, were targeted by a single drug. This highlights the imperative need to discover more effective drugs that target these proteins which may play a major role in therapeutics to alleviate disease conditions in patients.

Another notable finding in our analysis was that the drugs which showed a high degree in the network were mostly indicated for the treatment of autoimmune diseases and deregulated immune responses. One of them is etanercept that targets TNF, a major proinflammatory cytokine that affects various aspects of the immune response, and LTA as well. Etanercept is a genetically engineered decoy receptor that consists of the ligand-binding domain of TNFR2 and the Fc component of human IgG1. It competitively binds with high affinity to TNFR2 inhibiting the binding of both TNF-α and TNF-β to the cell surface receptors, consequently, inhibiting inflammation induced melanocyte death. It has been indicated to be clinically used for rheumatoid arthritis, psoriatic arthritis, ankylosing spondylitis, and Crohn's disease (Nanda and Bathon 2004). However, etanercept has been reported to be less efficient as a monotherapy

in vitiligo patients requiring the need of a combinative therapy (Rigopoulos et al. 2007). LTA, on the other hand, is involved in the follicular dendritic cells development and has been observed to induce signals leading to lymphoid neo-organogenesis driving the inflammatory responses in autoimmune diseases like rheumatoid arthritis (Takemura et al. 2001). This suggests that etanercept may suppress lymphoid neo-organogenesis and reduce the proliferation of mature dendritic cells in vitiligo lesions (Wang et al. 2011). The other drug, carfilzomib, is a tetrapeptide epoxyketone-based proteasome inhibitor that targets PSMB9 and PSMB8. Peptides generated from ubiquitin-tagged cytosolic proteins are presented to CTLs by MHC class-I molecules which are degraded by multi-catalytic, cytosolic immune-proteasome complex called LMP2 and LMP7 encoded by PSMB9 and PSMB8 genes respectively (Cresswell et al. 2005). This intrinsic enzymatic activity of immune-proteasomes may be altered by genetic variations which reduce the expression of PSMB8 and PSMB9 in vitiligo PBMCs after IFNG stimulation. This leads to defective proteolytic degradation and accumulation of ubiquitinylated proteins in the epidermis of vitiligo patients leading to ROS production and auto-inflammatory immune responses which may be detrimental for the manifestation of vitiligo (Dani et al. 2017). Carfilzomib targets the catalytic activity of immune-proteasomes and irreversibly inactivates the proteasome, thereby inhibiting aberrant immune function (Miller et al. 2013).

Drug–similarity network

The drug similarity tripartite network of protein targets, drugs, and interacting drugs comprised of 178 nodes and 1331 interactions (Fig. 13b). A drug and its interacting drug are considered to be connected if they share a common protein target. Interacting drug partners of a particular drug may enhance the efficacy of the drug or may even target the same protein. Such interacting drugs may represent themselves as potential drug repositioning candidates. With this concept, we constructed the drug–similarity network that displayed interconnections between drugs and their interacting drug partners.

Apart from the drugs etanercept and carfilzomib targeting more than one protein as shown in the drug–target network, we found two other drugs showing interaction with another protein target in the network. Both diethylstilbestrol and conjugated equine estrogens

Table 3 Solvent accessibility analysis of the mutated proteins by NetSurfP

Genes	Type	Class assignment	Relative surface accessibility (RSA)	Z-fit score for RSA prediction
MTHFR	Wild	B	0.027	0.737
	Mutant	B	0.026	0.781
TLR2	Wild	E	0.243	1.46
	Mutant	E	0.245	1.527
SOD2	Wild	B	0.2	− 0.736
	Mutant	B	0.166	− 0.705

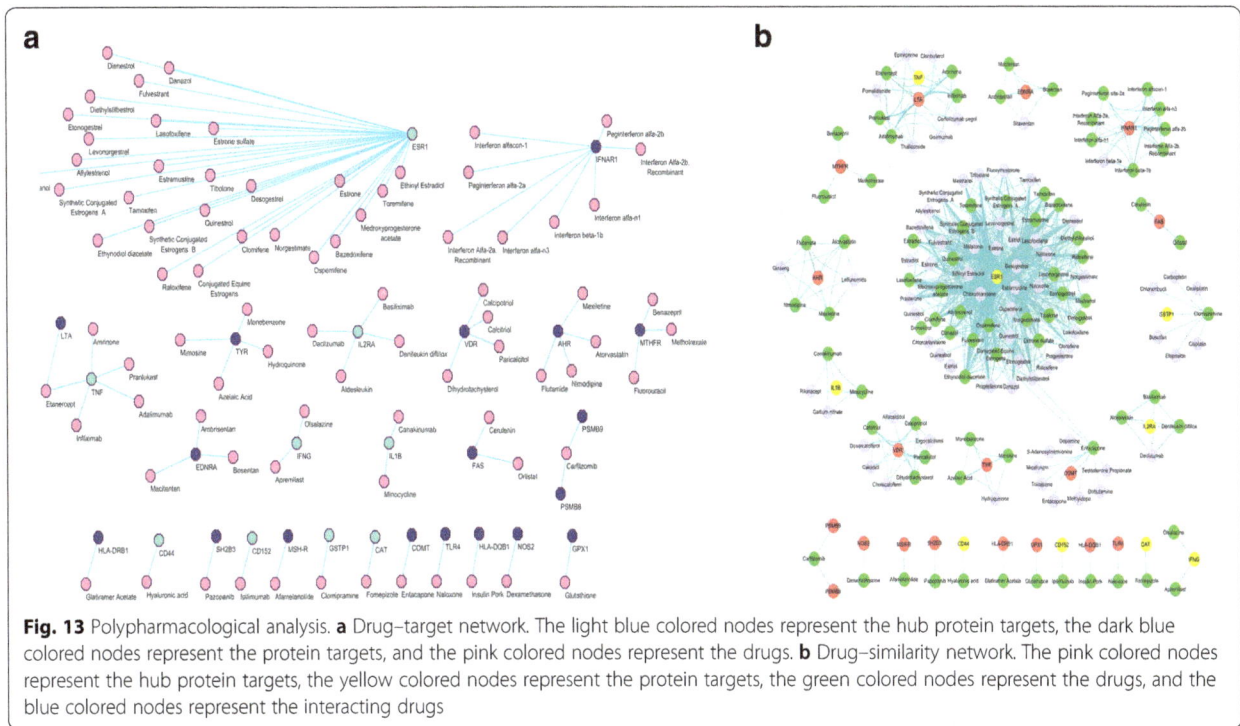

Fig. 13 Polypharmacological analysis. **a** Drug–target network. The light blue colored nodes represent the hub protein targets, the dark blue colored nodes represent the protein targets, and the pink colored nodes represent the drugs. **b** Drug–similarity network. The pink colored nodes represent the hub protein targets, the yellow colored nodes represent the protein targets, the green colored nodes represent the drugs, and the blue colored nodes represent the interacting drugs

targeting ESR1, which is one of the hub protein identified in the protein–protein interaction network analysis, were found to be interacting with the drug entacapone targeting COMT. This signifies that the two drugs interacting with entacapone might target COMT which is targeted by entacapone alone. Also, we found that there are no interacting drugs reported for etanercept targeting LTA and our drug similarity network analysis suggests that the interacting drugs for etanercept targeting TNF might as well target LTA. Etanercept has been less efficient as a monotherapy as mentioned earlier; therefore, the interacting drugs for etanercept as shown in the network might catalyze its efficiency when used in combination. Thus, further comprehensive study is required to validate the effectiveness of these drugs in combinative therapy. In addition, GSTP1, also a hub protein, was shown to be targeted by a single drug (clomipramine) in the drug–target network; however, seven interacting drugs were shown to be connected to this drug in this network. These interacting drugs can be further studied to investigate their potential as drug repositioning candidates for vitiligo treatment.

Protein modeling of TLR2

Among the three predicted functionally significant nsSNPs, we performed protein modeling of TLR2 since our drug–target network analysis showed TLR2 as a potential drug target for which drug information is currently not available. The G23D tool generated a full-length protein model for the TLR2 protein based on E-

value which was 0.001 by default as generated from the PDB library and ModBase hits. Since we did not perform any molecular dynamics simulation studies for protein structure optimization, therefore, the 3D homology model generated by G23D is a preliminary model implicating the disruptive role of the SNP (rs5743708) on TLR2 protein.

Figure 14a shows the cartoon representation of the modeled protein structure including both the wild-type (green) and the mutant (light blue) amino acid. It also displayed the other variants as reported in ClinVar, COSMIC, and dbSNP for TLR2 which is colored as red, yellow, and dark green respectively in stick representation in the 3D structure.

An A/G mutation (rs5743708) caused the substitution of the amino acid from arginine into glutamine at position 753 (R753Q) of the protein. The mutation was identified to be located within the TIR domain as annotated in UniProt. Since it is a membrane protein, it is exposed on the surface which is in agreement with the previous NetSurfP results. Analysis of the 3D structure suggests that the residue glutamine in position 753 is located in the middle of a helix. There was a difference in the size observed in the wild-type and mutant amino acids with the mutant residue being smaller than the wild-type residue causing conformational changes on the DD loop which might lead to loss of interactions. Also, the wild-type residue is positively charged, but the amino acid substitution leads to a decrease in the positive charge that changes the interaction surface within

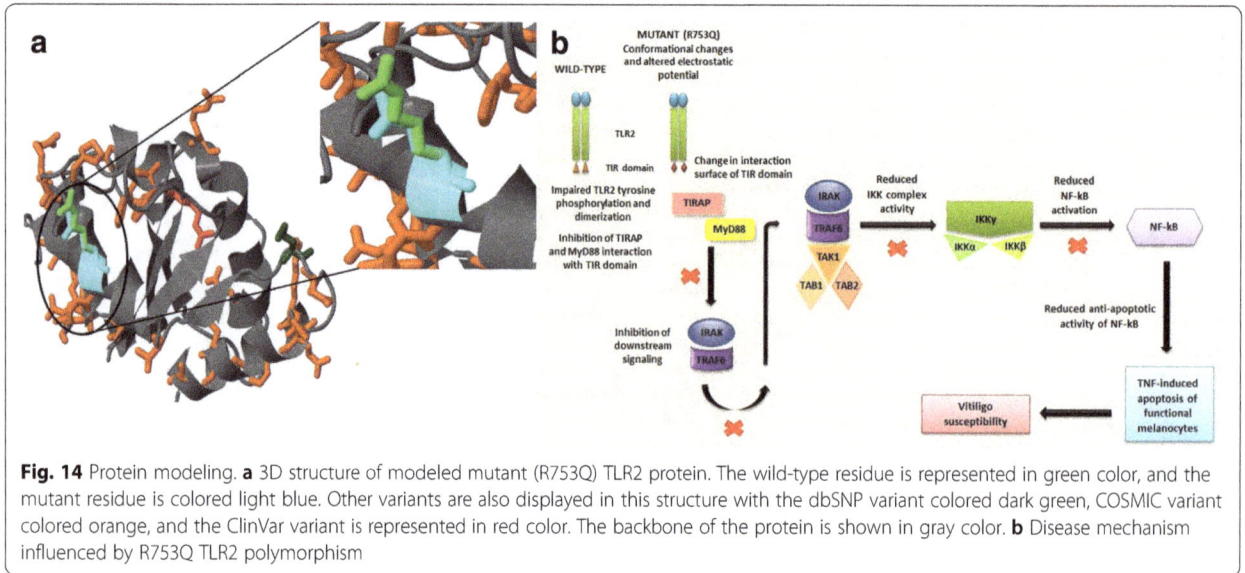

Fig. 14 Protein modeling. **a** 3D structure of modeled mutant (R753Q) TLR2 protein. The wild-type residue is represented in green color, and the mutant residue is colored light blue. Other variants are also displayed in this structure with the dbSNP variant colored dark green, COSMIC variant colored orange, and the ClinVar variant is represented in red color. The backbone of the protein is shown in gray color. **b** Disease mechanism influenced by R753Q TLR2 polymorphism

the TIR domain via altered electrostatic potential. These may affect TLR2 dimerization causing loss of interactions with other molecules or residues affecting the functional activity of the protein (Xiong et al. 2012). The R753Q polymorphism compromises the TLR2/1 or TLR2/6 assembly resulting in deficient tyrosine phosphorylation and impaired recruitment of MyD88. This reduces the phosphorylation of IRAK1 and diminishes the activation of MAPKs and NF-κB resulting in the deficient production of cytokines thus altering TLR2 signaling competence. Therefore, the compromised signaling is due to deficient tyrosine phosphorylation and not due to lower mutant receptor expression. The reduced activation of NF-κB signaling pathway results in melanocyte apoptosis suggesting their decisive role in the increased risk for the development of vitiligo (Karaca et al. 2013; Traks et al. 2015).

The protein–protein interaction analysis of TLR2 showed its interaction with TLR1, TLR6, LY96, MyD88, IRAK4, TRAF6, NFKB1, TIRAP, CD14, and HMGB1. All these proteins were found to have a fundamental role in regulating the innate immune responses. The amino acid substitution of arginine to glutamine at position 753 has been reported to be located in the TIR domain. TLR2 activates NF-κB in combination with either TLR1 or TLR6 by bringing together the TIR domains and triggering tyrosine phosphorylation. The TIR domain of TIRAP binds to the TIR domain of TLR2 which then extends a docking platform for MyD88 recruitment. MyD88 facilitates the recruitment of IRAK4 which activates TRAF6 leading to the translocation of activated NF-κB to the nucleus where it induces target gene expression generating inflammatory responses (Oliveira-Nascimento et al. 2012). Mutations in the TIR domain tend to have more severe impact on signaling than those affecting the extracellular domain

(Karaca et al. 2013). Genetic alterations in TLR2 might affect its interaction with both TLR1 and TLR6 consequently affecting NF-κB activation (Brown et al. 2006). It was also found that this mutation significantly reduced NF-κB activation by about 50 and 75% (Merx et al. 2007; Ben-Ali et al. 2011). In the case of vitiligo, altered NF-κB signaling may result in impaired melanogenesis inciting human melanocytes susceptible to TNF induced apoptosis (Shang et al. 2002) (Fig. 14b).

This implicates the possible detrimental effect of this mutation on the interaction of TLR2 with TIRAP, MyD88, IRAK4, TRAF6, and the consequent signal transduction. HMGB1 has been found to upregulate the expression of TLR2 of the NK cells and promote NK cell activation mediating inflammatory responses (Qiu et al. 2014), while CD14 (a co-receptor of TLR2) accelerates the microbial ligand transfer from CD14 to TLR2, resulting in an increased TLR2 signaling (Raby et al. 2013). LY96 have been found to enhance the expression of both TLR2 and TLR4 and vice versa enabling them to generate highly sensitive responses to a broad range of microbial lipopolysaccharide (LPS) structures (Dziarski et al. 2001). Altered expression of TLR2 will invariably affect the interaction of TLR2 with these proteins thereby influencing TLR2 signaling and inflammatory responses resulting in defective immune response to some antigens such as viruses in the case of vitiligo (Karaca et al. 2013).

VitmiRS

Currently, VitmiRS has information on 41 miRNAs and 134 associated SNPs for 84 unique genes. VitmiRS provides a user-friendly interface to detailed information on disease association of miRNAs and their target genes, SNPs and their position and location, the change in alleles and the resulting amino acid change due to such mutational events, and their respective literature reference. The users can search and access information for their respective query in the database browsing through query categories of miRNAs, SNPs, genes, and amino acid change. Further, the database interface also allows for the selection of particular attributes, such as PubMed ID, miRNA sequences, chromosome number, chromosome location, odds ratio, and p value; the geographical location and population in which the association of specific miRNAs and SNPs with vitiligo has been reported. Also, it incorporates the results of SNP analysis, thereby providing information on the pathogenic effect of the each SNPs as well. Thus, the database can be queried individually or in combination with any of the categories as mentioned above according to the need and interest of the user. The information available in VitmiRS may, therefore, be used for various associative studies relating to miRNAs and genetic variants to uncover their role and importance in vitiligo disease susceptibility and pathogenesis.

Discussion

An enhanced understanding of the disease causative genes and their relationship with other genes along with other diseases offers an improved resource for finding the candidate genes that mark the onset of a disease. Several unrelated diseases have been revealed to show common molecular mechanisms with strong association among them (Yu et al. 2015). As a result of such disease associations, the possibility of related diseases to occur together in an individual cannot be ruled out. Analysis of disease-gene bipartite network allowed the identification of several diseases which are under the influence of multiple genes wherein it highlighted vitiligo to be influenced by a multiplex of genes. Additionally, we also identified the genes which exhibit pleiotropy, thus accounting for multiple diseases and may play a crucial role in determining disease comorbidity. We explored some unique relationships with their previous published studies being non-existential which include the genetic association between rosacea and vitiligo, as caused by the gene BTNL2; the association between GM1-gangliosidosis and eczema, both being caused by GLB1 gene; and the association between piebaldism and urticaria pigmentosa as a result of a mutation in the KIT gene. This provides with a new perspective in understanding dermatosis opening new avenues for conducting genetic research. In the DSN analysis, we found shared SNPs between diseases xeroderma pigmentosum and keloid whose association has been previously unidentified. Also, our analysis shows a correlation between the diseases Beare–Stevenson cutis gyrata and Brooke–Spiegler syndrome. Our database, therefore, provides a fresh perspective to the possible association between these diseases, as no published literature source

indicating their correlation is available as of now. However, validation of our findings through wet-lab research can further strengthen our findings.

Based on our network analysis results of disease–gene association, we further carried out an integrative systems analysis of vitiligo. Vitiligo is a result of convoluted interactions of biological, environmental, and immunological events; hence, a single concept cannot be attributable to all the conditions of functional melanocyte loss. A large-scale analysis and integration of miRNA–disease associations will offer a platform to investigate the patterns of the miRNAs and its associations with diseases. Molecular signatures of miRNAs as reported in vitiligo patients suggest that these are actively involved and have a significant role in disease pathogenesis. Having a cardinal role in maintaining physiological homeostasis and disease development and progression, miRNAs are significant for melanocyte development and survival (Mansuri et al., 2016). Our miRNA–target gene network analysis revealed seven hub miRNAs, namely, hsa-miR-99b, hsa-miR-577, hsa-miR-9, hsa-miR-155, hsa-miR-211, hsa-miR-10a, and hsa-miR-145 implicating their role in vitiligo pathogenesis. The upregulation of hsa-miR-99b reduces the cytotoxic activity (cytokine effector functions) of NK cells which are crucial for the normal BCR signaling and proliferation of B cells. This causes deregulation of genes involved in B cell maturation and development resulting in the dysfunctioning of the immune system indicating them to be important players in vitiligo immunopathogenesis (Nandagopal et al. 2014; Šahmatova et al. 2016).

TYRP1 is targeted by hsa-miR-577, and its reduced expression as induced by miR-577 leads to increased sensitivity of melanocytes to oxidative stress causing early cell death of vitiligo melanocytes (Manga et al. 2006; Sturm and Duffy 2012). Also, the downregulation of PTPN22 was observed to be influenced by miR-577 which triggers the overexpression of T cells and suppresses anti-apoptotic AKT kinase inducing melanocyte destruction, thereby, rendering susceptibility to autoimmunity in vitiligo patients (Mansuri et al., 2016). Elevated levels of SIRT1 have been reported to protect cells from oxidative stress and inflammatory microenvironment (Han et al. 2008). Increased expression of miR-9 downregulates SIRT1 resulting in melanocytes apoptosis in vitiligo (Saunders et al. 2010). SIRT1 has been shown to regulate stress-activated MAPK pathway via Akt and ASK1 in vitiligo keratinocytes (Becatti et al. 2014). Previous studies have demonstrated the influence of miR-145 on the genes involved in the pigmentation process (Dynoodt et al. 2013). The genes targeted by miR-145 also regulate MAPK pathway along with JNK and TGFB signaling pathway and are related to the functional groups that might indirectly influence cellular processes in vitiligo wherefore they interfere with melanocytes function and viability (Šahmatova et al. 2016) suggesting the role of both miR-9 and miR-145 in the destruction of melanocytes in vitiligo.

TGFBR2 is targeted by miR-211, and downregulated miR-211 increases the expression of TGFBR2 which in turn downregulates MITF. MITF is a known primary regulator of melanocyte development and its survival (Levy et al. 2010); thus, deregulated MITF will considerably affect melanocyte development implying the role of miR-211 in vitiligo pathogenesis. Overexpression of miR-155 was found to modulate the levels of several interferon-regulated genes, such as SOCS1, IFITM1, and IRF1 that inhibits the expression of melanogenesis-associated genes, such as, TYRP1, YWHAE, SDCBP, and SOX10 in melanocytes and particularly YWHAE in keratinocytes. This suggests that upregulated miR-155 is associated with vitiligo pathogenesis which alters interferon signaling as well as targets melanogenesis-associated genes (Šahmatova et al. 2016). Both miR-155 and miR-10a are on their own largely dispensable for regulatory T cell (Treg) function and stability which is responsible for suppressing autoimmune pathology. Inhibition of miR-10a expression leads to reduced FOXP3 expression levels which subsequently decrease the stability of Treg cells (Jeker et al. 2012) resulting in the insufficient suppression of inflammation in autoimmune diseases which could likely happen in vitiligo patients.

Identifying the susceptible genes and their variants which drive the way to the onset of disease is fundamental to unravel their contribution in disease progression. Most of the vitiligo-associated genes are plausible biological candidate genes which when altered are responsible for stimulating melanocyte-specific immune responses. These candidate genes encode immunoregulatory and melanocyte proteins constituting a dense immunoregulatory network, an alteration in which highlights the systems and pathways mediating vitiligo susceptibility (Spritz 2013). Genetic variation alters or damages protein structure disrupting protein–protein interactions which are otherwise essential for regulatory processes constituting the pretext of disease development. Network-based studies of these interacting proteins may impart an insight into disease pathogenesis initiating better diagnosis and the feasibility of personalized treatment for vitiligo patients in the future. Our PPI network analysis results identified 15 hub proteins, namely, IL10, IFNG, IL4, CD44, IL1B, CTLA4, GZMB, FOXP3, TNF, IL2RA, CAT, ESR1, TLR2, HLA-A, and GSTP1 to be associated with vitiligo. The balance between pro- and anti-inflammatory cytokines plays a significant role in the pathogenesis of vitiligo. Higher concentrations of IFNG, a pro-inflammatory cytokine, enhance T cell-melanocyte attachment in the skin

initiating T cell-mediated apoptosis of melanocytes in vitiligo. On the other hand, reduced concentrations of IL-10, a potent regulator of anti-inflammatory immune responses, were observed in vitiligo patients (Singh et al. 2012). An increased IL-10 concentration with an increase in the IFNG levels exhibited a positive correlation with disease duration as reported in vitiligo patients (Ala et al. 2015). IL-4, an immunomodulatory cytokine, stimulates B cell proliferation and T cell development that leads to the elevation of baseline IgE levels inducing inflammation (Del Prete et al. 1988). Polymorphisms in the IL4 gene are known to increase its expression increasing the IgE levels thereby implicating its role in autoimmunity-mediated vitiligo susceptibility (Imran et al. 2012). CTLA4 expressed by Tregs is a negative regulator of T cell function and fosters tolerance to self-antigens. Decreased levels of CTLA4 mRNA and deregulated CTLA4 expression due to genetic variations have been found in vitiligo patients (Dwivedi et al. 2011) suggesting its involvement in susceptibility to vitiligo. Also, upregulated CD44 expression in response to naive T cell proliferation as induced by autoimmune melanocyte destruction concomitantly increases T cell development implicating the complex regulation of self-reactive T cells in vitiligo (Byrne et al. 2014).

Increased mRNA levels of IL1B increases SOD levels leading to increased H_2O_2 production as observed in vitiligo patients. Genetic variability in IL1B resulting in altered IL1B transcript levels might be associated with elevated NPY levels in patients with vitiligo whose synthesis is governed by IL1B (Laddha et al. 2014). Increased NPY levels lead to epidermal and dermal hypoxia which might potentiate melanocyte death in vitiligo (Tu et al. 2001). Alterations in CAT have been reported to result in the reduction of the catalase enzyme activity and consequently evoke excess H_2O_2 accumulation in the entire epidermis of vitiligo patients (Casp et al. 2002). Although the genetic mechanisms of estrogen in increased pigment cell activity are not largely known yet, ESR1 expression on human melanocytes has been demonstrated to have specific actions in human pigmentation (Im et al. 2002). Also, genetic variation in ESR1 gene has been reported to show its association with vitiligo (Jin et al. 2004). Additionally, GSTP1 is broadly expressed in defense against oxidative stress wherein they detoxify a variety of electrophilic compounds generated by ROS-induced damaged cells (Nebert and Vasiliou 2004). Altered GSTP1 expression fails to protect cells against chemical toxicity and stress contributing to melanocyte death in vitiligo patients (Dušinská et al. 2001; Liu et al. 2009).

Effector functions of IL2RA and GZMB in the target cell killing by cytotoxic T cells (CTLs) and NK cells activation-induced cell death terminate immune responses and mediate melanocyte killing in vitiligo (Spritz 2010). GZMB also have a role to play in cleaving melanocyte proteins that constitute vitiligo auto-antigens activating auto-antigens that initiate and propagate autoimmunity directed against melanocytes (Darrah and Rosen 2010). FOXP3, the master regulator of Treg cells, have a vital role in maintaining immune balance and its alteration triggers autoimmune diseases including vitiligo (Jahan et al. 2015). TNF downregulates MITF affecting melanocyte development and proliferation, and ultimately affecting melanogenesis. Also, TNF-α downregulates MSHR binding activity and reduces MC1-R expression, both of which are known inducers of melanogenesis (Camara-Lemarroy and Slas-Alanis 2013). TRAIL, a TNF family death receptor, activates caspases and cleaves melanocyte proteins and also promotes dendritic cell-mediated melanocyte death eliciting apoptosis of primary human melanocytes (Larribere et al. 2004). TNF, thus, acts as the central regulatory effector in the immunopathological mechanisms involved in vitiligo.

Among TLRs, TLR2 is fundamental for immune responses against mycobacterial infections, in sensing oxidative stress and cellular necrosis and, also in inducing apoptosis (Petry and Gaspari 2009). It also has the propensity to recognize a wide array of antigens evincing its instrumental role in the evolution of self-reactive diseases (Borrello et al. 2011). Altered expression and signaling due to TLR2 polymorphism have been proposed to be the reason for inadequate immune responses to viral or pathogenic antigens in vitiligo (Karaca et al. 2013; Traks et al. 2015).

The functional enrichment analysis result of the single large cluster consisting of 64 proteins demonstrated the vitiligo-associated genes to be primarily involved in immune response regulation by cytokines and oxidative stress, and apoptotic processes. Oxidative stress in the melanocytes stimulates local inflammatory responses whereby it leads to the activation of innate immune processes as a result of which melanocyte-specific cytotoxic immune responses are evoked in vitiligo patients. Vitiliginous melanocytes show increased surface expression of HLA-A, a class I MHC receptor, which enables it to present multiple autoantigens to T cells destroying skin melanocytes (Hayashi et al. 2016). Also, increased expression levels of HLA class II molecules triggers an increased production of immunostimulatory cytokines that may act as an adjuvant during the presentation of autoantigens (Cavalli et al. 2016), tying together with HLA class I molecules in the development of autoimmunity in vitiligo patients. Also, alteration in the concentration of various pro-inflammatory and anti-inflammatory cytokines such as IL-10, IL-2, TNF, and IFNG has been associated with many autoimmune disorders (Singh et al. 2012).

Apart from exhibiting pathways associated with immune responses and autoimmunity, our pathway analysis results also consisted of pathways corresponding to infectious diseases, particularly viral infections. Several studies have implicated the etiopathogenesis of vitiligo to multiple viral infections as epidermal melanocytes are important targets of viruses (Duvic et al. 1987; Grimes et al. 1996). Also, viral infectious diseases, in most cases, impair the body's systemic immune response. This explains the reason why the pathways associated with infectious diseases were also observed to be significant in the results. In the protein–pathway network, TNF was found to be involved in 24 out of 30 significant pathways indicating it to be a prime regulator of vitiligo immunopathogenesis (Birol et al. 2006).

Our SNP analysis predicted rs1801133 (MTHFR), rs5743708 (TLR2), and rs11575993 (SOD2) to be functionally significant for vitiligo susceptibility. Previous studies have shown these mutations to be associated with other diseases as well. The A222V variant of MTHFR has been reported to be associated with vascular diseases (Morita et al. 1997) and cancer (Hubner et al. 2007) The R753Q variant of TLR2 has been reported to be associated with colorectal cancer (Boraska Jelavić et al. 2006), atherosclerosis (Bielinski et al. 2011), and tuberculosis (Ogus et al. 2004). However, the L84F variant of SOD2 has only been reported in vitiligo till date (Laddha et al. 2013).

There is no definite cure available for vitiligo, and hence, the various treatment options available merely aim to improve skin appearance by repigmentation or stabilizing depigmentation without the assurance of reoccurrence or extension of depigmentation (Njoo and Westerhof 1999). Our drug–target network analysis revealed novel potential drug candidates which could be explored for improved therapeutics for vitiligo. It is noteworthy that most of the drugs defined for the protein targets, even a few hub protein targets, are not indicated to be used for the treatment of vitiligo as reported in DrugBank. This indicates a pressing need to evaluate these drugs and perform investigational studies to identify new indications and elucidate the efficiency of these drugs for the treatment of vitiligo. This would lead to significant contributions in drug discovery complementing the existing drug pipelines, thereby, improving the quality of life in vitiligo patients. Additionally, some of the hub proteins are targeted by a single drug which can be further examined to contrive better effective drugs to enhance the success rate of treatments. Interacting drug partners of a particular drug targeting a particular protein might either directly target that protein or enhance the efficacy of the drug. With this concept, we constructed the drug–similarity network and found interacting drugs for those proteins which were previously shown to be targeted by a single drug in the drug–target network. These interacting drugs might function as an alternative to the native drug with enhanced efficacy.

Polymorphism in TLR2 (rs5743708) was found to be deleterious in our SNP analysis results indicating its potentiality to induce vitiligo. TLR2 was also found to be one of the hub protein targets for which no drug information is available yet. The R753Q mutation was identified to be located within the TIR domain, an intracellular signaling domain, which compromises the signaling capacity of TIR domain impairing MyD88–TLR2 assembly. This inactivates NF-κB signaling pathway which can invariably influence the regulation of inflammatory processes and can even impair melanogenesis suggesting its role in vitiligo pathogenesis (Karaca et al. 2013; Traks et al. 2015). Our PPI network of TLR2 shows its interacting proteins suggesting that an altered TLR2 might have an impact on its interaction with other proteins essential for many biological functions and signaling processes. This indicates the need to analyze the structural details of the protein and the effect of mutation on its structure and function, and carry out further experimental studies to discover new drugs targeting the mutated TLR2 protein associated with vitiligo.

Conclusions

Investigating the patterns of miRNAs and its associations with diseases and identifying the susceptible genes variants triggering disease onset is significant for unraveling the key factors that underpin disease manifestation. We, therefore, identified vitiligo-associated miRNAs and their targets, and susceptible genes, and carried out a comprehensive network analysis of these data which revealed the association of significant hub miRNAs and proteins with disease susceptibility. We validated their functional role and carried out SNP analysis wherein we identified mutation in TLR2 (R753Q) as deleterious. Our drug–target network and drug–similarity network unveiled novel molecular determinants and drug repositioning candidates for vitiligo. Both our databases DermaGene and VitmiRS provide authentic and relevant information on the essentialities of disease association which may facilitate researchers in identifying dermatological disorder causation. We intend to regularly update both the databases, DermaGene and VitmiRS, respectively, through a bi-annual review to ensure consistency of data and to ensure it is maintained up-to-date. The procedure for regular update would rely on identification of latest entries which may be missing in our database and merging the new data with the existing data. Our approach can provide an insight into the regulatory mechanisms of disease manifestation, thereby, implicating its role in improved therapeutic and diagnostic interventions.

Additional files

Additional file 1: Disease co-morbidities and associated SNPs. Disease comorbidity arising from shared SNPs. (XLSX 9 kb)

Additional file 2: Disease co-morbidities and associated genes. Disease comorbidity arising from shared genes. (XLSX 10 kb)

Additional file 3: DAVID functional enrichment analysis. The 9 functionally enriched clusters as found by DAVID. (XLSX 13 kb)

Additional file 4: Hub protein–pathway analysis. The significant pathways of the hub proteins in the protein–pathway network. (XLSX 10 kb)

Additional file 5: SNP analysis. The results of nsSNPs analysis using six computational platforms. (XLSX 17 kb)

Abbreviations
DAVID: The Database for Annotation Visualization and Integrated Discovery; DGN: Disease–gene bipartite network; DSN: Disease–SNP bipartite network; G23D: Genomic variant to 3D protein data; HMDD: The Human microRNA Disease Database; KEGG: Kyoto Encyclopedia of Genes and Genomes; MCC: Maximum Clique Centrality; MCL: Markov Clustering Algorithm; PROVEAN: Protein Variation Effect Analyzer; SIFT: Sorting Intolerant From Tolerant; STRING: The Search Tool for the Retrieval of Interacting Genes

Funding
This work was supported by the Department of Biotechnology, Government of India [No.BT/PR5402/BID/7/508/2012].

Authors' contributions
YH conceived and designed the study. IS and RR collected data and performed the analysis for DermaGene and VitmiRS respectively. YH, RR, and IS evaluated the results and prepared the manuscript. LKG developed the web interface for both the databases. All authors read and approved the final manuscript.

Competing interests
The authors declare that they have no competing interests.

References
Adzhubei IA, Schmidt S, Peshkin L, Ramensky VE, et al. A method and server for predicting damaging missense mutations. Nat Methods. 2010;7(4):248–9.

Agarwal V, Bell GW, Nam JW, et al. Predicting effective microRNA target sites in mammalian mRNAs. elife. 2015;4:e05005.

Ala Y, Pasha MK, Rao RN, et al. Association of IFN-γ: IL-10 cytokine ratio with nonsegmental vitiligo pathogenesis. Autoimmune Dis. 2015; https://doi.org/10.1155/2015/423490.

Bansal S, Goel A. Chilblain lupus erythematosus in an adolescent girl. Indian Dermatol Online J. 2014;(Suppl 1):30–2.

Barabasi AL, Oltvai ZN. Network biology: understanding the cell's functional organization. Nat Rev Genet. 2004;5(2):101–13.

Barateau A, Vadrot N, Vicart P, et al. A novel lamin a mutant responsible for congenital muscular dystrophy causes distinct abnormalities of the cell nucleus. PLoS One. 2017;12:1–18.

Becatti M, Fiorillo C, Barygina V, et al. SIRT1 regulates MAPK pathways in vitiligo skin: insight into the molecular pathways of cell survival. J Cell Mol Med. 2014;18(3):514–29.

Ben-Ali M, Beatrice C, Jeremy M, et al. Functional characterization of naturally occurring genetic variants in the human TLR1-2-6 gene family. Hum Mutat. 2011;32(6):643–52.

Bielinski SJ, Hall JL, Pankow JS, et al. Genetic variants in TLR2 and TLR4 are associated with markers of monocyte activation: the Atherosclerosis Risk in Communities MRI Study. Hum Genet. 2011;129(6):655–62.

Birol A, Kisa U, Kurtipek GS, et al. Increased tumor necrosis factor alpha (TNF-α) and interleukin 1 alpha (IL1-α) levels in the lesional skin of patients with nonsegmental vitiligo. Int J Dermatol. 2006;45(8):992–3.

Boisseau-Garsaud AM, Garsaud P, Calès-Quist D, et al. Epidemiology of vitiligo in the French West Indies (Isle of Martinique). Int J Dermatol. 2000;39(1):18–20.

Boraska Jelavić T, Barisic M, Drmic-Hofman I, et al. Microsatelite GT polymorphism in the toll-like receptor 2 is associated with colorectal cancer. Clin Genet. 2006;70(2):156–60.

Borrello S, Nicolo C, Delogu G. TLR2: a crossroads between infections and autoimmunity? Int J Immunopathol Pharmacol. 2011;24(3):549–56.

Brown V, Brown RA, Ozinsky A, et al. Binding specificity of Toll-like receptor cytoplasmic domains. Eur J Immunol. 2006; https://doi.org/10.1002/eji.200535158.

Byrne KT, Zhang P, Steinberg SM, et al. Autoimmune vitiligo does not require the ongoing priming of naive CD8 T cells for disease progression or associated protection against melanoma. J Immunol. 2014;192(4):1433–9.

Camara-Lemarroy CR, Slas-Alanis JC. The role of tumor necrosis factor-α in the pathogenesis of vitiligo. Am J Clin Dermatol. 2013;14(5):343–50.

Capriotti E, Fariselli P, Rossi I, et al. A three-state prediction of single point mutations on protein stability changes. BMC bioinformatics. 2008;9(2):S6.

Casp CB, She JX, McCormack WT. Genetic association of the catalase gene (CAT) with vitiligo susceptibility. Pigment Cell Melanoma Res. 2002;15(1):62–6.

Cavalli G, Hayashi M, Jin Y, et al. MHC class II super-enhancer increases surface expression of HLA-DR and HLA-DQ and affects cytokine production in autoimmune vitiligo. Proc Natl Acad Sci U S A. 2016;113(5):1363–8.

Chin C-H, Chen S-H, Wu H-H, et al. cytoHubba: identifying hub objects and sub-networks from complex interactome. BMC Syst Biol. 2014;8(4):S11.

Choi Y, Sims GE, Murphy S, et al. Predicting the functional effect of amino acid substitutions and indels. PLoS One. 2012;7(10):e46688.

Conne B, Stutz A, Vassali J-D. The 3′ untranslated region of messenger RNA: a molecular 'hotspot' for pathology? Nat Med. 2000;6(6):637.

Cordell HJ. Detecting gene-gene interactions that underlie human diseases. Nat Rev Genet. 2009;10(6):392–404.

Cresswell P, Ackerman AL, Giodini A, et al. Mechanisms of MHC class I-restricted antigen processing and cross-presentation. Immunol Rev. 2005;207(1):145–57.

Dalamon VK, Buonfiglio P, Larralde M, et al. Connexin 26 (GJB2) mutation in Argentinean patient with keratitis-ichthyosis-deafness (KID) syndrome: a case report. BMC Med Genet. 2016; https://doi.org/10.1186/s12881-016-0298-y.

Dani P, Patnaik N, Singh A, et al. Association and expression of antigen processing gene PSMB8 coding for low molecular mass protease 7 (LMP7) with vitiligo in North India: case-control study. Br J Dermatol. 2017; https://doi.org/10.1111/bjd.15391.

Darrah E, Rosen A. Granzyme B cleavage of autoantigens in autoimmunity. Cell Death Differ. 2010;17(4):624–32.

Del Prete G, Maggi E, Parronchi P, et al. IL-4 is an essential factor for the IgE synthesis induced in vitro by human T cell clones and their supernatants. J Immunol. 1988;140(12):4193–8.

Dušinská M, Ficek A, Horská A, et al. Glutathione S-transferase polymorphisms influence the level of oxidative DNA damage and antioxidant protection in humans. Mutat Res Fund Mol Mech Mut. 2001;482(1):47–55.

Duvic M, et al. Human immunodeficiency virus—associated vitiligo: expression of autoimmunity with immunodeficiency? J Am Acad Dermatol. 1987;17(4):656–62.

Dwivedi M, Rapini R, Hoots WK, et al. Cytotoxic T-lymphocyte-associated antigen-4 (CTLA-4) in isolated vitiligo: a genotype-phenotype correlation. Pigment Cell Melanoma Res. 2011;24(4):737–40.

Dynoodt P, Mestdagh P, Peer GV, et al. Identification of miR-145 as a key regulator of the pigmentary process. J Invest Dermatol. 2013;133(1):201–9.

Dziarski R, Wang Q, Miyake K, Kirschning CJ, Gupta D. MD-2 enables Toll-like receptor 2 (TLR2)-mediated responses to lipopolysaccharide and enhances TLR2-mediated responses to Gram-positive and Gram-negative bacteria and their cell wall components. J Immunol. 2001;166(3):1938–44.

Griffiths-Jones S. miRBase: the microRNA sequence database, MicroRNA protocols. Methods Mol Biol. 2006;342:129–38.

Grimes PE, Sevall JS, Vojdani A. Cytomegalovirus DNA identified in skin biopsy specimens of patients with vitiligo. J Am Acad Dermatol. 1996;35(1):21–6.

Hafner C, Groesser L. Mosaic RASopathies. Cell Cycle. 2013;12 https://doi.org/10.4161/cc.23108.

Han MK, Song EK, Guo Y, et al. SIRT1 regulates apoptosis and Nanog expression in mouse embryonic stem cells by controlling p53 subcellular localization. Cell Stem Cell. 2008;2(3):241–51.

Handa S, Kaur I. Vitiligo: clinical findings in 1436 patients. J Dermatol. 1999;26(10):653–7.

Harman M, Durdu M, Ibiloglu I. Acrokeratosis verruciformis of Hopf exhibiting Darier disease-like cytological features. Clin Exp Dermatol. 2016;41(7):761–3.

Hayashi M, Jin Y, Yorgov D, et al. Autoimmune vitiligo is associated with gain-of-function by a transcriptional regulator that elevates expression of HLA-A* 02: 01 in vivo. Proc Natl Acad Sci U S A. 2016;113(5):1357–62.

Hedrich CM, Fiebig B, Hauck FH, et al. Chilblain lupus erythematosus—a review of literature. J Clin Rheumatol. 2008;27:949–54.

Howitz J, Brodthagen H, Schwartz M, et al. Prevalence of vitiligo: epidemiological survey on the Isle of Bornholm, Denmark. Arch Dermatol. 1977;113(1):47–52.

Huang DW, Sherman BT, Lempicki RA. Bioinformatics enrichment tools: paths toward the comprehensive functional analysis of large gene lists. Nucleic Acids Res. 2008;37(1):1–3.

Huang DW, Sherman BT, Lempicki RA. Systematic and integrative analysis of large gene lists using DAVID bioinformatics resources. Nat Protoc. 2009;4(1):44–57.

Huang KP, Mullangi S, Guo Y, et al. Autoimmune, atopic, and mental health comorbid conditions associated with alopecia areata in the United States. JAMA Dermatol. 2013;149(7):789–94.

Hubner RA, Lubbe S, Chandler I, et al. MTHFR C677T has differential influence on risk of MSI and MSS colorectal cancer. Hum Mol Gen. 2007;16(9):1072–7.

Im S, Lee ES, Kim W, et al. Donor specific response of estrogen and progesterone on cultured human melanocytes. J Korean Med Sci. 2002;17(1):58.

Imran M, Laddha NC, Dwivedi M, et al. Interleukin-4 genetic variants correlate with its transcript and protein levels in patients with vitiligo. Br J Dermatol. 2012;167(2):314–23.

Irvine AD, McLean WH. The molecular genetics of the genodermatoses: progress to date and future directions. Br J Dermatol. 2003;148:1–13.

Jahan P, Tippisetty S, Komaravalli PL. FOXP3 is a promising and potential candidate gene in generalised vitiligo susceptibility. Front Genet. 2015;6 https://doi.org/10.3389/fgene.2015.00249.

Jeker LT, Zhou X, Gershberg K, et al. MicroRNA 10a marks regulatory T cells. PLoS One. 2012;7(5):e36684.

Jin SY, Park HH, Li GZ, et al. Association of estrogen receptor 1 intron 1 C/T polymorphism in Korean vitiligo patients. J Dermatol Sci. 2004;35(3):181–6.

Karaca N, Ozturk G, Gerceker BT, et al. TLR2 and TLR4 gene polymorphisms in Turkish vitiligo patients. J Eur Acad Dermatol Venereol. 2013;27(1):e85.

Knox C, Law V, Jewison T, et al. DrugBank 3.0: a comprehensive resource for 'omics' research on drugs. Nucleic Acids Res. 2011;39(Database issue):D1035–41.

Krishnaram AS, Saigal A, Adityan B. Alopecia areata-vitiligo overlap syndrome: an emerging clinical variant. Indian J Dermatol Venereol Leprol. 2013;79(4):535–7. https://doi.org/10.4103/0378-6323.113100.

Kumar P, Henikoff S, Ng PC. Predicting the effects of coding non-synonymous variants on protein function using the SIFT algorithm. Nat Protoc. 2009;4(7):1073–81.

Laddha NC, Dwivedi M, Gani AR, et al. Involvement of superoxide dismutase isoenzymes and their genetic variants in progression of and higher susceptibility to vitiligo. Free Radic Biol Med. 2013;65:1110–25.

Laddha NC, Dwivedi M, Mansuri MS, et al. Association of neuropeptide Y (NPY), interleukin-1B (IL1B) genetic variants and correlation of IL1B transcript levels with vitiligo susceptibility. PLoS One. 2014;9(9):e107020.

Larribere L, Khaled M, Tartare-Deckert S, et al. PI3K mediates protection against TRAIL-induced apoptosis in primary human melanocytes. Cell Death Differ. 2004;11(10):1084–91.

Levy C, Khaled M, Iliopoulos D, Janas MM, Schubert S, et al. Intronic miR-211 assumes the tumor suppressive function of its host gene in melanoma. Mol Cell. 2010;40(5):841–9.

Lewis SN, Nsoesie E, Weeks C, et al. Prediction of disease and phenotype associations from genome-wide association studies. PLoS One. 2011;6(11):e27175.

Li Y, Qiu C, Tu J, et al. HMDD v2. 0: a database for experimentally supported human microRNA and disease associations. Nucleic Acids Res. 2014;42(D1):D1070–4.

Liu L, Li C, Gao J, et al. Genetic polymorphisms of glutathione S-transferase and risk of vitiligo in the Chinese population. J Invest Dermatol. 2009;129(11):2646–52.

Magesh R, Doss CGP. Computational pipeline to identify and characterize functional mutations in ornithine transcarbamylase deficiency. 3 Biotech. 2014;4(6):621–34.

Manga P, Sheyn D, Yang F, et al. A role for Tyrosinase-related protein 1 in 4-tert-butylphenol-induced toxicity in melanocytes: implications for vitiligo. Am J Pathol. 2006;169(5):1652–62.

Mansuri MS, Singh M, Begum R. miRNA signatures and transcriptional regulation of their target genes in vitiligo. J Dermatol. 2016; 84(1):50–8.

Marren P, Wilson C, Dawber RPR, et al. Hereditary hypotrichosis (Marie-Unna type) and juvenile macular degeneration (Stargardt's maculopathy). Clin Exp Dermatol. 1992;17:189–91.

Maruthappu T, Scott CA, Kelsell DP. Discovery in genetic skin disease: the impact of high throughput genetic technologies. Genes (Basel). 2014; 5(3):615–34.

Merx S, Neumaier M, Wagner H, et al. Characterization and investigation of single nucleotide polymorphisms and a novel TLR2 mutation in the human TLR2 gene. Hum Mol Gen. 2007;16(10):1225–32.

Mi H, Lazareva-Ulitsky B, Loo R, et al. The PANTHER database of protein families, subfamilies, functions and pathways. Nucleic Acids Res. 2005;33(suppl_1):D284–8.

Miller Z, Ao L, Bo K, Lee W. Inhibitors of the immunoproteasome: current status and future directions. Curr Pharm Des. 2013;19(22):4140–51.

Mir A, Wu T, Orlow SJ. Cutaneous features of crouzon syndrome with acanthosis Nigricans. JAMA Dermatol. 2013;149:737–41.

Mitra K, Carnuvis AR, Ramesh SK, et al. Integrative approaches for finding modular structure in biological networks. Nat Rev Genet. 2013;14(10):719–32.

Morita H, Taguchi J, Kurihara H, et al. Genetic polymorphism of 5, 10-methylenetetrahydrofolate reductase (MTHFR) as a risk factor for coronary artery disease. Circulation. 1997;95(8):2032–6.

Nanda S, Bathon JM. Etanercept: a clinical review of current and emerging indications. Expert Opin Pharmacother 2004. 2004;5(5):1175–86.

Nandagopal N, Ali AK, Komal AK, et al. The critical role of IL-15–PI3K–mTOR pathway in natural killer cell effector functions. Front Immunol. 2014;5 https://doi.org/10.3389/fimmu.2015.00355.

Nath SK, Kelly JA. Evidence for a susceptibility gene, SLEV1, on chromosome 17p13 in families with vitiligo-related systemic lupus erythematosus. Am J Hum Genet. 2001;69(6):1401–6.

Nebert DW, Vasiliou V. Analysis of the glutathione S-transferase (GST) gene family. Hum Genomics. 2004;1(6):460.

Njoo MD, Westerhof W. The development of guidelines for the treatment of vitiligo. Arch Dermatol. 1999;135(12):1514–21.

Ogus AC, Yoldas B, Ozdemir T, et al. The Arg753GLn polymorphism of the human toll-like receptor 2 gene in tuberculosis disease. Eur Respir J. 2004;23(2):219–23.

Oliveira-Nascimento L, Massari P, Wetzler LM. The role of TLR2 in infection and immunity. Front Immunol. 2012;3 https://doi.org/10.3389/fimmu.2012.00079.

Park J, Lee DS, Christakis NA, et al. The impact of cellular networks on disease comorbidity. Mol Sys Biol. 2009;5:262.

Pejaver V, Urresti J, Lugo-Martinez J, et al. MutPred2: inferring the molecular and phenotypic impact of amino acid variants. bioRxiv. 2017:134981. https://doi.org/10.1101/134981.

Petersen B, Petersen TN, Andersen P, et al. A generic method for assignment of reliability scores applied to solvent accessibility predictions. BMC Struct Biol. 2009;9(1):51.

Petry V, Gaspari AA. Toll-like receptors and dermatology. Int J Dermatol. 2009;48(6):558–70.

Picardo M, Dell'Anna ML, Ezzedine K, et al. Vitiligo. Nat Rev Dis Primers. 2015;1:15011.

Pinero J, Queralt-Rosinach N, Bravo A, et al. DisGeNET: a discovery platform for the dynamical exploration of human diseases and their genes. Database. 2015; https://doi.org/10.1093/database/bav028.

Qiu Y, Yang J, Wang W, et al. HMGB1-promoted and TLR2/4-dependent NK cell maturation and activation take part in rotavirus-induced murine biliary atresia. PLoS Pathog. 2014;10(3):e1004011.

Raby AC, Holst B, Le Boulder E, et al. Targeting the TLR co-receptor CD14 with TLR2-derived peptides modulates immune responses to pathogens. Sci Transl Med. 2013;5(185):185ra64.

Rigopoulos D, Gregoriou S, Larios G, et al. Etanercept in the treatment of vitiligo. Dermatology (Basel). 2007;215(1):84–5.

Šahmatova L, Tankov S, Prans E, et al. MicroRNA-155 is dysregulated in the skin of patients with vitiligo and inhibits melanogenesis-associated genes in melanocytes and keratinocytes. Acta Derm Venereol. 2016;96(6):742–8.

Saunders LR, Sharma AD, Tawney J, et al. miRNAs regulate SIRT1 expression during mouse embryonic stem cell differentiation and in adult mouse tissues. Aging (Albany NY). 2010;2(7):415.

Shang J, Eberle J, Geilen CC, et al. The role of nuclear factor-kappaB and melanogenesis in tumor necrosis factor-alpha-induced apoptosis of normal human melanocytes. Skin Pharmacol Physiol. 2002;15(5):321–9.

Shannon P, Markiel A, Ozier O, et al. Cytoscape: a software environment for integrated models of biomolecular interaction networks. Genome Res. 2003;13(11):2498–504.

Shen C, Gao J, Sheng Y, et al. Genetic susceptibility to vitiligo: GWAS approaches for identifying vitiligo susceptibility genes and loci. Front Genet. 2016;7:3.

Sherry ST, Ward M-H, Kholodov M, et al. dbSNP: the NCBI database of genetic variation. Nucleic Acids Res. 2001;29(1):308–11.

Singh S, Singh U, Pandey SS. Serum concentration of IL-6, IL-2, TNF-α, and IFNγ in vitiligo patients. Indian J Dermatol. 2012;57(1):12.

Smith FJD, Fisher MP, Healey E, et al. Novel keratin 16 mutation and protein expression studies in pachyonychia congenita type 1 and focal palmoplantar keratoderma. Exp Dermatol. 2000;9(3):170–7.

Solomon O, Kunik V, Simon A, et al. G23D: online tool for mapping and visualization of genomic variants on 3D protein structures. BMC Genomics. 2016;17(1):681.

Spritz RA. The genetics of generalized vitiligo: autoimmune pathways and an inverse relationship with malignant melanoma. Genome Med. 2010;2(10):78.

Srivastava I, Khurana P, Yadav M, et al. An integrative systems biology approach to unravel potential drug candidates for multiple age related disorders. Biochim Biophys Acta, Proteins Proteomics. 2017;1865:1729.

Sturm RA, Duffy DL. Human pigmentation genes under environmental selection. Genome Biol. 2012;13(9):248.

Takemura S, Braun A, Crowson C, et al. Lymphoid neogenesis in rheumatoid synovitis. J Immunol. 2001;167(2):1072–80.

Traks T, Keermann M, Karelson M, et al. Polymorphisms in Toll-like receptor genes are associated with vitiligo. Front Genet. 2015;6:278.

Tu C, Zhao D, Lin X. Levels of neuropeptide-Y in the plasma and skin tissue fluids of patients with vitiligo. J Dermatol Sci. 2001;27(3):178–82.

Vitkup D, Sander C, Church GM. The amino-acid mutational spectrum of human genetic disease. Genome Biol. 2003;4(11):R72.

Von Mering C, Jensen LJ, Snel B, et al. STRING: known and predicted protein–protein associations, integrated and transferred across organisms. Nucleic Acids Res. 2005;33:D433–7.

Wang CQ, Cruz-Inigo AE, Fuentes-Duculan J, et al. Th17 cells and activated dendritic cells are increased in vitiligo lesions. PLoS One. 2011;6(4):e18907.

Wang K, Li M, Hakonarson H. Analysing biological pathways in genome-wide association studies. Nat Rev Genet. 2010;11(12):843–54.

Werth VP, White WL, Sanchez MR. Incidence of alopecia areata in lupus erythematosus. Arch Dermatol. 1992;128:368–71.

Xiong Y, Song C, Snyder GA, et al. R753Q polymorphism inhibits Toll-like receptor (TLR) 2 tyrosine phosphorylation, dimerization with TLR6, and recruitment of myeloid differentiation primary response protein 88. J Biol Chem. 2012; 287(45):38327–37.

Yildirim MA, Goh KI, Barabasi AL, et al. Drug-target network. Nat Biotechnol. 2007; 25(10):1119–26.

Yu L, Huang J, et al. Inferring drug-disease associations based on known protein complexes. BMC Med Genet. 2015;8(2):S2.

Zonana J, Elder ME, Schneider LC, et al. A novel X-linked disorder of immune deficiency and hypohidrotic ectodermal dysplasia is allelic to incontinentia pigmenti and due to mutations in IKK-gamma (NEMO). Am J Hum Genet. 2000;67(6):1555–62.

30

MMP expression alteration and MMP-1 production control by syringic acid via AP-1 mechanism

Ji Young Ryu[1] and Eun Ju Na[2*]

Abstract

Background: Syringic acid is a phenolic compound that can be produced through selective hydrolysis of eudesmic acid containing 20% sulfuric acid. The acid is obtained by breaking down components, such as anthocyanin and lignin acid, present in the oils of acai berries and other fruits. Recently, the anti-inflammatory, selective toxicity, anticancer, and antioxidant effects of syringic acid have been studied, but few studies on the effects of syringic acid on human keratinocytes (HaCaT) cells have been published. The present study investigated the antioxidant effects of syringic acid, as a potential cosmetic ingredient, on matrix metalloproteinase (MMP) expression alteration and MMP production control through the activator protein-1 (AP-1) mechanism in HaCaT cells exposed to ultraviolet B radiation.

Methods: A reactive oxygen species (ROS)-scavenging assay using a luciferase reporter that utilizes the AP-1 response element, an enzyme-linked immunosorbent assay (ELISA), and quantitative reverse transcription polymerase chain reaction (qRT-PCR) were used. To confirm if ROS in HaCaT cells damaged by ultraviolet B are eliminated by syringic acid, 2'-7'-dichlorofluorescein diacetate was used to measure the ROS quantity. qRT-PCR analysis was used to measure the expressions of *SOD1* mRNA, *GPx1* mRNA, and catalase (*CAT*) mRNA, which are related to oxidation inhibition. To measure the anti-aging effects of syringic acid, qRT-PCR was used to measure the expression levels of *MMP* mRNA, *c-Jun*, and *c-Fos*.

Results: ROS were eliminated by syringic acid, and cell aging due to ultraviolet B was suppressed. Results of qRT-PCR analysis confirmed that syringic acid suppressed oxidation in HaCaT cells damaged by ultraviolet B. Further, syringic acid was found to suppress the expression of *MMP* mRNA, *c-Jun*, and *c-Fos* in a concentration-dependent manner. ELISA showed that MMP-1 production decreased in a concentration-dependent manner. The luciferase reporter analysis revealed a concentration-dependent decrease in the transcriptional activity of AP-1 promoter caused by syringic acid.

Conclusions: Syringic acid was shown to be involved in altering MMP expression and controlling MMP-1 production through the AP-1 mechanism. Thus, the antioxidant and anti-aging effects of syringic acid increased the survival rate of HaCaT cells damaged by ultraviolet B, suggesting that it can be used as a natural phytochemical in cosmetic products.

Keywords: Syringic acid, HaCaT , Ultraviolet B, ROS, Antioxidant, MMPs, Procollagen type I

* Correspondence: ejhk1010@naver.com
[2]Department of Biological Engineering, Konkuk University, 120 Neungdong-ro, Gwangjin-gu, Seoul 05029, Republic of Korea
Full list of author information is available at the end of the article

Background

External stimuli, including the sun's rays as well as direct and continuous exposure of keratinocytes to the external environment, lead to oxidative stress and skin aging. When the skin is in a continuous oxidative state with slow recovery, it becomes rough and dull, which causes skin aging characterized by loss of elasticity and wrinkles (Agarwal et al. 1988; Wong et al. 2007). Therefore, improving the body's antioxidant system is important for protecting keratinocytes and delaying cellular aging (Applegate et al. 1995).

Skin aging can be divided into two classes: intrinsic aging caused by natural genetics and extrinsic aging caused by exposure to the external environment (Naylor et al. 2011). Short-wavelength ultraviolet light (UVB) induces the production of matrix metalloproteinases (MMPs), which harm the skin (Pygmalion et al. 2010). The primary function of MMPs is to break down proteins and enzymes in the extra cellular matrix (ECM) (Egeblad and Werb 2002). Thus, MMPs have a destructive effect on the ECM and cause a decrease in fibrous collagen (Scharffetter-Kochanek et al. 2000). UCB passes through the skin keratin, causes DNA damage, and interacts with photosensitizers and chromatophores to induce oxidative stress (Ma et al. 2001). Consequently, UVB promotes the production of activator protein-1 (AP-1) and vitalization of nuclear factor kappa-light-chain-enhancer of activated B cells and induces the production of reactive oxygen species (ROS) on cell surface receptors, such as mitogen-activated kinases (MAPK) (Xu and Fisher 2005; Jiang et al. 2006). As such, UV is a major cause of skin aging. To delay aging, continuous research and development have been conducted in a variety of fields to normalize the signal systems within skin cells and prevent harm caused by UV and external stimuli.

Syringic acid, a type of phenolic compound, can be obtained through the selective hydrolysis of eudesmic acid containing 20% sulfuric acid (Bogert and Ehrlich 1919). It is contained in large amounts in oils of acai berries and other fruits (Pacheco-Palencia et al. 2008). Syringic acid is isolated from medicinal plants and biosynthesized through the shikimic acid pathway (Andrade et al. 2001; De Heredia et al. 2001; Dawidar et al. 2000). Studies on the selective effects of syringic acid (Shim et al. 1995; Goldberg et al. 1999; Ferguson 2001), such as strong anticancer and anti-inflammatory effects (Lü et al. 1998; Sun et al. 2002; Rekha et al. 2014), antioxidant effects (Srinivasn et al. 2014), and DPPH radical-scavenging activity, have been conducted. Compared with traditional chemical agents, natural ingredients extracted from plants are known to be less toxic to normal cells but are selectively toxic to cancer cells. Accordingly, there has been a growing interest in the mechanisms and extracted components of natural active compounds (Shim et al. 1995).

The present study investigated the antioxidant effects of syringic acid on MMP expression alteration and MMP production control through the AP-1 mechanism in human keratinocytes exposed to UVB radiation and confirmed the protective effects of syringic acid against cell damage and its potential as a cosmetic component.

Methods

Cell culture and sample treatment
Cell culture

A human keratinocyte (HaCaT) cell line was obtained from American Type Culture Collection (USA) and cultured Dulbecco's modified Eagle's medium (Hyclone, USA) containing HaCaT cells in 10% fetal bovine serum (Hyclone) and 1% penicillin/streptomycin (penicillin 100 IU/mL, streptomycin 100 μg/mL; Invitrogen, USA) and incubated at 37 °C in 5% CO_2.

Syringic acid treatment

Syringic acid was purchased from Sigma-Aldrich (USA) in refined powder form and was dissolved in dimethyl sulfoxide (Sigma-Aldrich) for the experiment. After culturing HaCaT cells (1×10^6 cells/well) in culture dishes for 24 h, syringic acid was added to the medium, and the culture was incubated for 6 h. The cells were then irradiated with a UVB lamp (UVP, USA). UVB wavelengths were measured using a USB 2000 fiberoptic spectrometer system (Ocean Optics, USA). To investigate the effects of UVB on HaCaT cells, the medium was removed from the culture plate and washed with phosphate-buffered saline (PBS; pH 7.4). To prevent the cells from drying, 1-mL PBS was added to the washed HaCaT cells, which were then irradiated with UVB with the lid open. After UBS irradiation, PBS was removed, fresh medium was added, and the cells were further cultured for 24 h.

Measurement of cell viability

The cell viability was measured using the principles of the water-soluble tetrazolium salts (WST)-1 assay, which measures the absorbance of formazan, a chromogenic material obtained by the reaction of mitochondrial dehydrogenase and soluble tetrazolium salts. The cells were inoculated into 96-well plates at a concentration of 3×10^3 cells/well in 100-μL amounts and incubated for 24 h. The cells were then treated with syringic acid at concentrations of 1, 2, 5, and 10 μM and incubated for another 24 h after exposure to UVB. Subsequently, 10-μL aliquots of EZ-Cytox cell viability assay kit reagent (ItsBio, Korea) was added to the cell culture plates. After 1-h incubation, a microplate reader (Bio-Rad, USA) was used to measure the absorbance at 490 nm to determine the cell viability; this process was repeated thrice to derive the mean and standard deviation of cell viability.

RNA extraction and cDNA production

After extracting RNA for a quantitative analysis of the changes in gene expression pattern in HaCaT cells due to syringic acid, cDNA was synthesized, and the expression level of the desired gene was determined through quantitative real-time polymerase chain reaction (qRT-PCR). After dissolving the incubated cells in TRIzol reagent (Invitrogen, USA), 0.2-mL chloroform (Biopure, Canada) was added, and the cells were kept at room temperature before centrifuging at 12000 rpm at 4 °C for 20 min. Subsequently, the supernatant fluid, including mRNA from the infranatant liquid with protein, was separated, and 0.5-mL isopropanol was added to it. The cells were kept at room temperature for 10 min and then centrifuged at 12000 rpm at 4 °C. After precipitating the RNA, it was washed with 75% ethanol, ethanol was removed, and the RNA was dried in room temperature. The dried mRNA was dissolved in diethylpyrocarbonate (DEPC; Biopure) water for use in the experiment, and only the extracted RNA that exceeded the purity level of 260/280 nm (1.8 ratio), as determined using nanodrop (Maestrogen, USA), was used in the experiment. After obtaining 10 µL of 1-µg RNA, 0.5-ng oligo dT18 with DEPC water was added in a PCR tube and kept at 70 °C for 10 min. After inducing RNA denaturation, RNA was incubated with M-MLV reverse transcriptase (Enzynomics, Korea) at 37 °C for 1 h to synthesize cDNA.

Measurement of gene expression

qRT-PCR is used to measure the amount of amplification products by measuring the real-time fluorescence of fluorescent material, such as double-strand DNA SYBR green, bound by PCR products. The threshold at which fluorescence can be detected was set to the threshold cycle (ct), and after measuring the number of cycles that were needed to reach the ct, the difference in expression levels was determined. If the expression level is high, ct is reached quickly. As the number of cycles decreases, expression decreases. Therefore, the difference in one cycle results in twice the expression.

qRT-PCR was performed using Linegene K (BioER, China) and mixing 0.2 µM of primers with 50 mM KCl, 20 mM Tris/HCl (pH 8.4), 0.8 mM dNTP, 0.5 U Extaq DNA polymerase, 3 mM MgCl, and 1× SYBR green (Invitrogen) in a PCR tube. The validity of PCR was verified by performing a melting curve analysis. The expression of each gene was normalized to β-actin expression in a comparative analysis. The primers used in the experiments were as follows (Table 1).

Measurement of AP-1 promoter activity

AP-1 promoter luciferase assay was used to determine the effects of syringic acid on the transcriptional activity of AP-1 promoter. In this experiment, expression was confirmed after transfection using a vector (BPS Bioscience, CA, USA) in which AP-1-responsive elements were located in front of the luciferase gene. The cells were placed in 96-well culture dishes at a concentration of 3×10^4 cells/well and incubated for 24 h. After stabilizing the cells, 1 µL of the reporter gene was mixed with 15 µL of the cell culture medium. Subsequently, after adding 0.35-µL lipofectamine 2000 to 15-µL cell culture medium, diluent DNA and lipofectamine 2000 diluent were mixed and reacted at room temperature for 25 min. After the mixture was added to the cell plates in 30-µL amounts, it was incubated for 24 h and treated with reagents and stimuli. After an additional 24 h of incubation, the transcriptional activity of AP-1 promoter was measured.

Production of MMP-1 and procollagen type I

The enzyme-linked immunosorbent assay (ELISA) is an enzyme-substrate binding assay that uses antigen-specific reactivity to detect an antigen. This method was used to measure the production of MMP-1 and procollagen type I. After seeding, the cells were incubated for 24 h. After stimulating the cells with the

Table 1 List of primers used in this study

Gene	Forward primer	Reverse primer
SOD1	GGGAGATGGCCCAACTACTG	CCAGTTGACATGCAACCGTT
GPx1	TTCCCGTGCAACCAGTTTG	GGACGTACTTGAGGGAATTCAGA
CAT	ATGGTCCATGCTCTCAAACC	CAGGTCATCCAATAGGAAGG
MMP1	TCTGACGTTGATCCCAGAGAGCAG	CAGGGTGACACCAGTGACTGCAC
MMP2	GGAATGCCATCCCCGATAAC	CAGCCTAGCCAGCCAGTCGGATTT
MMP9	GGGCTTAGATCATTCCTCTCAGTGCC	GAAGATGTTCACGTTGCAGGCATC
c-Fos	CGAAGGGAACGGAATAAGATG	GCTGCCAAAATAAACTCCAG
c-Jun	TCCTATGACGATGCCCTCAAC	GTGTTCTGGCTGTGCAGTTC

sample, the cells were cultured for another 24 h, and the cell culture medium was then separated. ELISA of MMP-1 and procollagen were performed using the MMP-1 ELISA kit (QIA55; Merck & Co., Inc., USA) and the procollagen type I C-peptide enzyme immunoassay kit (MK 101; Takara, Japan). A 100-μL aliquot of cell culture medium was added to the surface of each plastic cell culture dish well fixated with MMP-1 monoclonal antibody and incubated at room temperature for 2 h. The cells were washed five times with 1× washing buffer, 100-μL horseradish peroxidase-conjugated anti-MMP-1 antibody was added, and the cells were incubated at room temperature for 1 h. Subsequently, 100-μL of 3,3′,5,5′-tetramethylbenzidine (TMB) substrate was added and incubated in a dark room at room temperature for 30 min. The absorbance was measured at 450 nm.

Subsequently, 100 μL of the culture medium was dispensed into the anti-procollagen type I C-peptide (PIP) monoclonal antibody-coated plate and kept at room temperature for 2 h. The medium was washed five times with 1× washing buffer and procollagen type-IC-peptide (anti-PIP) monoclonal antibody, which was labeled with peroxidase, and hydrogen peroxide used to catalyze the dehydrogenation of substrates was added and reacted for 3 h. After adding 100-μL TMB substrate and incubating at room temperature for 15 min, the absorbance was measured at 450 nm.

Statistical analysis

All experiments were independently repeated ≥three times under the same conditions to obtain the experimental results. The results of each experiment were analyzed using the non-paired Student's t test. The p value was calculated, and any value < 0.05 was considered to indicate statistical significance.

Results

To examine the cytotoxicity of syringic acid and cytoprotective effects against UVB, HaCaT cells were treated with syringic acid at concentrations of 1, 2, 5, 10, and 20 μM and incubated for 25 h before WST-1 assay. We found that 1 μM of syringic acid resulted in a 105% cell survival rate, 2 μM resulted in a 108% cell survival rate, 5 μM resulted in a 104% cell survival rate, 10 μM resulted in a 96% cell survival rate, and 20 μM resulted in an 88% cell survival rate (Fig. 1). To investigate the cytoprotective effects of syringic acid against cell damage caused by UVB, the HaCaT cells were treated with syringic acid at concentrations of 1, 2, 5, and 10 μM and irradiated with 15 mJ/cm^2 UVB. Compared with the cell survival rate of 72% for the control group irradiated with UVB, that of cells treated with 1 μM of syringic acid increased to 78%, that of cells treated with 2 μM of syringic acid increased to 88%, that of the cells treated with 5 μM of syringic acid increased to 92%, and that of cells treated with 10 μM of syringic acid increased to 102% (Fig. 2).

In addition, we confirmed that ROS in HaCaT cells harmed by UVB were eliminated by syringic acid. After ROS produced by UVB were fluorescently stained with DCF-DA, flow cytometry (BD Biosciences, USA) was used to measure the change in values. It revealed that 15 mJ/cm^2 UVB caused a 2.6-fold increase in ROS, but after treatment with syringic acid at concentrations of 2, 5, and 10 μM, the ROS levels in the UVB-exposed HaCaT cells decreased by 2.1-, 1.5-, and 1.2-fold, respectively. In particular, 10 μM of syringic acid was more effective in eliminating ROS than the same concentration of N-acetyl-L-cysteine (NAC; Calbiochem, USA), which acts as a ROS scavenger (Fig. 3). We used qRT-PCR to verify that SOD1 mRNA, which decreased in response to UVB, had an antioxidant effect of superoxide anion radical elimination due to UVB and found that exposure to 15-mJ/cm^2 UVB caused the expression

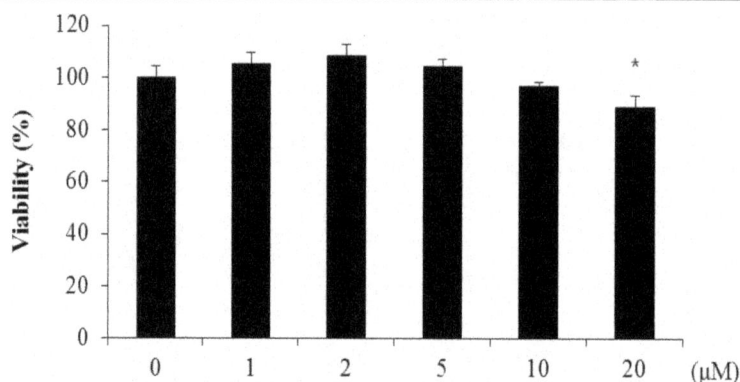

Fig. 1 Cellular toxicity of syringic acid in HaCaTs. Effect of syringic acid on HaCaT cell viability at the indicated concentrations. Results are expressed as the mean ± SD in triplicate; *$p < 0.05$ vs the non-treated group

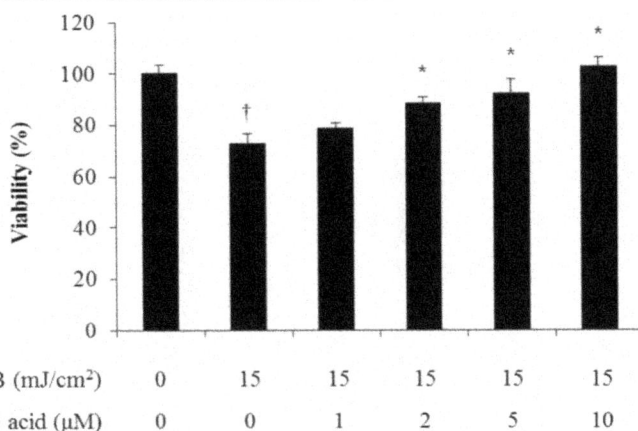

Fig. 2 Effect of syringic acid on the viability of UVB-irradiated HaCaTs. Data are expressed as the mean ± SD in triplicate; †$p < 0.05$ vs the non-treated group, *$p < 0.05$ vs the UVB-treated group without syringic acid

level of *SOD1* to decrease 0.7-fold, but after treatment with 2, 5, and 10 μM of syringic acid, the *SOD1* mRNA expression after exposure to 15 mJ/cm^2 UVB increased 0.9-, 1.1-, and 1.2-fold, respectively (Fig. 4). We also used qRT-PCR to verify that *GPX1* mRNA, which decreased in response to UVB, had an antioxidant effect of superoxide anion radical elimination caused by UVB and found that 15-mJ/cm^2 UVB caused the expression level of *GPX1* to decrease 0.2-fold, but after treatment with 2, 5, and 10 μM of syringic acid, the *SOD1* mRNA expression after exposure to 15 mJ/cm^2 UVB increased 0.8-, 1.4-, and 2.2-fold, respectively (Fig. 5). In this experiment, qRT-PCR was used to determine whether catalase (*CAT*) mRNA, which decreased in response to UVB, could be recovered to some extent by syringic acid and

found that 15-mJ/cm^2 UVB caused the expression level of *CAT* mRNA to decrease 0.2-fold, but after treatment with 2, 5, and 10 μM of syringic acid, *CAT* mRNA expression after exposure to 15 mJ/cm^2 UVB increased 0.4-, 0.7-, and 0.9-fold, respectively (Fig. 6).

To examine the changes in MMP expression and MMP-1 production caused by syringic acid through the AP-1 mechanism, qRT-PCR was used to determine the degree of reduction in *c-Jun and c-Fos* mRNA expression due to syringic acid after their increase in response to UVB. Our results revealed that 15-mJ/cm^2 UVB caused a 2.1-fold increase in the expression level of *c-Jun* mRNA, but after treatment with 2, 5, and 10 μM of syringic acid, *c-Jun* mRNA expression decreased 1.9-, 1.3-, and 1.1-fold, respectively. Exposure

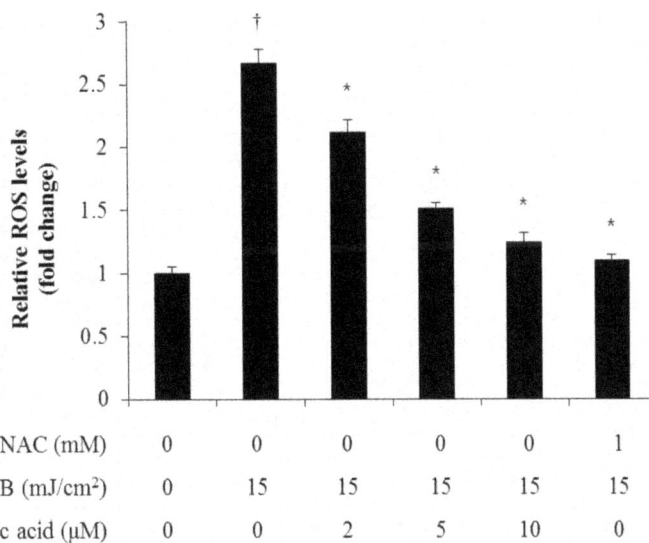

Fig. 3 ROS scavenging effect of syringic acid in UVB-irradiated HaCaTs. Results are expressed as the mean ± SD in triplicate; †$p < 0.05$ vs the non-treated group, *$p < 0.05$ vs the UVB-treated group without syringic acid

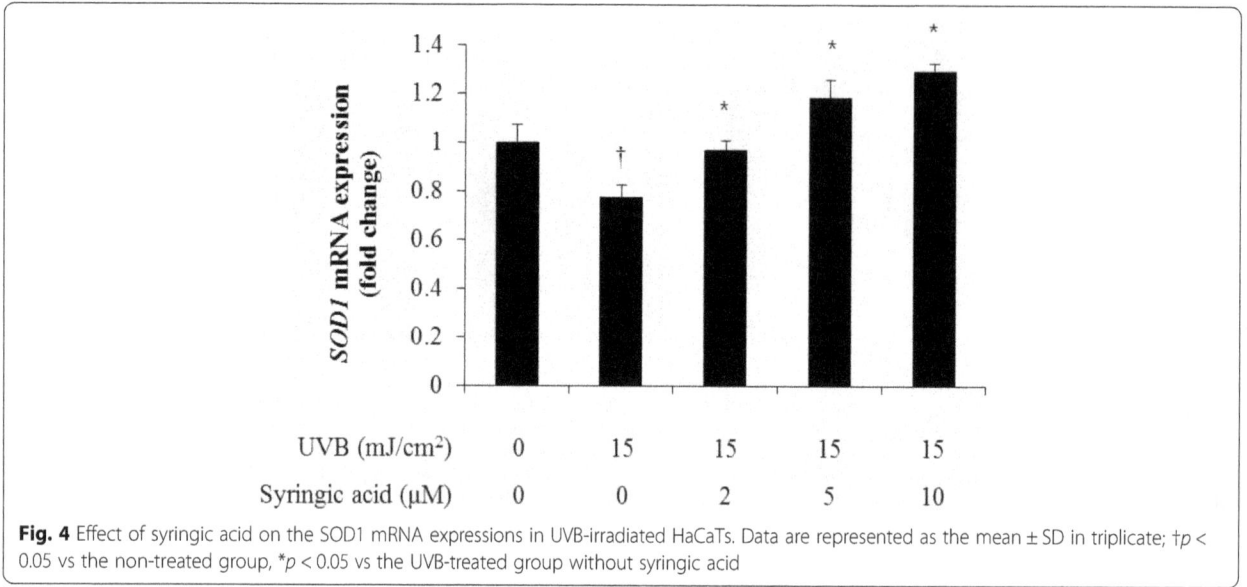

Fig. 4 Effect of syringic acid on the SOD1 mRNA expressions in UVB-irradiated HaCaTs. Data are represented as the mean ± SD in triplicate; †$p <$ 0.05 vs the non-treated group, *$p < 0.05$ vs the UVB-treated group without syringic acid

to 15-mJ/cm^2 UVB caused a 1.2-fold increase in the expression level of *c-Fos* mRNA, but after treatment with 2, 5, and 10 μM of syringic acid, *c-Fos* mRNA expression after exposure to 15 mJ/cm^2 UVB decreased 1.1-, 1.0-, and 0.9-fold, respectively (Fig. 7). In this experiment, AP-1 luciferase reporter vector (BPS Bioscience, CA, USA) with AP-1-responsive elements located in front of luciferase in the promoter region was used for transfection before luciferase gene expression was measured via luciferin luminescence measurement. The results confirmed the transcriptional activity of the transcription factor AP-1 promoter, which affects skin aging via inflammation, immune response, cell proliferation, and collagen degradation. The luminescence of luciferin increased twofold due to 15-mJ/cm^2 UVB, but after syringic acid treatment at concentrations of 2, 5, and 10 μM, it decreased 1.5-, 1.2-, and 1.0-fold, respectively, after exposure to 15 mJ/cm^2 UVB. We confirmed that the decrease in the luminescence of luciferin due to syringic acid was concentration-dependent. This finding confirmed that syringic acid inhibited the transcription activity of the transcription factor AP-1 promoter, which affects skin aging via skin inflammation,

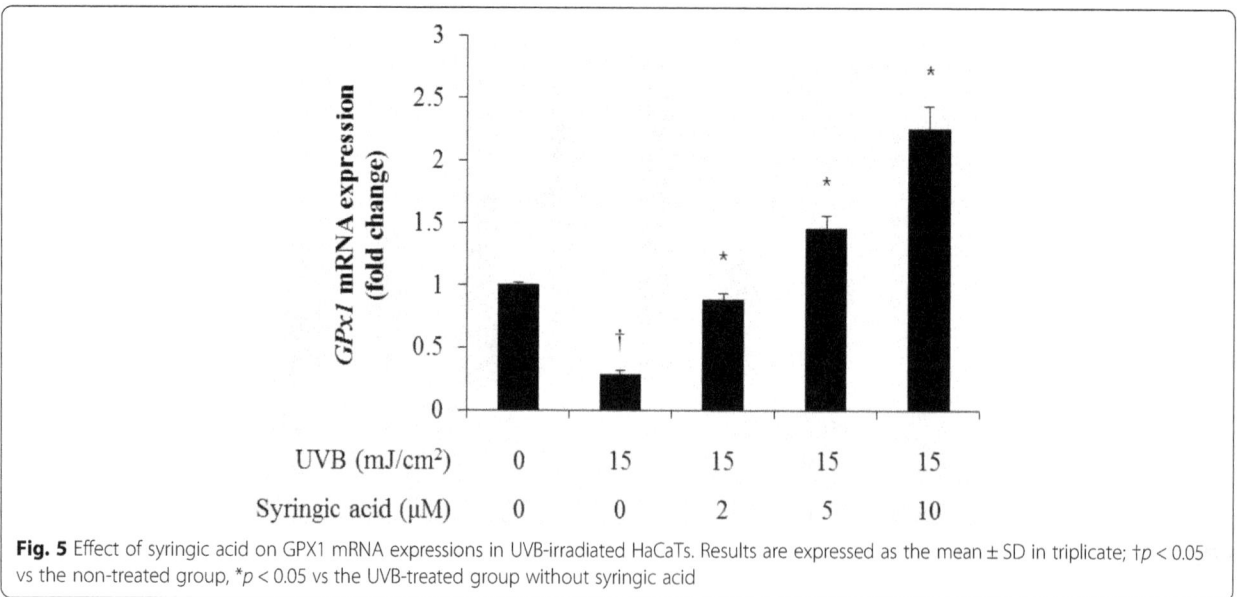

Fig. 5 Effect of syringic acid on GPX1 mRNA expressions in UVB-irradiated HaCaTs. Results are expressed as the mean ± SD in triplicate; †$p < 0.05$ vs the non-treated group, *$p < 0.05$ vs the UVB-treated group without syringic acid

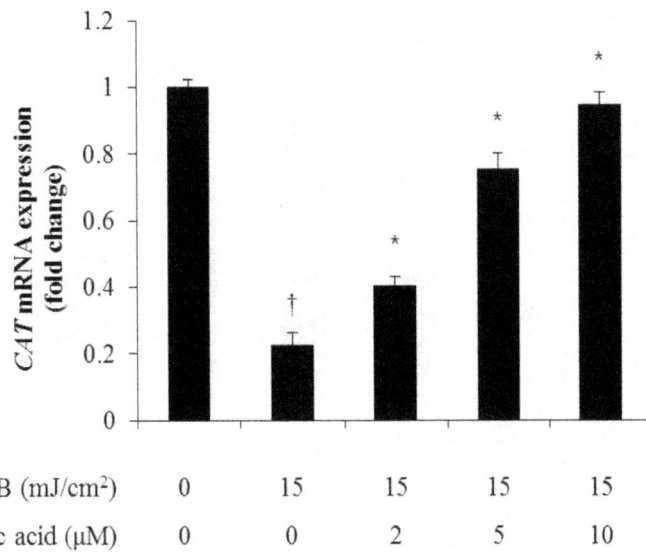

Fig. 6 Effect of syringic acid on CAT mRNA expressions in UVB-irradiated HaCaTs. Data are expressed as the mean ± SD in triplicate; †$p < 0.05$ vs the non-treated group, *$p < 0.05$ vs the UVB-treated group without syringic acid

immune response, cell proliferation, and collagen degradation (Fig. 8).

Change in *MMP* mRNA expression

The effect of syringic acid on *MMP-1*, *MMP-2*, and *MMP-9* expressions was confirmed by qRT-PCR. It demonstrated that after exposure to 15-mJ/cm^2 UVB, the expression levels of *MMP-1*, *MMP-2*, and *MMP-9* increased 2.5, 4.3, and 1.8-fold, respectively, but after treatment with 2, 5, and 10 μM of syringic acid, the *MMP-1* mRNA expression after exposure to 15-mJ/cm^2 UVB decreased 1.9-, 1.4-, and 1.06-fold, respectively. Because of syringic acid treatments at concentrations of 2, 5, and 10 μM, *MMP-2* mRNA expression after

exposure to 15-mJ/cm^2 UVB decreased 3.4-, 2.1-, and 0.9-fold, respectively, in a concentration-dependent manner, and *MMP-9* mRNA expression decreased to 1.0-, 0.9-, and 0.8-fold, respectively, in a concentration-dependent manner (Fig. 9). ELISA was used to determine the effects of syringic acid on the production of MMP-1, which is a collagen inhibitor that increases in response to UVB. It demonstrated that exposure to 15-mJ/cm^2 UVB caused a 1- to 1.9-fold increase in MMP-1 production, but after treatment with 2, 5, and 10 μM of syringic acid, MMP-1 production after exposure to 15-mJ/cm^2 UVB decreased 1.8-, 1.5-, and 1.3-fold, respectively (Fig. 10). Therefore, it seems that syringic acid has anti-aging effects in HaCaT cells.

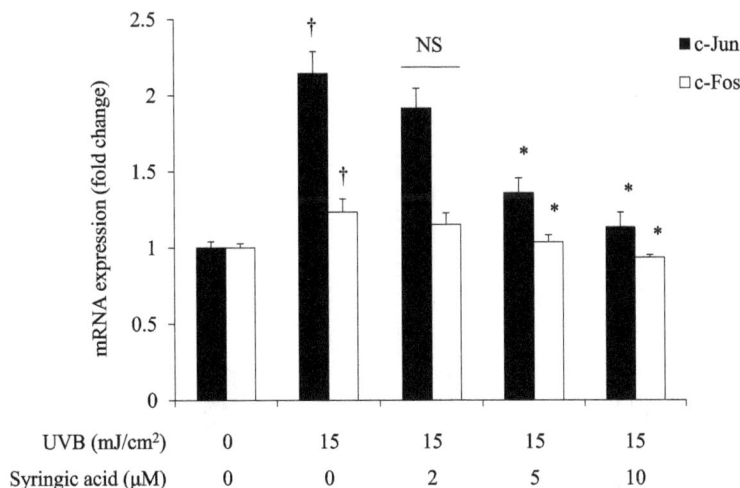

Fig. 7 Effect of syringic acid on c-Jun and c-Fos mRNA expressions in UVB-irradiated HaCaTs. Results are expressed as the mean ± SD in triplicate; †$p < 0.05$ vs the non-treated group, *$p < 0.05$ vs the UVB-treated group without syringic acid. NS means not significance

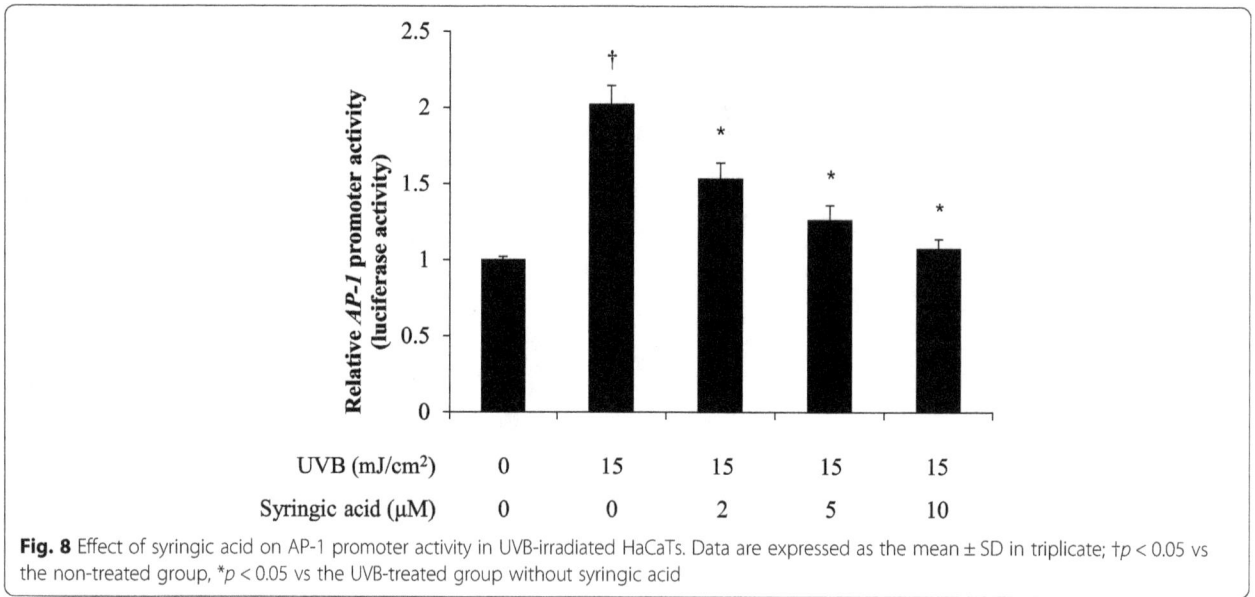

Fig. 8 Effect of syringic acid on AP-1 promoter activity in UVB-irradiated HaCaTs. Data are expressed as the mean ± SD in triplicate; $\dagger p < 0.05$ vs the non-treated group, $*p < 0.05$ vs the UVB-treated group without syringic acid

Discussion

This study demonstrated that 10 μM was the highest concentration of syringic acid used in the UVB cytoprotective experiments. We found that the cytoprotective effects of syringic acid and the cell survival rates in HaCaT harmed by UVB were concentration-dependent.

The oxidation inhibition effects of syringic acid on HaCaT cells harmed by UVB were examined. ROS decreased in HaCaT after pretreatment with syringic acid and also confirmed that syringic acid increased the expression of *SOD1* mRNA, an antioxidant gene, in a concentration-dependent manner. And found that syringic acid increased *GPX1* expression in a concentration-dependent manner, which reduced

oxygen-free radicals and suppressed cellular aging. This experiment confirmed the antioxidative effects of *GPX1*, where syringic acid increased the concentration of *CAT* mRNA, an antioxidant gene, in a concentration-dependent manner.

In this study, *c-Jun and c-Fos* mRNA, which are involved in the expression of proteins, such as MMP, increased in response to UVB but decreased in response to syringic acid in a concentration-dependent manner. Therefore, syringic acid is considered to have anti-aging effects in human keratinocytes, confirming the transcriptional activity of the transcription factor, AP-1 promoter, which affects skin aging due to inflammation, immune response, cell proliferation, and

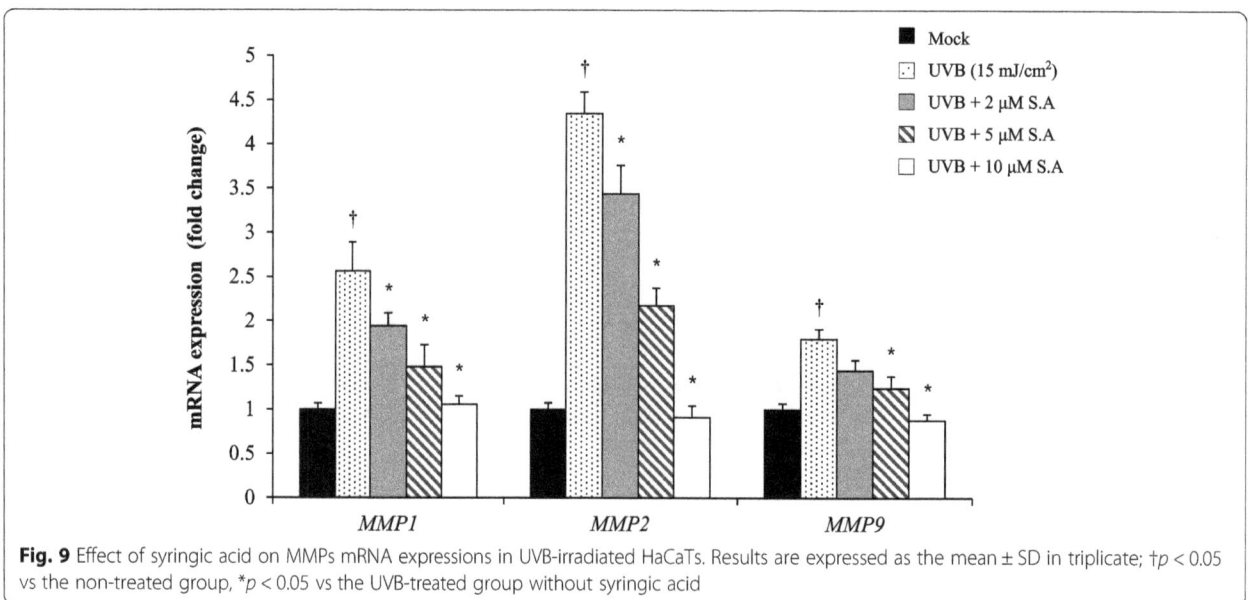

Fig. 9 Effect of syringic acid on MMPs mRNA expressions in UVB-irradiated HaCaTs. Results are expressed as the mean ± SD in triplicate; $\dagger p < 0.05$ vs the non-treated group, $*p < 0.05$ vs the UVB-treated group without syringic acid

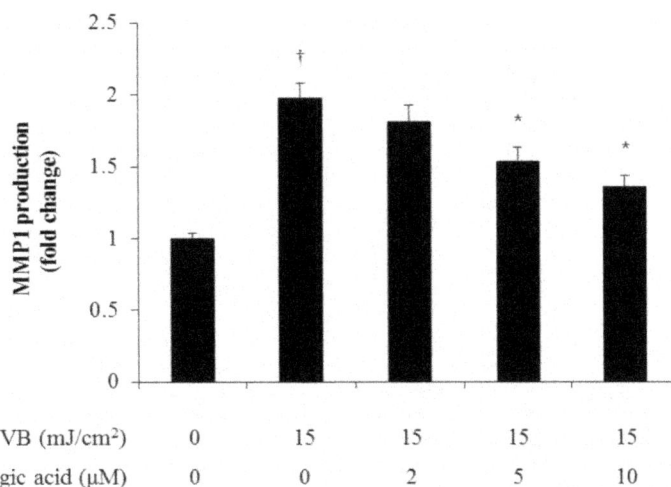

Fig. 10 Effect of syringic acid on MMP-1 production in UVB-irradiated HaCaTs. Data are represented as the mean ± SD in triplicate; †$p < 0.05$ vs the non-treated group, *$p < 0.05$ vs the UVB-treated group without syringic acid

collagen degradation. Therefore, syringic acid appeared to be an effective anti-aging agent in human keratinocytes.

Proteinases, such as MMP-1, play a crucial role in skin aging by abnormally suppressing collagen in dermal tissues (Chen et al. 2008). In the present study, we confirmed that syringic acid decreased the production of collagen-inhibiting enzyme MMP-1 in a concentration-dependent manner. Thus, syringic acid has an anti-aging effect in the human keratinocyte cell line HaCaT.

Therefore syringic acid was shown to be involved in altering MMP expression and controlling MMP-1 production through the AP-1 mechanism. Thus, the antioxidant and anti-aging effects of syringic acid increased the survival rate of HaCaT cells damaged by ultraviolet B, suggesting that it can be used as a natural phytochemical in cosmetic products.

Conclusion

Most studies related to syringic acid have focused on its antioxidant and anti-inflammatory roles in the fields of food, medicine, pharmacy, and life sciences. No study has been conducted on its role in anticancer treatments or cosmetics. In particular, no research on the effects of syringic acid in human keratinocytes has been published. The present study investigated the effects of syringic acid, which has been shown to protect against cell damage via anti-inflammatory, antioxidant, and anticancer effects. It examined antioxidative effects of syringic acid in HaCaT cells exposed to UVB and the effect on *MMP* expression alteration and MMP production control through AP-1 regulation. Syringic acid was tested for its cytoprotective effect and its potential as a cosmetic ingredient. Syringic acid was shown to be involved in

MMP gene expression and MMP production control through AP-1 regulation, thereby protecting human keratinocytes from damage and restoring the survival rate of the cells harmed by UVB. Syringic acid was shown to have antioxidant and anti-aging effects; therefore, it can potentially be used as a natural phytochemical ingredient in cosmetic products.

Abbreviations
Anti-PIP: Procollagen type-IC-peptide; AP-1: Activator protein-1; *CAT*: Catalase; *c-Fos*: Cellular-Fujinami OsteoSarcoma virus; *c-Jun*: Cellular-Jun; DEPC: Diethylpyrocarbonate; DMEM: Dulbecco's modified Eagle medium; FBS: Fetal bovine serum; GPX: Glutathione peroxidase; HaCaT: Human keratinocyte; MAPK: Mitogen-activated kinases; MMPs: Matrix metalloproteinases; qRT-PCR: Quantitative real-time polymerase chain reaction; ROS: Reactive oxygen species; SOD1: Superoxide dismutase 1; UV: Ultraviolet; WST: Water-soluble tetrazolium salts

Acknowledgements
Not applicable

Funding
Not applicable

Authors' contributions
Both authors contributed to all the research background such as the experiments, data collection, and statistical analysis as well as manuscript draft. Both authors read and approved the final manuscript.

Competing interests
The authors declare that they have no competing interests.

Author details
[1]Halla University, 28, Halladae-gil, Heungeop-myeon, Wonju-si, Gangwon-do 25404, Republic of Korea. [2]Department of Biological Engineering, Konkuk University, 120 Neungdong-ro, Gwangjin-gu, Seoul 05029, Republic of Korea.

References

Agarwal S, Drysdale BE, Shin HS. Tumor necrosis factor-mediated cytotoxicity involves ADP-ribosylation. J Immunol. 1988;140(12):4187–92.

Andrade PB, Oliveira BM, Seabra RM, Ferreira MA, Ferreres F, García-Viguera C. Analysis of phenolic compounds in Spanish Albrariño and Portuguese Alvarinho and Loureiro wines by capillary zone electrophoresis and high-performance liquid chromatography. Electrophoresis. 2001;22(8):1568–72.

Applegate LA, Noël A, Vile G, Frenk E, Tyrrell RM. Two genes contribute to different extents to the heme oxygenase enzyme activity measured in cultured human skin fibroblasts and keratinocytes. Photochem Photobiol. 1995;61(3):285–91.

Bogert M, Ehrlich J. The synthesis of certain pyrogallol ethers, including a new acetophenetide derived from the ethyl ether of syringic acid. J Am Chem Soc. 1919;41(5):798–810.

Chen W, Kang J, Xia J, Li Y, Yang B, Chen B, Sun W, Song X, Xiang W, Wang X, Wang F, Wan Y, Bi Z. p53-related apoptosis resistance and tumor suppression activity in UVB-induced premature senescent human skin fibroblasts. Int J Mol Med. 2008;21(5):645–53.

Dawidar AM, Ezmiriy ST, Abdel-Mogib M, el-Dessouki Y, Angawi RF. New stilbene carboxylic acid from Convolvulus hystrix. Pharmazie. 2000;55(11):848–9.

De Heredia JB, Torregrosa J, Dominguez JR, Peres JA. Kinetic model for phenolic compound oxidation by Fenton's reagent. Chmosphere. 2001;45(1):85–90.

Egeblad M, Werb Z. New functions for the matrix metalloproteinases in cancer progression. Nat Rev Cancer. 2002;2(3):161–74.

Ferguson LR. Role of plant polyphenols in genomic stability. Mutat Res. 2001; 475(1–2):89–111.

Goldberg DM, Hoffman B, Yang J, Soleas GJ. Phenolic constituents, furans, and total antioxidant status of distilled spirits. J Agric Food Chem. 1999;47(10):3978–85.

Jiang Q, Zhou C, Healey S, Chu W, Kouttab N, Bi Z, Wan Y. UV radiation down-regulates Dsg-2 via Rac/NADPH oxidase-mediated generation of ROS in human lens epithelial cells. Int J Mol Med. 2006;18(2):381–7.

Lü W, Shi J, Zhang S, Du Z. Determination of ferulic acid and peoniflorin in siwu decoction prepared by different methods of yellow rice wine. Zhongguo Zhong Yao Za Zhi. 1998;23(9):531–3. 575

Ma W, Wlaschek M, Tantcheva-Poór I, Schneider LA, Naderi L, Razi-Wolf Z, Schüller J, Scharffetter-Kochanek. Chronologicalageing and photoageing of the fibroblasts and thedermal connective tissue. Clin Exp Dermatol. 2001; 26(7):592–9.

Naylor EC, Watson Rachel EB, Sherratt MJ. Molecular aspects of skin ageing. Maturitas. 2011;69(3):249–56.

Pacheco-Palencia LA, Mertens-Talcott S, Talcott ST. Chemical composition, antioxidant properties, and thermal stability of a phytochemical enriched oil from acai (Euterpe oleracea Mart). J Agric Food Chem. 2008;56(12):4631–6.

Pygmalion MJ, Ruiz L, Popovic E, Gizard J, Portes P, Marat X, Lucet-Levannier K, Muller B, Galey JB. Skin cell protection against UVA by Sideroxyl, a new antioxidant complementary to sunscreens. Free Radic Biol Med. 2010; 49(11):1629–37.

Rekha KR, Selvakumar GP, Sivakamasundari RI. Effects of syringic acid on chronic MPTP/probenecid induced motor dysfunction, dopaminergic markers expression and neuroinflammation in C57BL/6 mice. Biomed Aging Pathol. 2014;4(2):95–104.

Scharffetter-Kochanek K, Brenneisen P, Wenk J, Herrmann G, Ma W, Kuhr L, Meewes C, Wlaschek M. Photoaging of the skin from phenotype to mechanisms. Exp Gerontol. 2000;35(3):307–16.

Shim JS, Kang MH, Kim YH, Roh JK, Roberts C, Lee IP. Chemopreventive effect of green tea (Camellia sinensis) among cigarette smokers. Cancer Epidermiol Biomarkers Prev. 1995;4(4):387–911.

Srinivasn S, Muthukumaranb J, Muruganathana U, Venkatesanb RS, Jalaludeenc AM. Antihyperglycemic effect of syringic acid on attenuating the key enzymes of carbohydrate metabolism in experimental diabetic rats. Biomed Prev Nutr. 2014;4(4):595–602.

Sun J, Chu YF, Wu X, Liu RH. Antioxidant and antiproliferative activities of commom fruit. Agric Food Chem. 2002;50(25):7449–54.

Wong T, McGrath JA, Navsaria H. The role of fibroblasts in tissue engineering and regeneration. Br J Dermatol. 2007;156(6):1149–55.

Xu Y, Fisher GJ. Ultraviolet (UV) light irradiation induced signal transduction in skin photoaging. J Dermatol Sci Suppl. 2005;1(2):S1–8.

31

Clinical application of a new hyaluronic acid filler based on its rheological properties and the anatomical site of injection

Won Lee[1], Jeung-Hyun Yoon[2], Ik-Soo Koh[3], Wook Oh[4], Ki-Wook Kim[5] and Eun-Jung Yang[6*]

Abstract

Background: Hyaluronic acid (HA) filler is the most commonly used filler for soft tissue augmentation. There are numerous commercially available HA fillers in the cosmetic market, and there are guidelines for each filler as determined by the manufacturing company. The successful use of injectable fillers requires an understanding of each option available so that the most appropriate form of hyaluronic acid may be selected for patients. The purpose of this study was to determine whether newly developed HA fillers are appropriate for forehead augmentation considering their rheological properties and the anatomical site of injection.

Methods: The rheological properties of new HA fillers were assessed e.t.p.q. S100, S300, S500 (Zetema®). Comparing the rheological properties, the authors chose e.t.p.q. S300® for forehead augmentation. The filler was injected into the foreheads of 40 consecutive patients for esthetic purposes.

Results: e.t.p.q. S300® was determined to be an appropriate filler for the forehead. The injection procedure employed was considered to be easy and safe when applied to the preperiosteal layer using a cannula. None of the patients had complications such as vascular compromise, infections, granulomas, or migration.

Conclusions: Understanding the physical properties of new fillers is necessary. As the preperiosteal layer of the forehead is an appropriate layer for the filler injection, physicians should consider injecting fillers with enough strength to withstand the shearing forces.

Keywords: Hyaluronic acid, Filler, Rheology

Background

The relationship between the forehead and nose is one of the most important factors for determining good external facial contours. In particular, a flat or depressed forehead makes it difficult to create a favorable side profile.

It is crucial to understand the anatomy to augment the forehead using hyaluronic acid (HA) as a soft tissue filler (Rohrich and Pessa 2007; Cotofana et al. 2017). An injection in the subcutaneous layer can lead to contour irregularities and a relative risk of vessel damage. The HA filler injection is recommended to be injected into the preperiosteal layer behind the frontal muscle. When injecting a soft tissue filler behind the frontal muscle layer, the filler must have sufficient lift to withstand the compressive pressure of the frontal muscle. Therefore, it is important to choose the appropriate filler to withstand compressive and shear forces.

Nevertheless, there is a shortage of objective data for all available fillers, and physicians generally choose fillers according to the doctor's experience or company guidelines. When new filler products are introduced for clinical use, it is important to determine the layer into which they can be injected and to consider whether the

* Correspondence: Enyang7@gmail.com
[6]Department of Plastic and Reconstructive Surgery, Cheil General Hospital and Women's Healthcare Center, College of Medicine, Dankook University College of Medicine, Yongin, South Korea
Full list of author information is available at the end of the article

physical and rheological properties of the product are appropriate for the target site anatomy.

We have studied the rheological properties of new hyaluronic acid fillers. Based on rheological studies, we selected HA fillers to improve the esthetics of the forehead and confirm if they have good lifting capacity.

Methods

Patient and methods

A total of 40 consecutive patients who underwent HA filler injection for esthetic reasons between March 2018 and June of 2018 at a private clinic were identified through a retrospective review of medical charts and evaluation of clinical photographs and were included in the study. All patients had opted for the injection for esthetic purposes. A single practitioner performed all procedures. The need for informed consent was waived by the institutional review board of Cheil General Hospital because of the retrospective nature of the study.

MCR 301 rheometer (Anton Paar Company, Graz, Austria) was used for the tests. The properties were measured from 1 to 0.02 Hz. The diameter of the plate of the rheometer was 2.45 cm, and the temperature was measured at 25 °C. A total of five fillers, Restylane®, Juvederm Volbella®, and e.t.p.q. S100®, S300®, and S500® were evaluated and compared for rheological tests (Table 1). Rheological test results are known to vary based on the different conditions of the materials. However, we evaluated each material in the same conditions and subsequently chose e.t.p.q. S300® for the procedures. e.t.p.q. S300® is a known monophasic filler (depends on its manufacturing process) and has a relatively high cohesiveness. The rheological test results of e.t.p.q. S300® are shown below (Fig. 1). The results were assessed subjectively by the patients by using a questionnaire, in which the patients were asked to rate their degree of satisfaction in terms of result and treatment convenience based on a 4-point scale (0, worse; 1, little satisfaction or not satisfied; 2, satisfied; and 3, very satisfied). The questionnaire was given to the patients at the end of the treatment, and again 15 days later.

Procedure

Patients underwent forehead augmentation with e.t.p.q. S300® (Zetema®). The amount of filler injection varied from 2 to 5 cc. The entry points were made above the eyebrow and laterally from the mid-pupillary line. Local anesthetics were injected in the supratrochlear and supraorbital nerve regions. The filler was injected with a 22-G cannula. The cannula was inserted through an entry point and was placed deep behind the frontalis muscle, and the end of the cannula was located at the region where the filler was supposed to be injected. The procedure was performed gently, especially around the medial portion. Preoperative and postoperative photographs were compared (Fig. 2). Patient satisfaction was determined through a questionnaire.

Results

During the study period, a total of 40 patients (all women, ages 31.3 years [21–55]) underwent forehead augmentation, and each of them received 2–5 cc of the HA filler. All patients were injected into the supraperiosteal layer. All patients were pleased with the esthetic results. Of the 20 patients, 18 rated the results with 3 points, and the remaining 2 patients scored 2 immediately after injection. The satisfaction assessment performed 1 month after the procedure revealed that 19 patients were very satisfied and 1 was satisfied. The new e.t.p.q. S300® HA filler was determined to be an appropriate filler for the forehead. None of the patients experienced bleeding, hematomas, bruising, or vascular compromise. In addition, no patients had delayed filler migration, granulomas, or delayed swelling. The average follow-up time was 3 months (range from 1 to 12 months).

Discussion

The purpose of this study was to determine if the newly developed HA filler was suitable for forehead augmentation considering the anatomy of the forehead and the properties of the filler.

HA fillers are the most commonly used soft tissue filler. Since HA has a dermal component, it was initially used as a dermal filler; however, it has gradually been used for augmentation purposes. There are several limitations of dermal fillers with respect to the augmentation purposes. The filler should be injected into the deeper layer of the dermis for augmentation. When injected into the subcutaneous layer, the risk of vascular

Table 1 Rheological property of hyaluronic acid fillers

Product	G′ (Pa)	G″ (Pa)	Complex viscosity (cP)	Cohesiveness (N)	Tan δ	Complex modulus	Elasticity (%)
Restylane	349	145	3,011,188	0.3509	0.4180	378	71
Juviderm Volbella	99	21	814,593	0.3046	0.2189	101	83
e.t.p.q. S100	37	15	323,859	0.4184	0.4269	40	71
e.t.p.q. S300	128	27	1,048,864	0.6102	0.2137	131	83
e.t.p.q. S500	224	57	1,847,607	0.8776	0.2551	231	80

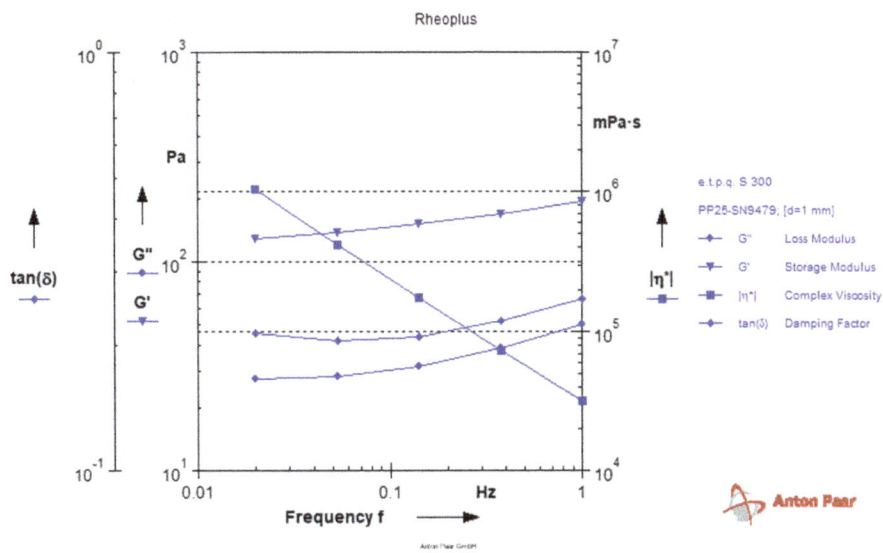

Meas. Pts.	Angular Frequency	Storage Modulus	Loss Modulus	Damping Factor	Complex Viscosity
	[rad/s]	[Pa]	[Pa]	[1]	[Pa·s]
1	6.28	1.94E+02	5.02E+01	0.258	3.19E+01
2	2.36	1.70E+02	3.89E+01	0.229	7.37E+01
3	0.889	1.52E+02	3.18E+01	0.209	1.75E+02
4	0.334	1.38E+02	2.84E+01	0.205	4.22E+02
5	0.126	1.29E+02	2.76E+01	0.214	1.05E+03

Fig. 1 Rheological results of e.p.t.q. S300®. e.p.t.q S300 has moderate cohesiveness and a higher cohesiveness than Juvéderm Volbella. The elasticity indicating the strength of the filler was also similar to that of Juvéderm

complications, such as vascular compression or occluding blood vessels, increases. Therefore, many doctors recommend injecting into a deeper layer than the subdermal layer to prevent such complications.

In the forehead, the filler can be injected in the subcutaneous layer in front of the frontalis muscle and in the preperiosteal layer in the back of the muscle. In the case of the subcutaneous layer, it is easier to make the desired shape in front of the muscle, but because of the vascular distribution, it is injected in the preperiosteal layer, which is mainly behind the muscle, thereby

reducing the risk of side effects. A recent topographical study regarding forehead filler injections also suggested that the supratrochlear and supraorbital arteries, which are critical anatomical structures, should be avoided during the injection procedure (Cong et al. 2017). Some doctors insist on injecting filler into the postperiosteal layer for forehead augmentation, but it is difficult to ensure the space for the filler injection between the periosteum and skull. It is equally difficult to inject the filler into the preperiosteal layer, but the preperiosteal layer is relatively safe and is clinically the most commonly used

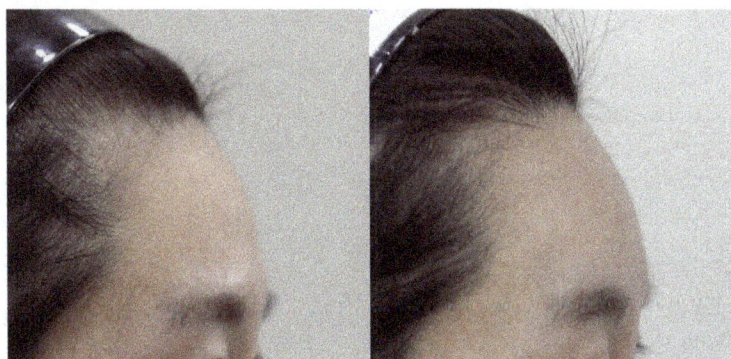

Fig. 2 24-year-old patient; pre-procedural and 3 months post-procedural photographs. A total of 3 cc of e.t.p.q S300 was injected

layer, as shown in the previous anatomical studies (van Loghem et al. 2017).

When injecting for augmentation purposes, the physical properties of the filler as well as the layer to be injected in should also be considered. Fillers used for lifting purposes should have enough lift capacity and longevity. Additionally, they should not migrate a few months after the injection. To understand the physical properties of fillers, physicians should consider the concentrations, injection forces, particle sizes, difference in the manufacturing processes, and rheological properties. Rheological properties are known as objective parameters for soft tissue fillers. Among the rheological properties, G′ is known for storage modulus and cohesiveness, which are important parameters for soft tissue filler properties (Pierre et al. 2015). Cohesiveness can be defined as a resistance to compression/stretching forces in a vertical plane once the product is implanted (Hee et al. 2015). When the physical properties of a filler are too soft, a filler can spread relatively, making it difficult to shape the target area. On the other hand, if a filler is too rigid, the projection can be represented well, but when applied to a relatively broad area such as the forehead, it becomes difficult to attain the desired shape. All the fillers could be used in the forehead, but the appropriate filler was determined on the basis of the results of the rheological study in this study. In the rheological study, the results of e.t.p.q. S300 were not too soft and not too rigid either, and the volume was maintained well when the filler was injected. Therefore, the rheological profile of S300 was deemed appropriate.

In addition, the characteristics of the site should be considered when injecting the filler for augmentation purposes. This includes the anatomic layer to be injected as described above, the difference in skin thickness along the face, and finally the desired shape of augmentation (Ha et al. 2005). For example, for chin augmentation, the post-implant chin should have a relatively limited area and should have its center raised. This implies that the filler must be injected into the deep layers, and a cohesive and rigid filler should be selected. However, augmentation in the forehead covers a relatively large area. A filler that spreads more widely is suitable for this purpose in contrast to a filler that remains limited to a specific area. We suggest that for patients considering a chin augmentation, a very rigid e.t.p.q. S500 would be a good candidate. For the forehead, we suggest the e.t.p.q. S300 as the purpose is to augment a relatively broader area. Based on the test results, the e.t.p.q. S300 exhibited sufficient cohesiveness and elastic moduli in our study. Considering only the G′ elastic modulus, S500 may be appropriate, but the forehead is different from the nose and chin, so projection is important, as is cohesiveness because it needs to be injected in a broader area. S300

has moderate cohesiveness compared with Restylane, one of the most commonly used HA fillers for forehead augmentation, and has a higher cohesiveness than Juvéderm Volbella.

When injected in the forehead, it has moderate cohesiveness, which makes the molding easier and migration less likely. The elasticity indicating the strength of the filler was also similar to that of Juvéderm. Therefore, it is considered to be a comparatively suitable filler for forehead augmentation.

Based on the rheological test, the e.t.p.q. S100 is also a good candidate for easy injection. However, since the HA modification value is high for e.t.p.q. S300, it can be maintained longer.

Conclusions

In cases of forehead augmentation, the preperiosteal layer is considered the most suitable layer for injection; thus, a sufficiently strong filler must be considered to withstand the shearing force.

Authors' contributions

WL contributed to the conceptualization, methodology, investigation, preparation, and writing of the original draft. JHY and ISK contributed to the conceptualization, writing, review, and editing of the draft. WO and KWK contributed to the formal analysis, preparation, and writing of the original draft. EJY contributed to the review and editing of the draft. All authors read and approved the final manuscript.

Competing interests

The authors declare that they have no competing interests.

Author details

[1]Yonsei E1 Plastic Surgery Clinic, Anyang, South Korea. [2]Yonseifams Clinic, Seoul, South Korea. [3]Kohlksoo Plastic Surgery Clinic, Seoul, South Korea. [4]Samsung Feel Clinic, Seoul, South Korea. [5]Regen Clinic, Seoul, South Korea. [6]Department of Plastic and Reconstructive Surgery, Cheil General Hospital and Women's Healthcare Center, College of Medicine, Dankook University College of Medicine, Yongin, South Korea.

References

Cong LY, Phothong W, Lee SH, et al. Topographic analysis of the supratrochlear artery and the supraorbital artery: implication for improving the safety of forehead augmentation. Plast Reconstr Surg. 2017;139:620e–7e.

Cotofana S, Mian A, Sykes JM, et al. An update on the anatomy of the forehead compartments. Plast Reconstr Surg. 2017;139:864e–72e.

Ha RY, Nojima K, Adams WP Jr, Brown SA. Analysis of facial skin thickness: defining the relative thickness index. Plast Reconstr Surg. 2005;115:1769–73.

Hee CK, Shumate GT, Narurkar V, Bernardin A, Messina DJ. Rheological properties and in vivo performance characteristics of soft tissue fillers. Dermatol Surg. 2015;41(Suppl 1):S373–81.

Pierre S, Liew S, Bernardin A. Basics of dermal filler rheology. Dermatol Surg. 2015;41(Suppl 1):S120–6.

Rohrich RJ, Pessa JE. The fat compartments of the face: anatomy and clinical implications for cosmetic surgery. Plast Reconstr Surg. 2007;119:2219–27. discussion 2228–2231

van Loghem JAJ, Humzah D, Kerscher M. Cannula versus sharp needle for placement of soft tissue fillers: an observational cadaver study. Aesthet Surg J. 2017;38:73–88.

Permissions

The contributors of this book come from diverse backgrounds, making this book a truly international effort. This book will bring forth new frontiers with its revolutionizing research information and detailed analysis of the nascent developments around the world.

We would like to thank all the contributing authors for lending their expertise to make the book truly unique. They have played a crucial role in the development of this book. Without their invaluable contributions this book wouldn't have been possible. They have made vital efforts to compile up to date information on the varied aspects of this subject to make this book a valuable addition to the collection of many professionals and students.

This book was conceptualized with the vision of imparting up-to-date information and advanced data in this field. To ensure the same, a matchless editorial board was set up. Every individual on the board went through rigorous rounds of assessment to prove their worth. After which they invested a large part of their time researching and compiling the most relevant data for our readers.

The editorial board has been involved in producing this book since its inception. They have spent rigorous hours researching and exploring the diverse topics which have resulted in the successful publishing of this book. They have passed on their knowledge of decades through this book. To expedite this challenging task, the publisher supported the team at every step. A small team of assistant editors was also appointed to further simplify the editing procedure and attain best results for the readers.

Apart from the editorial board, the designing team has also invested a significant amount of their time in understanding the subject and creating the most relevant covers. They scrutinized every image to scout for the most suitable representation of the subject and create an appropriate cover for the book.

The publishing team has been an ardent support to the editorial, designing and production team. Their endless efforts to recruit the best for this project, has resulted in the accomplishment of this book. They are a veteran in the field of academics and their pool of knowledge is as vast as their experience in printing. Their expertise and guidance has proved useful at every step. Their uncompromising quality standards have made this book an exceptional effort. Their encouragement from time to time has been an inspiration for everyone.

The publisher and the editorial board hope that this book will prove to be a valuable piece of knowledge for researchers, students, practitioners and scholars across the globe.

List of Contributors

In Jung, Aha Ryoung Jo, Yu Jeong Kwon, Seungbin Kwon and In-Sook An
Korea Institute of Dermatological Sciences, 6F, Tower A, 25, Beobwon-ro 11-gil, Songpa-gu, Seoul, Republic of Korea

Jung-Eun Ku
Department of Cosmetology, Kyung-In Women's University, 63, Gyeyangsan-ro, Gyeyang-gu, Incheon, Republic of Korea

Sang-Hun Bae and Jisook Moon
Department of biotechnology, College of Life Science, CHA University, Pangyo-Ro 335, Bundang-gu, Seongnam-si, Seoul, South Korea

Chun-Hyung Kim
Paean Biotechnology, Daejeon, South Korea

Pierre Leblanc and Kwang-Soo Kim
Molecular Neurobiology Laboratory, McLean Hospital, Harvard Medical School, 115 Mill St., Belmont, MA 02478, USA

Dahye Joo, Seonghee Jeong, Hyun Kyung Lee, Shang Hun Shin, Seong Jin Choi, Karam Kim and In-Sook An
Korea Institute of Dermatological Sciences, Cheongju-si, Chungcheongbuk-do 28160, Republic of Korea

Kyung-Yun Kim
URG Inc., URG Building, Seochogu, Seoul 06753, Republic of Korea

Jung-Eun Ku
Department of Cosmetology, Kyung-In Women's University, Incheon 21014, Republic of Korea

Sun-Hee Jeong
Department of Beauty Art, Faculty of Art, Suwon Women's University, Suwon-si, Gyeonggi-do 16632, Republic of Korea

Hwa Jun Cha
Department of Skin Care and Beauty, Osan University, Osan-si, Gyeonggi-do 18119, Republic of Korea.
Department of Skin Care and Cosmetics, Osan University, 45 Cheonghak-ro, Osan-si, Gyeonggi-do 18119, Republic of Korea

Song-Hyo Jin
Department of Pathology College of Medicine, Institute of Hansen's Disease, The Catholic University of Korea, Seoul 06591, Republic of Korea

Kyu Joong Ahn
Department of Dermatology, Konkuk University School of Medicine, Seoul 05029, Republic of Korea

Sungkwan An
Department of Cosmetics Engineering, Konkuk University, 120 Neungdong-ro, Gwangjin-gu, Seoul 05029, Republic of Korea

Yongwoo Jang and Jin Hyuk Jung
Molecular Neurobiology Laboratory, McLean Hospital and Program in Neuroscience, Harvard Medical School, 115 Mill St. Mail stop 149, Belmont, MA 02478-1064, USA

Kyung Yun Kim
URG Inc (2F, URG B/D), 28, Yangjaecheon-ro 19-gil, Seocho-gu, Seoul, Republic of Korea

Karam Kim, Dahye Joo, Seong Jin Choi and In Sook An
Korea Institute of Dermatological Sciences, 6F Tower A, 25 Beobwon-ro 11-gil, Songpa-gu, Seoul 05836, Republic of Korea

Hwa Jun Cha
Department of Beauty Care, Osan University, 45 Cheonghak-ro, Osan-si, Gyeonggi-do 18119, Republic of Korea

Sungkwan An
Department of Cosmetics Engineering, Konkuk University, 120 Neungdong-ro, Gwangjin-gu, Seoul 05029, Republic of Korea

Na Kyeong Lee
JEI University, 808 Main Building, 178, Jaeneung-ro, Dong-gu, Incheon 22573, Republic of Korea

William J. Sanders
Georgia Campus-Philadelphia College of Osteopathic Medicine (GA-PCOM), Suwanee, GA 30024, USA
Houston Medical Center, Warner Robins, GA 31088, USA

Antonella Savoia and Basso Di Pasquale
Promoitalia Group S.p.A, Pozzuoli, Naples, Italy

Angelica Perna Antonio De Luca Angela Lucariello
Department of Mental and Physical Health and Preventive Medicine, Section of Human Anatomy, Università degli Studi della Campania "L. Vanvitelli",
Caserta, Italy

Nicoletta Onori
San Giovanni Addolorata Hospital, Rome, Italy

Alfonso Baldi
Department of Environmental, Biological and
Pharmaceutical Sciences and Technologies, Università degli Studi della Campania "L. Vanvitelli", Caserta, Italy

Sungkwan An
Department of Cosmetics Engineering, Konkuk
University, 120 Neungdong-ro, Gwangjin-gu, Seoul
05029, Republic of Korea

Shang Hun Shin
Department of Cosmetics Engineering, Konkuk
University, 120 Neungdong-ro, Gwangjin-gu,
Seoul 05029, Republic of Korea
Korea Institute of Dermatological Sciences, 6F
Tower A, 25, Beobwon-ro 11-gil, Songpa-gu, Seoul
05836, Republic of Korea

Karam Kim and In-Sook An
Korea Institute of Dermatological Sciences, 6F
Tower A, 25, Beobwon-ro 11-gil, Songpa-gu,
Seoul 05836, Republic of Korea

Hwa Jun Cha
Department of Skin Care and Beauty, Osan
University, Osan-si, Gyeonggi-do 18119, Republic
of Korea

Kyung-Yun Kim
Inc., URG Building, Seochogu, Seoul 06753, Republic
of Korea

Jung-Eun Ku
Department of Cosmetology, Kyung-In Women's
University, Incheon 21014, Republic of Korea

Sun-Hee Jeong
Department of Beauty Art, Faculty of Art, Suwon
Women's University, Suwon-si, Gyeonggi-do 16632,
Republic of Korea

**Ian F. Burgess, Elizabeth R. Brunton, Nazma A.
Burgess and Mark N. Burgess**
Medical Entomology Centre, Insect Research and
Development Limited, 6 Quy
Court, Colliers Lane, Stow-cum-Quy, Cambridge
CB25 9AU, UK

**Li Li, Xiao-yue Wang, Hong Meng, Chang Liu and
Yin-Mao Dong**
Beijing Key Laboratory of Plant Resources Research
and Development, Beijing Technology and Business
University, Beijing 100048, People's Republic of
China

Guang-rong Liu
Infinitus (China) Company Ltd., Guangzhou
510665, China

Song-Hyo Jin
Department of Pathology College of Medicine,
Institute of Hansen's Disease,
The Catholic University of Korea, Seoul 06591,
Republic of Korea.

Kyu Joong Ahn
Department of Dermatology, Konkuk University
School of Medicine, Seoul 05029, Republic of Korea

Sungkwan An
Department of Cosmetics Engineering, Konkuk
University, 120 Neungdong-ro, Gwangjin-gu, Seoul
05029, Republic of Korea

**Hyun Kyung Lee, Seonghee Jeong, Shang Hun
Shin, Dahye Joo, Seong Jin Choi, Karam Kim and
In-Sook An**
Korea Institute of Dermatological Sciences,
Cheongju-si, Chungcheongbuk-do 28160, Republic
of Korea

Kyung-Yun Kim
URG Inc., URG Building, Seochogu, Seoul 06753,
Republic of Korea

Jung-Eun Ku
Department of Cosmetology, Kyung-In Women's
University, Incheon 21014, Republic of Korea

Sun-Hee Jeong
Department of Beauty Art, Faculty of Art, Suwon
Women's University, Suwon-si, Gyeonggi-do 16632,
Republic of Korea

Hwa Jun Cha
Department of Skin Care and Beauty, Osan University, Osan-si, Gyeonggi-do 18119, Republic of Korea.
Department of Skin Care and Cosmetics, Osan University, Osan-si45 Cheonghak-roGyeonggi-do 18119, Republic of Korea.

Ofonime M. Ogba, Patience E. Asukwo and Iquo B. Otu-Bassey
Department of Medical Laboratory Science, Faculty of Allied Medical
Sciences, University of Calabar, Calabar, Nigeria

Yeong Min Choi, Soo Young Choi, Hyonmin Kim, Jeongmin Kim, In-sook An and Jinhyuk Jung
Korea Institute for Skin and Clinical Sciences, Gene Cell Pharm Corporation, 6F, Tower A, 25, Beobwon-ro 11-gil, Songpa-gu, Seoul, Republic of Korea

Mun Sang Ki
NB Clinic, Ansan, Republic of Korea

Hee Jung Yong
Beauty People Beauty School, 68 Dolma-ro, Bundang-gu, Seongnam-si 13627, Gyeonggi-do, Republic of Korea

Jin Jung Ahn
Department of Cosmetology, Suwon Women's University, Suwon-si, Kyonggi-do, South Korea

Pragya Nagar and Yasha Hasija
Department of Biotechnology, Delhi Technological University, Shahbad Daulatpur, Main Bawana Road, Delhi 110042, India

Seeun Jeon
Management Division, Swinner, 5F, 441, Teheran-ro, Gangnam-gu, Seoul 06158, Republic of Korea

Mina Choi
Liberal Arts Department, Jangan University, 1182, Samcheonbyeongma-ro, Bongdam-eup, Hwaseong-si, Gyeonggi-do, Republic of Korea

Antonella Savoia
Buon Consiglio Hospital, Naples, Italy

Alfonso Baldi
Department of Environmental, Biological and Pharmaceutical Sciences and Technologies, Università degli Studi della Campania "L. Vanvitelli", Via Vivaldi, 43, 81100 Caserta, Italy

Hyun Jung Kim, Min Sook Jung, Jeong Min Shin and Yu Kyung Hur
Dasan Skin Clinical Research Center, Dasan C and Tech, 42, Eonju-ro 81-gil, Gangnam-gu, Seoul 06223, Republic of Korea

Kye Hwa Lim
Department of Beauty Care, Sangji Youngseo College, 84, Sangjidae-gil, Wonju-si, Gangwon-do 26339, Republic of Korea

Gyu Ri Kim
Department of Beauty and Cosmetic Science, Eulji University, 553, Sanseong-daero, Sujeong-gu, Seongnam-si, Gyeonggi-do 13135, Republic of Korea

Eman Salah
Dermatology, Venereology and Andrology department, Faculty of Medicine, Zagazig University, Zagazig, Egypt

Alshymaa A. Ahmed
Clinical Pathology department, Faculty of Medicine, Zagazig University, Zagazig, Egypt

Ji Hye Son
Department of Bioengineering, Graduate School of Konkuk University, Seoul 05029, Republic of Korea
Lemon Beauty Academy, Busan 47837, Republic of Korea

Soo-Yeon Kim
Department of Beauty Art, Doowon Technical University, Paju-si, Gyeonggi-do 10838, Republic of Korea

Hyun Hee Jang
School of Cosmetology, Kyungbok University, Namyangju-si, Gyeonggi-do, Republic of Korea

Sung Nae Lee
Department of Cosmetology, Kyungin Women's University, Incheon 21041, Republic of Korea

Kyu Joong Ahn
Department of Dermatology, Konkuk University School of Medicine, 120 Neungdong-ro, Gwang-jin-gu, Seoul 05029, Republic of Korea

Dhwani Rathod, Purna Pandya and Bela Padhiyar
Department of Dermatology, GMERS Medical College, Gandhinagar, Gujarat, India

Ishan Pandya
Department of Dermatology, SBKS Medical Institute and Research Centre, Piparia, Waghodiya, Vadodara, Gujarat, India

Gaurav Shah
Department of Oral and Maxillofacial Surgery, NIIMS Dental College, Jaipur, Rajasthan, India

Rima Shah
Department of Pharmacology, GMERS Medical College, Gandhinagar, Gujarat, India.

Razia Rahman, Isha Sharma, Lokesh K. Gahlot and Yasha Hasija
Department of Biotechnology, Delhi Technological University, Shahbad Daulatpur, Main Bawana Road, Delhi 110042, India

Ji Young Ryu
Halla University, 28, Halladae-gil, Heungeop-myeon, Wonju-si, Gangwon-do 25404, Republic of Korea

Won Lee
Yonsei E1 Plastic Surgery Clinic, Anyang, South Korea

Jeung-Hyun Yoon
Yonseifams Clinic, Seoul, South Korea

Ik-Soo Koh
KohIksoo Plastic Surgery Clinic, Seoul, South Korea

Wook Oh
Samsung Feel Clinic, Seoul, South Korea

Ki-Wook Kim
Regen Clinic, Seoul, South Korea

Eun-Jung Yang
Department of Plastic and Reconstructive Surgery, Cheil General Hospital and Women's Healthcare Center, College of Medicine, Dankook University College of Medicine, Yongin, South Korea

Eun Ju Na
Department of Biological Engineering, Konkuk University, 120 Neungdong-ro, Gwangjin-gu, Seoul 05029, Republic of Korea

Index

www.ingramcontent.com/pod-product-compliance
Lightning Source LLC
Chambersburg PA
CBHW061302190326
41458CB00011B/3743